SPORTS MEDICINE

CONTRIBUTORS

FRED L. ALLMAN, JR.

BRUNO BALKE

VEIDA BARCLAY

HARRY BASS

JOHN L. BOYER

E. R. BUSKIRK

J. A. DEMPSEY

ANN JEWETT

FRED W. KASCH

WILLIAM P. MORGAN

FRANCIS J. NAGLE

NEIL B. OLDRIDGE

SARAH M. ROBINSON

ALLAN J. RYAN

VOJIN N. SMODLAKA

GORDON STODDARD

KARL G. STOEDEFALKE

CLAYTON L. THOMAS

EDWARD W. WATT

SPORTS MEDICINE

Edited by

Allan J. Ryan, M.D.

University Health Service
University of Wisconsin Medical Center
Madison, Wisconsin

Fred L. Allman, Jr., M.D.

The Sports Medicine Clinic PC
Atlanta, Georgia

ACADEMIC PRESS   New York   San Francisco   London   1974

A Subsidiary of Harcourt Brace Jovanovich, Publishers

ACADEMIC PRESS, INC.
111 Fifth Avenue, New York, New York 10003

United Kingdom Edition published by
ACADEMIC PRESS, INC. (LONDON) LTD.
24/28 Oval Road, London NW1

Library of Congress Cataloging in Publication Data

Ryan, Allan J
    Sports medicine.

    Includes bibliographies.
    1.   Sports medicine.   I.   Allman, Fred L., joint
author.   II.   Title.   [DNLM: 1.   Sport medicine.
QT260 R988s 1974]
RC1210.R9   617'.1027   72-82639
ISBN 0–12–605060–0

Contents

Chapter 4.   THE LIMITS OF HUMAN PERFORMANCE
             ALLAN J. RYAN

PART II   MEDICAL SUPERVISION OF THE ATHLETE

Chapter 5.   MEDICAL QUALIFICATION FOR
             SPORTS PARTICIPATION
             FRED L. ALLMAN, JR.

Chapter 6.   CONDITIONING FOR SPORTS
             FRED L. ALLMAN, JR.

Chapter 7.   PSYCHOLOGY OF SPORTS COMPETITION
WILLIAM P. MORGAN

Chapter 8.   NUTRITION FOR THE ATHLETE
E. R. BUSKIRK

Chapter 9.   PROTECTIVE EQUIPMENT
GORDON STODDARD

Chapter 10.   ENVIRONMENTAL PROBLEMS AND
THEIR CONTROL
E. R. BUSKIRK

Chapter 11. ROLE OF SKILLS AND RULES IN THE PREVENTION OF SPORTS INJURIES

ALLAN J. RYAN

Chapter 12. THE IMMEDIATE MANAGEMENT OF SPORTS INJURIES

FRED L. ALLMAN, JR., AND ALLAN J. RYAN

Chapter 13. REHABILITATION OF THE INJURED ATHLETE

FRED L. ALLMAN, JR.

Chapter 26. TEAMWORK IN EXERCISE THERAPY
VOJIN N. SMODLAKA

Chapter 27. EXERCISE AND OBESITY
J. A. DEMPSEY

Chapter 28. EXERCISE AND CARDIOVASCULAR DISEASE
JOHN L. BOYER AND FRED W. KASCH

Chapter 29. EXERCISE AND RESPIRATORY DISEASE
HARRY BASS

Contents   xiii

List of Contributors

Numbers in parentheses indicate the pages on which the authors' contributions begin.

FRED L. ALLMAN, JR. (85,113,259,307,473), The Sports Medicine Clinic PC, Atlanta, Georgia

BRUNO BALKE* (505), Departments of Physiology and Physical Education, University of Wisconsin, Madison, Wisconsin

VEIDA BARCLAY (639), Nonington College of Physical Education, Nonington, Dover, Kent, England

HARRY BASS (619), Peter Bent Brigham Hospital, Harvard Medical School, Boston, Massachusetts

JOHN L. BOYER (595), Human Performance and Exercise Laboratory, California State University San Diego, San Diego, California

E. R. BUSKIRK (141,203), Laboratory for Human Performance Research, Intercollege Research Programs, The Pennsylvania State University, University Park, Pennsylvania

J. A. DEMPSEY (557), Department of Preventive Medicine, University of Wisconsin, Madison, Wisconsin

ANN JEWETT (407), Department of Physical Education—Women, University of Wisconsin, Madison, Wisconsin

FRED W. KASCH (595), Human Performance and Exercise Laboratory, California State University San Diego, San Diego, California

WILLIAM P. MORGAN (129,671), Department of Physical Education—Men, University of Wisconsin, Madison, Wisconsin

FRANCIS J. NAGLE (525), Department of Physiology and Physical Education—Men, University of Wisconsin, Madison, Wisconsin

NEIL B. OLDRIDGE† (525), Department of Physical Education—Men, University of Wisconsin, Madison, Wisconsin

* Present address: Aspen, Colorado

† Present address: Departments of Physical Education and Medicine, McMaster University, Hamilton, Ontario, Canada

SARAH M. ROBINSON (437), Department of Physical Education, Boston-Bouve College, Northeastern University, Boston, Massachusetts

ALLAN J. RYAN (3,13,31,57,235,259,375,417,463,487), University Health Service, University of Wisconsin Medical Center, Madison, Wisconsin

VOJIN N. SMODLAKA (541,551), Department of Rehabilitation Medicine, Methodist Hospital of Brooklyn, Brooklyn, New York

GORDON STODDARD (161), Head Athletic Trainer, University of Wisconsin, Madison, Wisconsin

KARL G. STOEDEFALKE (447), College of Health, Physical Education and Recreation, The Pennsylvania State University, University Park, Pennsylvania

CLAYTON L. THOMAS (347), Department of Population Sciences, Harvard University School of Public Health, Boston, Massachusetts, and Tampax, Inc., Palmer, Massachusetts

EDWARD W. WATT (473), Department of Physiology, Emory University School of Medicine, and Preventive Cardiology Clinic, Atlanta, Georgia

Preface

The concept of sports medicine as consisting of the medical supervision and care of the athlete, special or adapted physical education, exercise for the prevention of chronic degenerative disease, and exercise in the treatment of physical disorders or disease states is not original with the editors of this book. It developed gradually from the beginning of this specialty of medical practice in Europe in the early 1900's.

In this book, we have attempted to collate the best of modern thought in these four areas and to use them as a comprehensive basis for the practice of sports medicine. The names of the contributors indicate that specialists in the fields of physical education, physical therapy, exercise physiology, physical medicine, athletic training, internal medicine, and in diseases of women have major interests in this discipline. The list might be further expanded to include psychologists, sociologists, historians, as well as others. Still it remains a specialty of medical practice, and the physician who wishes to undertake it must familiarize himself with the contributions which these specialists from other fields have made and will continue to make.

Although the book was written with the sports physician primarily in mind, we hope it will be useful as a text and reference source for both instructors and students in medicine, physical education, physical theapy, and athletic training. University students who are active in sports or the graduate who continues to participate at an advanced level should find the work an invaluable source for the understanding of their own reactions to problems in sports and other physical recreation. Those physicians who are engaged in the rehabilitation of the physically or mentally disabled, whatever their specialty may be, should be able to profit especially from the fifth part of the book which deals with exercise as a mode of therapy.

We wish to acknowledge especially the outstanding efforts and co-operation of all those who contributed chapters; The Macmillan Company and the International Committee on the Standardization of Physical Fitness Testing for permission to reproduce in Part IV extensive portions of the sections on exercise testing from a forthcoming publication, "Fitness, Health and Work Capacity—International Standards for Assessment" (L. A. Larson, ed.); *Journal of the American Medical Association;* the Committee on Exercise and Physical Fitness for permission to quote extensively from "Is Your Patient Fit" and "Evaluation for Exercise Participation—The Apparently Healthy Individual"; The Rawlings Company for permission to reproduce and use the many pictures of sports protective equipment in Part II, Chapter 9; Elizabeth D. Robinton and the Cambridge University Press for permission to quote from her article "A quantitative and qualitative appraisal of microbial pollution of water by swimmers" which appeared in the Journal of Hygiene; and all those other persons and concerns who gave their permission for quotations and reproductions from their works.

Special thanks to Mrs. Barbara Hamilton for her painstaking care in preparing the manuscript in its final form and to Loren Seagrave for his preparation of the Subject Index.

ALLAN J. RYAN
FRED L. ALLMAN, JR.

SPORTS MEDICINE

PART I

INTRODUCTION

Chapter 1

SPORTS MEDICINE
IN THE WORLD TODAY

ALLAN J. RYAN

I. DEFINITION OF SPORTS MEDICINE

The strict definition of areas of medical practice is made difficult by the facts that many designations are historically rather than logically developed, and that there is considerable overlapping of research interests and clinical practice among the different fields. Since sports medicine has developed gradually, though sporadically, over a period of 2500 years, and since it draws upon many scientific and nonscientific areas of inquiry and practice, attempts to define it are considerably hampered by both factors. To add further to the confusion, although it includes the word "medicine," its practice is by no means restricted to physicians.

3

A. Origin of the Term

The first use of the term to describe an area of research and clinical practice centered around the performances of athletes appears to be in February, 1928, during the Second Olympic Winter Games at St. Moritz, Switzerland (Ryan, 1965). Doctors W. Knoll of Switzerland and F. Latarjet of France called together 33 physicians who were attending the Games with the teams of eleven nations. They established a committee to plan for the First International Congress of Sports Medicine, to take place in Amsterdam during the games of the IX Olympiad in August of the same year, and to propose and plan for an organization for a permanent International Assembly on Sports Medicine.

As a result of this committee's work, the first constitution of the Association International Medico-Sportive was adopted. Three principal purposes were outlined in this constitution: (1) to inaugurate scientific research in biology, psychology, and sociology in relation to sports; (2) to promote the study of medical problems encountered in physical exercises in sports in collaboration with various international sports federations and (3) to organize international congresses on sports medicine to be held during and at the site of the quadrennial Olympic Games. At the Second Congress, which was not held until 1933, the name of the organization was changed to the Federation International Medico-Sportive et Scientifique, and so it has remained, except for dropping the term "Scientifique," as the FIMS.

The first book to use the term was written by Dr. F. Herxheimer and published in Germany in 1932 under the title "Grundriss im Sportsmedizin" (Foundations of Sports Medicine). It dealt with exercise physiology and related topics as well as the medical problems of athletes. It is interesting that no book in English used this title until "Sports Medicine" by J. G. P. Williams was published in 1962.

Although sports medicine has been accepted as a specialty of medical practice in Europe for many years, and in some countries is recognized by the granting of diplomas and degrees, it has not yet reached this status in the English-speaking countries. Only the University of Wisconsin at Madison offers a certificate for an eight-month course that combines didactic with practical work in this field. One- to three-day postgraduate courses are now being offered regularly in the United States by various organizations, however.

B. The Four Areas of Activity

Based in part on these historical events and a modern conceptualization of the field of interests, sports medicine may be said today to comprise four principal areas of activitiy: (1) medical supervision of the athlete; (2) special (adapted) physical education; (3) therapeutic exercise; and (4) exercise in the prevention of chronic degenerative disease. Exposition of these topics make up Parts II–V of this book.

Part II, dealing with the medical supervision of the athlete, takes a very comprehensive view of the responsibilities of the physician in the total program of management. It demonstrates that concepts based on the clinical experience of physicians and on the experimental findings of scientists generally in the study of man's relationship to his environment can, and should, be applied to the sports situation. It emphasizes the importance of cooperative planning and execution of policies developed from these concepts by all those who are responsible for the supervision of athletes.

Part III focuses on the joint responsibilities of the physician and physical educator in special physical education. The purposes of physical education and the techniques that may be employed must be clear to the physician who is delimiting the type and amount of physical activity that his clinical observation indicates for the individual. The physical educator must be able to understand why these limitations are necessary and to interpret the restrictions in terms of a specific program of physical activity enabling the handicapped individual to realize his true potential.

Preservation of health and of that elusive quality that we call physical fitness are inextricably related. Part IV outlines for the physician and all other concerned persons the present status of the concepts that relate these two important subjects to each other. The correct prescription and evaluation of physical activity and its effects for the human individual are matters that must be familiar to every person who is interested in the preventive aspects of medicine, especially the physician.

Part V deals with an area that has only recently been rediscovered by most physicians, the role of exercise in the treatment of disease. Habitual inactivity tends to produce a disease state of itself. When abetted by further factors, such as overindulgence in food and drink, heavy cigarette smoking, and the pressures of a highly congested, competitive urban society, it may become lethal. The present state of knowledge regarding the significant concepts and possible approaches to therapy comprise the substance of these chapters.

C. The Practitioners of Sports Medicine

The practitioners of sports medicine may, within the scope of the given definition be physicians, coaches, trainers, exercise physiologists, psychologists, sociologists, physical educators, and others whose special interests are less well defined. The development of the field has come about chiefly as the result of the recognition of their mutual inter-dependence and of their cooperation. Their combination in multidisciplinary organizations and meetings offers the best possibility for the continued advancement of the field and of themselves as individual practitioners within its scope.

D. The Unifying Principle

If there is one theme that unifies the whole concept of sports medicine, it is that of the study and observation of man in motion. I propose as its typical symbol the running man (*Homo currens*). Descartes stated the proposition, "I think, therefore, I am" (Cogito, ergo, sum). Although valid philosophically, this statement is too static by itself to represent man's existence. Would it not be logical to extend it to say, "By moving I express my being"?

II. PRESENT ACTIVITIES IN SPORTS MEDICINE

A. The International Federation of Sports Medicine

At the time of the second International Congress of Sports Medicine in Turin, Italy in 1933, it was agreed that the general assembly of the new organization would meet every four years at the time of the summer Olympic Games. Because the interval seemed too long, French physicians organized the third International Congress at Chamonix, France in 1934 (V. N. Smodlaka, unpublished). Although this meeting was not official, it was attended by physicians from eight European countries. The topics that were discussed included (1) formation of a standard chart for the medical evaluation of physical fitness; (2) medical control of physical education and sports; (3) medical guidance in physical exercises; and (4) indications and contraindications for performing sports in the mountains at high altitudes. New proposals were made regarding the introduction of teaching of physical education into medical schools and licensing those who passed examinations in this subject as school physicians. Standardization of medical charts and an international system of medical licensing for athletes were also discussed.

The fourth International Congress at the Berlin Olympic Games in 1936 attracted 1500 physicians from 40 nations, an incredible number considering the embryonal state of development of the field. A fifth Congress was held in Paris the following year, at which time the Germans, who had gained a majority in voting power, elected Dr. Conti from their country as president. At the sixth Congress in Brussels in 1939, the German-dominated General Assembly succeeded in having the constitution and bylaws changed to assure their continued control. The occurrence of World War II soon halted any further activity, however.

After the War, Dr. Govaerts of Belgium, who was the last vice-president of the Federation, called a meeting of the surviving members of the executive committee. A revised constitution was approved by a new General Assembly that convened in Brussels on June 21, 1947. These statutes remained in effect with few changes until the fifteenth Congress in Tokyo in 1964, when they were again revised to create the following structure.

The membership is made up of honorary members, national associations, invited members, associate members, and representatives of the international sports federations. The membership consists of five bodies: (1) the Board of Representatives; (2) the Executive Committee; (3) the Plenary Assembly; (4) the Scientific Commission; and (5) the Interfederal Medical Commission.

The Plenary Assembly meets every four years on the occasion of the Olympic Games. It consists of (1) the members of the Executive Committee; (2) the members of the Board of Representatives; (3) the National Delegates; (4) the four members of the Scientific Commission designated by the Executive Committee; (5) three delegates of the International College of Sports Physicians; and (6) the delegates of the international groups of sports medicine recognized by FIMS and the delegates of the international institutions that have official dealings with FIMS. The Assembly is presided over by the president of FIMS. Its motions are submitted to the Board of Representatives.

The Board of Representatives meets every two years at the time and place of the International Congress. It is constituted of the delegates of the National Associations or Federations of Sports Medicine at the rate of one per country. The President of FIMS presides. The exact duties and responsibilities of this Board are not specified in the statutes.

The Executive Committee is elected for a period of four years by the Board of Representatives except for the Honorary President who is appointed for life. The retiring president remains a member ex officio. The Committee is composed of (1) an Honorary President; (2) the President of FIMS; (3) two Vice-Presidents; (4) a Secretary General; (5) a Treasurer; and (6) six members. This committee meets at least twice annually to debate and decide the general outlines of the activities of FIMS in accordance with the deliberations of the Board of Representatives.

The Scientific Commission is made up of the invited members and is directed by four members, chosen by the Executive Committee, who represent (1) the sciences of physiology and biology as applied to sports; (2) the practice of sports medicine and sports medical examinations; (3) sports traumatology and the prevention of sports accidents; and (4) prevention and treatment through physical activity. Its aims are to promote research in sports medicine, and to study of the adaptation of scientific data and issue opinions on questions submitted by the Executive Committee.

The Interfederal Medical Commission is made up of the physicians appointed by the International Sports Federations. Its purpose is to serve as a liaison to FIMS and to submit problems involving practical progress in sports medicine, especially those encountered in the medical examination of athletes.

It was also agreed at Tokyo to establish periodic courses in sports medicine at which participants could receive the title of Associate Fellow or Fellow of the FIMS. The first International Course was held at München–Grünwald in Germany in March 1965. It was organized by the Union of Bavarian Physicians for Sports Medicine. Delegates from 17 nations attended. The second International Course was held in Rome on September 1–8, 1966. Ninety delegates from many nations attended.

B. Other International Organizations

The number of other organizations interested and active in sports medicine has multiplied rapidly since 1945. The UNESCO organization includes an International Council of Sport and Physical Education. A Research Committee of this division was organized under the leadership of Professor Ernst Jokl in 1960 and has held many meetings in different countries since then. An International Committee for the Standardization of Physical Fitness Testing was organized in 1964 and has prepared a written set of standards to be used in the scientific studies of the functional capacities and anthropometry of the world's populations.

The Conseil International du Sport Militaire (CISM) was founded in 1948 to promote healthful recreation and sports activities in international competition for the world's armies. Its membership includes 37 nations. In 1970 it sponsored 21 international events, including 13 sports championships involving thousands of athletes. In 1961 an Academy was established which has undertaken research in diet, the medical control of athletes, physiology, philosophy and psychology of sports, coaching, training, and physical conditioning. It holds regular conferences and publishes its findings in "Sport International," the official CISM magazine, and leading research journals.

The Groupement Latin de Médecine Physique et Sport has held annual meetings in Europe since 1961. There is also an Ibero-American Confederation of Sports Medicine. The South American Congress on Sports Medicine was established in 1953. A first European Congress on Sports Medicine was held in Prague in 1963 but does not appear to have been repeated. An International Seminar on Sports Medicine was held in Bavaria, Germany in 1965.

Meetings of special interest groups in recent years have included the congresses of the International Association of Ski Traumatology and Winter Sports Medicine held annually in Europe since 1954, the annual meetings of the Medical Commission of the Association International Boxe Amateur, the International Meetings on the Hygiene of Sports Installations held in Europe since 1963, the International Symposia on Underwater Medicine held every two years in Europe since 1963, the International Congresses on Sport Psychology first held in Rome in 1965, the International Seminars on the History of Physical Education and Sport first held in Israel in 1968, and a series of International Symposia on Problems of Competition at Moderate Altitudes first held in Madrid in 1965.

C. Sports Medicine in the United States

The American College of Sports Medicine was founded in 1954 for the purposes of promoting scientific studies dealing with the effects of sports on humans through interdisciplinary meetings of scientists and educators, encouraging research, offering postgraduate education, and publishing a journal. Its membership is composed about half of physicians with physical educators, physiologists, and other scientists making up the remainder. Its journal, *Medicine and Science in Sport* was established in 1969. In 1971 it sponsored and coordinated the publication of "The Encyclopedia of Sports Sciences and Medicine" with more than 1000 contributors from all over the world (Larson, 1971).

The American Medical Association appointed an ad hoc committee on Injuries in Sports in 1954. This committee later became a standing committee under the name of the Committee on the Medical Aspects of Sports. This committee through its sponsorship of annual conferences on the Medical Aspects of Sports, through its publications, and through its consultations and communications with organized bodies regulating amateur and professional sports on all levels in the United States has greatly stimulated the activities of physicians and others to establish local, state, and regional conferences and organizations to promote education and research in sports medicine, especially with regard to the prevention of illness and injury in athletes.

A Committee on Exercise and Physical Fitness was also appointed by the American Medical Association in 1964. This committee has worked to establish standards for the determination of physical fitness, to encourage people of all ages to keep themselves fit through regular exercise, and to encourage the use of exercise for therapeutic purposes. Its publications and the conferences it has sponsored have been directed chiefly at improving the knowledge of physicians regarding physical fitness and its maintenance, but it has cooperated extensively with the President's Council on Physical Fitness and Sports in public education in this field.

The American Academy of Orthopedic Surgeons established a Committee on Sports Medicine in 1962. This committee has developed a series of three-day courses on various aspects of sports medicine, focused chiefly but not exclusively on orthopedic problems, which have been held at many different locations in the United States since 1969. The proceedings of the first conference were published under the title "A Symposium on Sports Medicine." In 1970 they published a "Bibliography of Sports Medicine."

A National Athletic Trainers Association was established in 1949 with the principal objective of "the advancement, encouragement and improvement of the athletic training profession in all of its phases; and to promote a better working relationship among those persons interested in problems of training." The membership at the present time numbers almost 2000. The *Journal of the National Athletic Trainers Association* is a quarterly publication containing original articles and reviews. The annual meetings of the Association feature a varied program of distinguished speakers from all areas of sports medicine.

The Association maintains close cooperation with all national organizations in the field of sports medicine and has been engaged in many collaborative projects. Among these might be mentioned cooperation with national cooperative committees on injury prevention and protective equipment and in the preparation of a manual for athletic trainers. After careful preparation, the Association has embarked on a certification program for athletic trainers, based on education and experience, and has established standards for courses to prepare athletic trainers in colleges and universities.

The President's Council on Physical Fitness and Sports originated as the President's Council on Youth Fitness under President Eisenhower in 1956. It was a cabinet level council as originally established with the Secretary of the Interior serving as chairman. A Citizen's Advisory Committee of 100 was appointed at the same time and held four meetings in the course of the next three years. An executive director was appointed on a full-time basis and was given a small office staff in Washington. This first council succeeded in stirring up national interest in physical fitness chiefly through advertising and personal contacts by the director.

The Council was reorganized under President Kennedy under the joint leadership of the Secretary of Health, Education and Welfare and a "special consultant to the President" who replaced the executive director. The name was changed to the President's Council on Physical Fitness. Under President Johnson, the name was again changed to the President's Council on Physical Fitness and Sports with a new "special consultant" and the Vice-President of the United States as Chairman. It was still a Cabinet-level body.

Finally, under President Nixon, the Cabinet-level council was abolished and replaced by a 15-member group drawn from many different walks of life and under the chairmanship of astronaut Captain James A. Lovell, Jr., USN. The new executive director was C. Carson Conrad, former chief of California's Bureau of Health Education, Physical Education, Athletics and Recreation. An advisory Conference of 100 persons prominent in the world of sports was appointed, reviving to some extent the original Citizen's Advisory Committee.

In the meantime, the President's Council had strengthened its position as a leader in the field through its many publications, regional clinics on Lifetime Sports, and Presidential Physical Fitness Awards. In cooperation with the American Medical Association, the National Industrial Recreation Society, and other organizations, it sponsored programs dealing with the role of exercise in the maintenance of health. With a number of colleges and universities, it established a National Youth Summer Fitness program for underprivileged boys and girls to teach them sports and give them an opportunity for recreation under skilled supervision.

The American Association for Health, Physical Education and Recreation is a gigantic combination of persons and organizations interested in the named topics which serves as the principal focus for all physical education related activities in the United States. Through its Research Council and its many publications it promotes scholarly production, and through the organizational activities of its Divisions, which include those on Physical Education, Girls' and Women's Sports, Men's Sports, and Safety Education, it facilitates the organization and administration of these areas in schools and colleges.

The American College Health Association includes representation from the majority of the nation's colleges and universities. Its section on sports medicine enrolls many of the college team physicians and provides a forum for discussion and interchange of experience which has helped to improve the standards of medical supervision of athletes at this level of education. It joins with the National Collegiate Athletic Association, the National Federation (high schools and junior colleges chiefly), the National Association for Intercollegiate Athletics, and the National Athletic Trainers Association to form the Joint Committee on Competitive Safeguards.

An increasing number of colleges and universities through their schools or departments of physical education and/or medical schools now maintain laboratories and other research facilities for research in sports medicine, especially in the areas of exercise physiology and therapeutic exercise and rehabilitation. There is no consistent pattern for the development or organization of such facilities as yet and they are dependent on a variety of sources for support. Such designations as human performance research and biodynamics are typical.

The first comprehensive postgraduate course for physicians in sports medicine in the United States has been offered at the University of Wisconsin at Madison since 1967. It begins each year on September 1 and concludes on the following April 30. Both didactic instruction in all phases of sports medicine and practical experience in working with the varsity sports teams are included in the course. A certificate is granted by the university to those completing the course. Beginning in 1971 a fourth-year elective course in sports medicine has been offered in the medical school of the university, the first formally organized course in this field for medical students in the United States.

Related activities that include in their membership other professionals such as engineers and manufacturers of sports equipment are exemplified by the International Committee on Protective Equipment for Sports, the F8 Committee of the American Society for Testing and Materials, and the Cooperating Committee on Protective Equipment for Sports.

It can be truly said that no field in medicine involves so many related disciplines or has experienced such a phenomenal growth in the past twenty years as sports medicine. And yet it is only beginning to explore the vast area that it has marked off for its special attention.

REFERENCES

Herxheimer, F. (1932). "Grundriss der Sportsmedizin." Greuthlein, Leipzig.
Larson, L., ed. (1971). "The Encyclopedia of Sports Sciences and Medicine." Macmillan, New York.
Ryan, A. J. (1965). *J. Amer. Med. Ass.* **194,** 643–645.
Smodlaka, V. N. (1974). "Short History of the International Federation of Sports Medicine." unpublished.
Williams, J. G. P. (1962). "Sports Medicine." Williams & Wilkins, Baltimore, Maryland.

Chapter 2

HISTORY OF SPORTS MEDICINE

ALLAN J. RYAN

The interest of physicians in the medical control of sports is almost as old as their recorded history. Although the art of medicine was highly developed along empirical lines in Babylonia, Egypt, and China as far back as the third millenium BC, we lack specific information as to whether special attention was given to sports. Medical practice in Egypt was specialized even at this early date, but we do not read of any sports physicians. Yet they must have been there to help guide and treat the boxers, wrestlers, archers, and other athletes, just as we know

13

they served the armies of the great kings and emperors. Therapeutic exercise was undoubtedly practiced, since in the "Ayur-Veda," a medical manuscript of Ancient India, dating from between 800 to 1000 BC, exercise and massage are recommended for chronic rheumatism (Guthrie, 1945).

I. THE GREEK PERIOD

Prospective competitors in the ancient Olympic Games were required to devote themselves to intensive training under supervision for a period of ten months during the year in which the quadrennial renewal took place (Schöbel, 1966). This training was ordinarily carried out at a gymnasium near the athlete's home under the supervision of the *gymnastes*, a physician who interested himself in all phases of the athlete's training. He, in turn, was assisted by the *paidotribes*, who was essentially a masseur, and the *aleiptes*, who anointed the athletes and also acted as a bath servant.

A. Therapeutic Exercise

Herodicus (born either in Sicily or Thrace about 400 BC), the teacher of Hippocrates, was the most famous, and perhaps the most able, of the *gymnastes* (Harris, 1966). Some of his medical writings that have survived in later texts indicate a serious concern about the diet of his patients, possibly a reflection of his interest in the diet of the athletes whom he supervised. He had a strong interest in exercise as a means of physicial rehabilitation, making such prescriptions even for patients suffering from fevers. His influence on his famous pupil was apparently great, since Hippocrates made many references to the therapeutic values of exercise, recommending it even for mental disease (Littré, 1839–1861).

Herophilus and Eristratus, both of whom taught at the medical school of Alexandria in the fourth century BC, also recommended moderate exercise as a treatment (Adams, 1844). Asclepiades (born in Bithynia and lived from 126 to 68 BC) treated his patients with diets and by massage, and recommended moderate exercise, including walking and running (Asclepiades, 1955).

B. The Training of Athletes

The best source of information available to us today is the "Gymnastikos" of Philostratus, which was not written until the third century

AD (Gordon, 1935). He describes the rigorous training of athletes of a former day who ate a Spartan diet, slept on animal skins spread on the ground, and bathed in cold mountain streams. He contrasts this with the practices of his own day, in which a more clear-cut separation had occurred between the physicians and the trainers. He blames the physicians for overstuffing the athletes, for encouraging them to eat fish, for failing to develop the endurance of the athletes, and for not enforcing generally more rigorous training.

Fish was readily available in Greece and usually eaten fresh (Harris, 1966). Cows and goats were kept for the milk and cheese they produced, but their flesh was seldom eaten by the average Greek except when they were sacrificed for the great festivals. Tradition tells us, however, that about the sixth century BC the heavyweight boxers and wrestlers began to add it to their diet. Milo of Croton, the only one to hold the all-Greece championship six times, is said to have consumed as much as 20 pounds of bread, 20 pounds of meat and 18 pints of wine in one day. For most athletes the basic food was barley or wheat made into bread or porridge. This was supplemented with milk, cheese, eggs, vegetables, and fruit. Olive oil was used for cooking and honey for sweetening.

Philostratus was very conscious of the dangerous admixture of high temperature and humidity and warned athletes to be cautious in their training when "the southern winds are humid, sluggish and oppressive beyond measure and are more likely to exhaust than stimulate." He was also aware that persons who are fat and stocky are less well able to radiate heat and should keep out of the sun, while those who are slender may tolerate exposure very well. It is interesting that athletes during the period of the Olympic Games exercised in the nude, although they wore shorts during the earlier Homeric period. It seems likely that the change occurred because of the advantage of being able to perspire freely in a climate that was characteristically warm and humid.

C. Medicine at the Olympic Games

A special enclosure was provided where the trainers could prepare and minister to the athletes. Quintus of Smyrna gives us a picture of typical medical services offered to the athlete in the fourth century AD (Harris, 1964). Sprained ankles were treated by bleeding, followed by the application of a lint dressing smeared with ointment. The wounds of a boxer were "sucked clean" and then sutured, and medicaments were applied to them externally. We have very little information about specific injuries or fatalities except in the description of some famous individual contests which survive. Although facial injuries were apparently common in boxing, and sometimes severe, only two deaths in the entire history of Olympic boxing are documented (Harris, 1964). A number of deaths took place in the *pankration*, a rough combination of boxing and wrestling, and in the chariot races.

II. THE ROMAN PERIOD

A. Galen

A forceful personality and a tireless worker, Galen of Pergamos left an enormous volume of writings that exerted a profound influence on medicine in Europe and Asia for more than 1200 years after his death at the close of the second century AD. For personal and political reasons he divided his life between Rome and Asia Minor. While there, after his first return from Rome, he administered to the gladiators who fought in the public exhibitions, becoming the first team physician of whom we have an exact record. He classified exercises for therapeutic purposes and recommended their use in moderation for many forms of disease (Galen, 1951).

Galen made and recorded more fundamental contributions to exercise physiology than any physician before or since (Galen, 1916; Singer, 1956; Duckworth, 1962). He was the first to develop systematic descriptions of the human body. He was also the first to recognize that muscle has but one action, contraction. He also observed that each muscle had only one direction of action, and that different muscle groups worked antagonistically. The stimulus to muscle contraction, he noted, came through the nerves from the brain. He developed the concept of muscle tone and related it to the erect posture. He described the connections and functions of the arteries and veins and showed that the arteries contained blood from the right side of the heart and air from the lungs. He described the formation of urine from the serous portion of the blood.

Galen was not in favor of the sporting practices of his day, however. In his "Exhortation on the Study of the Arts" he warned his readers

Take care not to be seduced by an imposter or charlatan who will teach you a useless or contemptible profession. Learn that an occupation which has no sensible end in life is not an art. Man stands between God and the animals, near the first on account of his intellectuality, with the second because he is immortal. When athletes miss their goal, they are disgraced; when they attain it, they are not yet even above brutes.

In his "Paraphrase of Mendotus" he says,

Athletes live a life quite contrary to the precepts of hygiene, and I regard their mode of living as a regime far more favorable to illness than to health. They lose their eyes and their teeth, and their limbs are strained. Even their vaunted strength is useless. They dig and plow but they cannot fight. They cannot endure heat and cold, nor like Heracles wear one garment winter and summer, go unshod and sleep on the open ground; in all this they are weaker than newborn babes. It is easy to discover they are always in debt. While practising their profession, and afterwards, they are never found richer than the high class servants of an opulent man. While athletes are following their profession, their body remains in a dangerous condition, but when they give up their profession they fall into a condition more parlous still; as a fact, some die shortly afterwards; others live for some little time but do not arrive at old age.

B. Other Roman Physicians

Aurelianus (fifth century AD) elaborated on the practice of medical rehabilitation, including the use of hydrotherapy and of weights and pulleys (Aurelianus, 1950). He was the first writer to recommend exercise during convalescence from surgery. Paulus Aegineta (seventh century AD) recommended exercise and defined it as violent motion which renders body organs fit for their functional action (Adams, 1844). This definition of exercise as an intensified movement of any sort he had apparently borrowed from Oribasius of Pergamon (fourth century AD). It was in contradistinction to the idea of Galen that exercise was a volitional activity and exerted its best effects when it was moderate in degree. Through the affirmation of Avicenna, it was Galen's idea which survived and continued to influence the thinking of physicians regarding sports of a very vigorous or violent character until modern times.

III. PERSIAN AND JEWISH PHYSICIANS

A. Avicenna

Beginning in about the tenth century, Muslim physicians translated the works of the Greek and Roman physicians, adding commentaries and observations of their own. The greatest scholar and most prolific author of this period was Avicenna (ibn Sina, born in Persia about 980 AD). He followed Galen's idea that medical gymnastics, the term by which therapeutic exercise came to be known in the Renaissance, should include all healthful and health-furthering exercises. In his Poem on Medicine (Kruger, 1962) he wrote,

> Among physical exercises, there are some moderate ones; it is to them that one ought to devote himself. They balance the body by expelling residues and impurities and are factors of good nutrition for adults and of happy growth for the young. Unmoderated exercise is an overload, alters the forces of the soul, leads to lassitude, consumes natural warmth, empties the body of its moisture, weakens the nerves through the violence of pain and causes the body to age before its time. . . . Do not give up hard exercise; do not seek rest too long; preserve a happy medium. Exercise your limbs to help them repel the bad humors by walking and struggling until you succeed in panting. . . . In summer decrease fatigue for perspiration is exhaustion.

B. Maimonides

Rabbi Moses ben Maimon (Maimonides) was the greatest of the medieval Jewish physicians, although he was born in Spain, spent most of his life in Egypt, and wrote his great medical and religious works in Arabic. As a follower of Galen, he believed in moderate exercise. In his Treatise of Hygiene (Galen, 1951) written in 1199 he said,

> A person should not eat until he has walked prior to the meal until his body begins to become warmed, or he should perform a physical task or tire himself by some other form of exertion. . . . Anyone who lives a sedentary life and does not exercise . . . even if he eats good foods and takes care of himself according to proper medical principles—all his days will be painful ones and his strength shall wane.

IV. THE RENAISSANCE

Through the discovery and translation of the Greek and Roman manuscripts by the Muslims, physicians and other scientists and educators in Europe became aware of the vast medical heritage of the past. One of the most important consequences was an intensification of interest in the values of exercise.

A. Italian Contributions

Vittorino da Feltre (1378–1446) established, under the patronage of the Marquis Gonzaga of Mantua, a school for children of the court which set a pattern that has influenced education in the Western World ever since (McCormick, 1943, 1944). Sports and physical exercises were conceived of as an indispensable and integral part of the educational process and were practiced daily by the children who entered the school at age four or five. Exercise activities were prescribed individually for each child and were varied according to the season, weather, and time of day. Vittorino had been influenced by his contemporary Vergerius, a professor of logic at Padua (Hackensmith, 1966a). In turn he influenced directly Maffeus Vegius (1407–1458) who wrote his beliefs in the obligatory introduction of gymnastics and sports into the educational process (Vegius, 1613).

Gerolamo Mercuriale (1530–1608) brought the appeal for regular and varied exercises to the general public with his publication of "Six Books on the Art of Gymnastics" (Mercuriale, 1569). This book, written in a popular style and beautifully illustrated, was reprinted for 150 years afterwards and had an enormous influence on medical as well as public opinion. He classified exercises into preventive and therapeutic forms and warned against strenuous military exercises and athletics.

Marsilius Cagnatus (1543–1612) of Verona in his "Preservation of Health" asked for specially educated physicians to supervise sports and games (Cagnatus, 1602). He led the way in recognizing the importance of knowledge and love of sports as well as a strong medical background in the problems of athletes as prerequisites for the sports physician. Girolamo Cardano (1501–1576), the physician-mathematician, conceived a theory of muscle movement from a mechanical standpoint which exerted a profound influence on the physiologists of the next century (Cardano, 1551).

B. French Contributions

Ambroise Paré was acknowledged to be the leading surgeon of his day. In his treatment of fractures, he emphasized the importance of exercise of the limbs following primary treatment. In his great "Surgery," he referred to the doctrine of Galen that the body needs exercise to maintain its health, and recommended specific exercises for different persons for special purposes (Paré, 1582).

Laurent Joubert (1529–1583) was professor of medicine at the University of Montpellier, and the first to introduce therapeutic gymnastics into the medical course because he considered physicians to be the only ones capable of prescribing it correctly. He was a great advocate of daily exercise (Joubert, 1582).

Joseph Duchesne (1546–1609) was the first to recommend swimming as a means of strengthening the body as well as a means of lifesaving. In his "Ars Medica Hermetica" (Duchesne, 1648) he wrote,

> The essential purpose of the gymnastics for the body is its deliverance from superfluous humours, the regulation of digestion, the strengthening of the heart and the joints, the opening of the pores of the skin and the stronger circulation of blood in the lungs by strenuous breathing.

Jean Canapé introduced a new era in exercise physiology with the publication of his essay, "The Movement of Muscles" (Canapé, 1546).

C. Spanish Contributions

The first printed book on exercise written by a physician was published by Christobal Mendez of Jaen in 1553 (Mendez, 1960). He wrote that

> The easiest way of all to preserve and restore health without diverse peculiarities and with greater profit than all other measures put together is to exercise well.

He advocated exercise for older and also handicapped persons. P. E. Gualtero, in 1644, wrote an essay entitled "Considerations to settle all doubts about the convenience of the art of swimming in order to keep healthy" (Camuñez, 1965).

V. THE SEVENTEENTH AND EIGHTEENTH CENTURIES

The great contributions to exercise physiology in the seventeenth century were the better understandings of muscular action which developed from the work of three Italian scientists. Fabricius in 1614, Aquapendente in 1614, and Aldrovandi in 1616 published works on the movements of animals which laid a foundation for the great work of Borelli (1608–1679). He applied his background of knowledge of physics and mechanics to an interpretation of all muscular action. He was able to expand and elaborate on Galen's descriptions of muscle tone and the antagonistic actions of muscles and to identify clearly the response of muscles to nerve impulses. He failed only in identifying the mechanism of contraction as a rearrangement of existing structure, and if better microscopes had been available to him he would have probably done that as well. His great work "On the Movement of Animals" was not published until after his death (Borelli, 1710).

Comenius (1592–1702), the great Moravian theologian and educator, suggested that as the human soul is nourished through books so must the body be nourished by movement (Joseph, 1949). He stated that a child's day should consist of sleep, intellectual development, and physical recreation in approximately equal parts. He suggested light exercises for pregnant women in order that they should produce offspring who were also lively and vigorous.

At the beginning of the eighteenth century, Ramazzini (1633–1714) wrote the first book on occupational diseases (Ramazzini, 1940). He pointed out that sedentary workers typically suffered from poor health and advocated that they be given regular exercises. Hoffmann (1708) in Holland and Stahl (1733) at Halle both wrote and lectured on the values of exercise in the prevention and treatment of disease. Andry (1658–1742) in Paris prescribed a variety of exercises for children to prevent and treat the diseases from which they suffered. He also recommended exercise for weight reduction. His great book "L'Orthopedie" gave the specialty of orthopedics its name (Andry, 1741). Robert Whytt (1714–1766), a neurologist of Edinburgh, established that reflex action was mediated through the spinal cord (Ackerknecht, 1955). In Russia, A. M. Protasov lectured in 1765 "On the Importance of Motion in the Maintenance of Health" (Vinokurov, 1959).

VI. THE NINETEENTH CENTURY

At the beginning of this century, Europe was engulfed in the Napoleonic wars. It became quite apparent to those countries who were resisting subjugation that the success of their efforts would depend on the physical abilities of their populations to undergo hardship and to endure on the field of combat. In spite of the development of artillery, it was still the foot soldier who determined the outcome of the battle. Modern physical education, apart from therapeutic exercise and no longer under medical direction, was developed by the work of Jahn in Prussia (Hackensmith, 1966a), Ling in Sweden (Westerblad, 1909), Nachtegall in Copenhagen (Hackensmith, 1966b), Clias in Berne (Clias, 1819), and Amoros in Paris (Hackensmith, 1966c). Exercise continued to be a mainstay of medical therapy since there were relatively few specifics that were effective in spite of the enormous empiric pharmacopeia.

As the century progressed, with the discovery of practical general anesthesia, the formulation of the bacterial origin of infectious disease by Pasteur, the development of antisepsis by Lister, and the foundation of modern chemotherapy by Ehrlich, physicians turned their attention away from exercise and toward the application of these new findings of therapy.

The enthusiasm for Ling's systematized Swedish gymnastics grew in the middle of the century until it swept the whole world. Because of a shortage of therapists trained in the system, machines were developed to provide active, assisted, and resisted exercise and even massage (Zander, 1879). Special hospitals were built in Russia for treatment by Swedish gymnasts. Gymnastics in America assumed a hybrid form as the result of influences of the Swedish system, the German Turnverein, and the Czech Sokols.

In France, Claude Bernard (1813–1878) laid the foundations for modern physiology with classic experiments in nutrition and study of the nervous system (Bernard, 1927). John Hughlings Jackson (1835–1911) developed the concept of a hierarchy of levels in the central nervous system (Taylor, 1932). William Einthoven (1860–1927) invented the string galvanometer and founded the new field of electrocardiography (Einthoven, 1903). In Russia, Chetyrkin, Pirogov, and other military surgeons developed programs of intensive physical exercise for the rehabilitation of wounded soldiers (Vinokurov, 1959).

What may have been the first English publication in sports medicine appeared in 1898 as a section on first aid in "The Encyclopedia of Sport" as written by J. B. Byles and Samuel Osborn (1898). In addition to describing practical measures of emergency treatment for hemorrhage, wounds, bites, bruises, fractures, dislocations, strains and head injuries, and transportation for the injured, its describes injuries commonly sustained in angling, boxing, cricket, cycling, football, hunting, lawn tennis, mountaineering, rowing and shooting and their management.

VII. THE TWENTIETH CENTURY

The first book to deal comprehensively with what we call sports medicine today was "Hygiene des Sports," written by Siegried Weissbein of Berlin and published in two volumes in 1910. He discussed not only the effects of sports activities on the body, including injuries and the appropriate emergency treatment, but also the importance of correct sports attire and sports suitable for very young children and the elderly. A monograph on sports injuries by G. Van Saar entitled "Die Sportverletzungen" was contributed to the "Encyclopedia of Surgery" edited by Professor P. Van Bruns of Tubingen and published by Van Saar in

1914. These two events helped to arouse sufficient interest so that a congress on physical therapy in sports and physiology of physical exercise was held in Paris in March 1913 (see Smodlaka, 1913). The progress of World War I terminated activities of this sort until the meeting at St. Moritz in 1928 which resulted in the establishment of the FIMS (LaCava, 1956).

In the meantime, the first steps in the establishment of modern concepts of exercise physiology and rehabilitative exercise had been taken with the publication of six remarkable and influential books. The first was "Exercise in Education and Medicine" written by Robert Tait McKenzie, M.D., Professor of Physical Education and Physical Therapy at the University of Pennsylvania, which appeared in 1909. In the first part of the book, exercise and its effects on the body are defined and a history of the development of physical education is presented. In the second part, practical applications of exercise to the treatment of injury and disease are laid forth.

The second and third were monographs by A. V. Hill of London, based on a series of lectures that he had given at the Lowell Institute in Boston and at the Chemistry Laboratory at Cornell University. The concept of the "steady state of exercise" was introduced in the first book which was entitled "Muscular Movement in Man" (Hill, 1927a). In the second, "Living Machinery" (Hill, 1927b)," neuromuscular coordination and cardiorespiratory function were related to the development of strength, speed, and endurance. Both were published in 1927.

A. B. Bock and D. B. Dill of the Harvard Fatigue Laboratory collaborated on a complete rewriting of Bainbridge's "The Physiology of Muscular Exercise" to produce the third edition of this fourth book in 1931 (Bainbridge, 1931). All aspects of training and conditioning as understood on the basis of the new concepts of exercise physiology developed in their own laboratory and abroad were discussed. In the same year, E. C. Schneider's "Physiology of Muscular Activity" appeared, presenting basic observations on exercise under a variety of conditions (Schneider, 1931). In 1935, Percy M. Dawson published "Physiology of Physical Education" based on his experiences as an investigator and teacher in Wisconsin and Maryland.

The biennial meetings of the FIMS, which had commenced in 1928, provided a continuing stimulus to the development of national federations of sports medicine so that there are now more than 40 around the world. The International Bulletin of the FIMS was established in 1934 and was published from 1947 until 1961 in the official organ of the Italian Federation of Sports Medicine. In that year the *Journal of Sports Medicine* was founded as the official publication of the FIMS and the Bulletin is now published therein on a quarterly basis. Many countries have now developed their journals emphasizing various phases of sports medicine. Books and monographs of all types have appeared in profusion during the past 15 years.

Education in sports medicine in Europe has progressed steadily from its beginnings after World War II. Degrees in the field are offered in Czechoslovakia and Yugoslavia, and speciality certification based on postgraduate study is offered in a number of countries. The FIMS has been offering short courses in sports medicine annually since 1965.

VIII. MEDICAL SERVICES FOR THE MODERN OLYMPIC GAMES

The development of medical services for the modern series of Olympic Games, which began in 1896, reflect, in general, the advances in sports medicine made during the twentieth century (Ryan, 1968). In the plans for the first revival of the Games, no medical element was included. Medical planning today for the care not only of the thousands of athletes and other team members but for the tens of thousands of spectators begins at least four years in advance and is extremely comprehensive.

Early medical interest centered around the marathon race, which was considered an extremely hazardous, and perhaps lethal, event. Greek physicians at Athens followed the race in ambulances and treated a number of contestants for exhaustion. At the Games in St. Louis in 1904, the air temperature in the shade was 90°F and the humidity very high. Only 14 of the 27 starters finished the race. The winner, T. J. Hicks of Cambridge, Massachusetts was treated during the race by a physician who followed him in a car and gave him several injections of strychnine as well as eggs and brandy by mouth. Suffering from severe heat exhaustion, probably aggravated by the treatment given him during the race, he required the services of four physicians who treated him in a nearby gymnasium after the race.

In Paris in 1906, ambulances and first-aid stations staffed with physicians and nurses were set out along the route of the marathon run. There were no serious incidents. At the Games in London in 1908, only 27 of the 58 starters were able to finish the race which was again run under conditions of great heat and humidity. The Italian runner, Dorando Pietri, had to be hospitalized for heat exhaustion and lay in a semicoma for two days before recovering. At Stockholm in 1912, another day of oppressive heat greeted the marathon race and a Portuguese runner named Lazaro died of heat stroke. This fatality led to a requirement that all marathon runners undergo a physical examination before the next Games in Antwerp in 1920. This was the first such medical requirement in the history of the Games.

The United States sent its first medical delegation to the Games when they were held in Paris in 1924. Doctor Graeme M. Hammond was chief medical officer. He was assisted by Drs. Milton A. Bridges and A. Franklin Carter and a nurse, Josephine Matthews. In the 10,000 meter cross-country race (an event no longer held), five runners were taken to the hospital suffering from heat exhaustion, but all survived.

Medical supervision of Olympic athletes was already well established by the second Winter Olympic Games at St. Moritz when 33 physicians were present representing 11 nations. The founding of the organization which became the FIMS and the establishment of the International Congresses on Sports Medicine which have been a feature of every summer Games renewal since then, except for 1932 and 1960, assisted greatly in providing better medical supervision for the Games.

An informal association has developed over the years between the International Olympic Committee (IOC) and the FIMS, which has served as a medical advisory body to the former through its executive committee and the Interfederal Medical Commission. It was only after receiving a favorable report from the FIMS executive committee that the IOC agreed to award the 1968 Games to Mexico City. Another product of this relationship has been the Olympic Medical Archives. This consists of the records of physical and other examinations of athletes submitted by the countries that participate in the Olympic Games, and which are maintained in the Olympic Museum in Lausanne, Switzerland.

The first Olympic village for athletes was erected at Los Angeles for the summer Games of 1932. It included a small hospital with complete equipment for laboratory and roentgenographic diagnosis and for physiatrics. Four hundred sixty-six persons were treated by the medical staff, including 130 who were admitted to the hospital in the village and six to general hospitals in Los Angeles. Each Games since then has had separate housing for athletes, although not always in a village as such, and some type of small hospital available to the members of all teams.

The second death of an althlete at the Games occurred in Berlin in 1936 when Ignaz Stiessohn of Austria was killed during a gliding exhibition. Two more deaths occurred during practice for the Winter Games at Innsbruck in 1964. Ross Milne, a member of the Australian downhill ski team went off the course out of control, struck a tree, and suffered a lethal head injury. A member of the British bobsled team, Kazimierz Kay-Skrzypeski, went off the run on his sled and suffered a rupture of his aorta when he struck a tree. Only one more death has occurred through the 1968 Games, that of the Danish cyclist Knud Enemark Jensen, who died of heatstroke aggravated by drugs, following the 100-km road race on an extremely hot day.

Organization of medical services at the Winter Olympics in Cortina d'Ampezzo, Italy in 1956, Squaw Valley, California in 1960, Innsbruck, Austria in 1964, and Grenoble in 1968 have been complicated by the tremendous increase in the number of spectators at sites remote from regular medical facilities and by the necessity of providing emergency care at venues of competition which are widely separated from each other. These services were organized under the Medical Department of the French Army at Grenoble and were probably the best seen so far for a Winter Games. A new hospital of a permanent nature was constructed for the Games.

There has been concern since two women medal winners for France at the European track and field championships at Oslo in 1946 subsequently declared themselves as men. Subsequently, examinations of the external genitalia were required prior to participation in the Olympic Games. With the advent of genotyping, interest in screening people for their basic sexual orientation has shifted to examination under the microscope of cells obtained in a smear from the buccal mucosa. This examination was required for the first time at the Winter Games in Grenoble in 1968. Interestingly, this requirement appeared to evoke a greater protest from women competitors than the external examinations.

Even taken together, these two screening examinations still ignore two other significant factors in determining sexual orientation, the phenotype, and the mental attitude of the individual. The buccal smear is not reliable in some individuals who exhibit a mosaic genotype pattern. The whole controversy ignores the question of men's sexual orientation, which has never been questioned at the Olympic Games. How many of these who were disqualified as women would be considered acceptable competitors as men? Should we provide a third category of competition for those who fall somewhere between the sexes?

Finally, the question of the use of drugs by athletes to improve performance, so-called "doping," has been a matter of continuing concern to officials at the Games. At Helsinki in 1952, the first unannounced check of athlete's living quarters, including personal clothing was carried out. Although testing methods on body secretions such as saliva and urine for drugs had been worked out many years ago and have been thoroughly evaluated at horse-racing tracks, such tests were not required at the Games until 1968.

One of the reasons that drug testing had not been carried out is that the legal implications of disqualifying an athlete on the basis of illegal use of drugs are such that an extremely elaborate protocol has to be set up in order to be sure that results are correct beyond any reasonable possibility of doubt. The time required, expense, and technical expertise needed are such that testing was limited to certain events and then only to medal winners and a few other contestants in final events selected at random. Only a few cases were detected and athletes disqualified: one pentathlon contestant had imbibed too much alcohol before the pistol shooting event (almost all competitors take some to steady their hands), a few cyclists for having used amphetamines, and a wrestler for inhaling some smelling salts during an interval in a match.

The IOC had appointed a five-member commission under the Prince de Merode in 1967 to supervise drug testing for the Olympic Games. This body was active at Grenoble, but three months before the summer Games in Mexico City responsibility for testing was transferred to the Interfederal Medical Commission. This had the effect of contributing to the natural difficulties already involved in overseeing the possible usage of drugs, thereby vitiating the effectiveness of the control. Certainly it left considerable room for improvement of surveillance of this important problem in 1972.

In the Olympic Games at Mexico City, four athletes were disqualified for unacceptable drug usage and several medals were forfeited. At Munich in 1972, six athletes, of whom three were medal winners, were disqualified for taking drugs on the forbidden list. Among them was Rick Demont, gold medal winner in the 1500-meter swim, who had taken a medication containing ephedrine for his asthma. A West German ice hockey player had been suspended by the International Hockey Association at the Winter Games in Sapporo the same year when ephedrine was found in his urine and his team had to forfeit a game in which he played.

REFERENCES

Ackerknecht, E. H. (1955). "A Short History of Medicine." Ronald Press, New York.
Adams, F. (1844). "Paulus Aegineta, The Seven Books of." Sydenham Soc., London.
Aldrovandi, M. (1616). "De Quadripedibus." Bologna.
Andry, N. (1741). "L'Orthopédie, ou l'Art de Prévenir et Corriger dans les Enfants les Deformités du Corps." Paris.
Aquapendente, F. (1614). "De Motu Animalium." Venice.
Asclepiades. (1955). "Asclepiades, His Life and Writing." (transl. by R. M. Green). Licht, New Haven, Connecticut.

Aurelianus, C. (1950). "On Chronic Diseases" (transl. by I. E. Drabkin). Univ. of Chicago Press, Chicago, Illinois.

Bainbridge, F. A. (1931). "The Physiology of Muscular Exercise," 3rd ed. (rewritten by A. V. Bock and D. B. Dill). Longmans, Green, New York.

Bernard, C. (1927). "An Introduction to the Study of Experimental Medicine" (transl. by H. C. Green). Macmillan, New York.

Borelli, G. A. (1710). "De Motu Animalium." Lugduni.

Byles, J. B., and Osborn, S. (1898). In "The Encyclopedia of Sport" (H. Peck and F. E. Aflalo, eds.), Vol. 1, pp. 394–398. Putnam, New York.

Cagnatus, M. (1602). "De Sanitate Tuenda." Padua.

Camuñez, S. C. (1965). *J. Sports Med. Phys. Fitness* **5**, 23–31.

Canapé, J. (1546). "L'anatomie du movement et des muscles Gallen." Paris.

Cardano, G. (1551). "De Subtilitate et du Rerum Varietate," Libri XXI. Paris.

Clias, P. (1819). "Cours élémentaire de gymnastique." Paris.

Dawson, P. M. (1935). "The Physiology of Physical Education." Williams & Wilkins, Baltimore, Maryland.

Duchesne, J. (1648). "Ars Medica Dogmatica Hermetica." Frankfort.

Duckworth, W. L. H. (1962). "Galen on Anatomical Procedures," Books X–XV. Cambridge Univ. Press, London and New York.

Einthoven, W. (1903). *Arch. Gesamte Physiol. Menschen Tiere* **99**, 472–480.

Galen (1916). "On the Natural Faculties" (transl. by A. J. Brock). Loeb Classical Library, Heineman, London.

Galen (1951). "De Sanitate Tuenda" (transl. by R. M. Green). Thomas, Springfield, Illinois.

Gordon, B. (1935). *Ann. Med. Hist.* **7**, 513–518.

Guthrie, D. (1945). "A History of Medicine." Nelson, London.

Hackensmith, C. W. (1966a). "History of Physical Education," p. 88–89. Harper, New York.

Hackensmith, C. W. (1966b). "History of Physical Education," pp. 88–89. Harper, New York.

Hackensmith, C. W. (1966c). "History of Physical Education," pp. 148–149. Harper, New York.

Harris, H. A. (1964). "Greek Athletes and Athletics," pp. 60–61. Hutchinson, London.

Harris, H. A. (1966). *Proc. Nutr. Soc.* **25**, 87–90.

Hill, A. V. (1927a). "Muscular Movement in Man; Factors Governing Speed and Recovery from Fatigue." McGraw-Hill, New York.

Hill, A. V. (1927b). "Living Machinery." Harcourt, New York.

Hoffmann, F. (1708). "Dissertationes Physico-Medicae." Hague.

Joseph, L. H. (1949). *Ciba Symp.* **10**, 1053.

Joubert, L. (1582). "Opera." Lugduni.

Kruger, H. C. (1962). "Avicenna's Poem on Medicine" (transl.), p. 24. Thomas, Springfield, Illinois.

LaCava, G. (1956). *J. Amer. Med. Ass.* **162**, 1109–1111.

Licht, S. (1961). "Therapeutic Exercise," 2nd ed., p. 456. Licht, New Haven, Connecticut.

Littré, E. (1839–1861). "Oeuvres complètes d'Hippocrate." Paris.

McCormick, P. J. (1943). *Cath. Univ. Bull., Wash.* **12**, 4–6.

McCormick, P. J. (1944). *Cath. Univ. Bull., Wash.* **13**, 6–8.

McKenzie, R. T. (1909). "Exercise in Education and Medicine." Saunders, Philadelphia, Pennsylvania.

Mendez, C. (1960). "The Book of Bodily Exercise" (transl. by F. Guerra, F. G. Kilgour, ed.).

Mercuriale, G. (1569). "De Arte Gymnastica." Venice.

Paré, A. (1582). "Opera Ambrosii Parei Regis Primarii et Parisiensis Chirurgi." Jacques du Puys, Paris.

Ramazzini, B. (1940). "De Morbis Artificiorum," (1713 transl. by W. C. Wright). Univ. of Chicago Press, Chicago, Illinois.

Ryan, A. J. (1968). *J. Amer. Med. Ass.* **205**, 715–720.

Schneider, R. C. (1931). "Physiology of Muscular Activity." Saunders, Philadelphia, Pennsylvania.

Schöbel, H. (1966). "The Ancient Olympic Games," p. 55. Studio Vista, London.

Singer, C. (1956). "Galen on Anatomical Procedures," Books I-VIII and 5 Chapters of Book IX. Oxford Univ. Press, London and New York.

Smodlaka, V. N. (1913). "Short History of the International Federation of Sports Medicine" (unpublished).

Stahl, E. E. (1733). "De Moto Corpori Humani." Erfurt.

Taylor, J., ed. (1932). "Selected Writings of John Hughlings Jackson." Hodder & Stoughton Ltd., London.

Van Saar, G. (1914). "Die Sportverletzungen," Enke, Stuttgart.

Vegius, M. (1613). "De Educatione Librorum." Lodi.

Vinokurov, P. A. (1959). "Lechebnaya Fizicheskaya Kultura." Moscow (quoted by Licht, 1961).

Weissbein, S. (1910). "Hygiene des Sport." Greuthlein, Leipzig.

Westerblad, C. A. (1909). "Ling, the Founder of Swedish Gymnastics." London.

Zander, G. (1879). "L'établissement de gymnastique médicale mécanique." Paris.

Chapter 3

THE CONCEPT OF PHYSICAL FITNESS

ALLAN J. RYAN

I. THE DEFINITION OF PHYSICAL FITNESS

A. American Medical Association

Physical fitness has been defined by the Committee on Exercise and Physical Fitness of the American Medical Association (1966) as "the general capacity to adapt and respond favorably to physical effort. The degree of physical fitness depends on the individual's state of health, constitution, and present and previous physical activity."

In amplification of this definition, the Committee has offered the following explanatory statements:

> An individual is physically fit when he is able to meet both the ordinary and the unusual demands of his daily life safety and effectively. These demands include working at either sedentary or active pursuits, meeting his social obligations to his family and to his community, and enjoying recreational activities of his choice without undue strain or exhaustion. The physically fit individual can return to his normal or rested state—repay energy costs— more readily than the unfit individual after physical exertion or sustained effort. Variations of acceptable levels of physical fitness exist among individuals.
>
> Levels of fitness necessary for proper and desired function and activity vary and many be limited by low levels of health or illness. Robust health enables an individual to attain a high degree of fitness as measured by the types of activities in which he can engage and the amount of effort he can expend in a given time as well as over a period of time. The permanently handicapped, but otherwise healthy, individual can develop high levels of fitness exclusive of the disabling condition. Those in ill health, with debilitating disease, chronic conditions or injuries, are unlikely to achieve maximum levels of fitness, but should strive for optimal personal goals. Sex and constitutional characteristics, such as body density, metabolic rate, and physical defects, will also affect the level of fitness attainable.
>
> Physical fitness is best attained by those who have earlier developed and maintained patterns of healthful living through the proper balance of diet, rest and exercise. Also included as a basic element is appropriate preventive and corrective medical and dental care. Fitness is further developed, maintained, and increased at any age, and even after illness, by a continuing program of regular, vigorous activity appropriate for the individual.

B. Other Definitions

Davis *et al.* (1961) have written, "physical fitness (which) is a product of many elements such as strength, endurance, skill and so on. It must be remembered, however, that physical fitness is only one component of total fitness of the individual which also includes mental fitness, social fitness, and emotional fitness. Total fitness is really a capacity for living."

Karpovich (1965) offered the following observations regarding physical fitness: "Strictly speaking, physical fitness means that a person possessing it meets certain physical requirements. These requirements may be anatomical (structural), physiological (functional), or both. . . . One should not forget that, at the present time, physical fitness measures merely the ability to pass physical fitness tests; and, therefore, the so-called degree of fitness possessed by an individual depends on the character of the test. . . . From an occupational point of view, physical fitness may be defined as the degree of the ability to execute a specific physical task under specific ambient conditions."

Åstrand and Rodahl (1970) have avoided any narrow definition of physical fitness, but wrote, "In a very broad sense, physical performance or fitness is determined by the individual's capacity for energy output (aerobic and anerobic processes), neuromuscular function (muscle strength and technique) and psychological factors (e.g., his motivation and tactics)."

DeVries (1966) has stated simply, "Physical fitness may be arbitrarily defined as the composite of at least five major components (motor fitness, physical working capacity, body weight, relaxation and flexibility), and each major component is composed, in turn, of measurable elements of physical performance of physiological function."

Although these definitions each emphasize different aspects of fitness, there is no fundamental disagreement among them. Fitness as an overall concept appears to have many components, including intellectual and emotional, as well as physical factors. These differ in relative importance from one period of life to another, depending on varying individual roles and responsibilities.

II. THE ATTAINMENT OF PHYSICAL FITNESS

A. The Components of Physical Fitness

The American Medical Association (AMA) definition of physical fitness states that physical fitness is the general capacity to adapt to physical effort. This means that, if no, or insufficient, physical effort is made, no adaptation will take place. The process of growth and development of the body is self-initiating, and continues spontaneously until it reaches its maximum, impelled by forces that are inherent in the body, and that are predominantly genetically controlled. At every stage of its growth, however, the body is responsive to its environment, and the final product represents the effects of this interaction. Identical twins raised in different environments from the time of birth may develop strikingly different physical characteristics as well as personalities. When growth has reached its maximum, the process of aging enters a phase in which those factors that lead throughout life to degeneration and decay of the body become predominant, very gradually at first and then more rapidly until senescence and death inevitably occur. Interaction with the environment is extremely important in its effects on the rate of this decay.

Our human bodies are so constituted that they are capable of adaptation to a wide range of environmental circumstances. Man can survive in the coldest weather of the Antarctic and in the hottest temperatures of the tropics. He can, in time, accommodate himself to living in either of these extreme conditions through a process of acclimation which helps him to compensate for the changes. He can hold an eggshell in his hand without crushing it, but he can also, with training, raise 400 pounds or more over his head. He can descend to the bottom of the sea and live there in a large tank in an atmosphere of compressed air for a month or more, and he can climb a mountain over 20,000 feet high without the use of oxygen equipment. He can jump over a bar over 7 feet high, and over a distance of 29 feet along the ground, impelled solely by the force of his own effort. He can run over 100 miles in one day.

When, and to the extent that, he fails to adapt to his environment, either through his innate inabiliy to do so, or through lack of the effort which may be necessary to secure this adaptation, he must then suffer the effects that the environment imposes on him. These may range from simple discomfort through illness and disability all the way to death. Life, in this sense, continues to be a struggle against the environment, whatever happy social or economic circumstances we may enjoy. Depending on which organ or body system is most affected by any failure of adaptation, we may develop disease affecting the central nervous system, the lungs, the heart, the gastrointestinal tract, and so on primarily, but ultimately, since all parts are interdependent, the functioning of the whole body.

1. Homeostasis and Adaptation

The AMA definition also states that physical fitness is the general capacity to respond favorably to physical effort. One of the characteristics of the human body is that it cannot remain continuously active, but periodically requires rest, which amounts to a cessation of all voluntary activity. This enables us to establish certain criteria of functioning for what we call a resting state of the body. We would naturally expect to find individual differences in these criteria, such as in the pulse rate, rate of respirations, blood pressure, and so on according to age, body size, and other variables, and we do. The remarkable thing is that these values on the whole lie within a rather narrow range for those persons who are free from disease or the immediate effects of injury. This is so because the body maintains a system of automatic controls that tend to preserve these ranges in spite of forces acting from outside and from within the body to change them, the principle which we call homeostasis. The greater the stress that is laid on the body, the more change there will be in the criteria that indicate the body's reaction to this stress, and the greater the effort must be for these criteria to be returned to their resting values. The repetition of stress increases the efficiency of the body in making the adaptation to effort, and, consequently, also facilitates the recovery from it.

The specific abilities of adaptation with which we are concerned in the development of physical fitness are basically those that allow the body to take more oxygen into the lungs, to utilize it more efficiently, to tolerate a greater than normal deficiency of oxygen during exercise, to increase the force with which the heart impels the blood into the circulation, to increase the size of the capillary bed in the lungs and the muscles, and to increase the size and strength of voluntary muscles. Some adaptation of the central nervous system is necessary for physical exercise. Extreme adaptations to permit highly skilled and coordinated motor performances are possible, but not essential to physical fitness. The differences between men and women in these adaptations should be only of degree.

2. Contributions of Health, Constitution, and Body Composition

In the second part of the AMA definition of physical fitness it is stated that the degree of fitness will depend on the individual's state of health and bodily constitution. If we consider a perfect state of health one in which an individual has no discoverable evidence of a physical defect, deformity, or disease, an ideal emotional balance, and no deficiency of his reasoning powers, then there must be very few indeed who could be said to be in such a condition, even for a very short period of time. The definition recognizes the relative importance of defects or diseases by referring to the "Degree of fitness." These may be of such trivial character as to exert no effect, or of such a serious nature as to impose considerable limitations on physical activity.

Any defect or disease that would impair the ability of the body to make the adaptations referred to in the previous section must inevitably reduce the general degree of fitness as long as it remains uncorrected. Bronchial asthma, for example, reduces the cross-sectional size of the air passages into the lung spasmodically to an extent that may greatly impair every effort of the body to increase its air intake per minute. A heart that has been damaged by disease so that it has little or no reserve capacity cannot increase its output substantially under the stress of exercise. Instead, it may become less efficient than when the individual is at rest.

It has been demonstrated by anthropologists that different body shapes and sizes tend to make their owners more or less suitable for certain types of physical activities. The person with a relatively light body and long legs (ectomorphic type) makes a good long distance runner. The man who is very short and stocky (endomorphic type) has the potentiality of becoming a good weight lifter. The individual who is generally well proportioned and of medium to tall height (mesomorph) may excel in a variety of sports, especially the team sports. In terms of functional capacity these three types as represented by individuals may exhibit a general state of fitness, but each one is more fit for certain specific performances than others.

This concept of a specificity of fitness may be further exploited by the athlete who undergoes practice and training for a particular sport. He places the emphasis in his conditioning process on the development of those physical and functional attributes and special skills that he hopes will enable him to gain mastery in that sport. In this way he develops the highly specific state of fitness suitable to a basketball player, fencer, weight lifter, or whatever other role in sport he may choose.

Although the individual's basic body constitution does not change during his lifetime, the relative composition of the body may be altered, usually by a change in the amount of body fat. This may make it appear that the constitution is altered due to the sometimes extreme alteration of the body contours. Normal reference man should have a body fat percentage of 12 to 14. The percent of body fat in any individual may be measured by underwater weighing, whole body counts of radioactive potassium, or by skinfold thickness measurements. For scientific purposes the first two methods are more reliable, but for practical clinical measurement the sum of six skinfolds, taken at the pectoral muscle, below the angle of the scapula, in the midaxillary line below the axilla, just above the elbow posteriously, at the umbilicus, and on the anterior surface of the thigh, will give a good estimate of the fat percentage. Any excess of body fat may be considered to indicate some degree of physical unfitness, since the individual is carrying dead weight that must affect his functional capacity unfavorably.

If a person suffers from an acute illness or injury, this has some immediate unfavorable effect on the general state of fitness of the body. If the illness is brief, a spontaneous recovery to the preexisting state of physical fitness may occur as the individual continues or resumes activity. If the illness is more prolonged, then a greater effort must be made to regain a state of fitness afterwards. The reasons for a loss of physical fitness during an acute illness may be single or multiple. Effects on the normal functioning of the endocrine system and the liver may be very important.

If someone is chronically ill, or has some defect that is not amenable to correction for whatever reason, it is possible to maintain a relatively high degree of physical fitness if he is willing and able to work for it. The wheelchair athlete is an excellent example of a person with a most severe physical handicap who, nevertheless, may demonstrate a very high level of physical fitness for certain sports or games activities. It will usually be more difficult for the chronically disabled person to reach his own optimal state of fitness than for the healthy but unfit person. If a person has been physically fit, and then becomes disabled, he may never achieve his former state if fitness, but may be able at least to approximate it.

B. Effects of Training

The last part of the definition of physical fitness says that "the degree of physical fitness will depend on . . . present and previous physical activity." We have described the ability of the human body to adapt itself to the circumstances of its environment. Physical activity brings adaptations, some of which have only a temporary, but others a lasting effect on the human body. Because of the former, the preservation of physical fitness in its entirety requires a continuity of activity.

Since we have already said that the specific adaptations with which we are concerned in the development and maintenance of physical fitness are those that allow the body to take in more oxygen, utilize it more efficiently, acquire a greater tolerance to a deficiency of oxygen, increase heart output and the size of lung and muscle capillary beds, and increase muscular strength, we must now discuss how these adaptations can be brought about and then maintained. Because many factors are involved, and all are to some extent interdependent, this is a very complex matter. Some aspects are well understood, but others present puzzles that are not yet solved.

The normal combustion of fat and carbohydrate in the body to produce energy requires the presence of oxygen. The body is able to utilize some glycogen that is stored in the muscles for very brief periods without oxygen. This is called anaerobic metabolism. When someone is resting or taking very light activity the amount of oxygen taken in by breathing shallowly and at a rate not in excess of 20 breaths per minute is adequate. Both fatty acids and glycogen are metabolized under these conditions. This is aerobic metabolism. As effort increases, more oxygen must be supplied. In the initial stages of vigorous exercise glycogen is burned preferentially since it requires less oxygen, but as time goes on the body burns more fatty acids and this further increases the oxygen demand. When oxygen cannot be supplied in quantities sufficient to meet the demand, the products of combustion, especially lactic acid, accumulate in the blood and muscle and are not recycled. The individual is then said to be in oxygen debt, since, according to present theory, he must still take in after exercise lessens in intensity or ceases enough additional oxygen to convert all the excess lactate into water and carbon dioxide, or to resynthesize it.

1. Cardiorespiratory Adaptations

The ability to increase energy expenditure can thus be seen to depend critically on the ability of the body to get oxygen in sufficient quantities to the muscle cells. It can do so in several ways: by increasing the rate of breathing; by increasing the depth of breathing; by increasing the rate at which oxygen is taken from the air in the lungs into the blood; by increasing the amount of hemoglobin available for oxygen transport; by increasing the rate of blood flow; and by increasing the rate at which oxygen is unloaded from the blood at the muscle cell.

The rate of breathing can be increased voluntarily, but in vigorous exercise the increase is largely involuntary, and is probably caused by the effect of increased blood lactate on the respiratory center. This mechanism probably also controls the depth of breathing. Whether a person can continue with an increased rate and depth of breathing depends on the strength of the respiratory muscles. These are primarily the diaphragm and the intercostal muscles. When these alone cannot satisfy the demand, the accessory muscles of respiration, the abdominal and certain of the neck muscles, must also act. The vigorous action of the neck muscles in a runner who is in the last stage of a long, fast race testifies to this.

In the physically fit person, then, these respiratory muscles must be well developed to allow a maximum intake of air. This means that they must be overloaded by exercise for the adaptation to take place. The possibilities of improving breathing efficiency by exercising greater voluntary control is one which has been explored by the practitioners of yoga. It has been applied to some extent in the training of runners, but there is not yet enough exact information to reach any definite conclusion.

The rate at which oxygen is taken into the blood from the lungs is determined by the pulmonary diffusing capacity. This depends on the partial pressure exerted by the oxygen in the alveoli as compared to the pressure due to the oxyhemoglobin in the blood. It also depends on the number and size of the capillaries in the walls of the alveoli. The effects of training are to increase the partial pressure in the alveoli by filling them with more and fresher air and to increase as much as twofold the volume of the capillary bed in the lungs.

The transport of oxygen in the blood is improved principally by increasing the amount of hemoglobin, since under normal atmospheric pressure the small amount of oxygen directly dissolved in the blood cannot be very much increased. Athletes in training show not only an increase in hemoglobin but also an increase in total blood volume. The rate of blood flow is increased by increasing the heart rate and the stroke volume. Slowing of the rate is now thought to be due to an increase in the acetylcholine content of heart muscle which favors a slower nervous response of the heart. The rate at which the heart is most efficient varies from individual to individual but in the young adult will be about 180 per minute. This rate of maximum efficiency decreases gradually in trained individuals after age 40, and even earlier in untrained persons. Increase in the stroke volume is due to dilatation of the heart chambers which accompanies hypertrophy of the heart muscle as an additional effect of training.

The rate at which oxygen is unloaded at the cell depends on the partial pressures of oxygen in the blood and in the cell. As the cell uses up its oxygen the drop in partial pressure makes the exchange from the blood take place more rapidly. The trained individual also appears to be able to utilize the oxygen in his cells more completely since he has increased the number of mitochondria in each cell. This helps to lower oxygen pressure in the cell even further, facilitating a more rapid exchange. These changes are reversible when training stops.

The efficient delivery of oxygen to the muscle cells and their adequate supply of nutritive elements derived from food substances make it possible for them to make their own adaptations to training. These must be forced by overloading, as in the case of the pulmonary and cardiovascular systems, and, in the same way, the majority of these adaptations are not permanent but may be reversed by physical inactivity.

2. Muscle Adaptations

Muscle activity has purposes other than to move the body on its parts from place to place. It is necessary to the growth and development of the child. If the bony skeleton is not subjected to the force of contracting muscles, it does not become strong and the long bones do not reach their maximum possible length. Muscle activity is also necessary to help the body adapt to the external forces that affect it, such as the force of gravity. Muscles that are not exercised lose that degree of normal tension that we call tone. Without muscle tone a person would be unable to sit or stand erect. Finally, a good general and symmetrical development of the body musclature contributes to overall fitness by demonstrating a body image that is esthetically pleasing, giving its owner a sense of pride and a continuing motivation to maintain this development.

Strength is an essential component of physical fitness, a strength adequate to meet the demands which the individual may make on his body for the activities of his daily life, physical recreation, and emergency needs. It may be defined very simply as the ability to produce tension in a muscle. It arises as the result of repeated muscular activity, from the process of learning the repeated action (skill development), and from the adaptation of the nervous system to the demands imposed on it. These three elements are inseparable, and the adaptations take place simultaneously over a measurable period of time, but this arbitrary division for purposes of analysis helps us to understand what takes place and how it may be influenced.

Once strength is developed, it may be maintained over a considerable period of time with much less effort, perhaps as seldom as twice or three times a week. With inactivity, however, strength falls off rapidly, at a rate of about 10% a week for most individuals. There is a natural tendency for strength to decrease with age in spite of continued physical activity. This falling off in an active person appears to begin about age 40, but may start earlier in the inactive. A person who has developed great strength in his early years may be able to retain a substantial proportion of it until the late years of life if he continues to enjoy good health and remains active, since, under these circumstances, the rate of decrease is very gradual.

The adaptations of muscle occur as the result of overloading, as has been pointed out, but appear to be specific to the method used. Almost any method used will obtain some results in terms of strength gain. The problem in training for physical fitness is to identify exactly the specific adaptations that are required for specific muscle groups and then to adopt those methods of exercise that will produce them most efficiently. It is possible to be deceived in the case of the untrained individual about the effectiveness of any method, since rapid gains occur at first due to the fact that muscle units that have not been previously used are brought into play. Progress must be observed over a period of months to determine the true results.

The classic description of how overload may be applied in the development of strength has been given by Lockhart (1959). There are four basic methods: (1) gradually increase the speed of the performance in a progressive manner; (2) gradually increase the total load; (3) progressively increase the time that a given position can be held and (4) with a constant resistance, progressively increase the total number of performances. The first two methods are more applicable to isotonic and the second two to isometric exercise. All systems of strength development up until recently were based on one or more of these methods.

Isotonic exercise occurs when the muscle shortens and moves the skeletal structure of the body in some way. Isometric exercise takes place when the muscle contracts against a resistance that does not allow it to shorten and to move the skeletal structure. There does not seem to be any difference in the firmness of muscles exercised by either method. Muscle bulk appears to increase to a greater extent when isotonic exercise is employed, but more rapid gains in strength may be possible with isometric exercise. There is no conclusive evidence that decay of strength following the exclusive use of one or the other method is more rapid in either case when the exercise is stopped.

Both isometric and isotonic exercises have their weaknesses, however, based on the ways in which the energy potentials of muscle are realized in the performance of functional activities from a mechanical standpoint. An improved rationale of this whole process has recently been offered by Perrine (1968), a consultant in bioengineering. In his viewpoint a muscle's capacity can be measured in terms of any one or a combination of three aspects of the mechanical energy it can transmit: (1) the maximum amount of force it can develop at all points in a range of joint movement; (2) the maximum amount of force it can develop at different speeds of joint movement; and (3) the maximum number of repetitions or total time duration the muscle can repetitively accomplish a given amount of work.

If strength is to be considered as the ability to produce tension in a muscle, it must be expressed in terms of some speed of contraction. If endurance is to be considered as the capacity of the muscle to produce work over a period of time, it must be expressed in terms of some rate of work. Isometric exercise has the disadvantage that the tension exerted by the muscle is at one length of shortening only, so that not all the fibers in a muscle are actively exercised. The improvement in strength that results falls in the very low speed category. Isotonic exercise has the disadvantages that the load lifted must be limited to that which can be moved through the weakest point in the range of motion, and that, because considerable acceleration may take place in some phase of the range of motion, the muscle is unable to develop its maximum power output.

According to Perrine (1968), an analysis of the energy requirements of almost all activities shows that these activities can be classified under four headings from the standpoint of the mechanics and energy output required:

1. A demand on a muscle's strength capacity where no shortening or very slow shortening takes place and the primary limitation is imposed by the ability of the muscle fibers to support the load statically. An example of this would be pushing a very heavy object.

2. A demand on muscle contraction at a very high speed of contraction, where the limitation on tension would be imposed by the ability of the muscle fibers to generate power. An example of this would be throwing a baseball.

3. A demand on the muscle's capacity for endurance in generating power at a high rate of contraction for a relatively short period. This could be in running a sprint race.

4. A demand on the endurance capacity of the muscles for production of power at a relatively slow rate but over an extended period of time. A long distance race would be an appropriate example.

An ingenious exercise device has been developed to overcome the disadvantages of isotonic and isometric exercise by a method which is called isokinetic exercise. It is called the Cybex exerciser.* The essential portion of this machine is a speed-controlling mechanism that regulates the rate at which the attachment through which energy is applied can move. When tension is applied, the attachment moves very rapidly to the preset speed and does not allow it to be exceeded. The resistance offered is proportional to the maximal tension exerted at any point in the range of motion. In this way the muscle works at maximum effort for all points in the range, but is never overstressed at any point. By allowing the exercising person to concentrate on generating more and more contractile force at a fixed rate of speed, the machine favors the development of maximum peak tension in the muscles used, and, therefore, the highest possible power output. It records the tension exerted throughout the entire range of motion on graph paper so that an objective record can be kept of any subject's progress.

According to DeLorme (1945), endurance in a muscle is related to strength according to the means used to develop it in an isotonic fashion. In working against weight resistance, four methods may be used to develop muscle strength:

1. Attempting to move a maximum weight one time
2. Making a series of repetitions against a resistance which is increased or decreased with each series

3. Making $\frac{2}{3}$ of a maximum number of repetitions against a fixed resistance

4. Making a maximum number of repetitions against a relatively low fixed resistance.

What has become known as DeLorne's axiom states that maximum strength can only be obtained by working against maximum resistance, and that maximum endurance in a muscle is developed by working a maximum number of times against a relatively low resistance. This has been challenged recently by DeLateur *et al.* (1968) in a study of healthy men aged 18 to 35 years. The muscle group tested was the quadriceps of the thigh and the subjects were divided into four groups who alternated in carrying out the assignments. The results were that those who trained for strength gained as much endurance as those who trained for it, while those who trained for endurance gained as much strength as those who trained for strength. All attained equal power, defined as work per unit time. Several criticisms can be made of this study, however. The previous physical activity experience of the subjects was not made known, the time of the study was very brief (only 20 sessions), and the weight differential was relatively small (25 versus 55 pounds).

One of the outcomes of strength development is increase in the bulk of the muscles exercised. The eventual size of the muscles appears to be a function of the intensity of the exercise and the resistance employed. Since both factors are apt to be greater in isotonic exercise, and since strength is roughly proportional to bulk of muscle, it would be expected that generally speaking isotonic exercises would result in greater average muscle sizes. Charles Atlas and his followers have succeeded, nevertheless, in producing remarkable increases in muscle bulk by the use of "dynamic tension," which is simply a form of isometric exercise. Increase in muscle bulk contributes to physical fitness by offering greater protection against injury to the bones and joints of the body.

3. Central Nervous System Adaptations

All of the strength that man can muster would be of no avail if it were not controlled and coordinated by a highly complex nervous system. Carrying out voluntary actions is probably the simplest task of the nervous system, even though it may involve rapid integration of perception and response. Much more complex are the involuntary responses, which involve reflex as well as direct pathways, and the autonamic regulatory mechanisms, which control posture, balance, and so on.

There is a great deal of variation in the degrees of proficiency reached by individuals in the nervous regulation of motor activity. Some very elementary responses appear to be inborn, since they can be demonstrated in the newborn child. Most of the complex ones are acquired as the result of experience. The baby is usually not able to stand unassisted until 6–8 months of age and it takes some further time until he is able to walk. All of the complex skills can be improved to a certain degree in each individual as the result of training. When they are inadequately developed the individual suffers from being unable to make an appropriate response to his environment. When they are developed to a high degree they improve the overall state of physical well-being and become components of physical fitness.

A skill is a learned pattern of performance that involves both voluntary and reflex actions. The individual sees a demonstration of the action or reads an instruction and then attempts to duplicate it. As the result of repeating the action, the pattern becomes fixed in the memory bank of the nervous system so that it can be called up at will. Gradually, refinements can be superimposed on the basic movement pattern to produce a more highly skilled action. The basic pattern has become so established that it is automatic, and only the refinements have to be willed. This means a higher state of physical fitness relative to the activity involved.

Since many skills have common elements in their basic patterns of movement, a certain amount of general as well as specific physical fitness results from their practice. The more individual skills a person masters, the more possible transfers can be made to other activities. The result is that such a person may appear to be generally gifted in the performance of physical activities, even those which may be quite new to him.

4. Speed and Reaction Time

Speed of motion and quickness of reaction are qualities that can be very different from individual to individual, and that, to some extent, appear to be constitutional. Anyone can improve the speed of his motions to some degree, even if he is not capable of achieving the same speed as some others. Reaction time can be shortened by training, but again only to individual limits. Whereas speed is highly specific for each action, reaction time appears to be a response characteristic of the nervous motor system as a whole.

5. Coordination

Coordination is essential to skill development. It requires a balance between opposing muscle actions which makes possible very fine movements and very rapid adjustments from one movement to another. It is a learned response, dependent on strength, speed, reaction time, and skills. It is highly specific for the particular action, but there is considerable carryover into actions that are similar. The person who acquires many skills easily may properly be said to be generally well coordinated, and, for that reason, more physically fit.

6. Posture

The postural reflexes that allow us to maintain an erect position against the force of gravity depend on muscle tone, stretch reflexes, kinesthetic sense, and balance. They are all susceptible to training, and we can therefore ascribe to the individual a certain degree of fitness, depending on how well they are developed. Poor habits relating to the maintenance of posture are as easy to develop as good habits, and may lead to a variety of physical complaints or disorders. Good posture is characteristic of a good state of physical fitness, and poor posture ordinarily goes with relatively poor fitness.

Muscle tone is that quality of muscle which keeps it in a state of partial contraction at all times in response to the sensory messages it receives from the nervous system. A muscle may be in a relatively poor state of tone if it is not exercised at all or very little. It does not lose its tone entirely unless its connections with the nervous system are severed completely. It is impossible to sit or stand unsupported without muscle tone. It is lost very quickly with confinement to bed.

The stretch reflex is important in maintaining the tone of the antigravity muscles. It originates in the receptors of any tendon that is stretched by the action of an opposing muscle. The reflex causes an involuntary contraction of the muscle whose tendon has been stretched. It is most completely developed in the extensor muscles since the force of gravity causes the joints of the spine, hips, knees, and ankles to move into flexion. The extensor reflex is one variety of stretch reflex that has cross-innervation.

7. Kinesthetic Sense

The kinesthetic sense of the body comes from a system of receptors and effectors in the nerve supply of voluntary muscles which enables us to judge our position in space relative to other objects, and to make comparisons of weights and pressures. This is highly susceptible to training. Where it is lacking, due to disease of the nervous system, the individual may be severely handicapped even if his other senses are intact.

8. Balance

Balance is regulated by impulses transmitted to the muscles from the organ of balance in the ears and from the stretch reflexes. It is highly developed in the juggler and the acrobat, but can be improved in anyone by training. A person whose organs of balance are not functioning cannot maintain an erect posture even if all other systems are working normally. It is dependent to some extent on visual input, but can be trained in the blind by using other senses.

9. Flexibility

Flexibility is an important component of physical fitness since it permits a full range of joint motion. It is favored by the symmetrical development of good strength in both the antagonistic muscle groups crossing the joints. Overdevelopment of one group will cause a decreased range of motion in the direction of pull of the opposing group. Inactivity causes a decrease of joint flexibility as the result of shortening of the fibers in the joint capsules. Failure of ability to relax muscle tension, due usually to a general increase in nervous tension, may also reduce general flexibility.

10. Varieties of Fitness

We see, then, that physical fitness has many components, and that it is not possible to speak of it as a general quality without acknowledging many individual variations that are dependent on constitutional factors, as well as experience and training. The person who manifests the highest degree of physical fitness is one who possesses all the qualities that have been discussed to the highest degree. Even so, for a specific task or skill there may be many others less generally fit who may exceed him in that performance. Varieties of physical fitness may thus be said to be almost infinite.

C. Formal Training Programs

Training programs that involve one type of exercise, such as calisthenics or isometric exercises, or which include several different types of exercises, such as a circuit training course, are offered in schools and colleges and other institutions whose primary objectives deal with sports and physical education. They are included in the training of members of the Armed Forces and are being made increasingly available to employees of business and industrial establishments. The quality and quantity of trained and untrained supervisors and instructors for these programs varies enormously.

Exercise programs have been offered to the public through radio instruction for many years, and now through television. Newspapers, magazines, books, and recordings contain a multitude of programs directed at men, women, children, or whole families. Local and national organizations of persons interested in attaining and maintaining physical fitness, such as the National Jogging Association, have appeared recently to supplement organizations of many years standing, such as the Turner societies.

Most of these programs, if used as the entire means of developing a compehensive state of physical fitness in any one individual, would fall short of the mark in different respects. Some put much more emphasis on the development of one component of fitness as compared to others. The chief deficiency is in failure to develop the qualities of increased capacity and endurance in the cardiopulmonary systems. Some of them actually recommend exercises and activities that could be detrimental to the development of physical fitness in some individuals. One example would be exercises putting unusual stress on the spine for persons who have unstable lower backs.

The success of these programs depend on the quality of instruction and supervision provided and the willingness of the participant to continue on a regular basis over an extended period of time. Both of these factors are seldom satisfied to a high degree. Two possible results are that participants may be deceiving themselves with regard to their state of fitness or become disillusioned in their quest for fitness and abandon it.

D. Informal Training Programs

As the result of being stimulated by friends or teachers or through the communications media, many individuals have embarked on their own personal training programs. These may include a wide variety of activities or may concentrate on one, such as walking, jogging, running, swimming, or cycling. Since these programs are largely dependent on self-motivation, they are more apt to be followed regularly over an extended program and to be based on activities that are enjoyable in themselves to those who select them.

In these programs, the tendency is to select activities that help to develop capacity and endurance. The danger is that without supervision, some individuals attempt to exceed their capacities too quickly with resultant injury, illness, or even a fatal outcome. Every person over age 40 who wishes to embark on such a program should seek medical advice before doing so.

E. Sports Activity

Participation in sports, even on a regular and continuing basis, does not provide any guarantee of physical fitness for the average person. The demands of sports on the functional capacity are so different that most of them can be relied on only for a very specialized type of fitness.

The best measure for the effectiveness of any sport in promoting a general state of physical fitness is the number of kilocalories consumed per hour in practice or competition. These energy expenditures have been calculated for all the commonly practiced sports activities. Even so, the intensity with which one practices is still an important variable. Although tennis is a sport in which energy expenditure on the average is fairly high, it can be played for recreation with very little work cost if one is content to stay at the baseline and not chase balls that are out of close reach.

Sports such as bowling and shuffleboard do not make sufficient demand on the average healthy person to produce any higher level of physical fitness. For a handicapped person, especially someone who was elderly with marginal heart function they might be rather strenuous. The question of improving the general state of fitness, therefore, depends on the baseline from which one starts. For this and other reasons (Chapter 18), sports and games are most useful in programs of adapted physical education and rehabilitation.

For sports that are not physically demanding in competition, coaches recommend training programs that include a greater stress on the body to develop the general state of fitness desirable for the sport, which would not be achieved in its practice alone. Football players, who cover only short distances in practice and play, run longer distances in training to develop their aerobic capacities.

III. THE MEASUREMENT OF PHYSICAL FITNESS

There is no general agreement today as to how the state of general physical fitness can be identified and measured. It was recognized as long ago as 1964 that these difficulties involve not only what steps should be taken in this determination, but also a lack of standardization of testing for physical fitness. At the Olympic Games in Tokyo in that year, a Committee on Standardization for Physical Fitness Testing was appointed and has worked since then to establish international standards for these studies. Standards have been agreed upon and are scheduled for publication with a supplementary volume of explanatory and interpretative material in 1974 (Larson, 1974).

Davies (1971) has stated that, "a person who is fit in the physiological sense will possess a complete integration between his functional and dimensional oxygen transporting components—his aerobic power and capacity will be high." Asmussen (1971) pointed out the most important criteria from the physiologist's point of view are "mobility, muscle strength, anaerobic power, aerobic power and endurance, and neuromuscular coordination." Measurement of a quality as general as "mobility" is obviously impossible. Some of its components, such as speed, agility, and reaction time may be measured with variable degrees of accuracy. Measurements of anerobic power have to be made indirectly, and present techniques do not permit a high degree of reliability.

A. Multiple Battery Tests

Physical fitness testing first became a subject of general interest in the United States with the publication of a study entitled "Minimum Muscular Fitness in School Children" by Kraus and Hirschland (1954). A comparison was made between the performances of European and United States school children on six simple exercise tests and the conclusion was drawn that European youth was far superior to American youth in general physical efficiency. This was given wide publicity and was one of the factors that led President Eisenhower to appoint a President's Council on Youth Fitness in 1956. The Kraus–Weber tests that were employed actually measured only two of many ability factors in physical efficiency and were applicable only to small children. The American Association for Health, Physical Education and Recreation subsequently proposed a more diversified test battery (1958). These tests have been widely used since then as a means of evaluating school children. The battery includes pull-ups, sit-ups, a 50-yard dash, a shuttle run, a 600-yard run-walk, a standing broad jump, and a softball throw for distance. The test was modified slightly on the basis of 10 years experience in 1969.

The concept of "motor fitness," which might be defined as the capacity for performing vigorous work, had already become popular during World War II for testing military personnel. The Army Air Force Physical Fitness Test (Larson, 1946), the Navy Standard Physical Fitness Test (1943), and the Army Physical Efficiency Test (Mathew, 1963) are examples of these multiple battery tests. Endurance, power, strength, agility, flexibility, and balance are the capacities measured by these tests. Similar test batteries designed for high school and college youth are the Indiana Motor Fitness Test (Bookwalter, 1943; Bookwalter and Bookwalter, 1953) and the DGWS Test (Metheny, 1945). Many of the tests employed in these batteries are the same or closely similar. The interested reader is referred to Mathews (1963) for the details.

Fleishman (1964), as the result of long study in the application of over a hundred different tests for different types of physical fitness, decided that no one test or battery of tests described up to that time gave a complete picture of the physical fitness of the individual. He performed a factor analysis of the 58 tests that he considered to be most significant and derived from this a battery of 14 tests which he called "Basic Fitness Tests." These were tested on children in 45 schools throughout the United States for validity. As the result of this experience he reduced the battery to 10 tests measuring 9 basic fitness factors (Table I).

B. Tests of Specific Fitness Factors

1. Strength Tests

Since the measurement of strength can be a highly objective process, strength testing as a measure of a person's overall fitness continues to be popular with physical enductators and coaches. When strength falls far below an expected level, one may well suspect the presence of some organic disease or severe emotional problem.

The strength index is a gross score obtained by measuring vital capacity with a wet spirometer in cubic inches and adding to it raw scores of grip strength in both hands to the nearest pound, back and leg lifts in pounds, and arm strength in pounds based on number of pull-ups and push-ups done. The Physical Fitness Index (PFI) is obtained by comparing the Strength Index (SI) with a norm based on the individual's age, sex, and weight.

$$PFI = \frac{Achieved\ SI}{Norm} \times 100$$

TABLE I

The Ten Basic Fitness Tests

Test	Primary factor measured
1. Extent flexibility The subject stands, with left side toward, and at arms length from wall. With feet together and in place, he twists back around as far as he can, touching wall with his right hand at shoulder height.	Extent flexibility
2. Dynamic flexibility With his back to the wall and hands together, the subject bends forward, touches an "X" between his feet, straightens, twists to the left, and touches an "X" behind him on the wall. He repeats the cycle, alternately twisting to the right and to the left, doing as many as possible in the time allowed.	Dynamic flexibility
3. Shuttle run 20-Yard distance, covered 5 times for 100 yard total.	Explosive strength
4. Softball throw The subject throws a 12″ softball as far as possible without moving his feet.	Explosive strength
5. Hand grip The subject squeezes a grip dynamometer as hard as possible.	Static strength
6. Pull-ups The subject hangs from bar with palms facing his body, and does as many pull-ups as possible.	Dynamic strength
7. Leg lifts While flat on his back, the subject raises his legs to a vertical position, and lowers them to floor as many times as possible in the time limit.	Trunk strength
8. Cable jump The subject holds, in front of him, a short rope held in each hand. He attempts to jump through this rope without tripping, falling, or releasing the rope.	Gross body coordination
9. Balance A The subject balances for as long as possible on a $\frac{3}{4}$-inch wide rail with his hands on his hips, using his preferred foot.	Gross body equilibrium
10. 600-Yard run-walk The student attempts to cover a 600-yard distance in as short a time as possible.	Stamina (cardiovascular endurance)

* The principles of the Cybex exerciser are described in "Isokinetic Exercise" (Perrine, 1968).

Cable-tension strength tests have been developed by Clark (1953) for 38 muscle groups using a tensiometer. A goniometer is also necessary to measure the joint angle at which the tension is exerted. Although these tests are used primarily for research purposes, there are many practical applications possible in adapted physical education, therapeutic exercise, and rehabilitation following illness or injury.

2. General Motor Ability Tests

There is no single test that can show adequately the ability of an individual to perform all of the skills of any one or more than one sport. Factors beside strength and endurance which contribute to a high level of performance in sports include speed, agility, balance, coordination, and power. Motor skills are highly specific to the task to be performed. Nevertheless, the person who exhibits a considerable number of specific motor skills may be rated high in motor ability generally since he demonstrates that he can adapt his basic qualities to any number of different performances.

Tests of motor ability consequently include a variety of activities which are then rated to produce a score. Examples of such test batteries are the Newton motor ability tests (Mathews, 1963), Scott motor ability test (Scott, 1969), Cozen's test of general athletic ability (Bovard *et al.*, 1949), and the Larson motor ability test (Larson, 1941), which has both indoor and outdoor versions.

3. Running Endurance

Probably the simplest and most reliable running test for cardiorespiratory function is Balke's 15-minute run (Balke, 1963). The criterion of performance is the distance covered on a measured track during 15 minutes. The individual makes his own pace. The raw score is compared to norms for age.

C. Body Composition

Reference man should have a body fat percentage of between 12 and 14 (Brozek, 1963). Any excess of body fat acts as a detriment to physical fitness because it is dead weight that has to be lifted or carried. Leanness is associated with high degrees of general physical fitness and athletes may have fat percentages as low as 4. An athlete with a body fat percentage in excess of 20 may be arbitrarily considered to be obese, even though he may otherwise manifest a high degree of physical fitness.

Body fat percentage may be determined by underwater weighing (Behnke *et al.*, 1942), the measurement of 1 to 6 skin fold thicknesses

(Brozek *et al.*, 1954) or by whole body counts of potassium (Allen *et al.*, 1960). For the practical purposes of assessment of athletes; the estimate based on skinfold thickness is satisfactory.

IV. MAINTENANCE OF PHYSICAL FITNESS

Once physical fitness is achieved, it is not maintained without a continuous effort. Any level of fitness may be maintained with less effort than is required to reach it. Regular vigorous activity at least 2–3 times a week is necessary for the maintenance of fitnesss. Many persons find it more enjoyable to continue a daily program of activity and can maintain their fitness with somewhat less intensity of work than those who exercise intermittently.

Strength that has been developed beyond the amount needed for daily living activities is lost at the rate of about 10% a week when training stops completely. Cardiorespiratory endurance is apparently lost somewhat less rapidly but steadily. Motor skills are rarely lost completely although they may deteriorate with the passage of time; usually they may be revived quickly on resuming the activity.

Control of excess fat weight is one of the most difficult problems in the maintenance of fitness since a reduction of daily energy expenditures with a continuation of the same caloric intake inevitably results in the deposition of fat.

The commitment to physical fitness should be lifelong, since the need to maintain optimum functioning of the body increases rather than decreases with age. Activity levels are gradually reduced consistent with age. They may be gauged by using the elevation of the pulse rate as a guide, since the most efficient heart rate decreases as a function of age, beginning in the late twenties or early thirties.

V. PHYSICAL FITNESS FOR THE HANDICAPPED

High levels of physical fitness may be attained by persons with relatively severe handicaps. Athletes lacking one or more limbs have been successful in amateur and even professional sports. Blind athletes have been excellent wrestlers. Sports programs for wheelchair athletes were introduced at Stoke–Mandeville Rehabilitation Centre in England after World War II and today involve thousands of persons all over the world.

The subject of physical education of the handicapped is dealt with extensively in Part III of this book. Although the production of competitive athletes is not the purpose of these programs, it may be an incidental result. The purposes do include establishment and maintenance of levels of physical fitness which are consistent with the handicaps present.

REFERENCES

American Association for Health, Physical Education and Recreation. (1958). "AAHPER Youth Fitness Test Manual." AAHPER-NEA, Fitness Department, 1201 Sixteenth St., N.W., Washington, D.C.

Allen, T. H., Anderson, E. C., and Langham, H. (1960). *J. Gerontol.* 15, 358–357.

Asmussen, E. (1971). Quoted by Fishbein (1971).

Åstrand, P-O, and Rodahl, K. (1970). "Textbook of Work Physiology," p. 6. McGraw-Hill, New York.

Balke, B. (1963). "A Simple Field Test for the Assessment of Physical Fitness," Bull. 63–6. Federal Aviation Agency Civil Aeromedical Research Institute, Oklahoma City, Oklahoma.

Behnke, A. R., Jr., Feen, B. G., and Welham, W. C. (1942). *J. Amer. Med. Ass.* 118, 495–498.

Bookwalter, K. W. (1943). *Res. Quart.* 14, 4.

Bookwalter, K. W., and Bookwalter, C. W. (1953). "A Measure of Motor Fitness for College, "Bull. No. 19a. School of Education, Indiana University, Bloomington.

Bovard, J. F., Cozens, F. W., and Hagman, P. (1949). "Tests and Measurements in Physical Education," 3rd ed. Saunders, Philadelphia, Pennsylvania.

Brozek, J. (1963). *Curr. Anthropol.* 4, 3–16.

Brozek, J., Brock, J. F., Fidanza, F., and Keys, A. (1954). *Fed. Proc., Fed. Amer. Soc. Exp. Biol.* 13, 19.

Clarke, H. H. (1953). "A Manual: Cable-Tension Strength Test." Brown-Murphy Co., Chicopee, Massachusetts.

Committee on Exercise and Physical Fitness. (1966). American Medical Association, Chicago, Illinois.

Davies, C. T. M. (1971). Quoted by Fishbein (1971).

Davis, E. C., Logan, G. A., and McKinney, W. C. (1961). "Biophysical Values of Muscular Activity," p. 51. W. C. Brown, Dubuque, Iowa.

DeLateur, B. J., Lehmann, J. F., and Fordyce, W. E. (1968). *Arch. Phys. Med. Rehabil.* 49, 245–248.

DeLorme, T. L. (1945). *J. Bone Joint Surg.* 27, 645–67.

deVries, H. A. (1966). "Physiology of Exercise for Physical Education and Athletics," pp. 220–221. W. C. Brown, Dubuque, Iowa.

Fishbein, M. (1971). *Med. World News,* p. 52.

Fleishman, E. A. (1964). "The Structure and Measurement of Physical Fitness." Prentice-Hall, Englewood Cliffs, New Jersey.

Karpovich, P. V. (1965). "Physiology of Muscular Activity," 6th ed., pp. 220–221. Saunders, Philadelphia, Pennsylvania.

Kraus, H., and Hirschland, R. P. (1954). *Res. Quart.* 25, 177–188.

Larson, L. A. (1941). *Res. Quart.* **12**, 3.
Larson, L. A. (1946). *Res. Quart.* **17**, 2.
Larson, L. A. (1974). "Fitness, Health and Work Capacity: International Standards for Assessment." Macmillan, New York.
Lockhart, A. (1959). Department of Physical Education, University of Southern California, Los Angeles (unpublished paper).
Mathews, D. K. (1963). "Measurement in Physical Education," p. 120. Saunders, Philadelphia, Pennsylvania.
Metheny, E., chm. (1945). *J. Health Phys. Educ.* **16**, 6.
Navy Standard Physical Fitness Test. (1943). Chapter IV. Bureau of Naval Personnel, Training Div. Phys. Sect. U.S. Govt. Printing Office, Washington, D.C.
Perrine, J. J. (1968). *J. Health, Phys. Educ. Recreation* pp. 40–44.
Scott, G. M. (1939). *Res. Quart.* **10**, 3.

Chapter 4

THE LIMITS OF HUMAN PERFORMANCE

ALLAN J. RYAN

Prediction of the potential for record performance in sports is probably as old as the custom of wagering on the outcome of sports events, that is, at least several thousand years old. The first attempt to put it on a scientific basis was apparently made by Professor Arthur Kennelly of Harvard University (1906) who based his predictions on studies that he made of the rate of exhaustion for horses running and for men running, skating, and swimming. He found the rates to be quite similar and used this apparent consistency as a basis for his calculations. Among other predictions he stated that the record for the mile run, which was at that time 4:12.8, would be reduced to 3:58.7.

Not all of the factors that affect human performance are susceptible to easy measurement. In addition to the physiological, there are anthropometric, psychological, environmental, technical, and social factors. To these may also be added the element of chance, or coincidence, which at some point allows some or all of the factors to exert a maximum influence at the same time to produce the record-breaking performance. Fortune favors the well-prepared, however, and it is seldom that a lucky circumstance produces a record performance by some one who had not already manifested the potential to achieve it.

It almost goes without saying that it is all but impossible to predict performances that cannot be measured in numbers, either of time or distance or repetitions. Scoring records, which are so commonly used as a basis for comparison of athletes in individual and team sports, are being broken regularly, but there is no basis on which predictions can be made as to how or when they might be broken. Bobby Orr is without doubt incomparable as a professional hockey player, but it is doubtful that he could have established the scoring records which he achieved in 1969–70 if it had not been for the expansion of the National Hockey League and the consequent formation of temporarily weaker teams.

I. ANTHROPOMETRIC FACTORS

Size is a factor in all types of sports performances that involve the athlete's accelerating his body, moving it over a distance, lifting it, turning it, exerting maximum force, and throwing. The relationships between body size and performance have been summarized very clearly and concisely by Åstrand and Rodahl (1970). Taller persons have greater strength in proportion to their size and also have greater respiratory capacities. They have an advantage in jumping events due to their higher center of gravity, and in throwing events, since they can launch their missile from a greater height. They are slower in accelerating their bodies than shorter persons, and are at a disadvantage in lifting them if their weight is greater, which it usually is.

Increases of height among the world's populations are observed to have occurred sporadically, but with increasing consistency during the past two centuries (Shapiro, 1963). This process has accelerated greatly in the last 50 years, especially in the United States. Studies of college populations in succeeding generations, where many of the subjects were in direct descent, especially at Harvard and Yale, have shown an increase in average height which in the case of Yale has reached a level of 1.0 cm every $12\frac{1}{2}$ years (Hathaway and Foard, 1960).

This increase in height has quite naturally been reflected in increases in average height among athletes in many sports, especially those sports where records of time and distance can be established. Khosla (1970) has pointed out that in only five sports or events in the Olympic program, excepting wrestling and weight lifting where the competitors cover a broad range of sizes by design, do the mean heights of the champion athletes fall below the median height for United States males of a comparable age (18–24): steeple-chase, marathon, gymnastics, soccer, and field hockey. Tanner (1962) showed that on the average, middle distance runners at the 1960 Olympic Games in Rome were 3 inches taller, and weight throwers were 4 inches taller than comparable groups in the 1928 Olympics at Amsterdam.

There is no question that the average increase in the height of athletes in recent years has contributed substantially through the increase in human power to the establishment of new world records. What remains in doubt is whether and how long these increases may continue to occur. We have some reasonable assurances that man's immediate progenitors averaged only about 4 feet 6 inches in height. Obviously the present rate of increase in height was not sustained from several million years ago. One thing that would help us to determine the future would be to know the causes of the recent growth spurt.

Scientists who have studied this problem are not in agreement as to the causes. Better nutrition, lower morbidity and mortality rates in the early years due to control of infectious diseases, more vigorous exercise in early years of life, earlier sexual maturity, and heterosis have all been implicated (Hathaway and Foard, 1960; Tanner, 1960; Ashcroft et al., 1966; Bakwin and McLaughlin, 1964). Although all these factors may have had some part in increasing the average height, the most significant role has probably been played by heterosis, the mixing of diverse populations. It has been demonstrated in other forms of life that the mixture of genes will produce increases in size in subsequent generations within the same species. There is certainly a tremendous variety of subspecies among *Homo sapiens,* and the improvements in travel and communications, trade, wars, etc., have produced a satisfactory mixture in the past 300 years, particularly. It has also been noted that groups that have remained isolated during this period of time have not apparently shared the same growth (Shapiro, 1963).

The prospects in the future seem good for increased mixing of the world's populations. The open question is how much further mixtures will provide additional growth increases. Somewhere there must be a limiting point where stability of growth is established. There are many examples of giantism occurring in subhuman species, notably the dinosaurs, the gorilla, and the giraffe, to name a few. In human populations we have tribes such as the Watusi and Dinkas, whose average height is well over 6 feet and individuals as tall as the late Robert Wadlow who reached the height of 8 feet 11 inches. Seven foot basketball players are no longer a rarity in the United States and in other countries. It seems that for the immediate future we are due for still further increases in average height.

II. PHYSIOLOGICAL FACTORS

Apart from those improvements that are inherent in the relationship of increased stature to increased power, it has been demonstrated possible by modern methods of training to improve for the average individual as well as the select athlete the capacities of the lungs and the cardiovascular system which increase the ability to take in air and to utilize its oxygen more efficiently and to increase muscle strength. With a greater understanding of all those physiological factors that affect performance, it is now also possible to utilize selectively those that are favorable and minimize those that are unfavorable, such as heat stress.

The scientific study of traditional training methods and the development of new systems based on physiological principles has revolutionized the teaching and practice of many sports, especially track and field (athletics) and swimming. Yet many persons feel that still more may be done along these lines. Still we lack detailed knowledge in many areas which would make these improvements even greater. How such knowledge may be obtained and applied is problematical, but the process has begun and will continue.

A. Respiratory Capacities

Human performance may be analyzed as far as the development of aerobic and anerobic capacities are concerned by studying the intake of air and the outflow of expired air. Through the compilation and correlation of the data involving gas exchange as recorded by instruments to measure the various lung volumes and the composition of expired air, it is possible to make statements regarding the state of training of the individual, and sometimes of his apparent potential as long as he has not already reached it to a maximum degree.

There is some disagreement among coaches and athletes as to the best training method to produce maximum respiratory capacities. Some favor long, slow, distance work and other interval training. Many athletes include both in their program. Very high capacities have been reached by athletes following all three approaches.

The determination of the maximum oxygen intake in liters per kilo of body weight per minute (max V_{O_2}) seems to give the most accurate estimation of an individual's respiratory capacity and endurance, although it also measures the efficiency of the cardiovascular system. The sum of the max V_{O_2} multiplied by the number of minutes working at maximum capacity plus the individual's ability to accumulate oxygen debt in liters gives the total respiratory requirement for a given piece of work. The average trained adult male is capable of reaching an oxygen debt of about 15 liters.

B. Cardiovascular Capacities

The efficiency of the heart depends on its ability to increase its output substantially during any bout of exercise. It does so by increasing its size, both in the thickness of its muscle wall and in the volume of its chambers. The former effect produces a permanent slight enlargement of the heart; dilation of the chambers is lost when training stops. Limiting factors in the enlargement of the heart are the dimensions of the chest, its fixation to the arteries and veins that leave and enter it, and the cross-sectional diameter of the aorta, which does not enlarge with exercise. Diseased hearts may become much larger than athletes' hearts, but they are inefficient because of the weak myocardium and its poor circulation.

An increase in the number of capillaries in the lung and in the muscles facilitates the exchange of oxygen and carbon dioxide. These changes occur in response to exercise. The limiting factor is uncertain, but it is estimated that the capillary surface may be doubled in both areas as the result of intensive training.

Other adaptive mechanisms that relate to cardiovascular capacities are increases in the total hemoglobin of the blood and increases in plasma volume. Hemoglobin increases under the stress of vigorous exercise, but especially when it is combined with decreased barometric pressure, as at moderate altitudes. The limiting factor appears to be increasing viscosity of the blood. The changes that take place are reversible at sea level, but provide a temporary advantage for performance at sea level for the three weeks or so that it takes for reversion to normal levels of hemoglobin. Plasma volume increases in response to heat stress but diminishes slightly at moderate altitudes. The advantage of increased plasma volume is to maintain adequate return to the heart and increase heat dissipation under conditions of elevated air temperature and increased relative humidity. The limiting factor is in the ability of the heart to handle the increased volume.

C. Muscle Strength

As pointed out in Section I, there is a close correlation between height and strength. Strength may be developed disproportionately, however, even in persons of relatively small stature by intensive training. Overloading muscles by isometric, isotonic, or isokinetic exercise may bring about enormous increases in strength over a period of time. Paul Anderson on one occasion raised 6270 pounds with a back lift.

With any type of training that increases strength, muscle size will also increase in the exercised muscles. Strength in any one muscle is found to be proportional to its cross-sectional areas. Maximum strength is achieved in the muscle when it is fully extended.

Limiting factors in increasing muscle are the ability of the circulation to supply the muscle and the strength of the skeletal structure with its ligaments to be able to resist the force exerted without breaking or tearing.

III. PSYCHOLOGICAL FACTORS

The factors preventing individuals from exerting their maximum strength or working to the absolute limit of their endurance are recognized but not well understood. Discomfort and pain are quite obvious reasons, but there are some situations where they are not involved and still the individual cannot extract the reserve energy present unless some other circumstance intervenes.

Excitement, cheering, loud noises, and other shocking or surprising events may cause an individual to exceed not only his previous best effort but to make an effort that afterwards seems wholly unreasonable, even to him. It is reported that a hysterical 123-pound woman, Mrs. Maxwell Rogers, lifted one end of a 3600-pound car which, after the collapse of a jack, had fallen on her son at Tampa, Florida on April 24, 1960 (McWhirter and McWhirter, 1971). She suffered compression fractures of several vertebrae.

Lack of self-confidence, fear of failure, and even fear of winning may act to prevent a competitor from realizing his best effort. The emotional factors that influence an athlete's performance may be so powerful that they nullify partially or completely physical abilities that are outstanding or even extraordinary (Ogilvie and Tutko, 1966).

Certain established records establish a mystique about them which create a psychological handicap for anyone attempting to break them. Babe Ruth's record of 60 home runs in one season stood intact for many years largely because of the impact of the personality of the man who set the record, as well as the fact that it was a round number with a magical quality. The four-minute mile was a psychological barrier that was finally overcome by a man, Roger Bannister, who was not only a world class runner but one who had convinced himself scientifically that he could do it.

The psychological characteristics of champion athletes have been described by several psychologists (Ogilvie and Tutko, 1966; Vanek and Cratty, 1970; Tutko and Richards, 1971). Neither complete self-control nor uncontrolled enthusiasm and/or aggression will satisfy the situation of a champion. There is a blend of drives, emotions, and controls which is different for each individual, even though certain common general characteristics are found. Motivation toward excellence is a characteristic that can be recognized in terms of an individual's continued dedication toward and success in sports, but is next to impossible to say what produces it, and why some persons have it and others of apparently equal ability do not.

One cannot define any limiting factors in the development of a perfect psychological set for record performance. Historical descriptions of the most outstanding performers in a variety of sports offer the only standards we have for comparison and prediction.

Fatigue is partially central and partially peripheral in origin. The exact mechanisms of both parts and their interrelationship remains obscure. A high degree of motivation can enable a person to carry on in a work task far beyond the point at which he would otherwise stop voluntarily with the feeling that he could no longer continue. The ability to ignore the pain which comes from long-continued effort can be cultivated by highly dedicated individuals. It is customary now to talk in training programs that emphasize endurance of "working through the pain."

IV. ENVIRONMENTAL FACTORS

The external circumstances accompanying sports performances or attempts to establish records may be a determining factor in the mark achieved. There are probably very few times when a set of completely favorable circumstances coincide with a state of almost perfect preparedness of an athlete who has the capability of a world record performance. Such a coincidence of critical factors occurred in the case of Bob Beamon's long jump of 29 feet 2½ inches at the Olympic Games in Mexico City on October 16, 1968.

Beamon's jump was made at 3:46 PM on a cloudy afternoon at an air temperature of 23.5°C, relative humidity of 42%, and a barometric pressure of 577.8 mm. From this it can be calculated that air density was 24% less than on a typical day at sea level, giving him a theoretical advantage of 3 inches for these conditions. Estimation of his probable speed in running (about 24 mph) gave him an additional 1% increase in speed over sea level, adding another 7⅛ inches to his jump. The decrease in gravititational pull is almost insignificant (0.1%) but may have added very slightly to his distance. The runway for the jump was fast, and when he made his first, and record-breaking jump, only three men had preceded him, so that it was in excellent condition. There was a slight following wind at 2.2 mile/hour, just 0.1 miles/hour below the velocity that would have disqualified any record. If he had had to jump one-half hour later it would have been in a heavy rain and the prospects of such a distance would have been highly unlikely.

The circumstances that may be controlling in any particular event include elevated temperature and humidity, cold, air resistance and movement, water resistance and movement, barometric pressure, gravity, the competition, and the audience setting.

A. Elevated Air Temperature and Humidity

Outdoors, moderate temperatures between 65° and 75°F are most suitable for peak human performance. As air temperature rises it becomes more difficult for the body to cool itself during exercise, with the result that extra energy is expended to facilitate the cooling process. As air temperature rises above mean body temperature the body begins to store heat, cutting down on the efficiency of its working processes, and posing the danger of heat exhaustion or stroke. Buskirk and Tait (1965) have pointed out that, at a work load of five times resting metabolism, the time to incipient collapse decreases steadily as the temperature and humidity increase. It is therefore highly unlikely that world records will be set under such conditions for any event requiring more than a relatively short time to complete. A high relative humidity, which favors the production of heat stroke through hydromeiosis, is more critical than the air temperature, since fatal heat stroke has occurred in a football player at an air temperature of 64°F when the relative humidity was 100% (Fox et al., 1966).

B. Cold

In a cold environment muscle viscosity increases and joints stiffen, impairing performance considerably. With minimal clothing, as in running or swimming costume, energy stores must be used at an increased rate available for running or swimming. Swimmers in marathon events frequently have to give up because of hypothermia.

The combination of cold air temperature and high wind velocity will induce hypothermia and frostbite rapidly in the person who is not well protected. Sky divers making delayed opening jumps from stratospheric altitudes must wear electrically heated clothing. Heavier clothing which must be worn by downhill and cross-country skiers in severe weather naturally mitigates against record performance by increasing both weight and resistance to the air.

C. Air Resistance and Movement

Decreased air resistance, as it is encountered at moderate altitudes due to the decreased density of the air, favors record performance in running and certain throwing events. The advantage is balanced by the disadvantage for any running event over 800 meters caused by decreased partial pressure of oxygen in the air. At high altitudes the advantage for even short distances disappears.

The most favorable condition for running on an oval track is still air, since the advantage achieved from a wind blowing the length of the oval or across it is outweighed by the greater work in running against it. A wind favoring a sprinter, hurdler or long jumper competing only in one direction on a straightaway may not exceed 2.2 miles/hour in velocity for a record to be acceptable in Olympic competition.

D. Water Resistance and Movement

The resistance of water to the swimmer is constant for the portions of the body which are submerged. The resistance may be decreased by greater buoyancy, which occurs in salt water. Not enough competitions with first-class swimmers have been held on closed courses to test whether more records would be set than in fresh water. Swimmers with a higher percentage of body fat are more buoyant and may be able to set records for endurance swimming but probably not for speed.

Waves act to impede the progress of a swimmer, tiring him and slowing him down. In long distance swimming in open water the best chances for record performance would be in still air with absence of waves. Wavelets occur in pools as the result of the water being stirred up by many swimmers. The sides of pools are constructed with troughs to dampen these wavelets, and the lane markers are now made with open baffles to reduce this effect even further.

Tides and other currents in the open water may aid or hinder the swimmer depending on his direction. By taking advantage of favorable ebb and flow of the tides swimmers are able to cross the English Channel in a V-shaped path which adds to the distance but decreases the work.

E. Barometric Pressure

With decreasing barometric pressure the partial pressure due to oxygen falls to a point where it begins to affect performance in any activity involving endurance at an altitude of a little over 4000 feet. It becomes increasingly difficult to support vigorous activity until the altitude exceeds 20,000 feet, at which point only very well acclimated persons do not require assistance from inhalation of oxygen. One team of alpinists climbed Mt. Everest (29,002 feet) without using oxygen equipment. A Colombian boy who stowed away in the wheel well of an airplane survived a flight of 4 hours at an altitude of 30,000 feet. This appears to be the absolute limit of human endurance at altitude without the use of oxygen.

At a medium altitude of 6000 to 7000 feet the decreased density of the air favors sprinters, jumpers, and throwers of the shot and javelin. At middle and long distances the advantage is counterbalanced by the decreased partial pressure of oxygen. Performance in distance running events may improve with acclimatization but not reach sea level values (Grover and Reeves, 1967).

Internal barometric pressures increase with the descent under water at the rate of 1 atmosphere for every 10 m. Depth in free diving is limited chiefly by breath-holding ability, which does not exceed 3 to 4 minutes even for most highly trained divers. The body is well able to stand the water pressure at depths much greater than can be reached because of the development of anoxic and hypercapnia (Chouteau and Corriol, 1971). In scuba diving, the limiting factors are the inability of the body to tolerate hyperoxia and the increased working of breathing against the inert gas in whatever mixture is used (Chouteau and Corriol, 1971). Helium is the best adjuvant. Hydrogen so far has proved to be too toxic. Greater depths are now being reached by using "saturation diving" which avoids the long decompression times.

F. Gravity

The force of gravity decreases slightly as one rises above the surface of the earth. This tends to favor jumpers and weight throwers at moderate altitudes. The advantage is very small compared to the other effects which are produced on performance by the decreased barometric pressure.

G. Competition

As efficient as men may become in learning to pace themselves correctly, the spur of competition leads most of them on to even greater efforts than they sometimes believe possible. Few world records are established in a noncompetitive setting. Where a record try is being made as the sole purpose of an event there are usually others involved in a simulated competition as pacesetters and in other roles.

The tendency of the body to stop somewhere short of its ultimate effort may be temporarily overcome by the excitement of competition. Bodily discomfort may be completely ignored in the heat of an important contest. The riddle of the "sick sports victor" has not yet been studied by sports psychologists and physicians. Many examples could be cited of previously successful athletes who rose from sick beds to enter and win sports contests, even setting records in the process.

H. Audience Setting

The cheers of the crowd and the tension generated by a large or enthusiastic audience has a powerful effect on some athletes, bringing out frequently their best performance. Feelings of apathy and disinterest on the part of spectators quickly communicate themselves to sensitive athletes who often respond in kind.

V. SOCIAL FACTORS

The social factors that are to some extent far extending human performance to the establishment of new world records have been pointed out by Craig (1968) and Buskirk and Tait (1965). They include a larger population from which to draw, greater number of persons involved in sports, greater prestige attached to sports participation, development of keener competitive attitudes, improved economic conditions, the effect of athletes marrying athletes, and the availability of better medical care. It seems likely that some of these factors may continue to bring about improvements for an extended period of time into the future, barring major changes in man's social organization.

A. Greater World Population

The total world population passed 3.5 billion in 1971, and if present rates of increase continue will reach 4 billion by 1980. Not only does this create a bigger base from which more outstanding athletes may appear but it inevitably brings about a greater genetic mix and brings more people together more times to create the situations in which sports competitions develop.

B. Greater Number of Sports Participants

Although sports are a universal phenomenon, even in the most primitive societies, the spread of European culture around the world in the last three centuries has been chiefly responsible for developing the type of sports and the attitude toward sports which has led to extending the apparent limits of human performance. Track and field sports and swimming has given us types of activities where achievements are measured in times and distances which can be compared from year to year and from generation to generation.

Perhaps the greatest single factor in the increase in sports participation has been the inclusion of physical education and sports programs in the programs of general education at all levels.

C. Greater Prestige for Sports Participation

The sportsman today, whether amateur or professional, does not have to apologize to anyone for spending ,a good part, or indeed all, of his time playing games. His exploits are recorded endlessly in newspapers, magazines, on radio and television, and in motion pictures. The successful athlete today is a cultural hero who is received by presidents and kings and honored with parades and medals. Professional athletes command some of the highest annual salaries paid in the United States today.

Sports in the socialist and communist countries have become important political factors in uniting populations at home, strengthening defensive forces, and promoting those countries in the international scene. Lenin recognized the value of sports and physical education and gave them a priority even over industrial and agricultural development in establishing the USSR. Cuba, with a tottering economy and an autocratic government holds its people to a common purpose through a comprehensive sports program.

D. Development of Competitive Attitudes

With an increasingly complex urban civilization, competition increases in its importance as a means of survival. The reflection of competitive attitudes developed in education, science, business, the professions, and even attaining social prestige is naturally felt in sports. This gives rise to such statements as that made by the late Vincent Lombardi, a successful football coach, who told his players that "Winning is not the most important thing; it is the *only* thing."

Keener competition means that better performance records will be established. When Paavo Nurmi and Willlie Ritola of Finland were setting world and Olympic running records in the 1920's, they had no worthy competition to push them to even greater efforts. As it is, the records of their achievements indicate that if they were facing today's record holders they would be equal if not superior to them in endurance.

E. Improved Economic Conditions

Improvement in average income levels and working conditions for many part of the world today mean that more time can be taken from the day for pursuit of leisure activities and more money is available to pay for them. As far as countries and communities are concerned, it means more and better facilities for sports participation and more professional instruction and supervision available. It also means greater income from spectators for both amateur and professional sports which helps to make more and better sports programs possible.

F. Athletes Marrying Athletes

Marriages between athletes, particularly among those who are most highly endowed physically, are becoming more common as the numbers of persons involved in sports increases and as women's sports are further developed. Such marriages tend to produce a relatively high percentage of athletically gifted children. In addition to the genetic effect there is the very important influence of growing up in a family where sports have a very high priority and where everyone participates in some type of sports activity.

G. Availability of Better Medical Care

The development of an athlete to the point where he is capable of a record-breaking performance takes many years. This progress may be delayed or stopped entirely by injury or intercurrent illness if either is not taken care of promptly and efficiently. Greater interest of physicians in sports as medical advisors and consultants has resulted gradually in cutting down the toll of disability and dropping out for athletes. The control of infectious disease especially has been important in this regard. Better treatment of acute injuries prevents many of them from becoming chronic. Advances in surgical management of sports injuries have resulted many times in complete rehabilitation of those who would formerly have been lost to sports competition.

VI. TECHNICAL FACTORS

The limits of human performance have been extended in the past, and will be further extended in the future, by technical factors which aid the athlete in his efforts. These include the development of improved apparatus and equipment, provision of better facilities, refinements of measurement techniques, and improvements in coaching techniques and systems.

A. Improved Apparatus and Equipment

An outstanding example of the effect of improving apparatus on extending performance limits is the development of the vaulting pole. Modern competitive pole vaulting began in 1853 when it appeared on the program of the Caledonian Games (Ganslen, 1965). From this time until about 1900, the poles were made of ash, spruce, oak, fir, or hickory and were relatively rigid. Bamboo poles were used sporadically by a few vaulters. The record height went gradually from 8 feet 6 inches to 12 feet. After the Olympic Games in Paris in 1900 most vaulters adopted the bamboo pole, and the record height advanced again to 14 feet in 1927.

Improvements in the technique of vaulting and in the vaulting box in which the pole was placed continued to occur and Warmerdam was able to raise the record vault with bamboo pole to 15 feet 7¾. In 1939 the aluminum pole was introduced, and in 1947 the steel pole. Both were rather rigid, and the latter was a little too heavy, so that no great advance was made as the result of using them.

The fiber glass pole was used first in 1948, but was not very dependable because it shattered easily. When the quality of these poles was improved, vaulters, led by the Finns, learned how to bend the pole to take advantage of its catapaulting action. The record was quickly moved to 16 feet and reached 18 feet in 1971. An additional technical factor that has made these greater heights attainable has been the use of beds of plastic foam for the landing pit. Whereas formerly the vaulter had to complete his vault in such a fashion that he would land on his feet, he can now come down safely and fairly comfortably flat on his back.

As far as personal equipment is concerned, the production of a very lightweight running shoe has played a considerable role in improving running times over medium and long distances. It is difficult to say what the percentage factor of improvement has been since many other variables have been operative during the period since this shoe was introduced after World War II. The theoretical advantage in having a lighter load to lift with each footstep over a mile or over must amount to an improvement of several seconds per mile.

B. Provision of Better Facilities

The improved design of swimming pools to cut down backwash has helped the reduction of swimming times. Faster track surfaces, resistant to the unfavorable effects of weather, such as the Tartan Track, have helped to make for better running times in indoor and outdoor meets. Improved design of indoor running tracks with wider surfaces, more scientifically banked curves, and fewer laps to the mile have also played a part.

C. Refinements of Measurement Techniques

The stopwatch with divisions of one-fifth, and then one-tenth of a second, was developed from the desire of coaches and officials to be able to separate the times of professional sprinters running at a distance of 150 yards. This made it possible to establish new records, since an accuracy of only one second or worse would not distinguish between the best and other performances at such a short distance.

This has now been succeeded by electrical timing systems for running, swimming, and downhill skiing which are accurate to one hundredth of a second. Since improvements tend to occur by smaller increments as the theoretical limits are being approached, it is now possible to follow more accurately the slight improvements that occur in extending the limits of human performance.

Techniques of linear measurement are just beginning to be improved, as by the device which was used to measure the distances in the long jump at Mexico City in 1968. This device, running on a rail fixed to the side of the jumping pit, failed only because no one had anticipated a jump of over 29 feet.

D. Improvements in Coaching Techniques and Systems

Improvements in running and swimming times at middle and long distances have resulted from the recognition by coaches that endurance is developed only by hard and intensive training. Covering more distance every week, whether by long, slow work or by interval training, has been the factor more responsible for improvement in times than any other. Whatever method has been used, it has brought the athletes who have used it closer to the ideal of maintaining a more even pace.

A second factor of great importance has been the recognition by coaches of the importance of developing the overall strength of the athlete for events such as running or swimming in which there is no deliberate physical contact. The use or isometric and isotonic exercises as part of the training for almost every sport has become a commonplace.

The development of attitudes that reject sensations of pain and fatigue through a psychological approach on the part of coaches has been a third factor in extending human performance limits. This is carried to a point where it could be described as being a state of self-hypnosis. The formal use of hypnosis, where the coach or hypnotist acts to control the situation directly, has so far not proved successful in extending performance limits in ways that cannot be duplicated by other means. The repeated use of hypnosis by unqualified persons who are not prepared to cope with the problems that may be raised is extremely dangerous and should not be permitted.

Further improvements in coaching techniques may be expected as the result of the increasing interest of coaches in exercise physiology and practical application of their findings.

VII. PREDICTING HUMAN PERFORMANCE LIMITS

Kennelly's initial report (1906), which started the whole series of speculations on human performance limits, was entitled, "An Approximate Law of Fatigue in the Speeds of Racing Animals." He compared the world racing records for horses, running, trotting, and pacing and for men walking, running, rowing, skating, and swimming. Adopting the symbols L for the distance covered in meters, T for the time in seconds, and V for the speed in meters per second, he plotted the records for each event on log paper, opposing each of the three variables in turn against each other. He found a linear relationship in each case, and when the records for one event were compared with the others he found that the lines were roughly parallel.

From these results he proposed the following equations:

$$T \cong \frac{L^{9/8}}{C}, \qquad \text{also } T \cong \frac{C^8}{V^9} \text{ seconds} \tag{1}$$

$$L \cong C^{8/9}T^{8/9}, \quad \text{also } L \cong \frac{C^8}{V^8} \text{ meters} \tag{2}$$

$$V \cong \frac{C}{L^{1/8}}, \qquad \text{also } V \cong \frac{C^{8/9}}{T^{1/9}} \text{ meters/second} \tag{3}$$

In these equations C stands for a constant and $\cong$ stands for approximately equal.

He concluded that there was "a certain approximate law of fatigue" which applied to all these events, and that "a record maker's best speed should be as nearly as possible uniform from start to finish, and just such as to bring him to muscular exhaustion at the goal." The records which appeared to him to be most open to attack were those which fell off the straight lines on the side indicating that the necessary average speed had not been maintained relative to performances on both sides of them.

In 1926 he reviewed the progress in record breaking during the preceding twenty years (Kennelly, 1926), and found that there had been an average increase in the racing speed of record-breaking running horses of 2.3%, a slighter but poorly defined improvement for trotting horses, but none for pacing horses. There had been no marked change in men's running speeds except at 100 m where average speed had increased from 9.8 to 9.9 m/second. Long distance running records continued to be weak. There were no improvements in race walking or rowing. In speed skating the times were too long and average speeds slow. This was due, although he did not note it, to the custom of skating the early stages of the race very slowly in a pack and sprinting only for the last part. An analysis of bicycle racing records showed similar inconsistency for the same reasons. In swimming, speeds had improved by 16% due to the introduction of the new free style in swimming by the Hawaiians. He observed that the law of distances and times related to average speeds is that a 1% increase in speeds reduces the running distance by 8% and the running time to exhaustion by 9%.

In the meantime, Meade (1916) had written "An Analytical Study of Athletic Records," in which he drew curves plotting the rate of running (per 100 yards in seconds for short distances) on the ordinate against the distance run in miles on the abscissa. For those distances that were run customarily, the records fell on a smooth parabolic curve from 220 yards to 5 miles. The rate for the 100- and 220-yard dashes was the same. For the less usual events the records fell on the defective side of the curve, as did the longer distances. He was not apparently aware of Kennelly's report since he called for a mathematical study of his findings. In a second report (Meade, 1934) he did not add anything to what had been reported up to that time.

Hill (1925) followed up Kennelly's lead with the first attempt to explain record performance on a physiological basis. He plotted speed on the ordinate against time on the abscissa and derived a relationship between the oxygen requirement and speed. He was limited by concepts that the maximal possible oxygen debt was 15 liters and the maximal oxygen intake possible was 4 liters/minute. He explained the physiological basis for the wastefulness of high speeds and reiterated Kennelly's caution that a uniform speed is the optimum for record breaking performance. He discussed some of the factors involved in high jumping and long jumping but did not analyze the records. He made no predictions of improvement, but laid a solid groundwork for those who were to follow.

In "The Dimensions of Animals and Their Muscular Dynamics" (Hill, 1950), he returned to considerations of performance limits in a discussion of the relationship between muscle loading and speed. Maximal power is developed at 0.3 maximal speed of muscle shortening and against 0.3 maximal loading. It is about $\frac{1}{10}$ of the product of maximum force and maximum velocity for the muscle in question. Maximum efficiency of muscle action is about 20% of the energy consumed and occurs at 0.2 maximum speed against an 0.5 maximum load. It is therefore possible to work at maximal power with nearly maximal efficiency. He calculated the maximum speed of human runners to be 12 yards/second. Due to the inertia of starting, it is not reached until 4 or 5 seconds have elapsed.

Brutus Hamilton, at that time track coach at the University of Southern California, proposed a table of human ultimates in track and field performance in 1935 and subsequently revised his estimates in 1952. These estimates were partly scientifically derived from the Finnish Decathlon scoring table, but were also based on his experience as a coach and were simply "informed guesses." All of the revised estimates have since been exceeded by a wide margin.

The forthcoming Olympic Games in Berlin stimulated Frederick Lewis Allen, a professional writer to discuss "Breaking World's Records" in Harper's Magazine (Allen, 1936). He charted record times for four running events on the ordinate against years on the abscissa. He stressed the importance of improvements in equipment, technique, and training, the greater size and greater numbers of athletes in competition each year, the emergence of Negro athletes and the effect of emotional psychological factors. He made a comparison between improvements in the record for running a mile and the gradual improvement in winning times each year at the AAU championship meet. Improvements in these times followed the setting of new records but also anticipated the setting of a new record.

Doctor A. W. Francis published a short article on "Running Records" in 1943. He plotted mean speed on the ordinate against the log of distance on the abscissa and derived a hyperbolic curve with a vertical asymptote at 1.5 and a horizontal one at 3.2 m/second. The equation was as follows:

$$(\log D - 1.5)(V - 3.2) = 6.081$$

The fit of the curve to the records was not a good one, however. He predicted ultimate records of 1.47.2 minutes for the 880-yard run, 2.04.7 for 1000 yards, and 3.58.7 for the mile. All of these marks have since been exceeded.

Lietzke (1952) studied world, Olympic, and American running records from 100 yards to 30,000 meters. He plotted rate per 1000 m against miles, and also made a semi-logarithmic plot of rate per 1000 m against time in seconds. He derived two curves which were fairly smooth, each of which had an initial upsweep due to the inertia of starting. They showed that a maximum rate was reached at 15 seconds (150 m). At 140 seconds (1000 m) the curves flatten out and then become steeper again beyond 10,000 m. Two years later Lietzke (1954), in "An Analytical Study of World and Olympic Racing Records," plotted the log of distance in miles against the log of time in seconds. From this he derived the equation

$$\log d = K \log t + \log a$$

where a represents a unit conversion factor, the y-intercept of the plot. He found that the slopes (K) for running, walking, swimming, horse running, bicycle racing (flying start, motor paced) and automobile racing (standing start) all have values between 0.8 and 1.0.

He drew rate curves plotting rate against distance and against time expressed in log seconds. He also calculated an exhaustion constant expressed in the following formulas where $\bar{r}$ is the average rate:

$$\bar{r} = d/t = at^{K-1} = a^{1/K}d^{(K-1)K}$$

since

$$d = at^K \ at = (d/a)^{1/K}$$
$$\log \bar{r} = (K - 1)/K \log d + 1/K \log a$$

or

$$\log \bar{r} = K^1 \log d + 1/K \log a$$

where

$$K^1 = (k - 1)k.$$

The constant K^1, which is the slope of the line obtained when $\log \bar{r}$ is plotted as a function of $\log d$, is a measure of how the average rates decrease with distance, and can be called "the exhaustion constant."

The values of K^1 can be calculated for each type of racing directly from k, the slope of the plot of log distance against log time. He gave it as 0.0941 for men running, 0.1136 for horses running, 0.858 for women running, and 0.0720 for men swimming. He stated that records that were "out of line" would be indicated by such calculations but offered no predictions regarding new records.

In 1954 and 1955, Henry studied records of men racing, plotting the log of velocity against linear time in seconds. By taking into account glycogen depletion and lactic acid metabolism, and including a subtractive term for loss due to internal resistance and the development of momentum, he derived an exponential expression of fatigue and was able to describe the speed and position of the runner as a function of.time with the following equation:

$$dy/dt = a_y e^{-k4t} + a_z e^{-k3t} + a_z e^{-k2t} + a_1 e^{k1t}$$

which gives the velocity of running in yards/second for any elapsed time between 5 seconds and 10,000 seconds.

On March 12, 1958, Karpovich (1958), basing his prognostication on the supposed limits of oxygen intake and oxygen debt capacity, predicted that the mile would be run in 3.56.6 minutes, which was only 0.6 seconds below Derek Ibbotson's world record at that time. After Jazy ran the mile in 3.53.6, eight years later, Karpovich (1966) predicted that it would be lowered only another 0.6 of a second. The following year Ryun lowered it by two seconds.

In 1960, Reindell reported on heart volumes of nonathletic persons as well as high jumpers, wrestlers, swimmers, football and tennis players, skiers, oarsmen, distance runners, and professional cyclists. He found the mean volume to range from 782 and 790 ml for nonathletes, jumpers, and wrestlers, through 876 for swimmers, football and tennis players, and 923 for skiers, oarsmen, and distance performers, to 1104 for professional cyclists. This confirmed earlier autopsy findings (Muller, 1883) and a later report by Gleason (1965). Since heart size plays an important part in determining cardiac output, if the muscle is not diseased, it became quite apparent that heart size was an important limiting factor in performance. In 1966, Dr. Reindell was quoted as saying at the Sixteenth World Congress of Sports Medicine in Hannover that the point was being reached where training techniques would no longer be able to overcome human biological limitations.

Craig (1963) constructed new velocity–duration curves with m/second on the ordinate and time in log seconds on the abscissa, based on then existing record performances in running and swimming. He made the assumption that the maximum rates of energy expenditure were equal for short distances (13.0–13.7 hp for runners and 14.1 for swimmers). The shape of the curves suggested that the swimmer could work closer to his maximum capacity for a longer distance than the runner. This might be due to a greater possibility for efficient heat exchange. He also constructed curves for individual swimmers and suggested that they should be comparable to world record curves although considerably below them. A failure of the curve to keep up in the longer distances would show lack of endurance in that swimmer. Curves of improvement in running and swimming times plotted against historical time showed that improvement is exponential, but the curves have to be reconstructed periodically to account for new records.

Five years later, Craig (1968) again examined record performances in men's and women's track and field and free-style swimming. When the curves were constructed on an ordinate of m/sec and abscissa of time in log seconds, two straight portions were noted in each curve corresponding to the sprints and distances requiring from 2 to 8 minutes for completion. He concluded that recovery takes place even while degradation of performance is occurring, and that the athlete must learn to balance these two forces. At maximum effort the anaerobic processes are exhausted in 40 seconds. In longer races, carbon dioxide production and heat dissipation are critical factors. At the middle distances, the ability to handle the imbalance of oxygen intake and carbon dioxide transport is critical. The essential process in fatigue may be metabolic acidosis, and endurance may involve chiefly the ability to buffer nonvolatile acids in the system. He further pointed out that horses are apparently capable of continuing to run at an average speed close to 85% of their maximum velocity, whereas man can do this only at about 71% of his.

In comparing increments in performance by decades and by percentage, Craig found that sprints had improved by 7.1%, middle distances by 9.4%, and long distances by 11.8% since 1900. Record performances in jumps improved 13.9%, and in throws (shot, javelin, discus, and hammer) by 55.8%. Swimming records improved 23%. In charting the increments of improvements and durations of records, the records that showed the biggest increments over the previous record actually lasted the shortest times. He concluded that it is impossible to say how long any given record may last. Plotting increments of performance as a function of historical time does not indicate that we have reached the point of progressively smaller increments as yet. Projecting record curves by time or distance against historical time is also an unproductive process.

Perhaps the only way to predict the occurrence of future records, Craig says, is to consider the record holder as part of a large population of competitors. In analyzing records in interscholastic and intercollegiate swimming he found that the mean times of winners in regular competitions tended to improve by decades. If the existing record in any event is not part of a normal distribution curve for the times or distances for all winning times or distances recently, and the curve is skewed far to the left, a new record can be expected at any time. Two standard deviations below the mean of winning times for champion intercollegiate swimmers is a parallel curve of the world records for the 100-yard freestyle as charted against historical time. This means, in effect, that the world record holder or breaker must be better than 95% of the other champion swimmers. The increase in the number of competitors is what continues to skew the curve to the left, since it can be shown by mathematical means that the mean of a larger group of competitors will be faster than that of a smaller group even though the means of the whole groups are the same.

Frucht and Jokl (1964) reported a "Parabolic Extrapolation of Olympic Performance Growth since 1900" in which they attempted to predict the results for the forthcoming Olympic Games in Tokyo. They constructed curves that were based on time for running and distance for jumping on the ordinate and historical time in years on the abscissa. These curves were parabolic and were based on a mixture of world's records and best Olympic performances. Their predictions were based on extrapolations of these curves. Their criteria for the success of their predictions was that they would lie within one standard deviation in 23 of 34 events and within 2.5 for the other 11. In a subsequent article (Jokl and Frucht, 1966) they claimed that 20 of 25 track and field events satisfied these criteria but were not able to explain the results in those that did not. They described some of the sociological factors that were producing changes in record performances.

Buskirk and Tait (1965) pointed out that there are many environmental limitations that may influence the limits of human performance. These include tolerance to peak G forces, the time to incipient collapse in sustained work in conditions of high air temperature and humidity, reduced partial pressure of oxygen at moderate and high altitudes, and water temperature in swimming. In describing record performances in men running and swimming and in horses and greyhounds running they plotted mean velocity in m/sec against historical time and also against time expressed in log seconds. They showed a change in the shape and slope of the curve for world running records between 1935 and 1965.

They discussed the many variables that could be responsible for improvements, including increased size and strength of athletes, superior skills, better facilities and equipment, more facilities and more competitors, better genetic selection, better nutrition, a more competitive environment, and better medical care. They emphasized the improvements in cardiovascular capacity which could result from training which is now producing maximum oxygen intakes as high as 81.7 ml/kg/minute which are related to increased heart size, increased cardiac output, increased diffusing capacity, a wider arteriovenous oxygen difference, and greater maximum anaerobic capacity. They did not offer any specific predictions.

Finally, Lloyd (1966) has produced the most elaborate mathematical analysis of all, based on physiological principles. He plotted records for male runners covering distances from 50 yards to 623 miles as of August 26, 1965 with log meters of distance on the ordinate and log seconds of time on the abscissa. He found an almost straight line which corresponds to a line with the equation

$$\log \text{ meters run} = 1.11 + 0.9 \log \text{ seconds taken}$$

Through an involved mathematical analysis supported by experimental evidence, chiefly from Margaria *et al.*, (1963a, b, 1964, 1965), he refutes Hill (1925, 1950), although he recognizes the importance of a relationship between the store of energy available and the rate at which it is expended.

The energy expended to cover a given distance, he says, is independent of the velocity. The power for fast sprinting is only twice that generated in marathon running. A comparison of the plotted slopes shows that there has been an increase in capacity for caloric usage in middle distance running of 15% in the past 90 years. The trend in record breaking is due to an increased ability to use oxygen efficiently, which in turn is related to greater cardiovascular capacity. His predictions are that the slopes of record plots can be expected to increase so that times for all running races up to 10,000 m should improve by 5.5% by the year 2000, and for longer races by 7.5%. This could mean times of 8.6 seconds for 100 yards, 42.4 seconds for 440 yards, 3.41 minutes for 1 mile, 26 minutes 8.4 seconds for 10,000 m and 2 hours 2 minutes for the marathon.

REFERENCES

Allen, F. L. (1936). *Harper's Mag.* 173, 302–310.
Ashcroft, M. T., Ling, J., Lovell, H. G., and Miall, W. E. (1966). *Brit. J. Prev. Soc. Med.* 20, 22.

Åstrand, P-O., and Rodahl, K. (1970). "Textbook of Work Physiology," Chapter 10. McGraw-Hill, New York.

Bakwin, H., and McLaughlin, S. M. (1964). Lancet 2, 1195–1196.

Buskirk, E. R., and Tait, G. T. (1965). Proc. Conf. Med. Aspects Sports, 7th, 1965 pp. 1–9.

Chouteau, J., and Corriol, J. H. (1971). Endeavour 30 (110), 70–76.

Craig, A. B., Jr. (1963). J. Sports Med. Phys. Fitness 3, 14–21.

Craig, A. B., Jr. (1968). J. Amer. Med. Ass. 205, 734–740.

Fox, E. L., Mathews, D. K., Bowers, R., and Kaufman, W. (1966). Res. Quart. 37, 332–339.

Francis, A. W. (1943). Science 98, 315–316.

Frucht, A. H., and Jokl, E. (1964). J. Sports Med. Phys. Fitness 4, 142–152.

Ganslen, R. V. (1965). "Mechanics of the Pole Vault" 6th ed., pp. 10–16. John Swift & Co., St. Louis, Missouri.

Gleason, D. F. (1965). Doctoral Thesis, University of Minnesota, Minneapolis.

Grover, R. F., and Reeves, J. T. (1967). In "The International Symposium on the Effects of Altitude on Physical Performance," pp. 80–85. Athletic Institute, Chicago, Illinois.

Hamilton, B. (1935). Amat. Athlete pp. 4–5, April.

Hamilton, B. (1952). Amat. Athlete pp. 6–7, May.

Hathaway, M. L., and Foard, E. D. (1960). "Heights and Weights of Adults in the United States," Home Econ. Res. Rep. No. 10. Human Nutr. Res. Div., U.S. Dep. Agr., Agr. Res. Serv., Washington, D.C.

Henry, F. M. (1954). Res. Quart. 25, 164–177.

Henry, F. M. (1955). Res. Quart. 26, 147–158.

Hill, A. V. (1925). Sci. Mon. 21, 409–428.

Hill, A. V. (1950). Sci. Progr. 38, 209–230.

Jokl, E., and Frucht, A. H. (1966). Abbottempo 1, 2–8.

Karpovich, P. V. (1958). Scope Weekly.

Karpovich, P. V. (1966). Med. Trib.

Kennelly, A. E. (1906). Proc. Amer. Acad. Arts Sci. 42, 275–331.

Kennelly, A. E. (1926). Proc. Amer. Acad. Arts Sci. 61, 487–521.

Khosla, T. (1970). Brit. J. Sports Med. 4, 270–277.

Lietzke, M. H. (1952). Sci. Amer. 86, 52–54.

Lietzke, M. H. (1954). Science 119, 333–336.

Lloyd, B. B. (1966). Advan. Sci. 22, 515–530.

McWhirter, N., and McWhirter, R., eds. (1971). "Guinness Book of World Records," 10th ed., p. 520. Stirling, New York.

Margaria, R., Cerretelli, P., Aghemo, P., and Sassi, G. (1963a). J. Appl. Physiol. 18, 367–370.

Margaria, R., Cerretelli, P., Mangili, F., and DiPrampero, P. E. (1963b). Congr. Eur. Med. Sports 1st, 1963 (cited in Margaria et al., 1964).

Margaria, R., Cerretelli, P., and Mangili, F. (1964). J. Appl. Physiol. 19, 623–628.

Margaria, R., Mangili, F., Cuttica, F., and Cerretelli, P. (1965). Ergonomics 8, 49–54.

Meade, G. P. (1916). Sci. Mon. 2, 596–600.

Meade, G. P. (1934). "Records and Record Breaking." New York University Alumnus New York.

Muller, W. (1883). "Die Massenverhaltnisse des Menschlichen Herzens." Voss, Hamburg.

Ogilvie, B. C., and Tutko, T. A. (1966). "Problem Athletes and How to Handle Them." Pelham Books, London.

Reindell, H. (1960). "Herz, Kreislaufkrankheiten und Sport." Barth, Leipzig.

Shapiro, H. L. (1963). *N.Y. Times, Mag. Sect.* p. 13, Dec. 15.

Tanner, J. M. (1960). "Growth at Adolescence." Oxford Univ. Press, London and New York.

Tanner, J. M. (1962). "The Physique of the Olympic Athlete." Allen & Unwin, London.

Tutko, T. A., and Richards, J. W. (1971). "The Psychology of Coaching. Allyn & Bacon, Boston, Massachusetts.

Vanek, M., and Cratty, B. J. (1970). "Psychology and the Superior Athlete." Macmillan, New York.

PART II

MEDICAL SUPERVISION OF THE ATHLETE

Chapter 5

MEDICAL QUALIFICATION FOR SPORTS PARTICIPATION

FRED L. ALLMAN, JR.

I. THE PURPOSES OF PREPARTICIPATION
PHYSICAL EVALUATION

Primary and foremost to be considered in any program designed to prevent athletic injuries is the preparticipation physical evaluation. The purpose of a complete physical evaluation is five fold: first, to determine the general state of health of the athlete; second, to disclose any existing defects; third, to uncover conditions that might predispose to injury; fourth, to institute treatment that will bring the individual to an optimum level; and fifth, to classify the individual according to his own qualifications. The evaluation must be thorough, with special consideration being given to rating the candidate on his level of maturation and physical development as well as his level of physical readiness.

Slocum (1959) has pointed out that the objective of such examinations is not only to determine which players meet all physical qualifications, and thus may participate with safety, but also to determine whether an individual may play safely in spite of definite recognized defects that appear detrimental on screening examination but on thorough study can be classified as not harmful.

II. TIMING OF THE PREPARTICIPATION EVALUATION

The preparticipation examination should be scheduled at least three weeks prior to the beginning of the season. By allowing an interval of at least three weeks, any condition that is disclosed during the examination may have necessary consultation and final evaluation prior to the beginning of the season. This time also allows for the correction of minor defects such as muscular weakness, skin disorders, minor infections, etc. The site of the examination should be, whenever possible, a preexisting health facility such as a student health service at the college, the public health clinic in the community, or, in case of the family physician, at his office. The commonly practiced habit of conducting the examination in the gymnasium, locker room, or coach's office is unsound because these facilities usually do not offer environments of quietness and privacy which are required for proper evaluation.

III. THE HEALTH HISTORY

It has been shown that the best and most complete examinations are the result of combined efforts of the family physician and a special

TABLE I

A Sample Health History Which Should Be Filled Out by the Parent and/or Athlete prior to the Physician's Examination

Do you know of any reason why this athlete should not participate in all sports? Yes ____ No ____

Has athlete been advised by a physician during the past five years to restrict activity? Yes ____ No ____

Is the athlete under a physician's care now? Yes ____ No ____

Has he been seen by a physician within the past year? Yes ____ No ____

Is he on any medication at the present time? Yes ____ No ____
Name of medication _____

Does athlete wear: Glasses ____ Contact lens ____ Dentures
Bridgework ____ Dental braces
Date of last visit to dentist _____

Has athlete ever had a surgical operation? Yes ____ No ____

Has athlete ever been confined to a hospital? Yes ____ No ____

Has he had any illness or infection lasting more than a week? Yes ____ No ____

Has he had any injuries requiring medical attention? Yes ____ No ____

Has he ever had any injury of muscle, bone, ligament, tendon or joint?
Yes ____ No ____
Was medical attention required? Yes ____ No ____
Was athlete temporarily disabled? Yes ____ No ____
How long diabled? _____

Has athlete ever had: Back pain ____ Shoulder dislocation ____
Ankle sprain ____ Knee trouble ____ Knee cap dislocation ____

Has athlete ever been knocked unconscious? Yes ____ No ____
How many times? ____
Was he evaluated by a physician? Yes ____ No ____
Was he hospitalized? Yes ____ No ____

Has athlete ever fainted? Yes ____ No ____
How many times? ____

Does athlete have frequent headaches? Yes ____ No ____

Has athlete ever had convulsions? Yes ____ No ____
How many times? ____

Has athlete ever become weak or ill when exposed to high temperature?
Yes ____ No ____

Does he have loss or seriously impaired function of any paired organ?
Eye ____ Lung ____ Kidney ____ Testicle ____

Does athlete have or has he ever had?

Asthma/hay fever	Yes ____	No ____
Allergies	Yes ____	No ____
To what? _____		
Diabetes	Yes ____	No ____
Heart disease (rheumatic fever, high blood pressure, murmurs)	Yes ____	No ____
Epilepsy	Yes ____	No ____
Abnormal bleeding tendencies	Yes ____	No ____
Kidney disease	Yes ____	No ____
Tuberculosis	Yes ____	No ____
Stomach/intestinal trouble	Yes ____	No ____
Arthritis	Yes ____	No ____

Please elaborate below on any of the above questions with a "yes" answer.

examination group of physicians. The family physician should be relied upon to provide information especially related to any injury or illness, old or new, that might have a bearing as to the physical fitness of the youth. This should include any history of past concussions, allergies, bleeding tendencies, chronic diseases, joint injury, whether healed or repaired, significant illnesses, surgical procedures, and pertinent family history. Previous or current immunizations, urinalysis, and blood count should also be included and sent with the previous information to the school physician or special examination group in writing. The special examinaiton group may be composed of voluntary or previously selected members of the local medical society and represent many different specialities. These might include the team physician, an orthopedic surgeon, an internist, a general surgeon, and an ear, nose, and throat specialist. Other specialists might be utilized initially or might be called upon at a later time should consultation be necessary.

The health history is extremely important and must be completed prior to the administration of the physical examination. Ideally, it should be completed by the athlete with the knowledge of the family physician and parent. Items which should be included in the health history are listed in Table I.

IV. PHYSICAL EXAMINATION

The physical examination must be thorough. It should include height, weight, blood pressure, examination of the head generally, eyes, ears, nose, throat, neck, lungs, heart, abdomen, liver, spleen, the musculo-skeletal system (with special emphasis being devoted to the neck, spine, shoulder, elbow, knee, and ankle), the genitalia, the abdominal wall, and skin. The examiner should be alert for any signs that might indicate an endocrine or metabolic disorder as he makes an overall appraisal of the general appearance of the candidate at rest and in motion.

V. DENTAL EXAMINATION

A complete dental evaluation should be an integral part of the pre-participation evaluation. In addition to the preparticipation evaluation, a team dentist is helpful in making arrangements for dental emergency treatment and has the major responsibility for the mouth protector program.

VI. LABORATORY EXAMINATIONS

These should include estimation of the hemoglobin or hematocrit and a urinalysis unless a recent report of the determinations is available from the family physician.

Special Laboratory Data

Special laboratory examinations should be obtained whenever indicated by the health history or physical examination. These might include a complete blood count, X-rays of a suspicious area, electrocardiogram, electroencephalogram, kidney function studies, vital capacity, or other tests that might be indicated by the special situation.

VII. IMMUNIZATIONS

Dates and reactions to previous administration of tetanus toxoid or antitoxin, poliomyelitis vaccine, diphtheria toxoid, smallpox vaccine, and other immunizing substances should be noted. If vaccination or booster doses of toxoid are needed due to the passage of many years since the original administration, they should be given at this time.

VIII. SPECIAL CONSULTATION

As mentioned previously, special consultation by a specialist should be obtained whenever doubt exists as to the extent of involvement of a disease process or condition, or where a condition exists for which no diagnosis has been obtained.

IX. ROLE OF PARAMEDICAL PERSONNEL

Nurses, physical educators, physical therapists, psychologists, dieticians, and other paramedical personnel may be called upon to help in evaluating the candidate for an athletic team. The nurse can provide assistance in vision and hearing tests as well as recording height, weight, blood pressure, pulse, respiration, and other clinical data. The physical educator and physical therapist can assist in performing fitness evaluations including step tests, one and one-half mile runs, body build, posture, flexibility, and strength evaluation. The psychologist is very helpful in determining the emotional stability of the individual and of the individual's psychic readiness for sports participation.

X. EVALUATION OF PHYSICAL READINESS FOR SPORTS

In order to evaluate full the candidate for sports participation, ascertaining the mere presence or absence of organic disease is not enough. It is necessary to evaluate his physical readiness for the particular sports event in which he plans to participate. Indications of the individual's physical readiness for sports may be found in many factors, including size, body build, flexibility, strength, cardiovascular and respiratory fitness, physical maturation, and emotional stability.

A. Body Build

Accurate evaluation of the body build of an individual may yield important facts relating to his physical readiness for sports participation. Factors to be considered are his age, height, weight, ponderal index (height in inches divided by the cube root of his weight), muscular development, amount of subcutaneous fat, somatotype, and posture. The importance of body build has not been given nearly as much attention in the medical literature as have simple height–weight relationships.

Weight is an inconstant measure of volume but volume increases according to the cube of linear dimensions. As an index of shape, it excludes body size, indicating the linearity and laterality more accurately than height–weight categories. Individuals in categories with ponderal indices of 11.6 or less are predominantly obese, extreme endomorphs, those whose physique is characterized by softness and roundness and in whom abdominal mass dominates thoracic bulk. In some cases they may be mesomorphs; that is, persons with massive muscular and bony development. Dominant ectomorphs, on the other hand, often have a ponderal index above 13. Normal ranges will vary somewhere between 11.5 and 14, according to the individual's age.

B. Somatotype*

The physique of an athlete reflects his physical fitness from two stand-points—that of heredity and that of his existing physical condition. An individual of given skeletal build should have sufficient muscular development to operate his skeleton effectively and to reflect good nutrition. A physically fit person should have relatively little adipose tissue under the skin and in the places where fat typically deposits. Too much fat is definitely detrimental to an athlete. The ideal physique demonstrates good muscular development with a moderate amount of fat and a proportionately well developed body. Some very odd body types are encountered such as those with strong legs coupled with a very weak upper body, those with excessively large bones and poorly developed muscles, and the very fat type who has poor musculature. While there may be many possible combinations, most physiques fall into one of four major categories (Fig. 1):

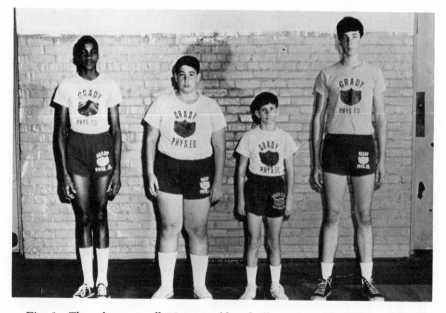

Fig. 1 These boys are all 13 years old and all members of eighth grade intra-mural sports teams in the same school.

* Reproduced by permission from Thomas K. Cureton, "The Physical Fitness Workbook."

1. Mesomorphic or Husky Type

This type has a relatively solid, muscular, big-boned physique. Such types are usually moderate in height or sometimes short, but with hard, heavy massive muscles. They are usually strong in weightlifting and carrying loads, and excel in hard collision or combat work in athletics. Their ligaments are usually strong. The measured girths are relatively large for the neck, upper arms, trunk, forearms, calves, and thighs.

2. Ectomorphic or Frail Type

This type has a relatively frail body with a short trunk and thin cross-sectional dimensions. The neck, arms, and legs are long with relatively undeveloped muscle bulk. This type suggests the lack of internal organic development. Injuries to such persons are frequent in contact sports. Notably there is a lack of strength for weightlifting and all kinds of maximum force work. These types may be frustrated or unduly exhausted with hard physical effort, but may be capable of sustained effort, as in long distance running.

3. Endomorphic or Soft, Fat Type

This type has a relatively fat and soft body, usually including a double chin, fat cheeks, and pads of fat on the backs of the upper arms, over the iliac crest, as well as over the abdomen, buttocks, and thighs. In events executed on the feet for speed or endurance, this type is ponderous and slow with poor agility and reaction. In events on the bars with the body supported by the arms, they are practically inept. This type floats well and sometimes will do well in long distance swimming.

4. Medial or Average Type

This type is not extreme in any of the previous characteristics. A majority of people are of this type. When well developed and conditioned, this type is most efficient on an all-around basis. The normal response to muscular effort and training is good if interest can be secured and the work gradually increased in dosage.

5. Dysplastic Type

A fifth, or unusual, type has been added for the unsymmetrical or dysplastic individuals. This includes those individuals mentioned previously with a weak upper body and strong lower body, the extremely tall and thin, those with a large skeleton but poor musculature, or any varying combination.

C. Posture

Postural evaluation is very important. Body alignment depends not only upon the integrity of the joints themselves but also upon the muscles acting upon the joints (Fig. 2). Lowman (1958) has pointed out that "a machine with properly aligned working members acts efficiently, and with care lasts much longer than one which is out of line. In a malaligned machine the wear and tear on bearings increases the stress and strain

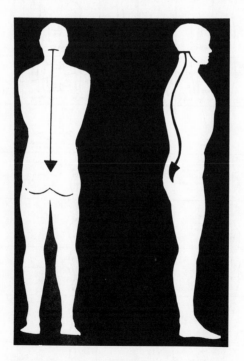

Fig. 2 These silhouettes show that for correct posture at any age following puberty the spine should not show any lateral deviation, but when viewed from the side should show gentle compensatory curves in the lumbar, thoracic, and cervical regions. The head should be held erect so that the eyes look straight forward. The pelvis should be rotated forward and the abdomen kept flat so that the shoulders can be held in a comfortably relaxed position without rounding forward.

TABLE II
A Type of Posture Score Sheet Which Is Commercially Available[a]

POSTURE SCORE SHEET	Name _____			SCORING DATES			
	GOOD - 10	FAIR - 5	POOR - 0				
HEAD LEFT RIGHT	HEAD ERECT GRAVITY LINE PASSES DIRECTLY THROUGH CENTER	HEAD TWISTED OR TURNED TO ONE SIDE SLIGHTLY	HEAD TWISTED OR TURNED TO ONE SIDE MARKEDLY				
SHOULDERS LEFT RIGHT	SHOULDERS LEVEL (HORIZONTALLY)	ONE SHOULDER SLIGHTLY HIGHER THAN OTHER	ONE SHOULDER MARKEDLY HIGHER THAN OTHER				
SPINE LEFT RIGHT	SPINE STRAIGHT	SPINE SLIGHTLY CURVED LATERALLY	SPINE MARKEDLY CURVED LATERALLY				
HIPS LEFT RIGHT	HIPS LEVEL (HORIZONTALLY)	ONE HIP SLIGHTLY HIGHER	ONE HIP MARKEDLY HIGHER				
ANKLES	FEET POINTED STRAIGHT AHEAD	FEET POINTED OUT	FEET POINTED OUT MARKEDLY ANKLES SAG IN (PRONATION)				
NECK	NECK ERECT, CHIN IN, HEAD IN BALANCE DIRECTLY ABOVE SHOULDERS	NECK SLIGHTLY FORWARD, CHIN SLIGHTLY OUT	NECK MARKEDLY FORWARD, CHIN MARKEDLY OUT				
UPPER BACK	UPPER BACK NORMALLY ROUNDED	UPPER BACK SLIGHTLY MORE ROUNDED	UPPER BACK MARKEDLY ROUNDED				
TRUNK	TRUNK ERECT	TRUNK INCLINED TO REAR SLIGHTLY	TRUNK INCLINED TO REAR MARKEDLY				
ABDOMEN	ABDOMEN FLAT	ABDOMEN PROTRUDING	ABDOMEN PROTRUDING AND SAGGING				
LOWER BACK	LOWER BACK NORMALLY CURVED	LOWER BACK SLIGHTLY HOLLOW	LOWER BACK MARKEDLY HOLLOW				
REEDCO INCORPORATED AUBURN, N.Y. 13021			**TOTAL SCORES**				

[a] Reproduced by permission of Reedco Incorporated, Auburn, New York. COPYRIGHT 1968

on the working members and produces general structural depreciation . . . [In the human machine], the maintenance of alignment is
effected by the balance of all muscles activating or acting on any joint
and the forces applied must be equated with age and structure of all
the parts of the human machine and adjustments made in accordance
with physiological age, musculoskeletal integrity and neuromuscular control." When the body is allowed to function in a position of poor alignment, postural strains are likely to occur. The extremes of muscular
effort and joint motion which are required in sports place certain implications on the interpretation of physical findings not ordinarily stressed
in those with more sedentary activity. Normal body alignment and muscle tonicity are interdependent. Opposing muscles should be equal in
length and tone with none being in a hypertonic or hypotonic state
(see Table II).

D. Flexibility

Flexibility is the ability to yield to passive stretch and to relax. Flexibility or suppleness is desirable to facilitate muscle action with a minimal
resistance of the tissues. It is necessary in order to obtain perfection
of movement. Recent studies have indicated that certain individuals
might have too much flexibility while others might have too little. Athletes
might thus be divided into tight or loose jointed individuals based upon
five simple tests. These five basic tests are as follows:
1. The ability to flex the spine so that the palms can touch the floor
with the knees fully extended.
2. The presence of backward curve of the knee of 20° or more with
the patient prone.
3. The demonstration with the knees flexed up to 15 or 30° and with
the hips, knees, and ankles turned out in maximum external rotation
so that the feet turn in a straight angle of 180° heel to heel with the
toes out.
4. The ability to lie or sit on the floor with the knees or ankles parallel
to the floor in external rotation or in internal rotation of a sufficient
degree to permit the legs and thighs to parallel the floor.
5. The presence of upper extremity laxity as demonstrated by exaggerated shoulder flexion, elbow hyperextension, and hypersupination of
the forearm to a position in which the hypothenar eminence is inclined
cephalad in a vertical plane with the elbows extended and the forearms
supinated.

Nicholas (1970), who has described these criteria, feels that any individual who cannot perform a single one of these five tests should be designated as a tight individual. Any individual who can accomplish one or more of these five tests is classified as a loose individual. His study to date indicates that, independent of many other factors responsible for injuries in athletics, an increased likelihood of ligamentous rupture of the knee may be present in loose jointed players, and muscle tears may occur more frequently in tight jointed players.

E. Skin Fold Thickness

Caliper measurements of skin fold thickness at preselected sites on the athlete's body may be used to determine the amount of subcutaneous fat. Many coaches, especially in football, like their athletes to be big, and often the athlete is encouraged to gain weight. This added weight is often fat, and if so may be more detrimental than beneficial to athletic performance. An estimate of the percent of body weight that is fat gives an indication of the individual's (detrimental) excess weight and

TABLE III

The Calculation of Body Fat Weight and Body Fat Percentage[a]

Fat-free body weight = body weight − body fat

$$\text{Body fat} = \text{body weight} \times \frac{T^b \times SA^b \times 0.739}{\text{body weight}} - .003 \times 0.7$$

$$\% \text{ Body fat} = \frac{\text{body fat}}{\text{body weight}} \times 100$$

[a] From Allen *et al.* (1956).

[b] $T = \dfrac{(\text{sum of 10 skinfolds} - 40)}{20}$; SA = body skin surface area. Calculation of skin surface area: SA (m^2) = Height$^{.725}$ × Weight$^{.425}$ × .007184. From DuBois and DuBois (1916).

Total skin fold measurements are based on the summation of 10 selected sites as follows: cheek, chest, chin, upper arm, abdomen, back, waist, calf, side, knee. All skin fold measures are in mm, height in cm, and weight in kg.

There are other formulas based upon six skin fold measures; however, it is the consensus of most investigatore that the above method is the more reliable and accurate prediction of percent body fat. This method correlates very highly ($r = 0.95$) with standardized densitometric procedures based on Archimedean principle. From Consolazio *et al.*, 1963.

thereby is a better indication of a desirable playing weight. See Table III for the formula and method of calculating the percent body fat.

F. Strength

Muscular strength and endurance are essential factors in athletic success. The hand dynamometer, a device to measure the strength of the hand grip, helps in evaluating young athletes for participation in competitive athletics. The gripping power is considered to be a fairly reliable index of an individual's physical maturity. See Table IV for the method and norms for various ages.

In addition to determination of the hand grip strength, some indication of lower extremity strength should be obtained. Minimal evaluation should include the determination of the bilateral quadriceps femoris strength in extending the knees against known resistance. Those individuals with unequal lower extremity strength or those with inadequate lower extremity strength must be considered to be high risk individuals and should be kept out of contact sports until the deficiency can be corrected.

G. Maturation

In order to classify individuals for safe and effective participation in certain athletic events, it is necessary to know their degree of physical maturity. Two of the best methods of evaluation physical maturity are by grading sexual and skeletal development.

1. Sexual Development

Sexual development rated according to the presence and character of pubic hair gives a reasonable estimation of how far a given individual has progressed through adolescence. (See Table V.)

2. Skeletal Development

The level of maturation of an individual may also be determined by the skeletal development, based upon the antero-posterior roengenogram of the wrist compared with norms in the Greulich–Pyle atlas (Greulich and Pyle, 1959).

TABLE IV
Hand Grip Strength Measurement and Norms for Boys and Girls of Ages 13–18[a]

Testing Arrangements

Equipment

All that is required is a Narragansett hand dynamometer.

Instructions

The dynamometer is placed in the palm of the patient's preferred hand. The dial should be facing away from the palm. The larger half of the grip is in the meaty part of the palm, with the fingers curled over the smaller half of the grip. Part of the fingers between the second and third knuckles should touch the grip, but the fingers should not curl far enough around to touch the dial and interfere with the pointer's movement.

The patient stands and holds his hand down his side, away from his body, palm facing his side. He is told that at the command "Squeeze," he is to squeeze the dynamometer once, sharply and steadily as hard as he can.

A demonstration of the proper grip and arm position should be given. During the test trial the examiner should make sure the patient's fingers do not hamper the dial, and that he does not rest or brace any part of his arm against his body.

During the first trial, correct any incorrect procedure. If the rules are violated, disregard the score, but count it as one squeeze. Emphasize the need for a short, sharp squeeze. If the student starts to squeeze slowly as soon as he takes the dynamometer, it will actually decrease his score due to muscle fatigue.

Each patient gets three trials separated by at least a full minute of rest. Without such rest he is likely to score lower each time he squeezes.

Scoring

Record the highest reading (the scale is read in pounds) of the three squeezes.

Hand Grip Norms[b]

Boys							Girls					
Age							Age					
13	14	15	16	17	18	Percentile	13	14	15	16	17	18
105	125	139	157	165	163	99th	65	83	84	90	99	101
102	120	130	149	156	156	98th	63	78	79	86	93	98
100	118	128	147	149	149	97th	62	76	77	83	90	96
95	115	121	140	144	144	95th	60	67	74	79	86	91
85	108	115	130	134	138	90th	58	60	69	76	79	86
80	105	111	126	129	134	85th	57	57	66	71	77	80
78	96	108	121	125	129	80th	55	56	62	69	75	78
75	93	106	118	120	125	75th	53	54	60	67	72	76
70	89	103	115	118	120	70th	50	52	59	66	69	73
67	84	98	110	115	117	60th	45	48	57	63	67	70
65	78	93	106	109	114	50th	42	43	55	59	63	67
57	75	88	101	106	109	40th	35	40	52	57	59	64
52	65	85	97	101	105	30th	33	38	49	55	57	69
50	59	81	93	98	101	25th	30	37	47	51	56	57
46	55	78	89	96	98	20th	28	36	46	49	56	56
43	50	76	86	92	96	15th	26	35	42	47	50	53
41	46	69	81	88	90	10th	24	32	39	45	47	49
39	41	61	76	82	86	5th	20	25	36	38	43	46
37	39	56	71	78	83	3rd	17	32	32	35	38	41
35	37	48	68	76	81	2nd	15	20	28	34	37	39
33	34	36	62	69	77	1st	10	15	20	31	31	37

[a] Fleishman (1964).

[b] Scores are in "pounds pressure."

TABLE V

Stages of Genital Development in Males

Stage	Pubic hair characteristics
I	No pubic hair. The vellus over the pubes is not further developed than that over the abdominal wall.
II	Sparse growth of long, slightly pigmented downy hair, straight or only slightly curled, appearing chiefly at the base of the penis or along the labia.
III	Considerably darker, coarser and more curled. The hair spreads sparsely over the junction of the pubes. (Hair shows up in black and white photo.)
IV	Hair now resembles adult type, but the area covered by it is still considerably smaller than in the adult. No spread to the medial surface of the thighs.
V	Adult in quantity and type with distribution of the horizontal pattern. Spread to medial surface of thighs but not up linea alba or elsewhere above the base of the inverse triangle.

[a] Larson (1973).

H. Cardiovascular Endurance

The direct association between increases in levels of fitness and increased circulation makes the measurement of circulatory capacity an effective and convenient measure of physical fitness. One of several tests that measures cardiovascular function is a modification of the Harvard step test, the "recovery index," which is as effective as any and requires little equipment or space (Gallagher *et al.*, 1967). The patient steps up and down on a bench at a rate of 30 times per minute for four minutes unless he stops earlier because of fatigue. Facing the bench or platform and starting with either foot at the signal "up," the patient places his foot on the bench and steps up so that both feet are on the bench, then immediately and in rhythm he steps down again and continues the exercise in a marching count, "Up, 2, 3, 4." The signal "up" comes every two seconds. On completing the exercise, he sits quietly. Pulse counts are then taken as scheduled: one minute after exercise for 30 seconds, two minutes after exercise for 30 seconds, and three minutes after exercise for 30 seconds. The patient's recovery index can then be determined by referring to a scale (Table VI).

I. Cooper One and One-Half Mile Field Test

Cooper (1968) noted a high correlation of field test data with laboratory determined oxygen consumption data. Due to the high correlation with maximal oxygen consumption, it might be assumed that the $1\frac{1}{2}$

TABLE VI

Determination of the Recovery Index from the Summation of Pulse Counts[a]

Total beats	Recovery index	Total beats	Recovery index	Total beats	Recovery index
110	109	142	85	174	69
111	108	143	84	175	69
112	107	144	83	176	68
113	106	145	83	177	68
114	105	146	82	178	67
115	104	147	82	179	67
116	103	148	81	180	67
117	102	149	81	181	66
118	102	150	80	182	66
119	101	151	80	183	66
120	100	152	79	184	65
121	99	153	78	185	65
122	98	154	78	186	65
123	98	155	77	187	64
124	97	156	77	188	64
125	96	157	76	189	64
126	95	158	76	190	63
127	95	159	76	191	63
128	94	160	75	192	63
129	93	161	75	193	62
130	92	162	74	194	62
131	92	163	74	195	61
132	92	164	73	196	61
133	90	165	73	197	61
134	90	166	72	198	61
135	89	167	72	199	60
136	88	168	71	200	60
137	88	169	71	201	60
138	87	170	71	202	59
139	86	171	70	203	59
140	86	172	70	204	59
141	85	173	70	205	58

[a] Gallagher *et al.*, 1967.

mile field performance test is an objective measure of physical fitness reflecting the cardiovascular status of an individual.

Procedure: If a measured track is not available, locate a flat, hard surface area and accurately measure a mile course. Place markers at the starting point, half mile mark and one mile mark. Using a stopwatch or watch with a sweep second hand, accurately record the time necessary to cover $1\frac{1}{2}$ miles. Do not hesitate to walk if undue breathlessness occurs. To determine the fitness category, refer to Table VII.

TABLE VII

Determination of the Degree of Physical Fitness by the
Time Taken to Cover One and One-Half Miles in
Running and/or Walking[a]

Fitness category	One and one-half mile time
I Very poor	Longer than 18 minutes
II Poor	15:01–18:00 minutes
III Fair	12:01–15:00 minutes
IV Good	10:01–12:00 minutes
V Excellent	10:00 minutes or less

[a] Cooper (1968).

XI. DISQUALIFYING CONDITIONS FOR SPORTS PARTICIPATION

The American Medical Association Committee on the Medical Aspects of Sports has published a guide for the medical evaluation of candidates for school sports (1966). In this guide, disqualifying conditions for sports participation have been listed and the various sports have been divided into three categories: Category I, Contact Sports; Category II, Noncontact Endurance Sports; and Category III, Noncontact, Nonendurance Sports. The contact sports include lacrosse, baseball, soccer, basketball, football, wrestling, hockey, and rugby. The non-contact endurance sports include cross country, track, tennis, crew, and swimming. The noncontact, nonendurance sports include bowling, golf, archery, field events, and other similar sports activities. See Table VIII for the AMA tabulation of disqualifying conditions.

A. Special Considerations

1. Eyes

In addition to the disqualifying conditions of absence or loss of function in one eye and severe myopia as given in the AMA table, there is a general consensus among ophthalmologists that all persons who have had previous retinal detachment repair should be excluded from all of the contact sports, but that persons who have simply had repair of retinal tears probably could engage in these sports with a qualifying letter from their ophthalmologists. In most instances, the athlete who

TABLE VIII

Disqualifying Conditions for Sports Participation[a]

Conditions	Contact[b]	Noncontact endurance[c]	Other[d]
General			
Acute infections: Respiratory, genitourinary, infectious mononucleosis, hepatitis, active rheumatic fever, active tuberculosis, boils, furuncles, impetigo	x	x	x
Obvious physical immaturity in comparison with other competitors	x	x	x
Obvious growth retardation	x		
Hemorrhagic disease: hemophilia, purpura and other bleeding tendencies	x		
Diabetes, inadequately controlled	x	x	x
Jaundice, whatever cause	x	x	x
Eyes			
Absence or loss of function of one eye	x		
Severe myopia, even if correctable	x		
Ears			
Significant impairment	x		
Respiratory			
Tuberculosis (active or under treatment)	x	x	x
Severe pulmonary insufficiency	x	x	x
Cardiovascular			
Mitral stenosis, aortic stenosis, aortic insufficiency, coarctation of aorta, cyanotic heart disease, recent carditis of any etiology	x	x	x
Hypertension on organic basis	x	x	x
Previous heart surgery for congenital or acquired heart disease	x	x	
Liver			
Enlarged liver	x		
Spleen			
Enlarged spleen	x		
Hernia			
Inguinal or femoral hernia	x	x	
Musculoskeletal			
Symptomatic abnormalities or inflammations	x	x	
Functional inadequacy of the musculoskeletal system, congenital or acquired, incompatible with the contact or skill demands of the sport	x	x	
Neurological			
History or symptoms of previous serious head trauma or repeated concussions	x		
Convulsive disorder not completely controlled by medication	x	x	
Previous surgery on head or spine	x	x	

TABLE VIII (Continued)

Conditions	Con-tact[b]	Noncontact endurance[c]	Other[d]
Renal			
Absence of one kidney	x		
Renal disease	x	x	x
Genitalia			
Absence of one testicle	x		
Undescended testicle	x		

[a] From Committee on The Medical Aspects of Sports (1966). Some of the disqualifying conditions listed above are subject to evaluation and consideration by the responsible physician with respect to anticipated risks, the otherwise athletic fitness of the candidate, special protective preventive measures which might be utilized, and the nature of the supervisory control. Disqualification, moreover, does not necessarily imply restriction from all sports at that time or from the sport in question in the future. If the decision is disqualification, however, the physician vested by the school with the authority to disqualify should not be overruled by any other person. This is a direct and unavoidable responsibility and needs the full support of the institution and all personnel involved.

[b] Lacrosse, baseball, soccer, basketball, football, wrestling, hockey, rubgy, etc.

[c] Cross country, track, tennis, crew, swimming, etc.

[d] Bowling, golf, archery, field events, etc.

has visual loss in one eye of 20/200 or greater from any cause probably should be excluded from contact sports in order to protect him from more serious injuries due to the lack of depth perception. There is a feeling among some ophthalmologists that they would not categorically disqualify a patient with high myopia from contact sports, but they recognize that a fair mumber of persons with or without high myopia have various types of retinal degeneration which make the danger of retinal detachment fairly great.

Athletes wearing contact lenses should be excluded from boxing and jumping events. Federal standards now require that the lenses of eye glasses must either be plastic or heat treated glass, making them more acceptable in athletic environments. For athletic participation, the plastic lenses are probably superior and safer in most instances.

2. Cardiovascular

There are two major pitfalls in screening for cardiovascular abnormalities. The first is overconcern with clinically insignificant findings, and the second is failure to recognize important disease. Between 50 and 60% of normal children have a systolic heart murmur at rest, and exercise and excitement will raise this proportion significantly. The finding of a systolic murmur on physical examination is far more often an insignificant finding than an abnormal one, with about 80% of the total representing a "harmless" functional systolic murmur.

Although most murmurs do not signify pathology that would exclude an individual from athletic participation, any cardiovascular abnormality recorded in the health history or detected by physical examination requires a very careful evaluation. The basic parameters for such an evaluation are pulse rate, cardiac rhythm, quality of heart sounds, location of murmurs, electrocardiogram, and functional capacity tests, observed at rest and after a standard exercise tolerance test.

Hyman (1967) has called attention to the following cardiovascular conditions as they relate to athletes:

1. Very slow and very fast pulse rates require instrumental studies. Normal sinus bradycardia is a regular slow rhythm with rates approaching 44 beats a minute; however, certain types of heart block may be present at this rate. A quick clinical test to differentiate these two types of slow rhythm is the so-called MacKenzie workout, a short spurt of physical activity. In sinus bradycardia, the pulse rate will rise whereas there is usually no change in heart block.

2. Normal sinus tachycardia is a regular rhythm with rates as high as 180 to 210 beats a minute while at rest. It is most often seen in young age athletes and is most frequently due to psychosomatic factors; however, a rate above 180 may have a pathological background and require more than a field physical examination. The hyperthyroid group and certain rheumatic valvular cardiac patients exhibit these findings. When the tachycardia is due to extracardiac factors, psychogenic, endocrine or toxic, the simple breathholding test of Parsonnet may be revealing. The subject is instructed to take a deep break and hold it as long as possible. During the first phase of the test the pulse rate may drop as much as 20 to 40 beats a minute but there is a prompt return to the former rapid rate. The vagal responsiveness is usually lost in organic or pathological types of tachycardia.

3. The most common irregularity in cardiac rhythm seen in athletes is all ages is the premature beat or extra systole. In the 10 to 18 age groups, sinus arrhythmia may be present in a marked degree but is easily diagnosed; the pulse rate speeds up on inspiration and slows down on expiration. Premature beats, on the other hand, are only occasionally influenced by the respiratory cycle.

4. Continuous irregularities of rhythm are important. Atrial fibrillation is the chief syndrome in this group. Paroxysmal atrial fibrillation is not uncommon in apparently normal hearts. The episode of fibrillation is

usually diagnosed by an irregular beating of the heart; the pulse rate may be very rapid, sometimes as high as 240 beats a minute. Paroxysmal atrial flutter has been relatively uncommon among athletes in the experience of Hyman. In case of paroxysmal atrial flutter, the rate is in the range of 180 to 240 beats a minute but more or less regular.

5. Cardiac sounds in well-conditioned athletes are heard without difficulty. Heart sounds that are difficult to hear, that seem to be distant or obscured, should be considered suspicious of underlying cardiovascular pathology until proven otherwise. Heart sounds that change their specific characteristic on change of body position or posture should likewise raise questions of cardiac integrity.

6. Heart murmurs require some respectful attention in evaluating a given athlete's ability to engage in stressful activities.

7. The upper limits of normal blood pressure in persons under 20 is 133/83 for males and 128/83 for females. Diastolic levels have the most clinical significance and in an individual with persistent diastolic pressure of 100 to 110 mm Hg, a thorough cardiovascular-renal study is indicated.

3. Skin

Acute infections, including boils, furuncules, impetigo, herpes simplex, and herpes gladiatorum should temporarily exclude an athlete from participation in a contact sport.

B. Chronic Conditions

In addition to the diseases and other conditions that have been listed previously, it is felt that an additional word needs to be said concerning certain chronic conditions. These conditions include convulsions, diabetes, asthma, and a history of multiple concussions. Schrode (1966) has stated that an explicit policy on how an athlete with a chronic condition should be handled has not been formulated because no policy could be sufficiently elastic or inclusive to apply to all cases. He has stated that judgments become highly individualized when based on total consideration of the circumstances involved in any given case, and that each athlete must be appraised, obtaining all the information possible about his medical, personal, and athletic background. Then, from the total appraisal, an estimate of the individual risk is made.

Schrode has suggested that athletes with chronic conditions be given a four-point evaluation. Medical evaluation entails a thorough history and physical examination with enough diagnostic studies to reach a specific diagnosis and to determine the extent of the condition. The frequency of episodes, the problem of control, routine medication, and activating circumstances must be considered. It then must be ascertained how well the patient understands his disorder. Is there insight into precipitating factors? Does he understand the medication schedule and the necessity of the medication? What are his personal interests? How important are sports to the individual? Does he understand the hazards of the disorder? The maturity and reliability of the patient is also important. From the athletic standpoint, is the individual a capable athlete with a promising future in athletics or is it something he simply wants to do in order to be a part of the team? Has he selected the sport that is best suited for his condition or are there other sports for which his physical capabilities would be better suited? The risk of participation with the given condition has to be evaluated based upon the particular sport and the athlete's competency for that sport. This risk should be thoroughly understood by all involved parties, including not only the athlete but also his parents, the coaching staff, and the medical staff. Only after all these factors have been considered should a decision be made as to whether or not an athlete with a given condition should be allowed to participate in a specific sport.

1. Convulsive Disorders

It is generally accepted by both physicians and educators that young people with convulsive disorders, once the seizures are under reasonable control, should be encouraged to lead as normal and active a life as possible. This applies to participation in sports as well as to other types physical activity. Each situation involving convulsive disorders is an individual one and cannot be classified under specific categories to which general rules apply. Therefore, in each instance, there should be a definitive diagnosis, a careful health history, review of the patient, and thoughtful planning of the medical and supporting management required. As a part of such management, the judgment should be made with respect to the individual's ability to participate without undue risk to either himself or his teammates. Three decisive factors in arriving at a reliable decision in this matter are (1) whether good control of his condition is maintained by medication, (2) whether extent and intensity of participation poses significant threat to his physical condition, and (3) whether the patient is cooperative and in control of any impulsiveness. When this judgment entails participation in sports, the athlete, the parents, and the athletic supervisory personnel should thoroughly understand the risks involved, preventive measures to be taken, and the values to be derived from competition in a suitable sport. Continuing medical and supporting supervision is imperative, with an informed person available to intercede for the protection of the player in both games and practice sessions.

A review of the literature on epilepsy in athletes has failed to demonstrate a case of convulsive disorder during an athletic event. Convulsive seizures have occurred, however, in postexercise states and hyperventilation may also precipitate an attack. A physician or other administrative personnel should be very reluctant to accept an individual with a history of convulsive disorders for participation in boxing, tackle football, ice hockey, diving, soccer, rugby, lacrosse, or, in other words, in activities where chronic recurrent head trauma or an unexpected fall carries the risk of serious injury and in situations where there would be swimming without supervision.

2. Diabetes

Diabetes that is poorly controlled is cause for exclusion from sports until such time as proper control has been achieved. Again, each situation is an individual one and cannot be classified under specified categories to which general rules apply. In each instance, there should be a definitive diagnosis, a careful health history, review of the patient, and thoughtful planning of the medical and supporting mangement required. As part of such management, a judgment should be made with respect to the individual's ability to participate without undue risk to either himself or his teammates. The two decisive factors in arriving at a reliable judgment of this matter are (1) whether good control of his condition is maintained by medication, and (2) whether extent and intensity of participation poses significant threat to his physical condition. The diabetic athlete should be encouraged to keep excellent records of his diabetic status, to report regularly for review, take his medication faithfully, and to watch his diet closely.

3. Asthma

Bronchial asthma is a chronic pulmonary disorder, frequently allergic in nature, characterized by paroxysms of dyspnea, wheezing, tightness in the chest, and bronchial spasms. Asthmatic attacks may be minor and short in duration with little discomfort or they may be very severe and of long duration, producing a characteristic picture of intractibility. Both physical and mental activities have been proven to be useful to asthmatic children and the majority of asthmatic children can participate in physical activities and athletics at school with minimal difficulty provided the asthma is under satisfactory control. Overfatigue and emotional upheaval in competitive athletic contests appear to be predisposing factors in precipitating asthmatic attacks in some instances. With proper medical management, the majority of asthmatic children in school can participate in physical education and athletics. In children with severe asthma, sports involving prolonged exertion should be prohibited. Noncontact, nonendurance sports should be encouraged, but each athlete must be evaluated on an individual basis depending upon his tolerance for duration and intensity of effort. There is evidence that swimming can be helpful (American Academy of Pediatrics Committee on Children with Handicaps, 1970). A periodic review of the health status of the asthmatic child should be made. Written records of annual and periodic evaluations by the physician managing the asthma should be on file in the office of the school nurse or physician. Certain sports such as basketball are not the ideal sport for an asthmatic whose attacks are precipitated by overexertion or inhalation of dust.

Graff-Lonnevig (1971) has indicated that some juvenile asthmatics in Sweden who formerly would have been excused from school sports are now playing ice hockey and basketball and following a strenuous physical training program. Early findings based on a preliminary study of the fitness of these children indicate high physical and psychological dividends as a result of the program.

4. Multiple Concussions

The athlete who has sustained two or more concussions must have a thorough appraisal of his status before further participation is allowed. All of the details of the risks involved, the extent of the previous injuries, and the possibility of sequelae with any subsequent injury must all be given careful consideration. There is an oft quoted rule that suggests that following three concussions an athlete should be disqualified from further participation. This is probably an oversimplification of a very complex condition and, as such, does not stand up to very close scrutiny. A careful estimate must be made in each case separately attempting to gauge the risk of occurrence of another injury and the damage possible therefrom. Extremely important in this consideration is the determination of the degree of severity of the previous concussions. A period of unconsciousness lasting from a few seconds to a few minutes without headache, retrograde amnesia, and objective neurological signs should not be given equal weight with the case involving prolonged unconsciousness with retrograde amnesia with objective neurological signs including tonic or chronic convulsions, prolonged mental confusion, prolonged unconsciousness, posttraumatic headaches, etc. After all factors have been considered, a thorough evaluation by a neurosurgeon or neurologist will probably offer the best chance of reaching the proper conclusion regarding the athlete's ability to return to participation.

Intensive research on the problems of head injuries in athletics has been conducted by Schneider et al. (1961), Reid et al. (1970), Gurdjian et al., (1962), and others. Through the efforts of these men, perhaps a more reliable method of determining which athletes should be disqualified following concussions will be available in the future. Until such time, however, every possible means of thorough evaluation should be utilized.

5. Musculoskeletal Disorders

Restriction of participation in athletics because of musculoskeletal disorders relates to three main factors: (1) likelihood of exacerbation of an existing disease, (2) probability of increasing an existing deformity, or (3) possibility of causing further bone or joint damage. The physical examination must determine the active and passive range of motion, the degree of stability, including both the dynamic and static stability, the symmetry about the joints as well as any joint incongruity, and any other signs that might suggest musculoskeletal pathology. In order for the indivudal to be eligible for athletic participation, the disease or process that involves the muscoloskeletal system of the athlete should not prevent him from competing fairly with normal persons and should not be aggravated by athletic competition. The physician who must make the decision regarding the playability of an individual with musculoskeletal involvement, as with other disorders, must at all times be aware of the skill and contact demand of the sport in question. Congenital disorders such as dislocation of the hip, club foot, and torticollis, if treated promptly and properly in infancy, seldom restrict the athlete in later life. Other conditions such as absence or abnormalities of spinal segments, including spina bifida and transitional vertebrae, are acceptable if the individual can compete satisfactorily and remain reasonably asymptomatic. Developmental conditions, such as hereditary multiple exostoses, enchondromatosis, fibrous dysplasia, and tumors such as nonossifying fibromas, chondromas, giant cell tumors, chondrobyastomas, and hemangiomas must be given careful consideration because their presence in the bone often diminishes the strength of the bone and predisposes to fracture.

Circulatory disturbances such as epiphyseal ischemic necrosis and osteochondritis dissecans, whether due to trauma or metabolic disturbances, often necessitate restriction from athletic participation during the active course of the disease. This is especially true for conditions such as Legg–Calve–Perthes and Scheurermann's disease, conditions that affect the contour of the proximal femoral epiphysis and the body of the vertebra respectively. Other osteochondroses of the traction epiphysis need not exclude the individual from athletic participation so long as they remain essentially asymptomatic. These include Osgood–Schlatter's, Severs, and other similar diseases of the traction epiphyses.

The presence of symptoms and/or joing incongruity in cases of osteochondritis dissecans, whether it involves the femur, humerus, or talus, should be considered as disqualifying conditions for many sports activities.

Infectious diseases of the bones and joints are disqualifying conditions until the process is completely under control and there is no chance of aggravation of the disease process or weakening of the musculo-skeletal system.

Nonunion and malunion following a fracture, due to the joint incongruity and lack of symmetry, will often exclude an individual from further participation, especially if a weight bearing limb is involved. Dislocations, especially of the shoulder and patella, when recurrent in nature are a hazard to athletes in most sports and both of these conditions should be given remedial treatment as soon as possible, and preferably before participation is allowed to continue.

In cases of static or mechanical problems such as pes planus, pes cavus, genu valgum, genu varum, genu recurvatum, lumbar lordosis, dorsal kyphosis, scoliosis, and leg length inequality, as well as conditions in which there is muscle group paralysis or atrophy, the athlete should be thoroughly evaluated and participation for the most part allowed or disallowed based upon the symptomatology present. The athlete who engages in contact sports is particularly vulnerable to injury if he has genu valgum or genu recurvatum. Lumbar lordosis, with the often accompanying tightness of the hamstring muscles, frequently leads to muscle strains in the running sports. Leg length inequality with a disparity in strength makes the individual more susceptible to muscle strains and to knee injuries.

In myositis ossificans traumatica, involving the shafts of the bones and not adjacent to the joint, once it becomes mature the athlete may resume participation in contact sports with proper padding to prevent further injury. A "qualified yes" may also be given to an individual with spondylolysis or spondylolisthesis for participation in athletics. Here again the decision must be based upon thorough evaluation and absence of symptomatology. The functional demands of athletics may cause symptoms to occur that otherwise would not be present, and if these symptoms cannot be controlled by a program of Williams flexion exercises and muscle strengthening, then the sport causing the symptoms must be avoided. Many athletes with spondylolysis or spondylolisthesis have found participation in athletics to be beneficial because muscular development and general body fitness essential to atheletics is also helpful in the prevention of back problems in many instances.

REFERENCES

Allen et al. (1956). *Metab., Clin. Exp.* **51**, 346–352.

American Academy of Pediatrics Committee on Children with Handicaps. (1970). *Pediatrics* **45**, Part 1, 1.

American Medical Association Committee on the Medical Aspects of Sports. (1966). "A Guide for Medical Evaluation of Candidates for School Sports." Amer. Med. Ass., Chicago, Illinois.

Consolazio, C. F., Johnson, R. E., and Pecora, L. J. (1963). "Physiological Measurements of Metabolic Functions in Man." McGraw-Hill, New York.

Cooper, K. H. (1968). "Aerobics," p. 54. Lippincott, Philadelphia, Pennsylvania.

DuBois, D., and DuBois, E. F. (1916). *AMA Arch. Intern. Med.* **17**, 863–871.

Fleishman, E. A. (1964). "The Structure and Measurement of Physical Fitness." Prentice-Hall, Englewood Cliffs, New Jersey.

Gallagher, J. R., Guild, W. R., Klumpp, T. G., Rose, K. D., Russell, J. C. H., Ryan, A. J., and Hein, F. V. (1967). *J. Amer. Med. Asso.* **201**, 117–118.

Graff-Lonnevig (1971). *Rep., Annu. Meet. Swed. Med. Soc. Med. Trib.*

Gruelich, W. W., and Pyle, S. (1959). "Radiographic Atlas of Skeletal Development of the Hand and Wrist." Stanford Univ. Press, Palo Alto, California.

Gurdjian, E. S., Lissner, H. R., and Patrick, L. M. (1962). **182**, 509–512.

Hyman, A. S. (1967). *14th Annu. Meet., Amer. Coll. Sports Med.*

International Committee on the Standardization of Physical Fitness Tests (ICSPFT). (1970). Conference, Oxford, England.

Larson, L. A., ed. (1973). "Fitness, Health and Work Capacity: International Standards for Assessment." Macmillan, New York.

Lowman, C. L. (1958). *J. Health Phys. Educ. Recreation* **29**, 14.

Nicholas, J. A. (1970). *J. Amer. Med. Ass.* **212**, 2236–2239.

Reid, S. E., Tarkington, J. A., and Petrovick, M. (1970). "Football Injuries—Papers Presented at a Workshop," pp. 83–94. Nat. Acad. Sci., Washington, D.C.

Schneider, R. C., Reifel, E., Crisler, H. O., and Oosterbaan, B. G. (1961). *J. Amer. Med. Ass.* **177**, 362–367.

Schrode, P. F. (1966). *J. Amer. Med. Ass.* **197**, 889–890.

Slocum, D. B. (1959). *Amer. Acad. Orthop. Surg.* **16**, 17–28.

Chapter 6

CONDITIONING FOR SPORTS

FRED L. ALLMAN, JR.

I. IMPORTANCE OF CONDITIONING

You can take a $5.00 piece of steel and make it into a horseshoe and sell it for $10.50, or you can make it into straight pins and get $25.00 for it. If you turn the steel into penknife blades, it is worth $440.00. If you craft it into tempered steel watch springs, that $5.00 piece of steel is worth $250,000.00.

When a coach, trainer, and team physician first begin to work with a young boy or girl, it is just as if they are starting out with a $5.00 piece of steel. What is done with that $5.00 piece of steel will determine its ultimate value. Time, effort, and thought in conjunction with proper leadership, guidance, dedication, and self-discipline will combine to form an end product of a highly toned precision athlete. Not every athlete will become the highly toned precision individual because one or more of the necessary ingredients will be missing. It is the responsibility of the coach, the trainer, and physician to make every effort to see that as many of the ingredients as possible will be provided to each boy, for it is then and only then that the $5.00 piece of steel will become the $250,000.00 highly toned precision form.

The role of conditioning in attaining top performance in atletics cannot be emphasized too much, yet too few physicians, coaches, and trainers fully understand the important components of a conditioning program. Also, it should be remembered that conditioning is a primary factor in prevention of injury.

In competitive athletics, there are no miracles. Top performance by an athlete requires coachability, dedication, and physical fitness. Other important factors are talent, effort, confidence, healthful living, and genetics. There is no known chemical agent that will both safely and effectively improve performance of healthy subjects. There is no gadget or gimmick that will be a panacea and produce top performance with just a few seconds a day. Top performance results from organization, study, application, and adaptation over a long period of time.

Hamilton (1935) made a list of ultimate track records that were regarded at that time as impossible to reach. They have all since been broken. Hamilton's recent comments (1963) are just as significant as were his predictions of 1935. He feels that all records presently on the books will eventually be broken. The shorter the race, the easier it is to tie the record, the harder to break it. The longer distance records may be broken by several seconds. He also speaks of the unwritten law of physiological compensation. Nature gives but she also takes away. Those with great height are denied great spring. Those with great strength and speed are denied great endurance. Those with great endurance never seem to have great speed. The brilliant starter in the sprints never seems to have a brilliant finish. The big shot putter never seems to have explosiveness. Yet, there seems to be almost no limit to man's physical capabilities.

Fifty-four and seven-tenths seconds have been reduced from the mile record since 1861 when it was run by N. S. Greene of Ireland in 4:46. Between Greene and Roger Bannister, who ran the first less than four minute mile on May 6, 1954, 25 other world records were established for the mile in just under 100 years. On July 17, 1966, Jim Ryun ran a mile in 3 minutes $51\frac{3}{10}$ seconds to set the world record. On June 23, 1967, he took another two-tenths of a second off that record. Between May of 1954 when Bannister ran the first less than four minute mile and May of 1971, nearly 100 runners have run a less than four minute mile 421 times—389 of these outdoors. Thus, between May 6, 1954, and May of 1971, nearly 100 runners were able to accomplish a feat 421 times that 26 world record holders could not accomplish in nearly 100 years. The first time Ryun ran a four minute mile, he finished eighth in the race.

In swimming, Johnny Weismuller held 67 of the world's swimming records up to and including the 400 meter mark for many years, with the 100 yard record standing for 17 years. Yet, as of this writing, of 26 world records in swimming for men, most were less than 18 months old.

The reasons for this unprecedented assault on the record books are varied and numerous. Each generation of athletes is bigger, stronger, and faster and performs under much better conditions than did its predecessors. Faster tracks, improved equipment, better diets, and new conditioning and training techniques are all factors in the ever increasing skills of our athletes. These things, combined with a growing social emphasis on physical fitness and an increased amount of leisure time for man to pursue athletic endeavors, have produced the healthiest, most physically capable generation in our country's history.

Top performance demands careful planning and self-discipline. All aspects of an athlete's life must be given careful consideration, and the athlete must devote himself to hard painful work and clean healthful living. Without equivocation, top performance by today's athletes is due to a very large measure to improved procedures for their conditioning. This has been especially true in track and field and swimming. The top performing athlete must train all year round, and must seek as a goal high standards of physical and mental readiness for the sport in which he is engaged.

II. PURPOSE OF CONDITIONING

Bilik (1941) has stated that the primary objective of intensive conditioning is to "put the body with extreme and exceptional care under the influence of all the agents which promote its health and strength in order to enable it to meet extreme and exceptional demands upon it. Training aims to condition the muscles, the heart, the lungs, the joints, the nervous system, the mind, the whole body, every tissue and every cell, to function at maximum possible efficiency and to stand up under the most gruelling stress and strain." The primary purpose of conditioning, then, is to promote physical fitness and sports fitness.

Physical fitness, while important for every individual, is essential for the athlete. Physical fitness helps the athlete to enjoy physical activity. Physical fitness sustains learning skills. Physical fitness enhances excellence. Physical fitness decreases the chance of injury, and physical fitness helps to speed recovery following injury.

III. GENERAL PRINCIPLES OF CONDITONING (Allman, 1969)

A. Establish a Goal

The goal of a conditioning program should be to achieve optimum or near optimum fitness.

B. Select the Proper Program

Select a conditioning program that will develop all parts of the body with special emphasis on areas of greatest need based upon the demands of the sport. Do not overemphasize any one area or aspect. No single sport, no single exercise, and no single piece of apparatus provides total balanced development for all parts of the body. Optimum fitness requires balance.

C. Warm-Up Principles

Always warm up. Calisthenics such as the side straddle hop and running in place are good warm-up exercises. The warm-up not only prepares the body for the forthcoming increased activity, but also is a good way to detect areas of stiffness and discomfort prior to beginning the exercise program. Darling and Downey (1971) have stated "the temperature of the muscles rises during work in spite of the efficient circulation. This is probably advantageous to muscular function. The optimum for the speed of chemical reaction and metabolism is 102°–103°F. There is some evidence that the speed, strength and efficiency of contractions are enhanced by a rise in the temperature of muscle toward this range. The only efficient method of raising muscle temperature is by work of the muscle itself."

D. Exercise Tolerance

Each training period should be adapted to the individual's tolerance level. Exercise tolerance is the level at which the body responds to exercise favorably. The exercise level should not be so high that the body has not fully recuperated in 24 hours or less. Alteration of work and rest is best and should be adapted to one's ability to recover. If the exercise is too easy it will fall short of the tolerance level; if too demanding it will exceed tolerance level and cause possible damage.

E. Progressive Overloads

The training plan must provide for progression until a high performance level or optimum fitness is achieved. In order to improve performance, overload is necessary. Overload is extending the work level beyond usual physical effort. This is achieved by exercising longer or with greater intensity than usual or both. In the early stages of conditioning, a higher proportion of slow, long-continued endurance work is favored over speed work. Later, as the physiological mechanisms adjust to the work load, the proportion of speed work to slow work is increased.

F. Dosage

In order to obtain a good cardiovascular response, the heart rate during the exercise period should reach a peak rate of at least 70% of its capable

range. Cooper (1968) has laid down two basic principles in this regard:
(1) "If the exercise is vigorous enough to produce a sustained heart
rate of 150 beats per minute or more, the training effect benefits begin
about five minutes after the exercise starts and continue as long as the
exercise is performed. (2) If the exercise is not vigorous enough to
produce or sustain a heart rate of 150 beats per minute but is still
demanding oxygen, the exercise must be continued considerably longer
than five minutes, the total period of time depending on the oxygen
consumed." It therefore becomes obvious that the dosage necessary to
produce a training effect will depend upon the state of the individual.
The poorly conditioned individual may obtain a training benefit with
relatively little intensity of exercise, whereas he increases the dosage
and intensity as he becomes better conditioned in order to achieve the
training benefit.

G. Recuperation

Following vigorous exercise, it is best to keep moving and not to
sit down. Sitting or assuming the recumbent position allows for pooling
of large amounts of blood in the lower extremity, thus depriving the
heart of sufficient return of blood. This, in turn, can lead to syncope and
other more serious disorders. It is much wiser to cool down slowly
while continuing with some upright movement such as walking.

H. Records

Records are essential if the individual is to progress optimally. Progress
should be noted to be rising and rhythmic although time trials should
not always indicate continued improvement. Even the gifted athlete
cannot peak each week. It therefore becomes necessary to select certain
key meets or events in which it is desirable to peak, and the conditioning
should be directed toward those particular events.

I. Motivation

Motivation is all important. Ultimate success in any conditioning program depends to a large degree on motivation. Those individuals and

teams who are able to maintain a high degree of motivation are likely to succeed. Those without motivation are almost certain to fail. Motivation is many things. It is the encouragement of a cheering gallery. It is a medal or trophy. It is the admiration of a friend or loved one, or of the coach or the teammates. However, the greatest motivation is the desire for improvement, the desire to be better tomorrow than today.

IV. GENERAL PRINCIPLES OF BASIC SPORTS FITNESS

Doherty (1963) has noted the following basic sports fitness principles.

1. The hard core of basic sports fitness cannot be gained completely through the action of the event itself.

2. The hard core of basic sports fitness develops gradually over a period of years.

3. The basic fitness work should always be supplementary.

4. The basic fitness work should always include the practice of skills of many sports, even though they seem unrelated to one's special event. This is especially important during the early years of training and during the months of "active rest" from each year of training. Other sports are basic training in skill learning.

5. Basic sports training must be continuous.

6. The intensity of basic sports training must be varied (rising and rhythmic).

7. Basic sports training must be individualized. Broer (1966) has stated, "The amount of daily exercise that is needed to reach and maintain physical efficiency at the highest attainable level is still determined mostly by observation or empirical methods. Experiments show that a daily amount of practice which is suitable for an individual is either too much or too little for others. They also demonstrate that regardless of the physical capacity of a given subject, there is a level of exercise which frequently repeated will lead to chronic fatigue 'staleness.'"

V. SPECIFIC FACTORS TO BE INCLUDED IN A BALANCED CONDITIONING PROGRAM

Conditioning work is both general and special. General conditioning refers to total body development. Special conditioning concentrates on

exercises and drills to develop the muscle groups for a special event
in which the athlete wishes to concentrate. There are a number of specific factors that are necessary to include in a conditioning program
if total fitness is to be achieved.

A. Endurance

Systemic or general endurance involves the sustaining of activity in
many of the large muscles of the body and is usually called cardiovascular
respiratory endurance. Local endurance refers to the ability to sustain
or repeat contraction in a single muscle or group of muscles. Cardiovascular endurance is the ability of the heart to perform more work than
is usual more economically for prolonged periods and the heart's ability
to recover quickly upon cessation of the activity. An efficient cardiovascular system is capable of adjusting the flow of blood in order to supply
oxygen to the necessary tissues and to remove chemical by-products
produced in muscle contraction. Aerobic exercises are those in which
there is adequate oxygen intake. Anaerobic exercises are those in which
there is inadequate oxygen intake or a gradual increase in oxygen intake
or a gradually increasing oxygen debt. Only when you extend yourself
is optimum effect from cardiovascular training achieved. Optimum effect
is not readily achieved, in other words, if all training efforts are within
the submaximal or aerobic capacity range. The body is capable of adapt-
ing specifically to imposed demands. In order to be of benefit in improving cardiovascular fitness, the organs need to be "stressed." Thus,
anaerobic work becomes a part of the aerobic training, and this is the
basis of a training which is known as "interval training" (alternately
stress and nonstress work). Improving endurance is primarily a matter
of building resistance to the many effects of fatigue (production of
lactic acid, lowered oxygen supply to the muscles, decreased sensitivity
of muscle fibers to stimuli, etc.). This is done by gradually increasing,
as the training effect improves, the amount of work that is done during
each exercise period. The upper limits of endurance training are still
unknown. Bannister, because of the disappointment of defeat at the
Helsinki Olympics in 1952, increased his work load severalfold and set
a world record when he ran the first less than four minute mile on
May 6, 1954. Snell's training included approximately five times the
amount of work that Bannister's training included and he soon lowered
the record.

Balke (1965) has reported on the seminomadic Tarahumara Indians
in the northwestern region of Mexico. These people have not only

adapted to the stresses of a relatively high elevation of their habitat, of rapid changes between hot and cold temperatures, and of their apparently inadequate nutrition, but have also accomplished unbelievable performances in running. Reports indicate that these people have run a distance of 600 miles in a five-day period. Actual observations have shown that the winners of the typical kick ball races ran 125 miles, nearly continuously. The energy expenditure in such a race should amount to more than 15,000 kilocalories over a 24 hour period.

B. Strength

Muscles must be put under tension in order for them to develop strength. Strength is obtained by loading muscles and pressing activity to the thresholds of fatigue. This may be accomplished by the use of isometrics, isotonics, or isokinetic exercises. Isometric contractions are those in which no shortening takes place in the muscle, the joints do not move in the direction of the contraction, and no actual work is done. Isotonic contractions are those in which the involved muscle shortens under load with resultant production of work. Isokinetic exercises are those in which joint motion occurs at a controlled rate. McCloy (1960) writing on the mechanical analysis of motor skills has stated that the first prerequisite for the economical learning of a skill is sufficient strength to perform the task. Hellebrandt and Houtz (1956), concerning the overload principle, have stated that the limits of performance must be persistently extended to improve muscle strength, and that the rate of improvement depends on the willingness of the subject to overload. The following conclusions have been drawn from their experimentation:

1. The slope of the training curve varies with the magnitude of the stress imposed, the frequency of the practice sessions and the duration of the overload effort.

2. Mere repetition of contractions which place little stress on the neuromuscular system has little effect on the functional capacity of the muscles.

3. The amount of work done per unit time is the critical variable upon which extension of the limits of performance depends.

4. The speed with which functional capacity increases suggests that the central nervous system changes contribute an important component to training.

5. The ability to develop maximal tension appears to be dependent on the proprioceptive facilitation with which overloading is associated.

In most athletic endeavors, the attainment of mere strength is often not enough. The attainment of explosive power is often necessary. Explosive power is the ability to release maximum muscular power in the shortest time.

C. Flexibility

Flexibility is the ability to yield to passive stretch and to relax. Flexibility training is designed to increase the range of motion of the joints. This process requires the stretching of the tissues, especially connective tissue, beyond the normal limit and sometimes to the point of discomfort. Flexibility or suppleness is desirable to facilitate muscular action with minimal resistance to the tissues. When connective tissue is not actively stretched, it periodically shortens. Flexibility is necessary in order to obtain perfection of movement and perfection of movement is necessary to achieve peak performance. Stretching should be done both before and after hard exercise as it helps to restore muscles to their normal functional capacity. Evidence seems to favor the slow controlled method of increasing flexibility over the ballistic (bobbing, lunging) type of exercise. Controlled movements are less likely to go beyond the extensibility of muscle tissue since pain would be the controlling factor. For the older athlete, flexibility exercises are even more important. Throughout life after age 25 there is generally a steady loss in flexibility in the principle joints. This is probably related to many factors, but most notably to dehydration and disuse of the tissues (similar to attrition seen in the rotator cuff, the long head of biceps, and the Achilles tendon). This decline is so parallel with aging that flexibility is one form of measurement of physiological aging.

D. Coordination or Rhythm Training

Rhythm training is utilized to promote a more precise coordination of movement. The athlete learns a sense of pace and achieves confidence in his ability to continue work in spite of the pain and discomfort of his prolonged effort. Coordination training refers to the process of superimposing new movement patterns over habitual ones. Through improvement of form, extra movements are reduced, thus producing precise, direct, stronger, and more economical motor function.

E. Reaction Training or Response Training

Reaction training is utilized to shorten the delay between a stimulus and response. This is accomplished by exercises to eliminate cerebral decision-making functions preceding the response. The objective in the process is to transfer from volitional to reflex control whole movement patterns. Although some reflexes are developed prenatally, most are learned. Armin Hary, the great German sprinter and winner of the 100 meter race at the Rome Olympics in 1960, gained his lead in the first 10 yards because of his phenomenal reaction time. In order to improve in reaction time, the athlete must practice movements characteristic of the sport in which he plans to participate, and each of these movements must be performed as rapidly as possible.

F. Relaxation Training

Most physicians, physical educators, and coaches understand muscle contraction and increased neuromuscular effort, but few have given much thought to relaxation and the reduction of neuromuscular tension. By relaxation is not meant playing golf. This is a diversion. Relaxation means reducing activity in the musculature as nearly as possible to the zero level. Thus, relaxation is a neuromuscular skill that must be learned as are other skills. As mentioned earlier in this chapter, Johnny Weismuller, one of the greatest competitive swimmers of all times, set world records in 67 different events ranging from 50 yards up to 880 yards. It has been said that half the secret of his success was skill and dedication and the other half was his ability to consciously relax.

G. Heat Training

Heat training is designed to induce favorable adaptation in temperature-regulating mechanisms. This improves resistance to the high temperatures of endurance efforts and induces increased salt retention and sweating. The adapted individual perspires more, but the perspiration contains less salt. If the organism is unable to adjust rather rapidly to the increased heat produced by effort, then fatigue is rapid to follow and performance is altered. Buttram (1968), after an extensive study of heat stress, has stated, "No one can study the deaths from heat stress as correlated with the climatic conditions of the time and place and type of activity involved without the firm belief that 98% of all such reactions are avoidable. A heat stroke is not a chance proposition like being struck by lightning. It is a predictable phenomenon."

H. Weight Control

The optimum weight for an athlete is best determined by assessing the lean body mass or body density. Accurate calculations of the lean body mass can be determined by assessing skin fold thicknesses at various levels and applying these determinations to existing formulas. A density less than 1.065 is generally considered a sign of obesity.

I. General Health Measures

1. Sleep

The athlete needs more sleep than the average adolescent. His extra activity makes restorative rest imperative. Eight hours of sleep is a good average minimum, but most athletes would be better off with nine. Sleep is intimately associated with one's ability to perform physical work and also with one's mental attitude.

2. Nutrition

Since two Greek athletes deviated from the chiefly vegetarian diet to one of meat in large quantities in the fifth century BC, the question of the proper diet for the athlete has been debated. Many claims have been made for "special diets" in the increased performance of athletes as much has been written concerning the "proper precompetition meal." Gordon (1958) has pointed out that muscles can operate indefinitely on fatty acids, and that this fat fuel produces more energy than glucose. He has postulated that, "second wind" may be the time at which the shift is made between sugar and fatty acid utilization. Cureton (1963) has suggested that the physical work of training may gradually exhaust certain critical nutritional ingredients in the athlete and that staleness may thus result with symptoms of fatigue, lassitude, and indisposition to hard work. Good nutrition is certainly necessary for top performance; however, there is no scientific evidence to indicate that unusual diets lead to improved performance.

3. Smoking

The ability to produce maximum effort and to build endurance for sports is related to the capacity of the athlete to take in and utilize oxygen. Performance in any athletic event that demands a maximum effort for even a brief period is adversely effected by impairment of ventilatory capacity. At least 10 different substances in cigarette smoke have been shown to reduce airway conductance to the lungs. The decrease may amount to as much as 50%. This decrease is related to obstruction of the air ducts which apparently results from muscle contraction, edema, and nervous reflex. Recent reliable studies have strongly linked cigarette smoking to lung cancer, emphysema, chronic bronchitis, and heart disease. The death rate from lung cancer among cigarette smokers is 10 times that of nonsmokers. Studies indicate that cigarette smoking is associated with nearly 80% of all cases of lung cancer.

4. Alcohol

Alcohol acts upon the central nervous system as a depressant, and, as a result, there is definite loss of skill and a marked drop in physical capacity following the use of even relatively small amounts. Mental and muscular efficiency are reduced and performance is altered. Prolonged alcohol intake may result in mental and physical deterioration as the result of inadequate nutritional balance.

J. Psychological Preparation and Mental Toughness

The late Vince Lombardi once stated, "The will to excel and the will to win are positive enduring factors. They are more important than any events that occasion them." The coach or trainer who devotes many hours to the previously mentioned phases of conditioning and neglects the mental attitude of his athletes will never attain high performance from his athletes. In order to succeed or win, an athlete must feel that he can win. He must feel like a champion and train like a champion. Most athletes put forth a physical effort of less than 50%, and seldom does this percentage go higher unless they are motivated by a proper mental attitude and spirit. Mental fatigue is usually present before physical fatigue. Courage, pacing, confidence, and the knowledge that one is physically well prepared help an individual to become mentally tough. Mental toughness and endurance capabilities are both essentials of stamina. Stamina means a more sustained work capacity, and this ability to continue to compete at a high level often determines the winner. Every competitor should read Walter O. Wintle's poem (1939), "It's All In The State of Mind." The last stanza reads, "Life's battles don't always go to the stronger or faster man. But sooner or later the man who wins is the fellow who thinks he can."

K. Agility, Speed, and Balance

Agility, speed, and balance represent other factors that are very important in preparation for sports participation. Like skill, these factors relate to the central nervous system, and the key to improvement in these areas is repetition. Skill is improved by the repetitive practice of the specific skill needed for the specific sport. The development of motor skills depends partially upon maturation. It, therefore, becomes necessary to utilize the potential that is associated with changes in the functional ability of an individual.

VI. SPECIFIC TRAINING PROGRAMS

A. Fartlek

Fartlek or marathon training is used early in the training program in an attempt to develop positive attitudes, confidence, and mental toughness while increasing endurance capabilities at a relatively leisurely pace.

B. Controlled Interval Training

Controlled interval training consists of a repeated series of underdistance efforts at a controlled speed with a controlled period of rest between each effort. The rest interval is long enough to permit partial but not complete recovery of the heart rate to normal. The distance is never longer than the distance that the athlete is training for.

C. Repetition Training

Repetition training is used in the training program to develop quality. Fixed distances are repeated in exactly the same amount of time. The rest intervals, however, are long enough to permit more complete recovery of the heart rate than allowed in interval training.

D. Overdistance Training

Overdistance training is that form of training that takes place at distances greater than the event being trained for, usually at a lower speed than that which will be possible in the event itself. This method of training is most often used in the early part of the season. This system helps to develop endurance that is more stable and longer lasting.

E. Circuit Training

Circuit training is the scientific arrangement of known and proven exercises designed to elicit maximum overall training effectiveness. Total balanced development for all parts of the body is the objective. Circuit training is based on sound, physiological principles and aims at providing various activities and a continuous challenge. A circuit utilizing proper exercise equipment will improve muscular strength and endurance, cardiovascular endurance and flexibility, apply the principle of "progressive overload," provide balanced development to the whole body, enable large numbers of performers to train at the same time, each according to his individual capacity, allow each individual to acquire a maximum workout in a short but adequate time, and inspire motivation through variety offered as well as by the application of new goals that become readily apparent almost daily.

F. Speed Training

The "speed principle" of training, as advocated by McGraw at the University of Texas and others, can be utilized with many other types of training programs. Utilizing the "speed principle," an athlete performs the movements in a given exercise as rapidly as possible within a prescribed time. For each exercise, a proposed range of "sets" and a time interval are given. For example, the recommendation for push-ups is one to three sets of 10 to 30 seconds each with a rest interval of 30 seconds. The athlete performs one set of push-ups for 10 seconds, rests for 30 seconds, then repeats. The time of exercising is gradually increased while the rest period is gradually diminished. As fitness improves, the number of sets of each exercise may be increased. Thus, the effort–recovery cycle, referred to previously as interval training, is again utilized.

VII. BALANCE AND INDIVIDUALITY

A good, properly selected conditioning program must be balanced and it must be individualized. It should not overemphasize any one aspect. No single sport, no single exercise, and no single piece of apparatus provides total balanced development for all parts of the body. The conditioning program for the quarterback or pitcher should vary from that of a tackle or outfielder. A stereotyped program will not offer maximum benefit to all athletes. Only when each athlete is individually evaluated and placed on his appropriate conditioning program will maximum benefits be derived. The optimum fitness required for top performance requires months of careful planning, self-discipline, and hard work.

REFERENCES

Allman, F. L., Jr. (1969). "Executive Fitness Desk Diary," p. 11. M. B. Productions, Inc., Dallas, Texas.
Balke, B. (1965). *Amer. J. Phys. Anthropol.* 23, 293–301.
Bilik, S. E. (1941). "The Trainer's Bible," 9th rev. ed. Atsco Press, New York.
Broer, M. R. (1966). "Efficiency of Human Movement," 2nd ed. Saunders, Philadelphia, Pennsylvania.
Buttram, W. R. (1968). "Physiological Aspects of Sports and Physical Fitness," pp. 45–46. Athletic Institute, Chicago, Illinois.
Cooper, K. H. (1968). *J. Amer. Med. Ass.* 203, 201–204.
Cureton, T. K. (1963). *Res. Quart.* 34, 440–453.
Darling, R. C., and Downey, J. (1971). *In* "Rehabilitation Medicine," p. 31. Saunders, Philadelphia, Pennsylvania.
Doherty, J. K. (1963). "Modern Track and Field," 2nd ed. Prentice-Hall, Englewood Cliffs, New Jersey.
Gordon, E. E. (1958). *Arch. Intern. Med.* 101, 702–713.
Hamilton, (1935). *Amat. Athlete* pp. 2–3.
Hamilton, (1963). "Sports Shorts," 6th ed. Djakarta, Indonesia.
Hellebrandt, F. A., and Houtz, S. J. (1956). *Phys. Ther. Rev.* 35, 371–383.
McCloy, C. H. (1940). *Res. Quart.* 11, 28–39.
Wintle, O. (1939). *In* "Verses are Light" (E. Bowes and G. Bowes, eds.). Garden City Publ. Co., Garden City, New York.

Chapter 7

PSYCHOLOGY OF SPORTS COMPETITION

WILLIAM P. MORGAN

I. OVERVIEW

Athletes, coaches, trainers, team physicians, and spectators alike commonly make reference to the psychological basis of athletic competition. For example, it is commonly felt that athletes, especially high-level performers, are a "special breed"; that is, they are thought to differ in various ways from the less successful athlete, as well as the nonathlete. Furthermore, most observers of sport feel that athletes from various subgroups differ from each other psychologically.

129

Motivation is thought to play a critical role in athletic performance, and attempts to facilitate performance have frequently been employed. For example, phenomena such as the pep talk, hypnosis, relaxation training, autosuggestion, music, and social facilitation have been used in attempts to improve training, as well as performance. In most cases these treatments have been directed toward *perceptual distortion* of the athlete's *perceived exertion* and *pain tolerance* for a given activity stimulus.

Despite the commonly advanced views regarding the psychological basis of sport and physical activity, such positions have not been corroborated by a wealth of objective psychometric data. The present chapter represents an attempt to synthesize the existing literature on the aforementioned points. The scope of the present chapter prohibits an exhaustive discussion of personality dynamics and motivation in the athlete. The reader, however, will find extensive coverage of these topics in Morgan (1970).

II. HISTORY OF SPORT PSYCHOLOGY

Investigators from various disciplines have been interested in the psychological foundations of sport and physical activity for many years, but the field of sport psychology has not been characterized by a formal orientation until rather recently. Workers in this rapidly developing field have been trained in disciplines such as anthropology, history, physical education, psychology, psychiatry, and sociology. Most workers in this field at present, however, are physical educators. In other words, *sport psychology* in the United States is not a specialized subfield subsumed under the rubric psychology.

The nature of sport psychology in Europe varies from the above description in several ways. European sport psychologists usually have been trained in either psychology or psychiatry. Also, sport psychology in countries such as Russia and Czechoslovakia is a specialized branch of psychology. As a matter of fact, Chairs of Sport Psychology exist at certain universities in Europe. It should also be emphasized that European sport psychologists are usually speaking of high-level competitive athletics when they use the term sport. Sport psycholgists in the United States, however, tend to view sport within a multidimensional context that includes physical activity of a recreational nature, as well as high-level athletics.

Vanek and Cratty (1970) have presented a history of sport psychology in Europe and the United States, and Hammer (1970) has described the nature of this field in Western Europe and the Far East. These discussions reveal that at least 25 volumes dealing with the psychological foundations of sport and physical activity have been published in the past five years. In addition, two international congresses dealing with sport psychology have been held, an *International Journal of Sport Psychology* is now being published, and the North American Society of Sport Psychology has met annually since 1966.

In many respects, the growth and development of sport psychology is similar to the emergence of other multidisciplinary fields such as bio-engineering, human factors, psychophysiology, and sports medicine. While there is considerable evidence that attests to the reality of sport psychology as an area of inquiry, the embryonic nature of this rapidly developing multidisciplinary field prohibits any forecasting of its ultimate direction. However, it is quite clear that contemproary workers in this field are concerned with the many specialized facets of psychology.

III. PERSONALITY DYNAMICS

The psychological characteristics of numerous athletic subgroups have been assessed by means of various personality inventories and projective devices. In addition, the psychological characteristics of athletes have been compared to those of nonathletes, and attempts to delineate the characteristics of high-level competitors have been made. More recently there has been moderate interest evidenced regarding the psychological study of female athletes. The purpose of the present section will be to synthesize these research findings.

A. Methodological Considerations

It is imperative that one realize from the outset that personality research with the athlete has been characterized by numerous statistical and design inelegancies (Morgan, 1972). For example, operational definitions of *independent* and *dependent* variables have varied greatly, sampling theory has been largely ignored, incorrect statistical analyses have frequently been employed, and there has been an absence of theoretical models in this research area for the most part. Therefore, it is recommended that one view the results presented in the subsequent sections in a tentative fashion.

B. Athletic Ability

Investigators have attempted to delineate the relationship between personality and athletic ability. For example, Johnson *et al.* (1954) tested athletes who were All-Americans or of national champion caliber and found them to possess (1) feelings of exceptional self-assurance, (2) high and generalized anxiety, and (3) extreme aggressiveness.

In another investigation of outstanding athletes, LaPlace (1954) found that major league and minor league baseball players differed on a number of psychological variables. In general, the major league players were better adjusted than the minor league players. However, neither group differed from normal on any of the variables examined.

On the other hand, Singer (1969) compared college baseball players ranked as high- and low-ability by their coach and found that they did not differ on any of the psychological scales used. However, these baseball players were found to differ significantly from the norm values on the *aggression, abasement, intraception,* and *autonomy* factors. Also, they differed on several factors from college tennis players.

Booth (1958) has reported that 22 items of the Minnesota Multiphasic Personality Inventory (MMPI) were found to discriminate between poor and good competitors. Also, athletes and nonathletes, as well as athletes from different subgroups, were found to differ on several MMPI scales. Furthermore, he reported that varsity athletes from individual sports were significantly more depressed than those from team sports. This observation has been confirmed in part by Carmen *et al.* (1968) who found a high incidence of depression in swimmers who, of course, are individual sport athletes.

Candidates for the 1960 Olympic Wrestling Team were evaluated by Rasch and Hunt (1960) and compared to norms for college men. These wrestlers did not differ from the norms, indicating that such athletes do not possess a unique profile. These findings were supported by Kroll (1967) who found wrestlers to only differ from established norms on one of sixteen psychological variables. Also, Kroll failed to observe any differences between wrestlers of differing ability levels. On the other hand, Morgan (1968) reported that performance in the 1966 World Tournament was significantly correlated with extraversion. Also, the United States wrestlers in Morgan's study were more extraverted than the published norms.

Morgan and Costill (1973) evaluated the relationship between marathoners' performance and various psychological variables. None of the psychological variables were found to correlate with marathon performance. However, these marathoners scored lower than the published norms on the extraversion and anxiety variables.

The personality profiles of winning and losing football teams has been evaluated by Kroll and Petersen (1965) who found significant discrimination between such teams. On the other hand, Kroll and Carlson (1967), using the same measure of personality, failed to observe significant differences in the profiles of karate participants who differed on ability level. Furthermore, contrary to popular views, these karate participants did not differ from the normal population.

Champion swimmers were reported by Parsons (1963) to differ from the average population on 15 of 16 personality factors. However, those swimmers from this same group who were selected to participate on a national team did not differ from those who were not selected. Newman (1968) evaluated the relationship between the swimming performance of high school athletes on seven traits from the Thurstone temperament schedule. The findings revealed that little relationship existed between swimming performance and personality. These findings have been substantiated by Rushall (1970).

On the basis of his research Kane (1964) has concluded that a positive relationship exists between "athletic ability and (1) Stability as opposed to Anxiety, and (2) Extraversion as opposed to Introversion [p. 89]." More recently, Andrews (1971) has concluded that "There is some evidence of a relationship between high level performance and stable extravert personality [p. 126]." While certain of the author's own work (Morgan, 1968) with wrestlers who participated in the 1966 World Tournament supports the view of Kane (1964) and Andrews (1971), there is an abundance of literature that is seemingly at odds with this position.

C. Athletes, Norms, and Nonathletes

While the previous section contained several comparisons of athletic groups with established norms, it was primarily concerned with the relationship between ability level and personality. The present section is concerned specifically with the question of whether or not athletes and nonathletes differ on various psychological states and traits.

In one of the earliest investigations dealing with this question, Henry (1941) compared student pilots, track athletes, physical education major students, and a group of weight lifters. The weight lifters were found to be more introverted and hypochondriacal than either the pilots or track athletes. These latter two groups were also significantly more neurotic than the physical education majors.

Thune (1949) compared 100 YMCA weight lifters and 100 YMCA athletes who did not participate in weight lifting. The weight lifters were found to be more concerned with their body build, lacked self-confidence, and were more shy. Also, the weight lifters exhibited a desire to be "strong, healthy, and dominant, to be more like other men [p. 305]." These findings are in agreement with the earlier report of Henry (1941). Also, Harlow (1951) found weight lifters to differ from non-weight-lifters on 13 of 18 psychoanalytically derived variables. The major difference was that the weight men were characterized by feelings of masculine inadequacy.

Slusher (1966) compared athletes who had won letters in baseball, basketball, football, swimming, and wrestling with nonathletes from the same population. The athletes were found to differ significantly from the nonathletes on all of the MMPI scales except the M and K measures.

The personality of ninth grade, twelfth grade, and college athletes was compared with nonathletes by Schendel (1965). He reported that the athletes and nonathletes at each educational level differed on numerous scales of the California Psychological Inventory (CPI).

The personality characteristics of Negro and white athletes and nonathletes has been examined by Hunt (1969) who reported that athletes tended to differ from nonathletes regardless of ethnic background. Also, the Negro and white athletes possessed similar personality types as did the nonathlete groups.

Fletcher and Dowell (1971) administered the Edwards Personal Preference Schedule (EPPS) to 950 male freshmen and compared those who had participated in high school athletics with those students lacking athletic backgrounds. The groups were found to differ on the Dominance, Aggression, and Order scales of the EPPS. In a somewhat related study, Berger and Littlefield (1969) found that freshman football players differed significantly from freshman nonathletes on the Scholastic Aptitude Test and composite CPI.

College wrestlers and experienced marathoners have been found to score appreciably lower than established norms on anxiety (Morgan and Hammer, 1971; Morgan and Costill, 1972). Also, these same marathoners were found to be more introverted than the normal population, as well as other athletic subgroups.

The majority of the investigations reviewed in this section demonstrate that athletes differ significantly from nonathletes and established norms on a number of psychological variables. Furthermore, it is also clear that athletes from various sport subgroups also differ on certain personality traits. One consistent finding throughout the sport psychology literature has been the observation that athletes score on the stability end of the neuroticism–stability dimension. As a matter of fact, it seems reasonable to propose that stability is a prerequisite for successful athletic performance. The author has proposed elsewhere (Morgan, 1972) that stability is an *antecedent*, rather than a *consequence*, of athletic performance; that is, there seems to be selective mortality taking place in which neurotic athletes drop out (Yanada and Hirata, 1970). This position is contradicted by the reports of Carmen *et al.* (1968), Pierce (1969), and Little (1969) which are reviewed in Chapter 31.

D. The Female Athlete

The preceding sections have been limited to discussions of the male athlete. Historically, sport psychologists have not directed their attention toward the female athlete. As a matter of fact, the investigations reviewed in this chapter have all been reported within the past four years.

Peterson *et al.* (1967) compared female athletes who had participated in individual sports at the 1964 Olympics with team sport athletes. The team sport athletes were members of either the 1964 Olympic volleyball team or one of the top ten AAU basketball teams for that same year. The two groups were found to differ on 7 of the 16 personality factors measured by the 16 PF. These groups were similar in that they were both characterized by emotional stability. Also, these athletes differed from established norms on several of the 16 PF factors. The findings of Peterson *et al.* (1967) were corroborated by Ogilvie (1968) who found that female swimmers possessed profiles similar to their individual sport athletes.

Malumphy (1968), who also used the 16 PF, compared college athletes in team, individual, team-individual, and subjectively judged sports, as well as nonathletes from the same population. The athletes differed from the nonathletes on various factors. Furthermore, the athletes from the various subgroups were also found to differ on a number of the 16 PF factors.

Female fencers who had participated in the 1968 National Championships were tested by Williams *et al.* (1970) with the 16 PF and EPPS. The high- and low-achievers, as measured by tournament success, were found to differ on only one of the 38 psychological variables. However, these female fencers were found to differ from established norms on a number of the 16 PF and EPPS measures.

IV. PERCEPTUAL FACTORS

Since athletes from various subgroups have been shown to differ on the dimensions of extraversion–introversion, it follows from Eysenckian theory (Morgan, 1972) that they should also differ on perceptual factors such as pain tolerance, augmentation and reduction, perceived exertion, and perceptual distortion. The purpose of the present section shall be to review investigations concerned with perception and physical performance.

A. Pain Tolerance

Contact athletes such as football players and wrestlers have been demonstrated to possess a greater tolerance for pain than noncontact athletes from sports such as tennis and golf (Ryan and Kovacic, 1966). Also, both the contact and noncontact athletes were found to have higher pain tolerance than nonathletes. Hence, athleticism must be added to a long list of physiological, psychological, and sociological determinants of pain tolerance (Sternbach, 1968).

B. Augmentation and Reduction

The observations of Ryan and Kovacic (1966) led Ryan and Foster (1967) to postulate that differences in pain tolerance of athletic groups were due to the tendency of certain athletes to "augment" and others to "reduce" sensory inputs. They compared contact athletes, noncontact athletes, and nonathletes on measures of pain tolerance and augmentation–reduction. The contact athletes were shown to (1) possess the characteristics of the "reducer" (i.e., greatest reduction of perceived size following stimulation), (2) tolerate the most pain, and (3) consistently judge time as passing more slowly.

C. Perceived Exertion

There is actually a lack of sufficient evidence pertaining to perceived exertion and athletic performance at this point in time to permit one to advance generalizations regarding this important aspect of sport. However, there is sufficient evidence to permit speculation.

First of all, it has been demonstrated that perceived exertion is related to the level of work, heart rate, oxygen consumption, and catecholamine production. This, of course, is in keeping with expectations derived from exercise physiology and psychophysics. However, at various points in training, athletes frequently report that standard training regimes become extremely difficult and previous performance levels are often no longer possible.

This phenomenon is often described as "staleness" and some coaches feel that it can be caused by "overtraining." At any rate, the athlete's perception of a given work load is just as important as the work intensity itself. The recent work of Morgan et al. (1973) is relevant here in that they have manipulated perceived exertion and metabolic costs of standard exercise by means of hypnotic suggestion. Since this was demonstrated in healthy adult males, it is reasonable to suggest that "staleness" is partially psychological. Also, one might speculate that athletes who are *presumably* training at 80% of maximum and complaining of complete exhaustion thereafter may, in fact, be working at or near maximum. The implication for coaches, trainers, and physicians is that baseline responses for standard exercise bouts be obtained in preseason or early season in order to facilitate the evaluation of "staleness" at a later point in time.

D. Perceptual Distortion

The question of whether or not it is possible to distort one's percept of an exercise task seems to have been answered in the affirmative by Morgan et al. (1973); that is, subjects exercising on a bicycle ergometer at a constant work load had higher and lower ratings of perceived exertion following hypnotic suggestions of heavy and light work, respectively.

Also, it has been demonstrated that weight-trained subjects who have presumably reached a training plateau can experience increases or decreases in muscular strength following perceptual distortion (Morgan et al. 1966). For example, these investigators demonstrated that the maximum bench press performance of subjects could be either increased or decreased by manipulating the subject's perception of the actual weight being lifted.

V. MOTIVATIONAL FACTORS

It is generally felt that a wide variety of motivational techniques are capable of evoking increases in muscular performance. Adequate discussion of this particular aspect of sport psychology is far beyond the scope of this chapter. However, the effect of factors such as anxiety, hypnosis, mental practice, physical warm-up, information feedback, music, and social facilitation on muscular performance has recently been reviewed in an edited volume by Morgan (1972). It is important to realize that attempts to facilitate muscular performance above "operational levels" should only be attempted where objective physiological evidence indicates that the athlete is clearly functioning at a pseudo maximum. Also, should the achievement of maximal levels be contraindicated from a psychodynamic standpoint, attempts to facilitate muscular performance should not be pursued.

For better or worse, the athlete should probably establish his own performance objectives. His decision on such a matter would obviously be influenced by input from his coach, trainer, team physician, teammates, and opponents. In the final analysis, however, whether it be intentional or unintentional, his decision to go for a record must be a highly personal and intellectual proposition. For example, following his recent world record in the high jump Pat Matzdorf explained that he had not shaved that morning because he wanted to "feel mean." This presumably played a role in his getting "psyched up." At any rate, his coach had established an objective that called for this performance to occur a year later. As with other great high jumpers, time will serve as the test of whether or not this performance was premature.

VI. SUMMARY

The present chapter has emphasized the role of personality dynamics in sport, and the influence of perceptual factors has been examined to a lesser extent. While there have been numerous methodological problems associated with the literature in this field, it seems reasonable to advance certain tentative conclusions.

The majority of investigations reviewed in this chapter support the view that athletes differ from nonathletes on a number of personality variables. Furthermore, these same investigations generally support the position that athletes from numerous sport groups differ on various personality dimensions, as well as pain tolerance and augmentation–reduction. Also, athletes have been found to differ from nonathletes on these same paramaters. Results of investigations designed to delineate personality correlates of athletic ability have been equivocal. On the other hand, investigators have consistently observed athletes to be stable as opposed to neurotic. It seems reasonable to propose that stability is a prerequisite for high-level athletic competition.

While there has been far less research directed toward an understanding of the female athlete, the limited research in this area is consonant with the results for males; that is, female athletes differ from nonathletes, athletes from different subgroups differ, and stability has been consistently observed in the female athlete.

Theoretical derivations from Eysenckian theory support the view that personality differences between athletic subgroups and between athletes and nonathletes represents an antecedent rather than consequent condition of sport.

REFERENCES

Andrews, J. C. (1971). *Educ. Rev.* **23,** 126.

Berger, R. A., and Littlefield, D. H. (1969). *Res. Quart.* **40,** 663.

Booth, E. G., Jr. (1958). *Res. Quart.* **29,** 127.

Carmen, L. R., Zerman, J. L., and Blaine, G. B., Jr. (1968). *Ment. Hyg.* **52,** 134.

Fletcher, R., and Dowell, L. (1971). *J. Psychol.* **77,** 39.

Hammer, W. M. (1970). *J. Sports Med.* **10,** 114.

Harlow, R. G. (1951). *J. Personality* **19,** 312.

Henry, F. M. (1941). *Psychol. Bull.* **38,** 745.

Hunt, D. H. (1969). *Res. Quart.* **40,** 704.

Johnson, W. R., Hutton, D. C., and Johnson, G. B. (1954). *Res. Quart.* **25,** 484.

Kane, J. E. (1964). *In* "International Research in Sport and Physical Education" (E. Jokl and E. Simon, eds.), pp. 85–94. Thomas, Springfield, Illinois.

Kroll, W. (1967). *Res. Quart.* **38,** 49.

Kroll, W., and Carlson, R. B. (1967). *Res. Quart.* **38,** 405.

Kroll, W., and Petersen, K. H. (1965). *Res. Quart.* **36,** 433.

LaPlace, J. P. (1954). *Res. Quart.* **25,** 313.

Little, J. C. (1969). *Acta Psychiat. Scand.* **45,** 187.

Malumphy, T. M. (1968). *Res. Quart.* **39,** 610.

Morgan, W. P. (1968). *J. Sports Med.* **8,** 212.

Morgan, W. P., ed. (1970). "Contemporary Readings in Sport Psychology." Thomas, Springfield, Illinois.

Morgan, W. P. (1972). *In* "Psychomotor Domain: Movement Behaviors" (R. N. Singer, ed.), Lea & Febiger, Philadelphia, Pennsylvania.

Morgan, W. P., ed. (1972). "Ergogenic Aids and Muscular Performance." Academic Press, New York.

Morgan, W. P., and Costill, D. L. (1972). *J. Sports Med.* **12,** 42.

Morgan, W. P., and Hammer, W. M. (1971). *Abstr. Amer. Ass. Health, Phys. Educ. Recreation, 1971,* Vol. 7, p. 28.

Morgan, W. P., Needle, R. H., and Coyne, L. L. (1966). *Abstr. Amer. Ass. Health, Phys. Educ. Recreation, 1966,* Vol. 3, p. 71.

Morgan, W. P., Raven, P. B., Drinkwater, B. L., and Horvath, S. M. (1973). *Int. J. Clin. Exp. Hypnosis.* **21,** 86.

Newman, E. N. (1968). *Res. Quart.* **39,** 1049.

Ogilvie, B. C. (1968). *J. Amer. Med. Ass.* **205,** 156.

Parsons, D. R. (1963). Unpublished Thesis, University of British Columbia, Vancouver.

Peterson, S. L., Weber, J. C., and Trousdale, W. W. (1967). *Res. Quart.* **38,** 686.

Pierce, R. A. (1969). *Amer. Coll. Health Ass.* **17,** 244.

Rasch, P. J., and Hunt, M. B. (1960). *J. Ass. Phys. Ment. Rehab.* **14,** 163.

Rushall, B. S. (1970). *Int. J. Sports Psychol.* **1,** 93.

Ryan, E. D., and Foster, R. L. (1967). *J. Personality Soc. Psychol.* **6,** 472.

Ryan, E. D., and Kovacic, C. R. (1966). *Percept. Mot. Skills* **22,** 383.

Schendel, J. (1965). *Res. Quart.* **36,** 52.

Singer, R. N. (1969). *Res. Quart.* **90,** 582.

Slusher, H. S. (1966). *Res. Quart.* **37,** 540.

Sternbach, R. A. (1968). "Pain." Academic Press, New York.

Thune, A. R. (1949). *Res. Quart.* **20,** 296.

Vanek, M., and Cratty, B. J. (1970). "Psychology and the Superior Athlete." Macmillan, New York.

Williams, J. M., Hoepner, B. J., Moody, D. L., and Ogilvie, B. C. (1970). *Res. Quart.* **41,** 446.

Yanada, H., and Hirata, H. (1970). *Proc. Coll. Phys. Educ., Univ. Tokyo, 1970,* Vol. 5, p. 1.

Chapter 8

NUTRITION FOR THE ATHLETE

E. R. BUSKIRK

I. INTRODUCTION

Nutrients obtained from ingested food provide the building blocks for the athlete's growth, development, and maturation, plus the fuel elements for routine energy expenditure and for initiation and maintenance of high level performance. Contracting muscle requires a continuing supply and replenishment of the substrates of fuels used to support contraction. It has been said that an athlete is no better than the adequacy of his nutrition.

Fortunately, with the many sources of good foods currently available there is no reason for the athlete to be inadequately nourished. The key for the athlete's nutrition as for everyone elses' is a balanced diet—balanced in all of the essential nutrients so that the body is provided the necessary fuels and building materials. In selecting a diet, the athlete can exercise considerable individuality. There is no "best" balanced diet, for one balanced diet is likely to be as good as another. But there is no substitute for proper planning of a balanced diet, for an unbalanced diet consumed for several weeks can have dire competitive consequences. Even faithful participation in an excellent physical conditioning regimen can not compensate for inadequate nutrition. Neither can a balanced diet alone compensate for poor skill development and training. Diet, conditioning, and training should be regarded as complementary. Similarly, a proper diet is no substitute for the will to win, but a nutrient may indirectly aid that will. If a good and essential food provides the athlete with a psychological edge, he should eat it but not to the excess of unbalancing his diet. Maintenance of a good diet is a year-round affair.

Established nutritional practices fortified by knowledge gleaned from current nutritional research should provide the basis for dietary planning. The athletic team physician and the local dietitians, i.e., hospital, school, etc., are the persons usually most knowledgeable in nutritional planning and who can provide sound nutritional advice. In addition, trainers who are well read and/or who have been associated with college programs are likely to have been exposed to discussions about good nutrition and should be able to provide nutritional counsel. Team physicians and trainers should be well aware of current dietary fads. Efforts should be made to clarify misrepresentation of nutritional facts in order to forestall initiation of costly and perhaps useless food habits.

II. ENERGY BALANCE

Daily caloric requirements vary with the athlete, his size and weight, his body build, the type of sport that he is engaged in, his frequency of competition, the type of practice and conditioning regimen he undergoes, his clothing worn, the surface he plays on, and the environment in which his sport is conducted. Since conditioning and training occupy 90% of the athlete's time available for the sport, the intensity and duration of training and/or conditioning are the factors largely responsible for the rate of energy turnover by the athlete. A rough caloric classification appears in Table I. While the classification is imprecise, the range in caloric requirements of from 3000 to 6000 kcal/day probably includes 95% of all athletes. Very large athletes training intensively for several hours will have the highest caloric requirements. The possible exception to this general rule is the smaller athlete who transports his body weight over long distances thereby using considerable energy, e.g., the cross-country runner.

A scheme for visualizing energy partitioning is depicted in Fig. 1. Our sustenance is provided by nutrients available in the food that we eat. Not all of the ingested foodstuffs are in the form of digestible items, e.g., cellulose is not digested by man as it is by cattle. The nondigestible, nonabsorbable material stays in the gastrointestinal tract to be excreted as a portion of the stool and exerts a bulk action for normal movements of the intestines. Of the nutrients that are digested, some are assimilated and incorporated into body storage pools including body tissue. Some are lost, some are secreted by special glands such as sweat, sebaceous, and tear glands, and some are excreted in the urine. A small amount of energy is lost via volatilized compounds in the expired air. The energy remaining is the stored or utilizable energy commonly called metabolizable energy. This energy provides the muscles and other tissues fuel for physical work. That portion of the energy not involved with physical work is lost as heat. Overall, the athlete

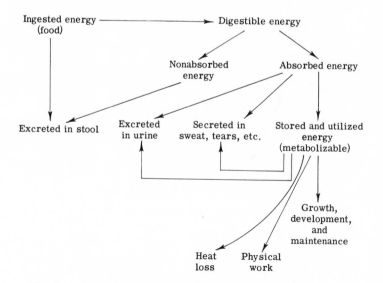

Fig. 1 Scheme for partitioning the energy available from food.

TABLE I

Classification of Activities by Type of Effort and Range of Probable Daily Caloric Requirements in Relation to the Demands of the Activity:
Effect of Length of Practice on the Daily Caloric Requirements

Duration of activity:	Short burst	Less than 1 minute	Sustained	1 to 10 minutes	10 minutes or more	Endurance
Intensity of activity:	Maximum effort	Strenuous effort	Low intensity	Sustained effort	Intense repeated effort	High intensity
Event	Discus Hammer throw Shot-put Javelin High jump Diving Ski jumping	Dashes including 440 yd Hurdles Long jump Hop, step, jump Pole vault Long horse vault 50 and 100 yd swimming events	Baseball Golf	880 yd run 1 and 2 mile runs Swimming events over 100 yd Wrestling Most gymnastic events Downhill, slalom skiing	Football Basketball Ice hockey Lacrosse Tennis Gymnastic all-round Fencing 3 mile run	Cross-country running 6 mile run Marathon running Soccer Cross-country skiing
kcal/day	3000 to 4000	3000 to 4000	3000 to 4000	3000 to 5000	3000 to 6000	4000 to 6000
Training	% Increase in daily caloric requirement in relation to length of practice					
≤1 hr	5	5	8	10	10	13
1–2 hr	10	10	17	20	20	25
≥2 hr	15	15	25	30	30	38

Remarks: It is assumed that body weight and size were approximately equal at each end of the kcal/day range for the participants in the events referred to in the above categories. Such an assumption is an oversimplification, e.g., shot putters are usually very large men and divers are usually small men. Note that an athlete in training requires at least 3000 kcal/day, and that additional training can markedly increase his daily caloric requirement.

is seldom more than 25% efficient in whatever he does, which means that at least 75% of his metabolizable energy is utilized for body temperature regulation and heat dissipation.

Gross Nutritional Status

An appraisal of gross nutritional status can be made by carefully following body weight and fatness. Measuring body weight is relatively easy if good scales are available. Assessing body fatness is more difficult and involves use of one of the several available procedures for measuring fat as a component of body composition. Weight gain may imply meeting normal growth and development requirements but it also may indicate the storage of excess energy as surplus fat. Other than for Sumo wrestling (inertial mass effects), channel swimming (thermal insulation), or football (protective cushioning), there appears little reason for the athlete to accumulate excess fat. In the healthy athlete, excess body water is not stored. Bone and muscle may be developed even in the mature athlete with an appropriate conditioning and training regimen. Weight loss may indicate a reduction in body fat stores, or, if the athlete is sick and confined to bed, body tissue including muscle mass may be lost as well. Thus, weight appraisal is a valuable guide to any athlete and to his physician in particular.

1. Estimation of Body Fat

Assistance from the team physician, trainer, and nurse in making the assessment of fatness as an indicator of gross nutritional status is also valuable. For example, skin fold thickness measurements can be used to check on body fatness. This simple method only measures subcutaneous fatness. Nevertheless, total body fatness can be calculated more accurately from the skin fold measurements than by use of height–weight ratios, total body weight, or the physician's or coach's eye appraisal. The latter methods are importantly affected by differences in body build and other components of body composition as well as by the stage of growth and development of the athlete. In relatively mature athletes, periodic body weight measurements would serve as a monitoring method of short-term changes in body fatness.

An athlete should not have over 15% body fat if he is preparing himself for competition (except as noted previously). In fact, 10% or even 7% body fat would be a better goal. Man needs fat in his body, for the structural and functional lipids in nerves, brain, and other tissues are

TABLE II
Simple Classification of Skin Fold Measurements for Athletes[a]

Classification	Triceps[a] (mm)	Scapular[b] (mm)	Abdomen[c] (mm)	Sum (mm)
Lean, <7% fat	<7	<8	<10	<25
Acceptable, 7–15% fat	7 to 13	8 to 15	10–20	25 to 48
Overfat, >15% fat	>13	15	>20	>48

[a] Skin fold location:

Triceps: back of the upper arm over triceps, midway on upper arm—skin fold lifted parallel to long axis of arm with arm pendant.

Scapular: below tip of right scapula—skin fold lifted along long axis of body.

Abdomen: 5 cm lateral from umbilicus—avoid abdominal crease—skin fold lifted on axis with umbilicus.

The scapular skin fold is the single best skin fold to measure. The triceps is next best. The skin fold thickness includes a double layer of skin and subcutaneous adipose tissue. It is not important to compute an absolute value for body fatness from the skin fold measurements unless it is felt necessary to do so.

The classification values can be adjusted depending on the coach's assessment of desirable limits of body skin fold thickness and fatness. For example, acceptable skin fold thicknesses will be less on runners than football players. Skin fold calipers are available from the following sources: (1) Cambridge Scientific Industries, Inc., Cambridge, Maryland; (2) H. E. Morse Co., 455 Douglas Avenue, Holland, Michigan.

vital. Nevertheless, excess fat is a burden that must be transported. Transport of excess weight reduces the athlete's efficiency.

A simple classification of skin fold measurements for athletes appears in Table II. The skin fold thickness is relatively independent of body size, for one only measures a double layer of skin plus the underlying fat.

2. Weight Control

Competitive weight maintenance should be the goal of the athlete in training. Weight fluctuations other than those associated with loss and replacement of body fluids means that inadequate attention has been paid to caloric consumption. The athlete's diet must conform to his energy expenditure. Fortunately, for most athletes the weight control process is close to self-regulating. The athlete with an overnutrition problem needs competent dietary counseling.

A comment should be made about weight control in wrestling. There are few sports in which weight categories are so rigorously defined. Weight reduction in wrestling is frequently undertaken to gain a competitive advantage. In the well-conditioned wrestler who has no more than 3 to 5% body fat, his body fat stores are already at a low level. Thus, further weight reduction must involve loss of his body water and tissue. Withholding water, inducing sweating, or undernutrition are the methods employed to achieve weight loss. Fortunately, the body can take tremendous abuse without serious penalty. Nevertheless, chronic water loss or undernutrition over several days may serve no useful function. The body becomes dehydrated, and highly concentrated urine is voided. There is the distinct possibility of developing calculi or concretions in the kidney; uremia may develop, and nephritis or nephrosis ensue. Temperature regulation may become abnormal along with other debilitating effects of dehydration. Through such drastic weight reduction procedures, the wrestler certainly gets no stronger or smarter—he is gambling that on a relative basis he will retain an edge over the competitor in the lower weight class. The gamble may pay off, but the preparation is physiologically unsound.

III. BALANCED DIET

A balanced diet provides not only the required energy in calories but proper dietary composition with respect to protein, carbohydrate, and fat. In general, it would seem desirable to use a diet providing as a percent of caloric intake the following mixture:

Protein	10–20%
Carbohydrate	50–55%
Fat	30–35%

The athlete in training who requires 3000 kcal/day or more may find it easier to take extra calories as fat than from the other food sources. Fat is more "dense" calorically than protein or carbohydrate, for fat provides approximately 9 kcal/g, whereas protein and carbohydrate provide about 4 kcal/g. In contrast, the efficiency of energy supply in terms of kcal per liter of oxygen utilized is greater for carbohydrates (5 kcal/liter O_2) than for fat (4.6 kcal/liter O_2). Increasing the fat content of the diet may later prove injurious to the athlete, for his dietary habits may continue and a high dietary fat intake (particularly the saturated fats) has been importantly associated with the development of atherosclerosis and coronary heart disease.

In the growing and developing athlete, high quality protein intakes are critical, for some of the dietary protein is incorporated into his increasing mass of body tissue including muscle. Protein intakes as high as 20% of ingested calories may be appropriate. The mature athlete can remain in nitrogen balance with as little as 1 g protein per kg body weight per day, whereas the growing, developing athlete may require up to 2 g/kg.

Carbohydrate intake should be high enough to ensure complete filling of muscle and liver glycogen stores. This is usually no problem on common diets. Fat is also readily available, and with our penchant for bacon, steak, and other fatty meats the problem is usually one of trimming excess fat from the available meat cuts.

The composition of the ingested protein is important, for protein provides the nitrogen and amino acids for synthesis of various body tissues, and these same amino acids are involved in numerous metabolic functions. Protein in excess of requirement serves only to provide energy, and the associated organic acids must be excreted, which means obligatory work for the kidneys. Twenty-two amino acids have been shown to be physiologically important, but some of these are synthesized by the body. Eight are not synthesized and must be provided in the diet, hence the term "essential amino acids." They are isoleucine, leucine, lysine, methionine, phenylalanine, threonine, tryptophan, and valine. There is increasing evidence that arginine and histidine should also be regarded as essential in growing and developing children. Good quality protein of high biological value contains these essential amino acids. Milk, cheese, poultry, eggs, meat, fish, and whole grain cereals when supplemented with milk supply such protein.

Certain types of athletes such as football and hockey players are subject to tissue damage brought about by the battering and bruising they undergo. This damaged tissue requires repair which means synthesis of new tissues. The protein requirement in these athletes is higher than normal. The growing, developing athlete subjected to tissue damage may well have a daily protein requirement of up to 2.5 g/kg per day.

Vegetarians have a problem since they must exercise great care to ensure an adequate intake of high quality protein and essential amino acids. A mixture of nuts, whole grain cereals, roots, and seeds should provide protein of adequate quality, but vegetarians should consult appropriate nutritional tables to assure proper protein nutrition.

Current literature refers to the dynamic state of equilibrium of all nutrients and their subunits. Each nutrient has a specific subunit that is digested. This subunit may be immediately metabolized following its delivery by the circulation to the metabolizing tissue. Similarly, the subunit may be temporarily stored or converted into an entirely different compound for utilization in a specific metabolic process. Even the socalled inert tissues such as bone and adipose tissue are subject to constant change or turnover. The processes of digestion, utilization, and

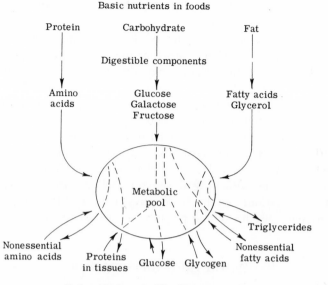

Fig. 2 Components of nutrients, following digestion of subunits, enter metabolic pool and are interconverted into end products. Storage time in any form is short because all components and subunits are continuously cycled and recycled.

turnover by virtue of cycling and recycling through a metabolic pool is depicted in Fig. 2.

Food guides are important in the development of a balanced diet. The Institute of Home Economics of the Agricultural Research Service, USDA, has prepared a daily food guide. The essential foods for athletes are listed in Table III. The guide is simple but has limitations in that

TABLE III

Guide to Good Eating for Athletes: Servings for Daily Consumption[a]

Food groups	Food	Number of servings
Milk	Milk, cheese, ice cream, and other milk-made foods	4 or more glasses or equivalent
Meat	Meats, fish, poultry, eggs, dry beans, peas, nuts	3 or more servings
Vegetables	Dark green, light green, yellow, potatoes	4 or more servings
Fruits	Citrus fruits, apples, juices, tomatoes	3 or more servings
Breads and Cereals	Whole grain, enriched	4 or more servings

[a] This will provide a well-balanced diet that is adequate in all nutrients. Servings in any category except fruits can be increased to add more calories.

wise selections must be made and the word "serving" must be interpreted.

The mothers of most athletes hopefully start them in the right nutritional direction by preparing meals that provide a balanced diet. When this is not the case, the athlete may develop poor nutritional habits and frequently select foods of marginal nutritional value. Teen-aged athletes, in particular, who eat on their own without benefit of a knowledgeable mother or a well-run training table, are likely to select foods of appeal to them but without regard to nutritional value. Hamburgers, french fries, pizzas, cokes, etc., make up the familiar list. Obviously, this repetitive diet is unbalanced and does not provide the nutritional counseling, but the athlete will seldom seek counseling on his own. Appropriate questions by the team physician should establish if there is a nutritional cause for subpar performance by an athlete.

IV. DIETARY SUPPLEMENTS

A. Minerals

While minerals are not really dietary supplements because adequate quantities are provided in a balanced diet, they are essential as building materials and for body regulatory reactions. Each mineral listed in Table IV may have one or more known function of nutritional importance. Only a few uses will be mentioned. Phosphorus and particularly calcium are needed for bone development. Sodium and potassium are required for maintenance of the extracellular and intracellular fluid volumes, respectively. Iron and copper are necessary for formation of normal hemoglobin and myoglobin. Female athletes may need more of these two elements. Many of the elements are important in acid–base regulation because they form compounds which are acids, bases, salts, or buffers.

Some of the important minerals in the body, the assumed requirements (if known) for athletes, and the source of the element are listed in Table IV. A separation is made into those elements known to be required in relatively large amounts, i.e., more than 1 g, and those necessary in trace or very small amounts. Note that the daily requirement of many of the elements is unknown.

Most of the trace elements are required for proper physiological functioning largely by participation as catalysts in metabolic reactions. Since many of the trace elements appear to be stored in the liver, they may accumulate to toxic levels if taken in larger than required amounts as dietary supplements.

TABLE IV

Minerals: Suggested Daily Requirements and Nutritional Sources[a]

Element	Symbol	Requirement	Source
Sodium	Na	7.5 g	Salt, cereals, meats
Potassium	K	1 g	Cereals, fish, shellfish, meats
Phosphorus	P	1.5 g	Meat, eggs, vegetables, nuts
Calcium	Ca	1 g	Milk, dairy products
Magnesium	Mg	300 mg	Meat, cereals, fruits, vegetables, nuts
Sulfur	S	Unknown	Meats
Chlorine	Cl	7.5 g	Salt, cereals
Trace Elements:			
Copper	Cu	5 mg	Liver, kidney, shellfish, nuts
Iodine	I	0.1 mg	Iodized salt, seafoods
Fluorine	F	Unknown	Fluoridated water, meat, seafood, milk
Iron	Fe	15 mg	Liver, other meats, fruits
Zinc	Zn	10 mg	Meat, vegetables
Manganese	Mn	5 mg	Cereals, vegetables
Molybdenum	Mo	Unknown	Legumes, cereal, organ meats, yeast
Cobalt	Co	Unknown	Common foods
Selenium	Se	Unknown	Meats, legumes
Chromium	Cr	Unknown	Common foods
Bromine	Br	Unknown	Salt, common foods

Acid and Base Forming Mineral Elements

Acid forming	Base forming
Sulfur	Sodium
Phosphorus	Potassium
Chlorine	Calcium
	Magnesium
	Iron

[a] Minerals help maintain body fluid neutrality (slight alkalinity) by forming acids, bases, buffering compounds, and salts.

B. Vitamins

Attention has recently been refocused on vitamins as nutrients with emphasis on vitamin C. Currently, a wide variety of vitamin and/or mineral preparations are available. A well-balanced diet contains adequate vitamins as it does minerals. In general, the excess water soluble vitamins ingested are excreted in the urine, and the excess fat soluble vitamins appear to be stored in the liver. Thus, no requirement for extra vitamins appears to exist. The proponents of vitamin usage cite the example of animals, which when exposed to stress, manufacture extra vitamin C, something that man can not do. The reasoning goes that exercise, and particularly competition, is a stress and the athlete therefore needs supplementary vitamin C. Unfortunately, data to defend or refute this argument are not available. The toxic effects of fat-soluble vitamins A and D when ingested in extremely high quantities are well documented.

A listing of vitamins, their name, and the suggested upper limits for daily allowances for college athletes is provided in Table V. As with minerals, the daily requirement for many vitamins is unknown.

Several of the vitamins, including those of the B complex and C, E, and K, are intimately involved in metabolic reactions. The requirement for these vitamins could well be increased as a result of the high metabolic turnover in athletes. Both vitamins A and D are required for proper bone ossification which is of vital importance to the growing athlete. Vitamins also play an important role in the regulation of ap-

TABLE V

Recommended Vitamin Allowances for College Athletes[a]

Vitamin	Other designation	Recommended daily allowance[b]
Water soluble		
B Complex		
Vitamin B_1	Thiamine	0.4 mg/1000 kcal
Vitamin B_2	Riboflavin	0.6 mg/1000 kcal
Vitamin B_6	Pyridoxine (and 2 related compounds)	2–3 mg
Niacin	Nicotinic acid or its amide	6.6 mg/1000 kcal
Pantothenic Acid	Pantothenic acid	10 mg
Biotin	Biotin	300 γ
Choline	Choline	900 mg
Folic acid (Folate)	Pteroylglutamic acid	100 γ
Vitamin B_{12}	Cobalamin	5 γ
Vitamin C	Ascorbic acid	1 mg/kg body wt.
Fat soluble[c]		
Vitamin A	Retinol	5,000 I.U.
Vitamin D	Calciferol and 7-dehydrocholesterol	400 I.U.
Vitamin E	Tocopherols	30 mg
Vitamin K	Phylloquinones	Questionable

[a] Milk, yellow and green vegetables, fruits, eggs, meats, butter, and whole grain cereals are good natural food sources for the vitamins.

[b] Recommended allowances are given as the upper suggested limit of young male allowances. I.U., international unit; mg, milligrams; γ, gamma or micrograms.

[c] Food fat serves as a carrier for the fat-soluble vitamins.

petite, digestion and utilization of foods, resistance to certain infections, and maintenance of nervous stability. Both vitamins and minerals have related functions as cofactors in enzymatic reactions.

The body has a built-in regulator for directly providing additional vitamins and minerals. As more energy is utilized, appetite is increased and satiety modified. Along with increased food intake more vitamins and minerals are consumed and made available for use by the body.

C. Water

Water can be treated separately. Water is made available by drinking, by consumption of water that is an integral part of a food, and by the oxidation of foodstuffs. Water is lost from the body in urine, stool, sweat, insensible perspiration, diffusing through the skin, and by humidification of expired air. The athlete may regularly incur a short term negative water balance of from 2 to 3% during each daily exercise session with regular adherence to his conditioning and training regimen. This water is replaced as soon as he has had adequate rest and has consumed food and fluids. Regular losses in excess of 5% of body weight indicate that a water replacement program should be instituted because of the debilitating effects of dehydration which set in at about this level. Fortunately, the athlete's thirst mechanism usually prevents him from reaching the critical 5% dehydration level. The exception is the athlete who works hard in a hot environment. He will usually lose more water and will become partially dehydrated. Increased water and salt intake should be encouraged under hot conditions, for the salt helps hold the water in the body. In addition, the salt intake replenishes that excreted in urine and secreted in sweat.

V. NONFOOD SUPPLEMENTS

A. Alcohol

A variety of chemicals and other drugs have been used as aids ostensibly to improve performance capabilities. Among the most common of these is alcohol. But alcohol deserves no consideration as a food to be consumed by athletes. Ethyl alcohol is rapidly absorbed in the stomach and small intestine and can be readily oxidized by the liver and other tissues. There is evidence that alcohol has a direct toxic effect on the liver and promotes accumulation of fat. Alcohol can also do irreparable central nervous system damage and has a depressing effect on the central nervous system as well. With consumption of fairly small amounts of alcohol, coordination, judgment, and consequently performance are all impaired.

B. Caffeine

Caffeine is used widely in our culture, for it is contained in substantial quantities in tea, coffee, and cola drinks. Because caffeine acts as a central nervous system stimulant, a variety of concentrated caffeine preparations have been made available. Although caffeine ostensibly improves attention and alertness and delays fatigue, there is no known evidence that it improves the performance of athletes. In fact, use of caffeine by the athlete is contraindicated except in moderation, for it increases the work of the heart of athletes and produces a very strong diuretic effect.

C. Anabolic Steroids

Anabolic steroids of the androgenic type have been used extensively by some athletes to increase muscularity, body size, and bulk. Evidence exists in the literature that such may be the case if these steroids are appropriately administered at certain ages and stages of development. Nevertheless, the evidence is not clear-cut, and the side effects of these hormones should definitely preclude their use for other than clinical therapy. For example, in the prepubertal athlete, bone development may not occur normally with premature closing of the epiphyses. In older athletes, production of testosterone may be curtailed, the testicles may atrophy, and metabolically related conditions may ensue such as jaundice (liver damage) and edema. Abnormal breast development may begin. Thus, the metabolic and other consequences of use of anabolic steroids are too serious to warrant their consideration as performance aids by athletes.

D. Other Substances

A variety of other nonfood supplements have also been employed. These range from sodium bicarbonate and sodium citrate to aspartic acid. A rational case can be made as to why they are important in metabolic processes and why, with the increased metabolism of extensive exercise, increased available amounts of these compounds should aid performance. Proof of these assumptions is difficult at best, and the available experiments are not conclusive, showing that this type of supplementation is of little, if any, value to the athlete on a balanced diet.

In the hands of the experienced team physician who uses his drug arsenal for medical treatment, athletic management procedures are enhanced and the well-treated athlete finds himself better able to cope with the rigors of competition. Unfortunately, athletes themselves actively seek illusive performance aids including drugs. Drugs that have been employed in athletics to improve performance form a list too long for this chapter. Only the categories of drugs and their most important actions are listed in Table VI. It should be reemphasized that all of these drugs are dangerous if not medically prescribed for specific treatment.

Metabolic inhibitors are substances known to block or alter normal metabolic reactions. Nicotine from inhalation of tobacco smoke, DDT,

TABLE VI

Drugs Commonly Used to Enhance Performance General Drug Categories and Important Actions

Drug category	Important action
Amphetamines	Central nervous system stimulant which supposedly promotes alertness and confidence. Stimulates action of the naturally occurring catecholamines on heart, arterioles, nerves and metabolic reactions.
Barbituates	Central nervous system depressant most commonly used to lessen pain or produce sleep. A hypnotic or sedative.
Hallucinogens	Central nervous system activator or inhibitor depending on person and area of CNS predominantly influenced. Creates bizarre effects for normal thought processes are changed and reality avoided.
Local anesthetics	Peripheral nerve depressant which relieves pain and can prevent muscle swelling and spasm.
Metabolic inhibitors	Interferes with normal metabolic reactions.
Narcotics	Central nervous system depressant that produces stupor, insensibility or sleep. Use can lead to dependence and addiction.
Peripheral vasodilators	Dilate peripheral arterioles and coronary arteries to presumably supply more blood to working muscle.
Tranquilizers	To calm or sedate without producing stupor or sleep. Used to enhance recovery from fatigue.

and other chemicals commonly used for pest and weed eradication by the farmer and home owner fall into this category. If inhaled, eaten, drunk, or absorbed through the skin, these inhibitors can cause physical weakness, weight loss, general disability, and even death. These effects are not usually seen as a result of a single exposure but most commonly reflect chronic exposure. Thus it behooves the athlete to avoid the offending chemicals by not smoking and by staying out of areas where pesticides and herbicides are employed.

Periodically new fads evolve in the nonfood supplement category. It is the nature of athletes to explore the unknown to seek a competitive advantage. The natural course for a fad is for it to go through a period of popular utilization to be followed by a period of evaluation and, finally, a period of rationality which largely discredits the fad. This pattern has been repeated many times through the years. The athlete is well advised to avoid the fads and concentrate on conditioning and training plus good nutrition.

VI. SPECIAL DIETARY PLANNING

A. Increasing Glycogen Stores

The glycogen story began many years ago. It has been recognized for some time that the circulating substrates utilized for fuel by the muscle are glucose, glycogen, and free fatty acids. Utilization of these substrates is not a mutually exclusive affair, but a "mix" is oxidized and this "mix" changes with the level of physical activity. The "mix" may also be dependent on prior nutrition, genetically controlled enzymatic endowment, etc. Only recently has it been shown that glycogen is preferentially utilized at high rates of energy expenditure and that glycogen and creatinine phosphate depletion in muscle is associated with reduction in performance capacity, particularly in endurance events lasting 30 minutes or more. Glycogen reserves in muscle can become "supersaturated" which provides adequate glycogen to sustain high level performance if the glycogen stores in muscle are depleted by hard training accompanied by a high protein and fat but relatively low carbohydrate diet 3 to 4 days prior to competition. Following depletion, muscle glycogen stores can be built up to higher than normal values by keeping the level of activity relatively low and by consuming a high carbohydrate diet. Most sports do not require larger than normal glycogen stores, so that the combined training and dietary manipulations are probably unnecessary. In endurance sports such as marathon running, cross-country skiing, or channel swimming, the combined training and dietary program could well provide the competitive edge to the winner.

B. Avoiding Flatulence

Flatulence or overproduction of flatus can be disturbing to the athlete and detrimental to peak performance. Various beans and other legumes are notorious for their gas producing ability as are sauerkraut and other cabbage preparations. Flatus is comprised of a mixture of gases but predominantly nitrogen, methane, and carbon dioxide with hydrogen sulfide responsible for the objectionable odor. While jet propulsion may be desirable in a vehicle, the energy released in flatus is negligible. Thus, the elimination of flatus serves only the useful purpose of ridding the gastrointestinal tract of stored gas. Foods that stimulate gas production should be avoided, particularly prior to competition.

C. Training Table

The training table can be one of the most beneficial and rewarding experiences of an athlete's career if the training table is well run and if the food is excellent tasting and nutritious and is served in an atmosphere conducive to the enjoyment of food. Meals well planned by a competent nutritionist serve as a teaching device, for the training table provides guidance as to what constitutes a balanced diet. Thus, food habits can be formed by the athlete which will serve him in good stead throughout his lifetime. The athlete can socialize with his teammates in an atmosphere conducive to the development of *esprit de corps*. Use of the training table simplifies supply of special foods and preparations such as a honey mix, salt solution, etc. Proper meal timing is insured. Calorically controlled diets can also be administered via the training table to the athlete with a weight problem.

In the final analysis, the burden of providing good nutrition is on the athlete himself. The athlete on his own must attempt to gain nutritional experience so that he makes intelligent selection of foods. He must be nutritionally aware. Fortunately, several sources of nutritional guidance are open to him, chief among which is the team physician.

VII. CONTESTS AND MEALS

Precontest nutritional preparation has received renewed attention in recent years because of the extensive work on glycogen and its utilization during strenuous activity. Thus, dietary preparation for an endurance contest should begin at least 48 hours before competition. Adequate carbohydrate should be taken to saturate the glycogen storage capacity of liver and muscle. Conditioning and training should be curtailed at least 30 hours prior to competition so that the muscles have an opportunity for full recovery including a buildup of their glycogen content.

The precontest meal, if made up of conventional foods, should be consumed a minimum of three hours, but preferably four to five hours, prior to the contest. This allows adequate time for nutrient passage from the stomach to the intestines and for some digestion and absorption to take place. Otherwise, there is a good possibility that the "keyed-up" athlete will compete with food in his stomach. Even so, large amounts of protein or fat should be avoided, for proteins stimulate gastric secretion and yield organic acids which will be retained and not excreted when kidney blood flow is reduced during exercise. Fat is so slowly moved by the stomach and absorbed from the intestinal tract that very little of the energy available from the ingested fat can be utilized. Bland, nongreasy, easily digested foods and fluids which contain higher than the normal amounts of carbohydrates should be consumed in the precontest meal. Foods that tend to irritate the lining wall of the intestine or produce stool bulk or excessive gas should be avoided. Thus, cabbage, cucumbers, nuts, beans, salads, oils, spices, plus rough or seedy vegetables should be avoided. The athlete, in order to achieve his full competitive potential, must eat to avoid abdominal cramps, slow stomach emptying, inadequate glycogen reserves, and diarrhea.

There is much to recommend a liquid precontest meal because a liquid meal will pass through the stomach much faster than a solid meal. Liquid meals can be tasty and contain sufficient carbohydrate. An intelligent practice would be to follow a light breakfast of toast, jelly, and a fruit such as peaches, by a liquid meal an hour or so later, but the latter should be fed at least two hours before the contest. The cost of the liquid meal is low and the result quite satisfying to the athlete who understands its purpose.

Before or during prolonged contests, many athletes have found that simple sugar solutions, dextrose tablets, and sugar-base candy bars are satisfying. There is no reason why these easily digested and absorbed sugar sources should not be used. Similarly, a sugared salt solution may be an invaluable aid when competing in a hot environment. Attention should be paid to the postcontest meal which is frequently a rushed and poorly planned affair. Competition is over and the athlete may have a date or a travel commitment or otherwise shortchange his nutritional requirements. In addition, the athlete may not be relaxed nor be ready to eat. Ideally, the athlete could well use a dinner type meal of 1500 to 1800 kcal served in a quiet, relaxed, congenial atmosphere an hour or two or perhaps several hours after the contest, providing the athlete is ready to take on the job of digesting food. Since the athlete may still be tense, beverages containing caffeine or other stimulants should be avoided. One of the joys of competition is the postcontest camaraderie. A well-planned meal can add further enjoyment to the gathering.

SELECTED REFERENCES

Åstrand, P. O. (1968). *Nutr. Today.* 3:9–11.

Bergstrom, J. (1967). *Circ. Res.* **20/21**, Suppl. 1, 1 and 91–98.

Bogert, L. J., Briggs, G. M., and Calloway, D. H. (1966). "Nutrition and Physical Fitness," Saunders, Philadelphia, Pennsylvania.

Bourne, G. H. (1968). *In* "Exercise Physiology" (H. B. Falls, ed.), pp. 155–171. Academic Press, New York.

Bullen, B., Mayer, J., and Stare, F. J. (1959). *Amer. J. Surg.* **98**, 343–352.

Buskirk, E. R. (1971). *In* "Administration of Athletics in Colleges and Universities" (E. S. Steitz, ed.), pp. 186–205. NEA, Washington, D.C.

Hultman, E. (1967). *Circ. Res.* **22/21**, Suppl. 1, 1 and 99–114.

Novick, M. M., and Taylor, B. (1970). "Training and Conditioning of Athletes." Lea & Febiger, Philadelphia, Pennsylvania.

Pike, R., and Brown, M. L. (1967). "Nutrition an Integrated Approach." Wiley, New York.

Rose, K. D., Schneider, P. J., and Sullivan, G. P. (1961). *J. Amer. Med. Ass.* **178**, 30–33.

Steggerda, F. R., and Dimmick, J. F. (1961). *Amer. J. Clin. Nutr.* **19**, 120–124.

Van Ittalie, T. B., Sinisterra, L., and Stare, F. J. (1956). *J. Amer. Med. Ass.* **162**, 1120–1126.

Van Ittalie, T. B., Sinisterra, L., and Stare, F. J. (1960). *In* "Science and Medicine of Exercise and Sports" (W. D. Johnson, ed.), pp. 285–300. Harper, New York.

Yoshimura, H. (1966). *Nutr. Requir. Survival Cold Altitude, Proc. Symp. Arctic Biol. Med., 5th, 1965,* pp. 85–120.

Yoshimura, H. (1971). "Nutrition for Athletes: A Handbook for Coaches." Amer. Ass. Health, Phys. Educ. and Recreation, Washington, D.C.

Chapter 9

PROTECTIVE EQUIPMENT

GORDON STODDARD

I. THE PRESENT STATUS OF PROTECTIVE EQUIPMENT DESIGN
AND MANUFACTURE

In every sports activity, there is an opportunity for trauma. Some injuries are not entirely preventable, since they arise from the nature of the actions performed in the sport, even when it is conducted under the most ideal conditions and with careful and prudent supervision. Some sports injuries occur as a result of completely unpredictable events. This still leaves a large group of accidents in sports which may be prevented or at least minimized by the proper use of protective equipment.

In the last decade, significant advances have been made in the improvement of protective equipment, although few dramatic changes have been made in design. Although manufacturers of sports equipment are continually attempting to improve the quality of their products, efforts in the past have been guided more by individual suggestions from coaches, athletes, and other interested persons, rather than by a planned approach to the problems in protection in sports. Deficiencies or failures of protective items have also had their influence on the manufacturer.

Today's application of new materials, increased knowledge of what equipment is desirable, and advanced engineering principles have contributed overwhelmingly to the vast improvements made in the development of protective devices. The scientific explosion is responsible for the creation of thousands of new materials. The majority of the new materials are not applicable to the unique requirements of sports protective equipment. Unfortunately however, many new materials have not been applied, because they are unknown to those who might be able to use them.

Basic marketing and equipment performance analysis has contributed to the advances made in protective equipment. Data on laboratory and field performances of equipment is increasingly important to the manufacturer, as well as to the wearer for obvious reasons. However, laboratory tests of protective equipment leave much to be desired. In order to conduct an authoritative test it is necessary to simulate the exact conditions under which the equipment will be used. The process of developing new additional protective equipment has not been without its particular problems. There has been a lack of a systematic approach to the various problems of protection of the participant. Not enough concentrated gathering of data relative to the performance and injury preventing qualities of the products has been initiated. One can find in the literature few studies relative to a comprehensive approach to all protective situations. Not enough new materials have been adopted and applied in the production of sports equipment. At present, major manufacturers have recognized the need for adaptation of new materials and the importance of employing a product design team. The immediate future will see an explosion of competition among manufacturers and a trend toward a more comprehensive approach to product design, durability, and safety.

Two of the very basic problems in the development of protective equipment fall into the categories of (1) deceleration of various forces and (2) standards whereby the product can be judged. It has long been a challenge to manufacturers to wrestle with the problems of decelerating rapidly forces characterized by a high mass and low velocity, as well as those of low mass and high velocity. In addition, there is still a lack of definitive standards by which the quality of protective products can be judged. Heretofore, a protective device has been evaluated or judged primarily on an individual or institutional basis. If the equipment performs to the satisfaction of the coaching staff and is economical, then it is judged and accepted on that basis. Ironically, the same brand and make of equipment, acceptable and judged adequate by some, is not necessarily acceptable to others.

The first attempt in the United States to develop national standards for sports protective equipment was made on December 9, 1960 when the Sports Car Club of America requested that the American Standards Association initiate a project to prepare specifications for road-user's helmets. A conference was held at ASA headquarters in April, 1961 which resulted in the establishment of Sectional Committee Z-90 with a charge to establish a safety code for vehicular head protection. The scope of the committee was to establish safety requirements for head protection for automobile drivers engaged in high hazard activities or occupations and for motorcyclists. The specifications for Protective Headgear for Vehicular Users were published in 1966 (American Standards Association, 1966).

In 1968, the Z-90 Committee agreed to take into consideration the development of standards for the football helmet. A separate committee was formed under the title of Z-90.2, comprising representatives of football helmet manufacturers, engineers, and other interested persons, and under the sponsorship of the United States of America Standards Institute, the new name of the American Standards Association. A set of standards were proposed, discussed, and revised for the last time in 1970 but not accepted. They were based in great part on the original Z-90.1 standards, but it was eventually conceded that the tests required were not consistent with the actual football situation.

A conference on football injuries was held by the American Society for Testing and Materials on November 18 and 19, 1968. This resulted in the establishment in June, 1969 of the F-8 Committee on Protective Equipment in Sports. This committee includes representatives of manufacturers, consumers, and other interested parties. The scope of the committee was stated to be, "Standardization of specifications, test methods and recommended practices for protective equipment for sports and related materials for the purpose of minimizing injury. Promotion of knowledge as it relates to protective equipment standards. Coordination of this work with other ASTM technical committees and other organizations in this area (Hale, 1969)." The F-8 Committee is organized into subcommittees on Statistics, Game Rules, Playing Surfaces, Body and

Extremities, and Head and Neck. Editorial and Definitions subcommittees will be established when they are needed.

In 1970, a National Operating Committee for Specifications and Standards for Athletic Equipment was organized cooperatively by the National Collegiate Athletic Association, the National Football Alliance, the Athletic Goods Manufacturers Association, the American Medical Association's Committee on the Medical Aspects of Sports, the National Athletic Trainers Association, and the Section on Sports Medicine of the American College Health Association. It has provided some research grants for studies in protective sports equipment.

II. GUIDELINES TO FOLLOW IN THE SELECTION OF ATHLETIC EQUIPMENT

A. Factors Affecting Choice

The types and quality of equipment available to the coach pose a major dilemma especially at the secondary school level. The choice is determined primarily by the following factors: (1) the size of the institution; (2) the budgetary structure; (3) the philosophy of administrative officials toward athletics; and (4) the knowledge of the buyer. Many institutions place a great deal of emphasis on providing the best possible quality protective equipment available, rather than to rely entirely on quantity purchasing because of limited funds.

The selection of protective equipment is a basic hurdle faced by all in sports. Experience, knowledge, and common sense will help to minimize the task. Every individual has definite personal guidelines in mind when selecting equipment. In many cases, selections are made wisely, but in some the experience is a traumatic one. Quality should never be sacrificed for quantity in the purchasing of equipment. It is far more desirable to purchase more equipment buying fewer items each year, than to buy in large quantities and expect the equipment to last for a long period of time. The fantastic looking deals are often misleading and should be avoided. The salesman often wants to unload equipment that is outdated and will soon be replaced by a newer, more protective item. Before purchasing a protective item in quantity, it is necessary to evaluate the ability of the product to perform for a period of time. Sample items are generally available from a salesman. A few pieces of equipment should be purchased initially when possible. If the product then performs up to expectations, a larger quantity can be purchased safely in the future.

B. Guidelines for Purchase

Most coaches admit to a certain degree of uncertainty when purchasing equipment, and must rely heavily on the advice of the salesman or manufacturer in making their selection. The following information should be considered before a purchase is made (Novich and Taylor, 1970): (1) design and material; (2) cost of maintenance and utility of the product; (3) safety factors; (4) quality and workmanship; (5) availability of the supplier and service; and (6) price.

1. Design and Material

The design of equipment and the material used in it influence each other considerably. Both should contribute to the serviceability of the product. The design should be practical, fitting the needs of the athlete. The flashy looking item certainly will have eye appeal, but, one should be skeptical of the frills and extras, as they serve little valuable purpose. The quality of the material is perhaps the most difficult to judge. Experience, consultation with manufacturing representatives, dealers or salesmen, and conversations with colleagues can provide the buyer with enough basic insight to judge and analyze various materials. The buyer's judgment, when also based on field testing, will assure an intelligent evaluation of the product. One should never be reluctant to try new products. Only after a trial period, however, should one consider, in most instances, a large quantity purchase.

2. Maintenance and Utility

Protective equipment must be practical to maintain and have a high utility ratio. It must be capable of being cleaned and repaired easily and economically, and of being reconditioned economically when this is needed. The cost of maintenance should always be considered in purchases of equipment if all other factors are equal, since the yearly expense may outweigh initial cost savings.

3. Safety Factors

One of the cardinal principles in the athletic code is that the athlete is entitled to the best possible protective equipment available. In buying equipment, the first consideration must be the safety factor. Through careful selection, with assistance from others, the buyer can be relatively certain of purchasing the equipment which embodies most closely the maximum protective requirements for the part or area to be protected. It must be capable of multiple reuse without appreciable loss of its protective factors.

4. Quality and Workmanship

Quality should never be sacrificed for quantity in athletic equipment. The buyer should look for consistent quality in a line regardless of the material used. Workmanship is an equally important feature. The purchasing of a single item initially, to compare with the workmanship and quality of present equipment, is good business.

5. Availability of Supplier and Service

Reputable equipment dealers will show and demonstrate products on request, and offer a large variety of items from which to choose. Service must be prompt and reliable, in order to insure complete satisfaction with the equipment. A buyer should seek out those dealers in an area who are reputable and dependable before making a decision as to the source of supply.

6. Price

Generally, the athletic equipment of finest quality is the most expensive. Quality must never be sacrificed for price. A careful analysis of the basic design, construction, and utility of a product generally provides a basis for evaluating its cost. Good equipment will cost slightly more. The dividends in the long run are well worth the initial investment.

III. FACTORS TO BE CONSIDERED IN THE ALLOCATION OF EQUIPMENT

There are several important factors to be considered in regard to the allocation of athletic equipment. The size of the institution, the number of teams, and the administrative philosophy will all influence the decision making process. The following axioms are applicable:

1. A hand-me-down routine of distribution should be discouraged.
2. Each athlete is entitled to and should be provided with the maximum amount of protection possible.
3. Regardless of other factors, proper fitting of equipment is of paramount importance.

4. The team physician, athletic trainer, equipment personnel, and coaching staff must work as a team to insure the best possible outcome.

5. Budgetary provisions for clearing, repairing, and reconditioning must be made on an annual basis.

6. The squad size, in relationship to available funds for quality equipment, must be considered.

IV. THE NEEDS FOR PROTECTIVE EQUIPMENT IN SPORTS

Each sport has its specific, and even unique, hazards and requirements. Protective equipment is designed according to the nature of the sport. We can divide the protective needs into three distinct categories, those for the collision, the noncollision, and the combat sports. There are distinctive physical qualities associated with the environment of each sport. Consequently, the type of equipment worn must be suitable to the environment. Naturally, athletes in the collision and combat sports require a greater degree of protection. The various anatomical areas must be considered in specific terms of their basic needs. Hazards of player interaction in sports are numerous. Interaction with an opponent or an opponent's equipment is a chief source of sports injury. Hazards, which are inherent in the nature of the playing environment, are obvious. The hockey player colliding with the boards poses a protective problem in this area. Protective demands reflect the combativeness of the sport and the hazards thereby imposed. The shape, weight, and body density of the player and the amount of impact expected are factors affecting protective demands in collision sports.

Injuries of characteristic type, frequency, and severity are seen in collision sport, noncollision sports, and endurance events. Some injuries are common to all sports, i.e., abrasions, contusions, strains, and sprains. The severity of any injury depends on many factors. Maximum protection is not guaranteed the athlete by equipment alone. His physical condition is of extreme importance in preventing injury. Coaching techniques offer a wide range of variables, which may influence the occurrence of injury. Questionable coaching techniques in some cases have unfortunately contributed to an increased number of injuries, especially in the collision sports. Proper wearing and careful fitting of equipment is essential in protection from injuries. The equipment must fit as tightly as possible without impairing movement or function. Ill-fitting equipment will reduce the athletes chances for maximum protection considerably.

In many cases, modification of existing equipment to prevent reinjury is essential. Special injury pads are available from the manufacturer for added protection of various anatomical areas and can easily be adapted to reinforce the injured area. Modifications by the coach, trainer, or team physician can be accomplished by using a selection of one of the nonresilient materials now available. Foam or sponge rubber can be utilized to pad a specific anatomical area.

The disregard for protective equipment in some sports even though the number and severity of injuries has increased presents a specific problem. This is traditional in some sports, where a considerable chance of injury is involved, because of the speed of the game, the physical contact between players, the number of players involved, the implements used in the game, or the surface on which the game is played. Rugby, soccer, and hurling are examples of such sports. In ice hockey, where protection is vital, we still have professionals who refuse to wear a protective helmet or goalie mask, because of a desire to exhibit their manliness or pressure from their peers. This attitude remains even though the ice hockey player knows that serious or fatal head injury can be the result.

A. Protective Equipment in the Collision Sports

The term "contact sport" is no longer a descriptive term. In our modern sports era, the strength, size, speed, and agility of the participants and the installation of artificial playing surfaces has produced an increased violence in athletics. A collision sport today may be described as one which involves an interaction of players with players, a player with the environmental hazards, or a player with a projectile.

1. Football

To the layman, the risk of injury from participation in football is great. Because of the nature of the sport, many injuries do occur. Permanent disabilities and fatalities in football are minimal, however, in relationship to the number of participants each year. The competitive nature of football and the benefits that can be derived from it certainly far outweigh the risk of serious injury.

a. HELMET. The present football helmet is the product of 75 years of evolution. From a soft glove shell padded lightly with felt it has become a hard plastic shell capable of resisting very high impacts and lined with a suspension system containing highly shock-absorbent synthetic materials. At every stage of development it has had its detractors, who eventually lived to defend the existing model against subsequent innovations. Today it faces a paradoxical double indictment: that it offers insufficient protection against the forces generated in the modern game; and that it is a hazard to the safety of the players, against whom it may be used accidentally or deliberately as an offensive or defensive weapon.

It is interesting that the wearing of a helmet did not become mandatory until 1939, 65 years after the first game between Yale and Harvard, although it had been introduced in 1896, and had assumed roughly its present form in 1925. Unfortunately statistics to tell us what were the rates of occurrence of concussions and other head injuries were not collected during the period when no or very few players wore helmets. Interviews with players and coaches of the early days, however, indicate that head injuries were not considered to be much of a problem and fatalities were extremely rare from this cause. Players wore their hair long until about the time of World War I.

The qualities sought by manufacturers in the modern helmet have been decided upon by laboratory experimentation, field testing, and conceptual reasoning. One source of dissatisfaction to all concerned is that the laboratory test mechanism, typically the dropping of a weight on a helmet held on a metal head form, does not nearly approximate the actual conditions in which the helmet is worn. Developments based exclusively on such test results are considered somewhat suspect by those who are working to improve the helmet today. On the other hand, the findings of field testing have been largely anecdotal, and testimonials have been influenced by factors such as styling and comfort as much as by safety records. Conceptual reasoning has been hampered by the lack of information regarding human tolerances.

At the present writing there are helmets in which the shell is merely padded, in which the padding is worked into a sort of suspension system (Fig. 1 and 2), in which there is a strap suspension system and minimal padding or a great deal of padding (Fig. 3 and 4), and in which the strap suspension is supplemented by an interconnecting system of air and fluid cells whose function is to distribute shock more evenly over the head. High impact plastic is the most popular material for shell construction but fiberglass has been used in a helmet closely resembling those used for racing. Padding on the outside of the shell has been discarded after some years of experimentation.

The main principles involved in helmet construction have been to prevent insofar as possible "bottoming" of the shell on the head, and distributing forces transmitted through the helmet as widely as possible

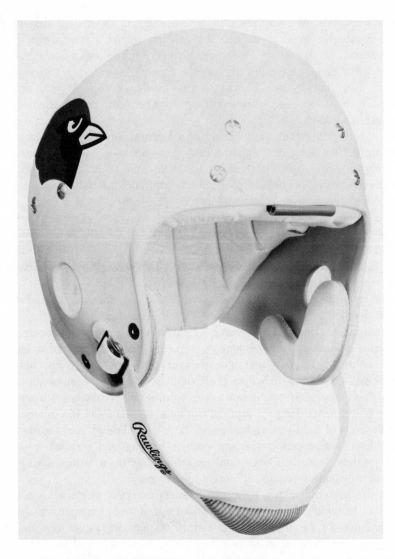

Fig. 1 Football helmet with padding and padded suspension system, three-quarter front view. Courtesy Rawlings Co.

around the head. The most vulnerable area of the skull lies in a band running across the forehead, back over the temples and around the occiput posteriorly. Other considerations have been to extend protection down over the occiput, but at the same time to avoid having a sharp edge of the helmet cut across the neck when the head is fully extended, and to keep the helmet in place so that it would not rotate

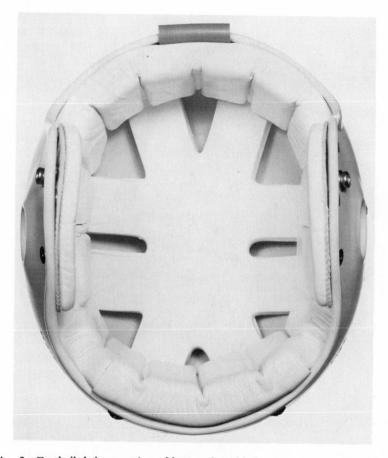

Fig. 2 Football helmet with padding and padded ·suspension system, interior view. Courtesy Rawlings Co.

on the head when struck, either circumferentially or in a sagittal plane.

The chief purpose of the chin strap is to hold the helmet on the head. If it is properly adjusted it should also resist circumferential rotation. A strap attached to the helmet at four points rather than two is more secure, and may help to prevent rotation in the sagittal plane if the second point of attachment is low on the helmet behind the ear.

Proper fitting of the helmet to each player is important to make sure that it stays in place and is not excessively uncomfortable. Since shell sizes are limited, and head shapes as well as sizes manifest a great variety, fitting of the conventional helmet involves adjusting the suspension system and adding pads or shims of appropriate sizes. Padding that is designed to protect should not be subtracted in order to help

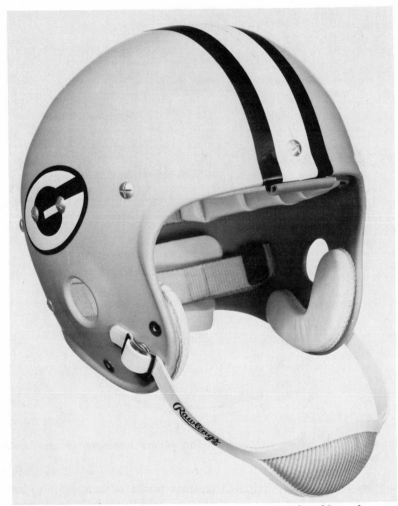

Fig. 3   Football helmet with strap suspension system and padding, three-quarter front view. Courtesy Rawlings Co.

fit a helmet. Air helmets can be adjusted while on the player's head by inflating the air sacs through tiny holes in the helmets outer surface. Helmets should be rechecked for their fit periodically during the season and readjusted as necessary.

  b. FACE MASK AND DENTAL GUARD. Although these are two separate and distinct pieces of equipment they may be considered together because of the obvious effect of the face bar or mask in reducing dental

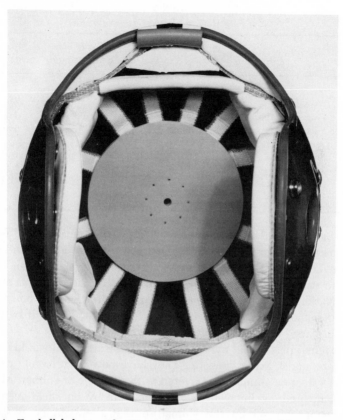

Fig. 4 Football helmet with strap suspension system and padding, interior view.
Courtesy Rawlings Co.

as well as facial injuries. The classic and often-quoted study that demonstrates the effect of these two pieces of equipment in reducing the numbers and severity of dental injuries was reported by Wisconsin Interscholastic Athletic Association (1967). The results of the introduction of this equipment, as can be seen in Table I, was gratifying not only to the players and their parents, but to the administrators of the Association since it kept their insurance plan against injuries from financial disaster. A similar experience was encountered in New York State where from 1960, the last year in which wearing a mouthguard was not mandatory, to 1968 there was a 69% decrease in claims for dental injuries and a 54% decrease in cost to an average of only $29.47 per claim. In the latter year, 69% of the claims were for dental injuries in physical education and intramural sports, and only 7.5% for football.

TABLE I
Effect of Face Mask and Dental Guards on Injuries

Year	Protection	Players	Facial and dental injuries	Incidence/100
1954	No face masks or dental guards	15,714	356	2.26
1955	Face masks introduced	15,714	288	1.83
1959	Face masks mandatory; few dental guards	22,969	275	1.20
1963	Face masks and dental guards mandatory	30,357	143	0.47
1966	Face masks and dental guards mandatory	34,298	115	0.33

Paul Brown, at that time coach of the Cleveland Browns football team, was the first to put a curved plastic bar across the face and attach it to the helmet. He did it because he had a player with an injured nose. The style caught on quickly and in 1955 the face bar was adopted by the National Football League as official protective equipment. Colleges and schools picked it up quickly and began modifying it by adding additional bars, eventually making its use mandatory.

The original plastic and nylon bars were too fragile and would collapse on the face under heavy pressure. They have now been largely replaced by metal (steel or aluminum) covered with a plastic or rubber. Multiple bars are favored by linemen and double bars by backfield men (Fig. 5). Some are hinged on the helmet so that they can be raised like the visor of a knight's armor helmet. Crossbars were inserted for extra strength but also to prevent elbows and fists from getting between the bars themselves or the upper bar and the brow of the helmet.

An article from the University of Michigan in 1961 (Schneider *et al.*, 1961) blamed the faceguard for fatal and nonfatal spinal cord injuries. Although the number of cases cited was extremely small, and all of them were not fully documented, the article created a sensation. The thesis was that when the face mask was grabbed and pushed up, accidentally or deliberately, pressure was exerted on the neck and spinal cord by the rear edge of the helmet. Most manufacturers cut down the back of the helmet and some added a shock-absorbent pad at the lower edge. Face guards were moved in closer to the face to reduce leverage. A penalty of 15 yards for grasping the mask was introduced at all levels of play. The furor subsided and the guard has remained.

It has been demonstrated by Schneider and Antine (1965) and others that the face guard tends to reduce the visual field somewhat at and

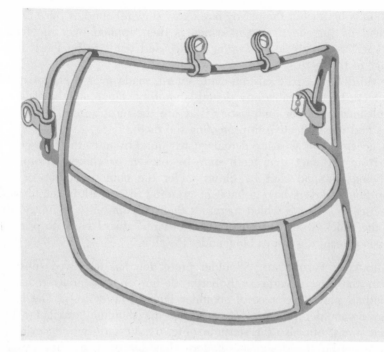

Fig. 5 Football face guard for backfield player without central vertical cross-bar to allow better visibility. Four points of fixed attachment to the helmet. Courtesy of Rawlings Co.

below the level of the knees. This can be hazardous to the player who cannot see clearly the blocker or tackler who is coming in low. The torsion exerted on the face guard also has a tendency to crack the helmet at the points where it is attached.

Dental guards for use in the mouth are of three general types. The first, and most commonly used is already roughly formed in plastic to fit over the upper or lower teeth. When heated in boiling water the plastic softens and can then be molded by the player to the shape of his teeth before plunging it into cold water to harden it again. These provide reasonable protection but do not stay in place well and are so thin that they are bitten through easily.

The second type is formed in the mouth. One brand has a firm outer rubber shell and a soft material inside which softens on boiling and can be fitted in the same way as the stock type. These tend to be thick, to interfere with speech, and do not stay in place well. A second brand has a plastic outer shell and an inner shell formed by mixing a powder and liquid, which is then molded to the shape of the teeth.

Retention is better but the plastic has a very slow rebound. A third brand is formed of silicone in a tray which is then applied over the teeth. This type has too thick a chewing surface and tends to be short in its coverage of the teeth.

The third type is the custom-made guard, made over a plaster mold of the teeth by the dentist or a dental laboratory. These may be of latex, soft vulcanized rubber, or plastic. They are the most acceptable to the players and most effective in protecting the teeth.

The necessity for wearing dental guards in addition to the face guard arises from the fact that teeth may be broken or chipped from the jaws being snapped shut by blows under the chin or on top of the helmet. Some players have a habit of grinding their teeth in the tension of practice or a game which increases their susceptibility to injury. Finally, the shock absorbent quality of the dental guard helps to prevent concussions resulting from a blow under the chin.

c. SHOULDER PROTECTION. Shoulder protection has improved substantially in the past decade, with better design and materials reducing the football player's chance of shoulder injury considerably. The large cantilever shoulder pad protects not only the shoulder, clavicular and scapular areas, but also the sternum (Fig. 6). Versatility and flexibility are apparent in the design of modern shoulder pads, as they can be individually fitted and come in an assortment of models and sizes to suit the individual position. Optional snap-in accessories can be added

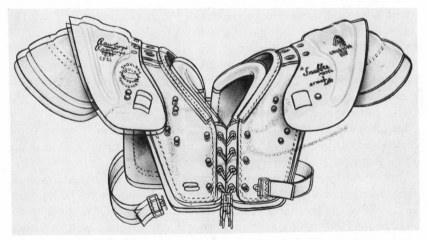

Fig. 6 Football shoulder pad of intermediate size with double cantilever construction. Courtesy Rawlings Co.

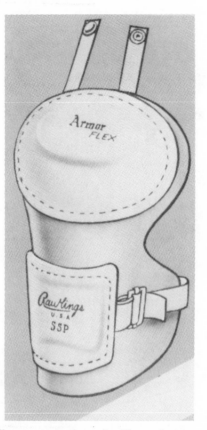

Fig. 7   Football snap-on auxiliary shoulder pad. Courtesy Rawlings Co.

for greater protection of the acromioclavicular joint (Fig. 7) the biceps, and the sternum.

   d. HIP PROTECTION. The snap-in-style type of hip pad is popular with today's athletes with the girdle style (Fig. 8) sharing some if its popularity. The snap-in type offers excellent protection to the ilium and coccyx, provided the pads remain in place, are fitted properly, and are faithfully worn. Some manufacturers have made modifications to basic hip pad design for specific institutions on request for hip protection which they feel better meets their needs. Most hip protection in football is adequate if pads are worn properly and kept in good repair.

   e. FOOTBALL ACCESSORY PADS. The playing position and the size of the individual are important to the protection of the participant with accessory pads. Some football positions require less bulky equipment,

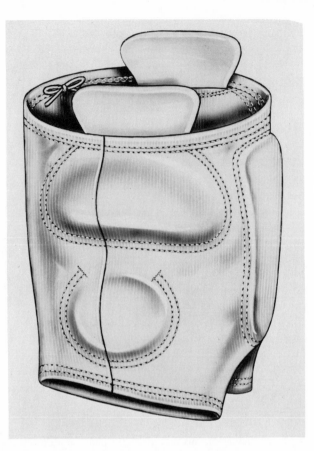

Fig. 8   Football hip and sacral pads built into a girdle. Courtesy Rawlings Co.

while participants who play in the combat zone from tackle to tackle, must have larger more bulky items of equipment. Rib pads (Fig. 9) are not worn uniformly today because of the nature of the modern game and the extra protection now provided by the shoulder and hip pads. Thigh pads, knee pads, forearm pads, hand pads, and elbow pads are important protective items in offering total protection. Thigh pads and knee pads especially must remain in place to be effective.

f. JERSEY. A football jersey is designed not only for eye appeal, but it must perform the protective task for which it was intended, to keep the shoulder pads from excessive movement. A loose fitting or torn jersey will only lead to shoulder injury. If the athlete does not need help in getting his jersey over his shoulder pads, then it is likely it does

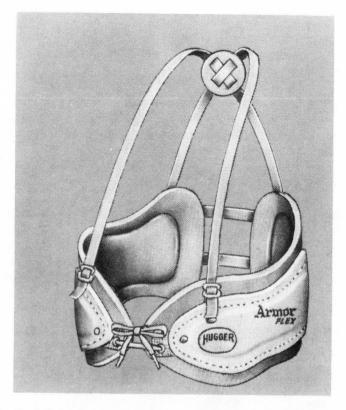

Fig. 9 Football blocking vest supported by shoulder straps. Courtesy Rawlings Co.

not fit properly. The majority of football jerseys are made of nylon, cotton, or a combination of materials, and are preferably light in weight. Fishnet or porous jerseys allow cooling of the wearer, which is essential during hot, humid weather in preventing heat stress.

g. FOOTBALL PANTS. The football pants must fit as snugly as possible to hold the thigh, knee, and hip pads in place. Stretch materials allow for a perfect fit and freedom of movement.

h. FOOTBALL SHOES. The high-top shoe was standard for many years in football because most men wore shoes of this style when football began, but also because it was felt that the high-laced shoe helped to protect the ankle from injury. Professional players introduced the low shoe after World War II because the backs and ends were looking for lighter weight to allow them greater speed. College and high school

players soon began to demand and wear the low-cut shoes and they
have now become standard. High-topped shoes are still worn by a few
of the older players and by some interior linemen who feel more secure
in them.

The New York State High School Study by Hafner *et al.* (1968)
showed that the occurrence of ankle injuries was no greater in low-cut
than in high-top shoes, providing the ankles were wrapped or taped.
This is in agreement with the experience of the great majority of football
coaches and trainers.

The modern shoe is very light in weight and is made typically of
kangaroo leather. A series of slits around the top of the shoe in some
models allows the introduction of a nylon strip which is tied into the
laces at the front of the shoe to hold the shoe tightly on the foot
(Fig. 10). It contains five detachable cleats of a conical shape on the
fore part of the sole and two on the heel. The number, location, length,
and shape of the cleats have all been adjudged at one time or another
as factors in the occurrence of ankle and knee injuries in football.

Early football shoes had strips of leather tacked across the soles and
heels to aid in securing a footing on the grass. These gradually evolved
into oblong and then into conical cleats. In recent years they have been
3/4 inch long, but some cleats for use on wet or muddy fields have

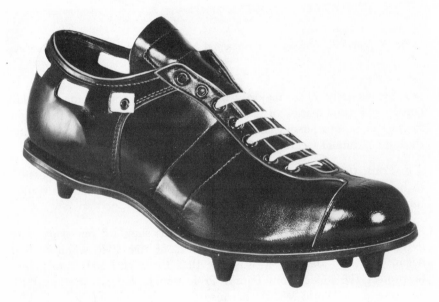

Fig. 10 Football shoe with conventional cleat system. Courtesy Rawlings Co.

been as long as one inch. In 1955, Dr. Daniel Hanley (1969) became concerned about the number of kneee injuries on the Bowdoin College football team. He began to study the factors relating to their occurrence with the athletic trainer and reviewed many films of games in which he attempted to visualize the mechanisms involved in the production of these injuries. He found that guards and tackles on defense suffered the greatest number of knee injuries. Thirty-three percent of all knee injuries occured in the act of being blocked, 23% in pile-ups, 23% in the open field without any apparent contact, 11% while tackling, and 10% while carrying the ball.

From his observations, Dr. Hanley decided that four factors were involved ordinarily in producing a knee injury: the foot was planted with the body weight placed on it; the long cleats were digging into the ground and fixing the foot; the knee was being flexed as it moved forward; and a torsion was applied to the knee by a fast twist or a blow. He also noticed that the rear cleats on the shoe were not used ordinarily in blocking and tackling. The one factor which it appeared could be influenced was the length of the cleats. He decided to remove the cleats from the heel of the shoe, replacing them with a flat $\frac{3}{8}$ inch rubber heel. He also replaced the long conical cleats with $\frac{1}{2}$ inch flatter soccer-type cleats. By 1966 these shoes were being used for all games as well as practices. During this period of development he had elicited the interest and cooperation of 75 professional, college, and high school teams. When he surveyed their results for the 1965 season by questionnaire he found that knee and ankle injuries had occurred in only 6% of those wearing rubber heels and short cleats against 14% for those wearing the regular cleated shoe.

Dr. Joseph Torg (1971) studied the occurrence of knee injuries in 18 public high school teams in Philadelphia over three seasons and of 16 Catholic high school teams over two seasons of play. Comparisons of their experience with players wearing regular cleated shoes with $\frac{3}{4}$ inch cleats one year and soccer-type shoes with a molded sole of 14 to 15 $\frac{3}{8}$ inch cleats the next showed that knee injuries were reduced by more than 50%, and injuries severe enough to require surgery by 85%.

The advent of artificial turf has created new problems as far as the shoe is concerned. When dry, all the artificial turfs appear to provide greater traction than grass. Long cleats cannot be used, and the $\frac{3}{8}$ inch plastic cleat in arrangements of 14 or 15 seems to provide the best footing. Although the cleats cannot become fixed in the surface, the greater gripping area provides so much holding power that many more toe sprains are being seen. The first shoes provided for this turf had a rather thin sole, which contributed to the big toe problem and also took up too much heat from the turf when it was exposed to the hot sun of late summer and early fall. These problems are being corrected, but we do not as of this writing have enough information to say whether ankle and knee injuries are more or less on artificial turf than on grass.

2. Ice Hockey

In the game of ice hockey, a variety of forces are involved. The interaction of the players, the players with the opponent's equipment, and the players with the environment each present distinctive protective problems. It is evident that a great deal of force through body contact is generated in ice hockey. Unfortunately, hockey protective equipment is still in its infant stage. The low mass of the puck, which can be propelled at speeds of over one hundred miles per hour, compounds the risk of injury. The hazards imposed by use of the stick and the sharp skates are obvious. The ridigity of the present elbow pad is a problem, as the player is tempted to use his elbows in retaliation to an opponent's challenge.

a. HELMET. The hockey helmet should be made mandatory for all players. When one considers the speed and impact capabilities of the puck and the chance of receiving a blow from a misdirected stick or a high speed collision with the boards, the helmet becomes exceptionally important. Most hockey helmets offer some protective qualities but are still inadequate at present. The basic problem is one of protecting the temporal areas and the base of the skull, while still allowing for adequate ventilation and minimal impairment of peripheral vision. Recently, manufacturers have developed more acceptable helmet designs (Fig. 11), but we still must overcome the traditional reluctance of the professional players to wear them.

b. SHOULDER PADS. A variety of models of shoulder pads are available to the hockey players; most are inadequate. The majority do not give enough protection to the acromioclavicular joint; consequently, we see numerous sprains or contusion injuries to this area. In the future, a lightweight, yet energy absorbent material similar to the football pad, must be developed to replace the classic felt and foam rubber combination being used at present.

c. ACCESSORY PADS AND GLOVES. The hip, thigh, elbow, shin, and knee protectors are made of a combination of felt, foam rubber, and plastic; all, with the exception of the elbow pad, seem adequate. The elbow pad is too rigid and eventually must be made of a softer material (Fig.

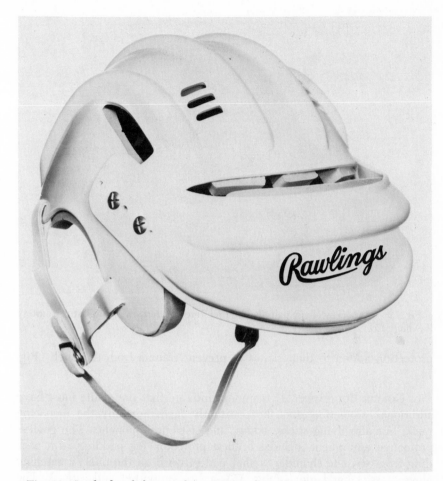

Fig. 11 Ice hockey helmet with two-piece adjustable shell and Ensolite padding. Courtesy Rawlings Co.

12). The hockey gloves are made of leather with protective reinforcement over the knuckles, wrist, and padded except on the palm of the hand (Fig. 13).

d. SKATES. The skates of the hockey player are a hazard, as well as a liability. The rear tips of the skates are covered with a plastic or rubber tip, preventing the sharp points from becoming a major hazard. The toe of the skate is reinforced to make it firm. The Achilles tendon is protected by a reinforced leather strip which extends up 3 inches from the back of the shoe. The goalies and defensemen have additional

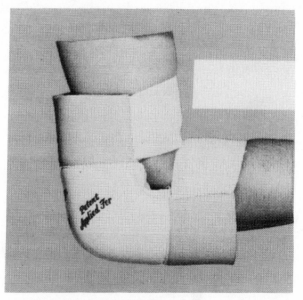

Fig. 12   Ice hockey elbow pad. Padding reinforced externally with plastic. Courtesy Rawlings Co.

protection added to their skates to prevent trauma from the puck (Fig. 14).

   e. GOALIE EQUIPMENT. It is understandable that the goalie must have additional protection since he constantly faces not only the menacing puck, but also flying sticks, skates, and snarling opponents. The goalie's protective equipment includes a chest protector, leg padding, arm padding from wrist to shoulder, a shot pad to ward off the puck, a catching glove, a stick-hand glove (Fig. 15), a cup supporter, and a mask. The goalie mask is mandatory in all organized leagues, except in the National Hockey League. Some professional goalies are reluctant to wear a mask because of tradition and a complaint of impairment of vision, especially when the puck is close to their feet. The mask must protect the vital skull areas, especially the frontal, temporal, and occipital areas and give as wide a field of vision as possible. Most masks are individually molded from the face with plaster which then becomes the base for the fiberglass product, but new plastics and other materials are being used experimentally. For a goalie not to wear a protective mask is comparable to a soldier going into combat without a weapon.

   f. MOUTH PROTECTION. Mouth protection in ice hockey is not mandatory except in high school and the Western Collegiate Hockey Association, but should be. The classic hockey player's grin, exhibiting a toothless smile, has been traditionally accepted but, hopefully, will be eliminated with the wearing of a mouth protector. Mouth protection not only protects the dentures, but equally absorbs a blow received to the chin or mouth before it is transmitted to the skull. The external

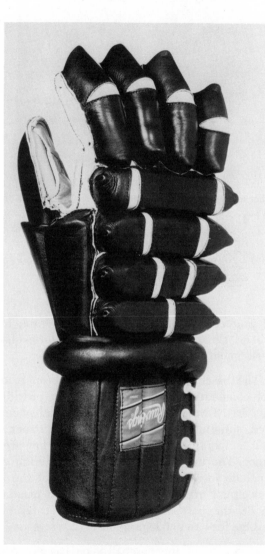

Fig. 13 Ice hockey glove with leather palm, reinforced back hand rolls, three-piece curved thumb (fiber reinforced) and double-stitched thumb and first finger. Courtesy Rawlings Co.

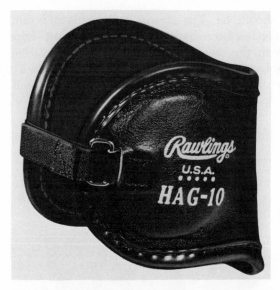

Fig. 14   Ice hockey ankle guard. Plastic reinforced leather with foam padding and stretch nylon band. Courtesy Rawlings Co.

protector is essential for the younger players, to whom it is difficult to fit a satisfactory guard over the teeth.

3. Baseball

Adoption of protective devices and equipment through the years in baseball has been slow. Historically, serious injuries have preceded mandatory development and use of protective equipment.

a. HELMET. The baseball batting helmet has been made mandatory on all levels of competition, yet is still lacking in providing maximum protection (Fig. 16). In recent years, some baseball players have been seriously injured, suffering permanent injury when struck with the ball in the facial or temporal areas, despite the fact they were wearing a protective helmet. The use of more absorbent materials and a change in design to include more protection for the top of the head and the temporal and occipital areas seem inevitable. The mandatory wearing of the helmet on the basepaths should receive careful consideration by those responsible for baseball legislation.

b. SHOES. The design of the baseball shoe has not been altered in years. The steel cleats represent a hazard to the opponent as well as the wearer (Fig. 17). Lacerations in baseball are too frequent as a result of a player being spiked during the sliding sequence. In the future, the present steel cleat may give way to a more resilient nonpenetrating material. The use of multiple track spikes has not met with favor. Foot traction in baseball is essential, but a reduction in stress from foot fixation is a necessity.

  c. CATCHING EQUIPMENT. The position most vulnerable to injury in baseball is that of the catcher, followed closely by that of the pitcher. The modern catcher's face mask with its magnesium bars has performed its function well (Fig. 18). Consideration for increased protection to the catcher and the plate umpire is in the experimental stage (Fig. 19). The chest protector, shinguards, and cup supporter have proven highly protective to the catcher. Protecting the nongloved hand is a

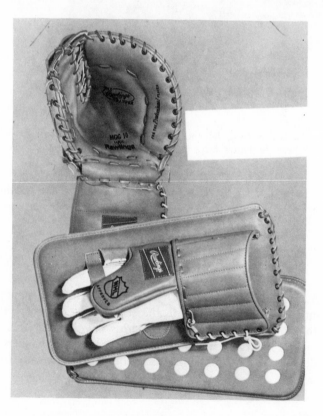

Fig. 15 Ice hockey goalie gloves. The mitt for the catching hand resembles a baseball glove but has a closed back. The glove for the stick hand has a protector pad and a removable glove. Courtesy Rawlings Co.

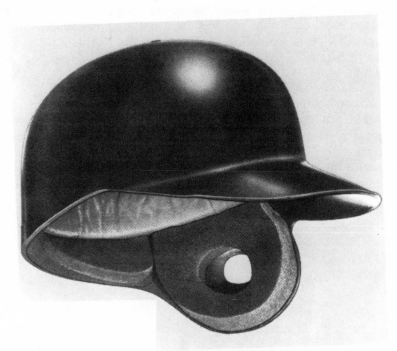

Fig. 16 Baseball batting helmet. One-piece molded plastic with ear protector on the side where the batter faces the pitcher, padded with plastic foam. Courtesy Rawlings Co.

dilemma, and is a basic problem of concentration and chance rather than equipment.

4. Rugby

Rugby players use little, if any, protective equipment. Valid injury statistics are nonexistent, yet injuries do occur, and some are quite serious. As rugby gains in popularity in the United States, new protective equipment may evolve. Players in the scrum wear a light leather head harness to protect the ears. Some forwards have a light felt pad sewn into the jersey over the point of the shoulder. The hooker may, but usually does not, wear shin guards. Shoes are similar to those worn for soccer.

5. Lacrosse

Significant injury data on lacrosse injuries has not been collected in spite of the increasing popularity of the game. As with all other collision sports, the opportunity for injury does exist in lacrosse. The lacrosse helmet is made of a light plastic with a suspension and has a mask of thin metal bars to ward off the stick. Elbow pads and padded gloves are used. The goalie wears pads which cover his chest, thighs, and legs. A lightweight cleated shoe is used.

6. Basketball

In the past, basketball has not been considered a collision sport but modern experience would indicate otherwise. As the game of basketball has become increasingly physical, the chances of injury have been comparably increased. Injuries resulting from flying elbows, general body impact with the opponent, and rebounding agressiveness are evident. The basketball shoe market is highly competitive with new materials and designs capturing the buyer's attention. The controversy still exists regarding the protective qualities of the oxford model and the high-top model. The oxford model is by far the most popular because of its

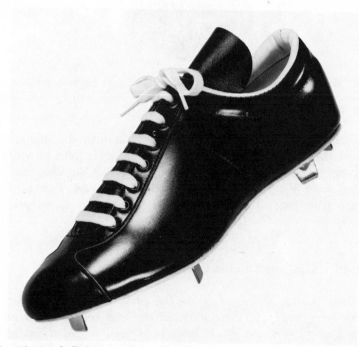

Fig. 17 Baseball shoe. Leather with molded nylon outsole and padded soft collar. Pro split spikes. Courtesy Rawlings Co.

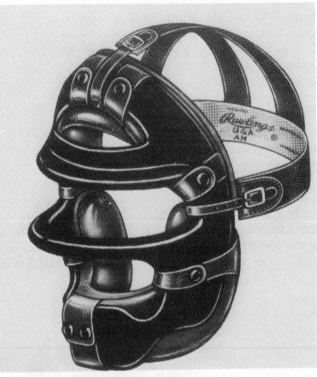

Fig. 18   Baseball catcher's mask. Vinyl coated lightweight magnesium frame, snap-on padding, black vinyl covering and Polypropylene Cradle web harness. Courtesy Rawlings Co.

eye appeal, yet only weighs a few ounces less than the higher shoe. Many feel that the additional canvas over the ankle joint provided by the high-top model gives it more protective qualities. Padding has been eliminated from the shorts in most modern uniforms. Fewer players wear knee pads today than 20 years ago, unless they have had some knee injury.

B. Protective Equipment in the Combat Sports

Wrestling, boxing, and fencing are the combat sports of western society. We have added to these judo, karate, and kendo. Although the techniques of all of these sports have been used in individual serious combat and in warfare to maim and even to kill the adversary, the objectives when they are practiced as sports is to score points or to temporarily disable the opponent without injuring him. Specialized protective equipment has been developed, partly by tradition and custom, and partly in response to demand.

1. Wrestling

Wrestling costume has consisted traditionally of a pull-over sleeveless jersey with a low neckline, athletic supporter, jersey tights, and shoes. Many young wrestlers today prefer to wear shorts rather than tights. The introduction of the smooth-surfaced plastic foam mats with a reduction in abrasions, or "mat burns," has made this feasible. The greater ability of these mats to absorb shock has also made elbow and knee pads less necessary except to protect the wrestler if he goes off the mat. There is no practical method of protection against the torsional injuries to the fingers, wrist, elbows, shoulder, neck, rib cartilage, knees, and ankles which occur so commonly.

a. HEADGEAR. This is now mandatory for high school and college wrestlers. Its sole purpose is to protect the ear from injury which causes a hematoma between the skin and the cartilage of the pinna. The chief problem is not to cushion the ear but to keep the headgear in place during the action, a good deal of which centers around the head. The number of different designs available is the best indication that this

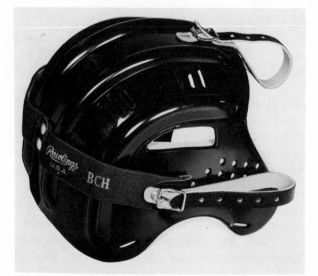

Fig. 19 Baseball catcher's helmet. Cy-co-lite plastic with Ensolite padding. Courtesy Rawlings Co.

problem has not been satisfactorily solved by any of them. It should be comfortable as well as stable and should not be so extensive as to prevent normal radiation of heat. Its surface should be minimally abrasive to an opponent.

b. KNEE AND ELBOW PADS. These pads are made to slip over the extremity and are held in place by their elasticity. There is no way to keep them from being displaced occasionally in the course of a match, however. The pad is usually a closed-cell plastic foam today.

c. SHOE. Most wrestlers wear the high shoe since it stays on the foot better and provides some external support as well as resistance to abrasion for the ankle. It is usually made of canvas and/or leather and has a sole made to give good gripping power.

2. Boxing

The boxing costume consists in a headgear (except in professional fights), trunks, supporter with protective cup, and high-topped shoes. Over this on his way to and from the ring the fighter wears a bathrobe tied with a sash to prevent chilling. While sparring or boxing he wears a mouthpiece. On his hands he wears gloves which vary in size and weight, chiefly according to the amount of padding, from 8 to 16 ounces. Beneath the gloves his hands and wrists are wrapped with gauze and some adhesive tape.

a. HEADGEAR. The purpose of the headgear is to prevent lacerations, especially around the eyebrows, and contusions of the ear cartilage. Consequently, it is constructed with an open crown, crossed by four straps, heavy padding all around the ears (but in some models exposing the ear itself within a built-up circle of padding), extending over the temples and the forehead and barely exposing the eyebrows (Fig. 20). In some models the padding is extended down along the chin, and, in one, entirely across the chin to make a complete frame for the face. The covering is leather and the padding may be plastic foam, latex foam, or a combination of either of these with hair.

b. MOUTHPIECE. The usual mouthpiece is double, so that it protects both upper and lower teeth in a hinged fashion, decreasing the diameter of the breathing area considerably. Fighters may, however, wear single mouth pieces which are custom-fitted to both upper and lower rows of teeth. The materials used are either plastic or latex rubber.

c. HAND BANDAGING. Limits are placed by law in each state where boxing is legal on the length of hand bandaging which may be used

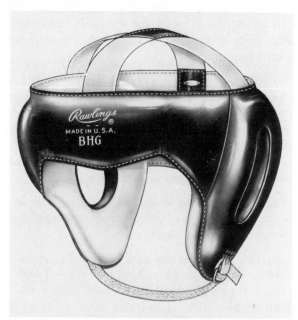

Fig. 20 Boxing headgear. Padded and leather covered with adjustable straps. Courtesy Rawlings Co.

and the amount of adhesive tape which may be attached to hold it in place. There is little or no uniformity in these laws and little regard appears to be paid in practice to how much is actually used. Crinoline gauze is usually employed and a typical allowable length is five yards. The combination of tape and gauze adds considerable rigidity to the fist under the gloves so that it tends to become a club.

d. Gloves. The surface is leather and the padding plastic or latex foam with or without some admixture of hair. The term glove is a misnomer since it is actually a mitten, with the thumb rather widely separated from the other fingers and especially reinforced. The heavier gloves (12–16 ounces) are used for training and sparring, and the lighter ones (8–10 ounces) for fighting. Gloves are available in laced or slip-on style with elastic wrists. The laced models hold some danger to the opponent if the laced portion, which extends over the palm, is drawn accidentally or deliberately across his face.

The ostensible purpose of the gloves is to protect the hands, just as the bandaging of the hands is designed to hold the metacarpals together for strength. The result, however, especially when the gloves have become wet from the sweat of the fighters or the water thrown on them by the seconds, is to convert the hands into lethal weapons with which to attack the head of the opponent. Thus given courage, the boxer bangs away at the unprotected (professional) head and sometimes breaks his hand anyway.

e. SUPPORTER. A conventional supporter, but often with a somewhat wider waist band, is worn with a plastic or aluminum padded cup. The padded cup was first introduced by "Foul-proof" Taylor and was largely responsible for the rule that eliminated the possibility of a fighter claiming a fight on the grounds that he was hit a blow "below the belt." The referee may warn a fighter for consistently hitting low, however, and take points away from him in professional fights.

f. SHOES. The high-top shoe is made of leather and laces down to the toes. The soles are made of some nonskid material to give a firm footing but one that will release easily.

g. THE RING. The ring posts are padded and the "ropes" (which are now really cables) should also be padded and covered with a soft material. The floor of the ring should be covered with a shock-absorbent pad overlaid with either canvas or a plastic.

3. Fencing

Fencing costume consists in a long-sleeved jersey, cup supporter, and trunks under a padded jacket, trousers which come just below the knee, long stockings, and shoes. The fencer wears a glove on his sword hand and a mask.

a. MASK. The mask is composed primarily of a heavy steel mesh, with interstices small enough to prevent penetration of the tip of the sword, and a band that passes over the top of the head to the occiput to hold the mask in place. It is padded on the inside at the points of contact with the head. A protective apron extends down from the front of the mask to cover the upper part of the neck. The top and back of the head are exposed except for the band already described.

b. GLOVE. This is usually a gauntlet, padded on the back and over the thumb to protect against blows from the sword. The sword itself has a guard which varies in size and shape between the three weapons of foil, epee, and saber. The gauntlet is made long enough to overlap the sleeve of the sword hand.

c. JACKET. The jacket is padded on the front and in the sword arm. Padding is heavier for the saber fencer since he has to ward off or accept the slashing blows used with this weapon. The jacket is long, extending down to the crotch, and close-fitting. It is made of either heavy cotton or a synthetic combined with cotton. The sleeves extend to the wrist.

d. TROUSERS. The trousers are made of the same materials as the jackets and extend down just over the knee where they are fastened closely to the leg, usually by an elastic material. They are not padded.

4. Judo, Karate, and Aikiddo

The costume for these three related sports is essentially the same. There is a long loose-fitting white cotton trousers and a jacket of the same material with three-quarter sleeves and wide lapels. The jacket is held closed by a belt, the color of which indicates the wearer's rank in proficiency. Shoes are not worn. No protective equipment other than the clothing is worn, but because of its length and character it does serve to protect the wearer against floor or mat burns.

Judo and aikiddo especially are practiced on mats. In Japan, the tatami mat is used. It is composed essentially of bundles of tightly bound straw fitted closely together to form a firm but resilient surface. Outside of Japan ordinary wrestling mats of shock absorbent material are used.

5. Kendo

This is a combat sport in which wooden sticks five feet long are wielded in the manner of the ancient Japanese long sword to score points by striking prescribed areas of the opponent, namely on the head and across the ribs. The costume is a pair of loose fitting cotton trousers and a long jacket with half sleeves that are lightly padded.

a. HELMET. The modern helmet covers the head on all sides and surrounds a mask which allows the same visibility as that used for fencing. The materials and construction of the helmet, which is padded, are designed to resist sharp blows of the stick without allowing a concussion.

b. RIB PROTECTOR. A broad, padded protector of heavily lacquered fiber fastens around the lower ribs to take the blows of the stick which are directed there.

C. Protective Equipment in Other Sports

In other sports the needs for protective equipment are much less, with very few exceptions. Rather than to treat them sport by sport it is more convenient and significant to group them according to the areas of the body which require protection, comparing and contrasting the requirements for each particular activity. These groups include head-gear, overall clothing, gloves, and special cushioning devices.

1. Headgear

a. The equestrian sports were late in adopting headgear although they are among the oldest of all.

i. Polo was the first, with its modified topee, to protect the head of the rider. The player had not only to be protected in the event of a fall, and from the added possibility of a horse stepping on his head, but from the possible blows by the wooden mallet and ball used in the game. As racing helmets have been improved, some of their features have been adopted in the design and material of the polo helmet.

ii. Flat racers and steeplechasers wore a cap but did not have a protec-tive helmet until the introduction of the fibreglas cap for harness racing drivers and the so-called Caliente palstic helmet for jockeys in 1956. These are now mandatory throughout the United States and have saved many lives and prevented serious disabling injuries.

iii. Jumping horses in amateur competition over a closed or cross-coun-try course produces falls off and on the horse. Many of the riders wear protective helmets, although they are not mandatory. The classic derby hat of the hunter and show rider had a relatively hard, high crown which served to cushion the shock of falls to some degree.

b. MOTOR SPORTS. It is quite obvious that racing an airplane, car, or boat requires some type of headgear for protection in crashes, whether or not the driver is ejected from the vehicle. Standards for such headgear have been developed by the United States Air Force and by the USA Standards Institute through contracts with universities, such as Cornell, and private organizations, such a the Snell Foundation. The Z-90.1 stan-dard is now well recognized for vehicular users. The principle employed in constructing these helmets is to use a replaceable liner capable of absorbing very high impacts one time but with no or very poor rebound capabilities.

Because of the need to keep wind pressure off the face and to cut off flying objects which achieve the velocity of missiles at high speeds, a mask of transparent high-impact plastic is attached to these helmets. This creates an additional problem of cooling the head, especially in the cockpit of a racing car where air temperatures may go very high in hot weather.

c. PARACHUTING. The parachutist's helmet should have the same general construction as the motor vehicle users. When used at very high altitudes it must be electrically heated, not only for comfort but to prevent clouding of the face mask.

d. WINTER SPORTS. Downhill skiers wear crash helmets because of the high speeds that they may reach and the frequently hard surfaces on which they fall. The helmet is essentially the same as one for motor vehicles. Similar helmets and masks are used for snowmobiling, tobogganing, and ice boating. Masks have almost completely replaced protective goggles except in downhill skiing.

e. SURFING. A plastic helmet with a slow-rebound liner has been developed for surfing and is being taken up gradually by competitive surfers

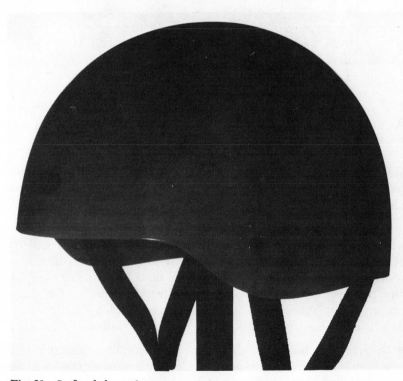

Fig. 21 Surfing helmet, three-quarter side view. Plastic with nylon straps. Courtesy Bell Toptex Co.

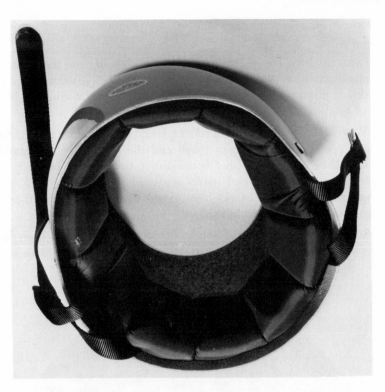

Fig. 22 Surfing helmet, interior view. Nylon-covered foam padding over a crushable liner. Courtesy Bell Toptex Co.

(Figs. 21 and 22). The risk is not only from being driven down onto a hard rocky bottom by the breaking waves, but from being hit on the head by one's own or another's surfboard.

f. SWIMMING AND SCUBA DIVING. Helmets are used for undersea exploration and industrial work. They are tied into a dry suit and connected to an air hose. Masks are used by skin and scuba divers, but covering the eyes only. Ear plugs may be used by swimmers and skin divers but may not be used by scuba divers because of the danger of external ear "squeeze." Water polo players used a light rubber or plastic helmet whose chief purpose is to prevent lacerations.

g. SHOOTING SPORTS. The danger of deafness from shotgun blasts or the accumulation and echoes of rifle fire in closed ranges is very real. Ear plugs or large baffles (which are more effective) are therefore worn by shooters and officials. The best ear plugs are made of finely spun Fiberglas. Waxed cotton is used but is less effective.

2. Overall Clothing

In certain sports where protection from heat loss and chilling are important and in others where there is a hazard of fire, special overall protective clothing must be worn.

a. OUTDOOR WINTER SPORTS. In toboganning, snowmobiling, and ice sailing, high speeds are reached, often in conditions of extreme cold. Waterproof and windproof materials are used with light foam linings to prevent chilling.

b. MOTOR SPORTS. Racing cars, boats, and planes are fueled for the most part now with highly explosive high test gasoline. Racers therefore wear flameproof coveralls, underwear, socks, and gloves.

c. UNDERWATER ACTIVITIES. Since water absorbs heat pound for pound four times as much as air, on a volume basis 1600 times as much, it is necessary to insulate the body for any extended underwater activity. This may be done with a dry or a wet suit. The principle of the wet suit is that the water between the skin and the suit is rapidly warmed by the body and the rubber is a poor conductor of the heat that has been exchanged.

d. SPORTS PARACHUTING. A windproof coverall is worn. In jumps from high altitudes electrically heated clothing should be worn.

3. Gloves

Athletes now use gloves to protect the hand from the grip of some object used in a game to avoid blistering and excessive callous formation as the result of intensive, extended, and year-round practice. Gloves are now used by the majority of golfers, many baseball (for batting) and tennis players, archers, bowlers and others. Mittens are used for outdoor winter sports, since they are more effective than gloves in keeping the fingers warm. Many scuba divers use gloves to protect the hands from contact with sharp objects under water.

4. Special Cushioning and Other Devices

There are many examples of such protective pieces, such as the wrist protector used by the archer and the heavy leather pads used on the forearms and legs of the rider on the skeleton bobsled. Shoulder harness is used for restraint in motor racing vehicles. Lifejackets should be worn in water-skiing and by motor boat racers. Automatically inflatable life jackets should be worn by sports parachutists jumping over water.

V. STANDARDS AND SPECIFICATIONS FOR PROTECTIVE
EQUIPMENT

In the past there has been a definite lack of standards pertaining to protective equipment. Presently, a trend exists to provide a uniform code of standards and specification for sports equipment. The manufacturer and user would benefit equally if such a code were in existence. Standardization is critically needed since competition and demand dictate to a great degree the type and quality of equipment manufactured. Great variance exists in the design, construction, and materials employed in the production of protective items. The development of standards has been severely hampered, however, by lack of specific information regarding the nature and occurrence of injuries and the factors in sports which produce them. Legal and economic pressures to standardize equipment will perhaps result in an increased uniformity of quality among manufacturers, and still allow for a certain degree of individuality.

A. Development toward Standards

Development of protective equipment standards has been long overdue, but invariably forthcoming. To be effective, a code of standardization should contain the following minimal provisions:

1. A definition and basic terminology regarding the product
2. A specification of design and material
3. The safety requirements
4. Product expectation and minimal performance expectations
5. Usefulness of the product
6. Practicability of the product
7. Establish product authority, i.e., NCAA, AMA, and NATA
8. Must contain buyer and user information
9. Include performance quality

B. Specifications

Specifications for modern protective equipment should contain the following (University Extension, University of Wisconsin, 1968):

1. The ability of the product to be able to absorb shock without rebound
2. Be designed to distribute the impact forces to the stronger parts of the body
3. The product must be flexible and nonrestrictive
4. It should be nonabsorbent of perspiration
5. Have energy absorbing qualities, not affected by change in thermal conditions
6. Be designed not to endanger the opponent or wearer
7. Must be resistant to heat or flame

Impact protective equipment must have distinctive characteristics of energy absorbing protection against severe impact. Impact equipment must also be cushioned to minimize discomfort from minor impact. Materials being used are rigid or nonresilient foamed plastics, cellular polystyrene, cellulose acetate, or polyesters. Foam rubber and soft foamed synthetics offer a cushioning effect. Fiberglass, styrofoam, and air cap compositions are materials applicable to the present and future in a combination of uses.

REFERENCES

American Standards Association. (1966). Protective Headgear for Vehicular Users. UDC 614.891:629.82 (New USA Standards Institute, New York, New York).

Hafner, J. K., Callahan, W. T., Crowley, F. J., and Kamber, G. M. (1968). New York State Public High School Athletic Association and The Educational Council for School Research and Development, Albany, New York.

Hale, C. J. (1969). "Report of Committee F-8 on Protective Equipment for Sports," ASTM XXX-2 MISC. Amer. Soc. Test. Mater., Philadelphia, Pennsylvania.

Hanley, D. (1969). N.Y. Times, February 9.

Novich, M., and Taylor, B. (1970). "Training and Conditioning of Athletes," pp. 27–28. Lea & Febiger, Philadelphia, Pennsylvania.

Schneider, R. C., and Antine, B. E. (1965). J. Amer. Med. Ass. 192, 616–618.

Schneider, R. C., Reifel, E., Crisler, H. O., and Oosterbaan, B. G. (1961). J. Amer. Med. Ass. 177, 362–367.

Torg, J. S. (1971). J. Amer. Med. Ass. 218, 1504–1506.

University Extension, University of Wisconsin. (1968). Nat. Conf. Protect. Equip. Sports, 1968.

Wisconsin Interscholastic Athletic Association. (1967). "Football Mask and Dental Guard Study," Wisconsin Interscholastic Athletic Bull., p. 36. Stevens Point, Wisconsin.

Chapter 10

ENVIRONMENTAL PROBLEMS AND THEIR CONTROL

E. R. BUSKIRK

I. INTRODUCTION

A variety of environmental problems confront athletes as they prepare for competition indoors and outdoors, on land, in water, or at altitude. Preparation and conditioning in one environment does not necessarily convey an advantage in another. Adaptation to prevailing conditions and acclimatization to environmental stress have real physiological sequelae of importance to the athlete gearing for top performance. In this chapter several environmental problems will be dealt with including heat, cold, hypoxia, water and air quality, gravity, special indoor facilities frequented by athletes, and the interaction between environmental stress and the athlete's physiological status. This list is only a partial one, and many of the topics are dealt with somewhat superficially because of necessary space restrictions. The references provided were selected for the interested reader so that he could explore in depth topics of importance to him.

II. TEMPERATURE REGULATION AND THERMAL BALANCE

A. Appraising the Thermal Environment

If the athlete is to intelligently interpret guidance about the thermal environment, he must understand it and the impact it has on him. There are several environmental variables bearing on his heat transfer that can be readily measured. These include:

Measurement	Measuring devices
Dry bulb air temperature	Ordinary thermometer
Wet bulb air temperature	Thermometer with bulb covered by wetted wick and exposed to constant high rate of air movement
Radiant energy at several wavelengths	Radiometers of several types including black globe thermometer
Air movement or air velocity	Anemometer
Water temperature	Ordinary thermometer
Barometric pressure	Manometer

The athlete can vary the impact of these variables on his body by varying his clothing, his energy expenditure, his posture, his speed of progression, etc. Usually the athlete working in any natural environment finds himself in a complex heat exchange situation where his heat transfer or rate of heat storage or loss (S) is governed by the following processes:

Heat production:	Energy expenditure associated with activity, M
Heat loss or gain to environment:	Convection and conduction, C
	Radiation, R
	$R + C$ represents the dry heat exchange with the environment
Heat loss:	Evaporation, E
	Mechanical work, W

where $S = M + C + R - E - W$

In terms of calculating the athlete's heat exchange in air or water, convection and conduction are lumped together and one deals with combined heat transfer. Radiation can be treated separately. Consideration of both combined heat transfer and radiation is complicated if clothing is worn or clothing is switched during activity, or the athlete's metabolic rate is changed. Thus, the athlete trains or competes within a microclimate created by his clothing (and other special circumstances) that is hard to assess outside the laboratory. The laboratory is, however, not the athlete's real world, and approximations must be made if appropriate guidance is to be provided. It is important to recognize also that the three avenues of heat exchange seldom operate independently, but as the algebraic sum of the interacting forces. Similarly it is important to realize that convective heat transfer within the body by the circulating blood and lymph is the most important mechanism for transferring heat and balancing temperatures within the body.

Although increased attention has been placed on measurement of the thermal environment for the athlete, he at times is subjected to considerable thermal stress. As long as the thermal stress is not hazardous no harm results, but thermal extremes can be hazardous, as can the combination of moderate temperatures and high humidities, and special precautions need to be taken. These precautions are discussed in the succeeding sections.

The athlete's body appraises the thermal environment through a variety of thermal sensors. Thus far, thermal sensors have been identified in the hypothalamus (presumably a major center for body temperature regulation), brain, skin, muscles, spinal cord, and large blood vessels including veins. Apparently many of the receptors are neurally connected with the brain, since cold and warm sensation and perception are important for voluntary behavioral thermoregulation. Thus, we seek sun or shade, put on or take off clothing, move out of or into the wind, etc.

A variety of effector organs are activated as a result of thermally initiated stimulation. These include the heart, skeletal muscles, smooth muscles in the walls of arterioles that control the supply of blood to the muscles and skin, endocrine glands, sweat glands, and kidneys.

B. Protection against Heat Injury

The high metabolic demands of peak and sustained high level performance in a hot environment can create critical strain on the athlete's body including his temperature regulation mechanisms and his thermal balance. The stimulus of competition, the insistence of coaches, and the enthusiasm and encouragement of spectators all add to the stress of the moment. Thus, the athlete's rate of heat storage may become excessive perhaps because one or more of his mechanisms for heat loss may become virtually overwhelmed. Obviously, precipitating conditions leading to heat illness and injury should be avoided if at all possible.

It is nearly impossible to state precise limiting conditions for different types of athletes training and competing in different sports in different locations. Thus, only general guidelines can be provided. It is hoped that an effort will be made by those responsible for the education of team physicians, trainers, and coaches to provide basic information on avoidance of heat injury. The ultimate goal is the prevention of all heat injury, and only those actively working with athletes can exercise the required supervision. These "supervisors" should understand the physiology of heat exposure, the acclimatization process and the concepts behind preparation of guides for limiting conditions, as well as the signs and symptoms of developing heat strain.

A schematic representation of the interacting mechanisms involved in development of heat disorders is shown in Fig. 1. Metabolic heat generated by physical activity together with environmental heat stress and hypohydration (partial dehydration) synergistically interact to produce the various listed signs of heat strain. Simply physiological measures of heat strain include pulse rate, peripheral vasodilation or constriction, sweating, and body core and skin temperature. If the body's compensatory mechanisms are overwhelmed or compromised in some way, then strain increases rapidly and heat injury may result. It should be remembered that the athlete can effectively lose heat from his body surface only by convection and evaporation. Clothing effectively reduces

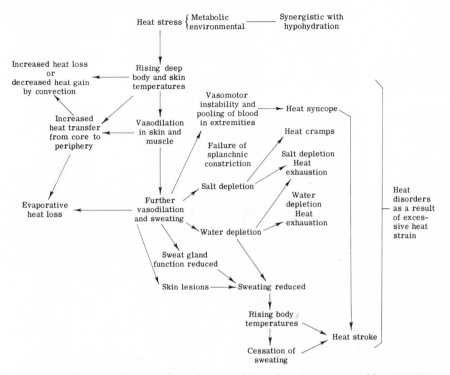

Fig. 1 Schematic diagram of heat stress and heat disorders. From Belding (1967) and Leithead and Lind (1964).

the body's ability to lose heat by both mechanisms. Conditions of high humidity curtail evaporation even further.

When conditioning, training, or competition is conducted in a hot environment, there are preventive measures that can be taken to reduce the impact of heat stress on the body. The various heat disorder possibilities are listed in Table I in terms of the clinical diagnosis, the treatment involved, and the method employed to prevent the heat stress. In Table II, environmental and related considerations in the conduct of athletics (particularly football) are presented. It should be reemphasized that most heat injury is preventable. The management suggestions presented in Table II should provide a rational basis for development of a prevention program.

A simple heat stress index has been developed that combines the effects of temperature, humidity, and the radiant heat for an air environment. The index is obtained by combining the dry bulb temperature (T_a), wet bulb temperature (T_{wb}), and matte black globe temperature (T_g) as indicated in Table III. Note that the globe temperature measurement is omitted for an indoor environment. Murphy and Ashe have

TABLE I

Heat Disorders: Treatment and Prevention

Disorder	Cause	Clinical features and diagnosis	Treatment	Prevention
Heat cramps	Hard work in heat Heavy and prolonged sweating Inadequate salt intake	Low serum sodium and chloride Muscle twitching, cramps and spasms in arms, legs, and abdomen—usually after mid-day	Severe case: intravenous administration of 500 ml of normal saline Light case: oral administration of saline Rest in cool environment Salt foods used Delay 24 to 48 hours before reentering hot area	Insure acclimatization Provide extra salt at meals Drink saline when working
Heat syncope	Peripheral vasodilation and pooling of blood Circulatory instability and loss of vasomotor tone Cerebral hypoxia Hyperventilation Inadequate acclimatization Infection	Weakness and fatigue Hypotension Increased venous compliance Blurred vision Pallor Syncope Elevated skin and deep body temperatures	Place supine and lower head Rest in cool environment Provide oral saline if conscious and resting Keep record of blood pressure, pulse rate, and body temperature	Insure acclimatization Lighten work regimen with sudden rise in environmental temperature or humidity Avoid maintenance of upright static work conditions Comment: predisposes to heat stroke
Water depletion and heat exhaustion	Heavy and prolonged sweating Inadequate fluid intake Polyuria or diarrhea	Reduced sweating, but excessive weight loss Elevated skin and deep body temperatures High hematocrit, serum protein, and sodium Dry tongue and mouth Excessive thirst Hyporexia Weak, disconsolate, uncoordinated, and mentally dull Concentrated urine	Bed rest in cool environment Replace fluids by intravenous drip if drinking is impaired. Increase fluids to 6 or 8 liters per day Sponge with cool water Provide small quantities of semiliquid food Keep record of body weight, water and salt intake, and body temperature	Provide adequate water Provide opportunity for intermittent cooling and adequate rest

Condition	Cause	Signs and symptoms	Treatment	Prevention
Salt depletion and heat exhaustion	Heavy and prolonged sweating Inadequate salt intake Inadequate acclimatization Vomiting or diarrhea	Headache, dizziness, and fatigue Hyporexia Nausea, vomiting, diarrhea Muscle cramps Syncope High hematocrit and serum protein, but low plasma volume Uremia and hypercalemia Low sodium and chloride in sweat and urine	Bed rest in cool environment Replace fluids and salt by intravenous saline drip if drinking is impaired Provide small quantities of semiliquid food Keep record of urinary osmolarity or specific gravity, blood pressure, pulse rate, hematocrit, blood urea, and serum sodium or chloride Keep record of body weight, water and salt intake, and body temperature	Provide adequate salt and water, 10 to 15 g of salt per day may be necessary Provide opportunity for intermittent cooling and adequate rest Insure acclimatization Comment: develops more slowly (3–5 days) than water depletion heat exhaustion
Heat hyperpyrexia leading to heat stroke	Thermoregulatory failure of sudden onset	Generalized anhidrosis and dry skin Elevated skin and deep body temperatures frequently over 40.5°C (105°F), may have chills Irrational Muscle flacidity Involuntary limb movements Seizures and coma Spotty cyanosis and ecchymosis Vomiting and diarrhea frequently with blood Tachycardia and tachypnea	Lower body temperature to 38.9°C (102°F) within 1 hour with cold rinse or spray 7.2°C (45°F). Use cool air fan or place in ice water bath. Use alcohol rinse if nothing else is available Use suction equipment to clear airway and perform tracheotomy if necessary Inject 25 to 30 mg chloropromazine every 30 minutes Bed rest in a cool environment Keep record of skin and deep body temperatures	Insure acclimatization Adapt activities to environment Screen participants with infection or past history of heat illness
Skin lesions	Constantly wetted skin Over exposure to sun	Erythematous papulovesicular rash Itchy skin Obstruction of sweat ducts	Treat secondary disorders Maintain shaded and dry skin Rest in cool environment	Dry skin when possible and keep shaded Examine skin regularly Provide opportunity for intermittent cooling and adequate sweat free periods

TABLE II

Environmental and Related Considerations in the Conduct of Athletics, Particularly Football

I. General warning
   A. Most adverse reactions to environmental heat and humidity occur during first few days of training
   B. It is necessary to become thoroughly acclimatized to heat to successfully compete in hot and/or humid environments
   C. Occurrence of a heat injury indicates poor supervision of the athletic program
II. Athletes who are most susceptible to heat injury
   A. Individuals unaccustomed to work in the heat
   B. Overweight individuals, particularly large linemen
   C. Eager athlete who constantly competes at his capacity
   D. Ill athlete, one with an infection, fever, or gastrointestinal disturbance
   E. Athlete who receives an immunization injection and subsequently develops a temperature elevation
III. Prevention of heat injury
   A. Provide complete medical history and physical examination. Include:
      1. History of previous heat illnesses or fainting in the heat
      2. Inquiry about sweating and peripheral vascular defects
   B. Evaluate general physical condition
      1. Type and duration of training activities for previous month
         a. Extent of work in the heat
         b. General training activities
   C. Measure temperature and humidity on the practice or playing fields
      1. Make measurements before and during training or competitive sessions
      2. Adjust activity level to environmental conditions
         a. Decrease activity if hot or humid (see attached recommendations)
         b. Eliminate unnecessary clothing when hot or humid
   D. Acclimatize athletes to heat gradually
      1. Acclimatization to heat requires work in the heat
         a. Recommend type and variety of warm weather workouts for preseason training
         b. Provide graduated training program for first 7 to 10 days and other abnormally hot or humid days.
      2. Provide adequate rest intervals and salt and water replacement during the acclimatization period
   E. Replace body water and salt losses as they are lost
      1. Supply cold saline—thoroughly mix one teaspoon salt in six quarts of tap water—give 3–4 ounces every 15 minutes or 8 ounces every half-hour; flavor if desired
      2. Allow additional water as desired by player
      3. Provide salt on training tables and encourage salting of food
      4. Weigh each day before and after training or competition
         a. Treat athlete who loses excessive weight each day
         b. Treat well-conditioned athlete who continues to lose weight for several days
   F. Clothing and uniforms
      1. Provide lightweight clothing that is loose fitting at the neck, waist, and sleeves. Use shorts and T-shirt at beginning of training.
      2. Avoid excessive padding and taping
      3. Avoid use of long stockings, long sleeves, double jerseys, and other excess clothing
      4. Avoid use of rubberized clothing or sweatsuits
      5. Provide clean clothing daily—all items
   G. Provide rest periods to dissipate accumulated body heat
      1. Rest in cool, shaded area with some air movement
      2. Avoid hot brick walls or hot benches
      3. Loosen or remove jerseys or other garments
      4. Take saline and/or water during the rest period

TABLE III

Approximate Limiting Conditions for a Well-Conditioned, Heat-Acclimatized Athlete Performing One Hour of Sustained Running[a]

$WBGT$[b]	T_a[c]	T_{wb}[d]	rh[e]	Pw[f]	T_g[g]
29.4 (85)	27.7 (82)	27.7 (82)	100	27	36.1 (97)
28.8 (84)	28.3 (83)	26.6 (80)	76	25	36.6 (98)
28.8 (84)	32.2 (90)	25.0 (77)	55	20	40.6 (105)
27.6 (82)	33.3 (92)	22.8 (73)	37	15	41.7 (107)
26.7 (80)	35.5 (96)	20.5 (69)	25	11	43.9 (111)

[a] Athlete minimally clothed. Temperatures given in both degrees centigrade and (fahrenheit).

[b] $WBGT$, wet bulb globe temperature index; where $WBGT$ (outdoors) = $0.1\ T_a + 0.7\ T_{wb} + 0.2\ T_g$ and $WBGT$ (indoors) = $0.3\ T_a + 0.7\ T_{wb}$.

[c] T_a, dry bulb temperature of the ambient air.

[d] T_{wb}, wet bulb temperature.

[e] rh, relative humidity in percent.

[f] Pw, vapor pressure in mm Hg.

[g] T_g, black matte globe temperature.

provided a table for football based exclusively on the wet bulb temperature (see Table IV). Since football players usually wear a full uniform, their covered body surface reduces their effective skin surface area participating in evaporative cooling. Use of the wet bulb temperature measurement is more critical for the clothed than for the unclothed man. Various devices are currently available for making the environmental measurements. Some of these devices are shown in Fig. 2. While data secured from the nearest Weather Bureau is better than none, the on-site climate surrounding the athlete (i.e., from ground level to seven feet

TABLE IV

Wet Bulb Temperature Guide for Planning and Conducting Football Practices[a]

Wet bulb temperature	Plan
15.6°C (60°F)	Normal practice possible
16.1°C to 18.4°C (61° to 65°F)	Pay close attention to all squad members particularly those who have lost considerable body weight
18.9°C to 21.1°C (66° to 70°F)	Insist that water or salt solution be given on the field; observe players carefully as above
21.6°C to 23.9°C (71° to 75°F)	Schedule rest periods every 30 minutes; follow above
24.4°C (76°F +)	Conduct practice in shorts or delay or postpone practice until conditions improve

[a] Whenever relative humidity is 95% or higher, precaution should be taken and close observation employed. Use as a guide only—it is no substitute for good clinical judgment.

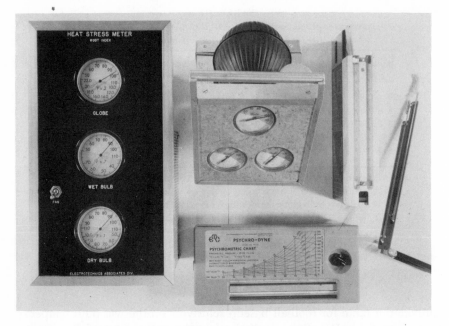

Fig. 2 Devices for measuring climatic variables on athletic fields. The heat stress meter on the left, made by Electrotechnics Associates measures the dry-bulb, wet-bulb, and black globe temperatures. Proportional scales are provided to calculate the WBGT index. A similar but smaller heat stress meter built at Penn State appears in the upper center. A Psychro-dyne or the dry-bulb wet-bulb measuring device made by Environmental Technology Associates is in the lower center position. A similar unit made by the Bendix Corp. is at the upper right and a conventional sling psychrometer is at the far right.

above ground) is the climate of importance. Deviations of several critical degrees can exist between on-site and weather bureau readings.

C. Heat Acclimatization

Heat acclimatization renders the athlete more capable of dealing with heat. For equal physical effort, the heat acclimatized athlete shows less heat strain than the nonacclimatized athlete when working in a hot environment. Heat acclimatization is brought about by several important body adjustments which allow the athlete to work with: a lower body temperature, lower heart rate and cardiac output, more precise regulation of sweat rate and peripheral blood flow, and a more stable blood pressure.

In general, acclimatization to heat may be characterized by the following summary:

1. It begins with the first exposure, progresses rapidly with subsequent exposures, and is well developed in about seven days.

2. It can be induced by short intermittent bouts of exercise in the heat, e.g., of from two to four hours daily. Physical inactivity in the heat results in but slight acclimatization.

3. Athletes in good physical condition acclimatize more rapidly than nonconditioned people and are capable of more work in the heat. Nevertheless, tip-top physical condition does not confer heat acclimatization, and the athlete is at a competitive disadvantage in the heat if not heat acclimatized.

4. Daily work, if progressively increased in the heat, leads to early development of maximal performance capacity. Overexertion on the first exposure may result in disability, which in turn inhibits the acclimatization process.

5. Acclimatization to warm conditions will facilitate acclimatization to hot conditions but will not confer complete acclimatization to hot conditions. Acclimatization to hot conditions will facilitate performance under warm conditions.

6. The general pattern of acclimatization is similar for work of different intensity and duration.

7. Acclimatization to hot dry climates enhances performance capabilities in hot wet climates and vice versa.

8. Inadequate water and salt replacement can retard the acclimatization process.

9. Acclimatization to heat is retained for about two weeks with no exposure. Thereafter, loss of acclimatization is highly individual. Athletes who stay in good physical condition should retain heat acclimatization best.

It was said in regard to the 1960 Olympics in Rome that heat was such an important debilitating factor that the best competitors were not necessarily the winners unless they were heat acclimatized. In summary, it is important to remember that proper acclimatization greatly reduces the possibility of heat injury.

D. Protection against Cold Injury

Cold poses few special problems for the athlete familiar with cold environmental conditions in the northern hemisphere. Frostbite and freezing of tissues must be avoided as well as excessive drying of the skin and airways. The athlete must keep his body warm enough to avoid shivering which can interfere with finely coordinated muscular action. Clothing that is too warm only precipitates unnecessary sweating, and bulky clothing adds a hobbling effect that reduces efficiency of body movement. Fortunately, improved clothing materials and designs enable the athlete to wear protective clothing of sufficiently light weight and small bulk to prevent cold injury without unduly hindering normal movement.

Areas of the body that may need special protection in the cold are the airways, ears, nose, chest, hands, and feet. During cross-country running or skiing under severe cold conditions, the athlete may find it convenient to use a nose and mouth cover that provides negligible resistance to air movement but retains a fraction of the warmed and humidified expired air for rebreathing. Some athletes find this type of cover comfortable and useful, particularly during training. The nose and ears are susceptible to frostbite more readily than other areas of the face and should be protected if frostbite is likely. Because of the increased air movement across the chest with sustained forward progress, the chest can cool rapidly and the nipples can dry out and crack. This excessive drying and cooling can be avoided with proper covering of the chest. Similarly the hands can cool rapidly if held up and forward, good gloves can provide needed protection. The feet should be kept warm and reasonably dry so that "feel" and balance is easy to maintain. Sure footing is an asset under icy and otherwise slippery conditions. The loss of finger dexterity and tactile sensitivity can be a real handicap to athletes who must use their bare hands. Keeping the hands warm between events is of the utmost importance. Handwarmers are useful for this purpose, and down muffs also provide excellent protection.

III. ALTITUDE AND HYPOXIA

The Mexico Olympics in 1968 refocused attention on the relationships between altitude (hypoxia) and physical performance capacity. The impetus provided by the Olympic games was valuable for both the athletic and scientific communities. One of the important conclusions from these efforts was that even relatively acute adaptation to altitude, i.e., 3 weeks or less, proved to be useful. The athlete who trained at an equivalent altitude knew what to expect, i.e., he benefited from an educational experience and gave his body time to partially adapt to altitude. Nevertheless, such partial adaptation enhances performance capability to a lesser extent than natural acclimatization to altitude. Athletes born and trained in a similar environment, e.g., the runners from Kenya, did exceedingly well in the Mexico Olympics.

A. Work Capacity

It has been conclusively shown that in athletes who utilize high rates of aerobic metabolism their performance is adversely affected by reduction of the oxygen content of the ambient air at altitude. The reduction in oxygen partial pressure with reduction in barometric pressure results in reduced oxygen partial pressure in the athlete's alveolar air and arterial blood. The decrement in running and swimming performance is related to the decrement in the maximal oxygen intake. Maximal oxygen intake decreases with increased altitude from sea level approximately 3% per 305 m (1000 feet) (see Fig. 3). There is little apparent value in attempting to adapt sea level athletes to altitudes over 3810 m (12,500 feet) in order to improve their performance at a lower altitude. The reason

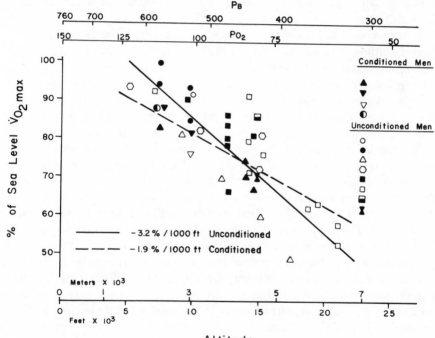

Fig. 3 Effect of reduced partial pressure of oxygen on the maximal oxygen intake (V_{O_2} max) expressed as a percent of sea level V_{O_2} max for conditioned and unconditioned men. Modified Figure 2 from J. Kollias and E. R. Buskirk. Exercise and Altitude. In "Science and Medicine of Exercise and Sports" (W. R. Johnson and E. R. Buskirk, eds.). Reproduced with permission of Harper and Row, Inc., New York, 1974.

for this is that the intensity of conditioning and training must of necessity be reduced at the higher altitude, and even though some adaptation to altitude may occur the relative deconditioning cancels the improved adaptation. Thus, performance may not change and may even be reduced at the lower altitude.

In general, the more time spent at altitude and the more demanding the conditioning and training regimen the better the adaptation and performance capability. One possible exception might be the athlete who can fly to the site of competition at altitude and then compete immediately before his body starts to adapt. This athlete might compete quite favorably. Although some team games such as soccer are played at altitudes up to 5486 m (18,000 feet) in the Andean communities of South America, international competition is seldom scheduled above 3048 m (10,000 feet). Teams from low land areas simply have no desire to compete at these high altitudes. Thus, mountain climbing and downhill skiing are virtually the only sports conducted at higher terrestrial altitude.

It is not well known that on a per kilogram body basis well-conditioned natives resident to high altitude have high aerobic capacities, i.e., higher than well-trained athletes who were newcomers to altitude. This relatively large aerobic capacity in the native is associated with a high oxygen saturation of arterial blood coupled with a large circulating red cell mass which insures a greater oxygen content of arterial blood perfusing working muscle. Together with a more favorable acid–base balance, and perhaps a more favorable chemical adaptation favoring oxygen transport in red blood cells, e.g., increased amount of 2,3-diphosphoglycerate, the naturally acclimatized native has a distinct physiological advantage over his more poorly acclimatized competitor. There is also some evidence that muscle capillarity may be increased by hypoxia. This may mean that the working muscle is more adequately perfused in the naturally acclimatized native. Similarly the native's oxygen transport mechanisms within muscle may be relatively superior, i.e., his muscle myoglobin content, DPNH oxidase, TPNH cytochrome c reductase, and transhydrogenase are increased. There may also be an increased number of mitochondria in the muscles of those chronically exposed to hypoxic conditions.

Despite short term or acute adaptation and/or acclimatization to altitude the following conclusions seem warranted: (1) performance times for distance events are subnormal (with respect to sea level) at all altitudes above 1524 m (5,000 feet), while sprint events are unaffected below 3108 m (10,200 feet) and (2) on return to sea level from altitude, aerobic capacity and performance times are not significantly different from prealtitude values assuming the level of conditioning has not changed. The latter point requires further research, for it is unclear whether hypoxia is the common and perhaps exclusive stimulus for adaptation to altitude and physical conditioning.

B. Gastrointestinal Distress and Physical Collapse

An important factor limiting performance at any altitude is gastrointestinal distress and diarrhea. Whether hypoxia interacts with the offending organisms is unknown, but the incidence seemed to be higher at the Mexico Olympics than in the Olympics conducted elsewhere. Although prophylactic medication (e.g., succinylsulfathiazole) and strict sanitary supervision were available, it is reported that 40% of the USA competitors developed diarrhea.

Fortunately the expressed fear of an overwhelming number of physical collapses and even deaths in Mexico City was unfounded. Postcompetition collapse involving physiological and psychological components was no more frequent than at lower altitudes. Apparently the body's protective mechanisms can cope with the severe hypoxia wrought by the combination of hard work at moderate altitude.

C. Protection against Mountain Sickness

Mountain sickness is frequently brought about by exposure to a natural hypoxic environment for periods of two hours or more. It is associated with headache, dyspnea, fatigue, drowsiness, insomnia, and perhaps nausea, vomiting, and loss of appetite at higher elevations. The greatest evidence of symptoms occurs within two to twelve hours following arrival at altitude. Within five to seven days most people become symptom free. Discomfort has been observed as low as 1524 m (5000 feet), and more people are affected at 2133 m (7000 feet). Still more are affected at 3108 m (10,200 feet), and only a fortunate few are symptom free above 4511 m (14,800 feet). An overnight or longer stay at an intermediate altitude generally reduces the symptoms at a higher altitude. Although well-conditioned athletes are probably as susceptible as less well-conditioned men, their familiarity with toleration of unpleasant physical stress presumably allows them to accomplish physically demanding tasks which the less well-conditioned will not undertake or which will make them violently ill if they do.

Several drugs have been employed to reduce the severity of acute mountain sickness. Pretreatment with acetazolamide or benzolamide was found to be effective at 4300 m (14,110 feet). Both drugs act as carbonic anhydrase inhibitors and increase renal excretion of bicarbonate, a process normally brought about later with the development at altitude of respiratory alkalosis. The effects of these drugs on the athlete's performance have not been thoroughly evaluated.

D. Protection against Pulmonary Edema

Pulmonary edema, perhaps with associated pulmonary hypertension, is the most serious problem at high altitude. One would arbitrarily suspect that the athlete competing at altitude would be a prime candidate because of his elevation in blood pressure with intense physical effort. Nevertheless, there is little evidence to confirm this suspicion. There is a decided individual susceptibility to development of the syndrome, for symptoms such as coughing and dyspnea usually develop within 24 to 72 hours after the arrival at altitude in excess of 3108 m (10,200 feet). Later, rales develop, and the presence of fluid in the chest can be detected. Emergency treatment, including oxygen therapy, should be applied immediately and the patient moved to lower altitude. The precise mechanism for development of pulmonary edema is unknown, but pulmonary hypertension secondary to increased resistance of the pulmonary arterioles brought about by the hypoxic stimulus has been implicated.

IV. WATER AS A SPECIAL ENVIRONMENT

A. Surface Swimming and Thermal Protection

Most water sports are conducted at the water surface, although the popularity of scuba as a recreational and occupational activity has put large numbers of people beneath the surface of the water for short periods. (The use of underwater habitats increases diving time considerably.) With surface swimming, frequent medical problems include resuscitation, sunburn, dermatosis, outer and middle ear infections, plus the usual assortment of common athletic injuries such as: abrasions, contusions, sprains, etc. The well-managed competitive swimmer usually has easy access to good medical care, but the age-group club swimmer is frequently under the direct supervision of only a part-time coach who may be ill equipped in the medical area.

Swimming poses a special temperature regulation problem because evaporative heat loss cannot occur in water, and heat transfer is largely by combined convection and conduction. The range in temperature for pool water varies considerably and has been found to vary from 20.0° to 34.5°C (68° to 94°F), even in pools used for competition. Some coaches use water temperature to "psych" the competition, but also many water conditioning facilities are inadequate and one takes the conditions one gets. Evaluation of the effect of water temperature on performance indicates that only times in the longer swims are lengthened by water above 26.6°C (80°F). As the pool water nears that of body temperature, deep body temperatures tend to rise in the competitive swimmer. Temperatures of 39.7°C (103.5°F) have been recorded in a 1500 m competitor after his race in 34.4°C (94°F) water. Under circumstances such as these, the relatively large skin blood flow is reduced to support working muscle. An explosive rise in deep body temperature can then occur because of the small rate of convective and conductive cooling. In water temperatures over 35°C (95°F) heat would be gained by the body from the water and only very short events could be swam without danger of heat injury.

In cold water near freezing, survival becomes a problem because of the high rate of convective and conductive cooling. Skin temperatures tend to approach those of the water, and heat loss is ultimately reduced to a relatively low rate. It is difficult for the swimmer to keep his metabolic rate high enough to avoid hypothermia and possible death. The highest resistance to heat loss is developed by marked cutaneous and extremity vasoconstriction, which results in reduction in peripheral blood flow plus the establishment of pronounced countercurrent heat exchange between the larger arteries and veins in the extremities.

Fortunately no athlete other than the channel swimmer must cope with cold water conditions. The channel swimmer utilizes several factors to successfully compete in this rigorous event. Most of these swimmers have ample subcutaneous fat which, when the skin blood flow is reduced, serves well as peripheral insulation. It is suspected that their countercurrent heat exchange mechanisms are superior. In addition, they are sufficiently well conditioned to sustain high metabolic rates for several hours and are very efficient swimmers.

At the present time, the greatest deterrent to extending deep diving capabilities is excessive body heat loss. Only the availability of superior insulated clothing plus a small individual body heater will solve the problem of prolonged work in cold water at great depth.

Diving from one and three meter boards or platforms poses special injury problems. The team physician would be well advised to check various safety features such as board mounting, spacing between boards, nonslip surfaces, etc., to try to have the best possible installations so as to avoid injury. Rules for equipment use should be agreed upon with the coach and adhered to.

B. Scuba

A variety of medical problems are associated with the use of self contained underwater breathing apparatus (scuba). Chief among these is lack of knowledge by the user. Because water pressure increases approximately one atmosphere for every 9 m (30 feet) of depth, the scuba user is in a dangerous environment whenever he descends to depths of 3 m (10 feet) or more. No one should undertake scuba diving without going through at least a 20 hour course with competent instruction. In addition, supervised use of scuba at various depths to 9 m (30 feet) should be part of this instruction. A safety maxim of scuba is to never dive without a buddy and preferably with surface support personnel.

The problems with SCUBA are numerous and include:

1. Use of improper air tanks with contaminating gases or oil droplets in the compressed air. Inadequate filling of air tanks. Use of leaky tanks.

2. Failure to equalize pressure in the airways during the dive and the return to surface.

3. Failure to follow an established decompression schedule.

4. Failure to observe rate of air utilization and to return to the surface with a safe amount of air remaining.

5. Failure to observe proper safety precautions and to use common sense. Failure to avoid underwater hazards, to dive in safe water, to avoid sharks, jellyfish, and other dangerous forms of marine life.

Treatment following injury presupposes that the physician knows diving medicine and is familiar with the various forms of barotrauma, such as decompression sickness, ear and sinus squeezes, thoracic squeeze, etc., and is familiar with tables of decompression. The physician should also know about the availability of pressure chambers.

C. Water Quality

A variety of pollutants including debris, silt, herbicides, pesticides, mine drainage wastes, sewage effluent, and a host of other organic and inorganic chemicals degrade water quality and make swimming hazardous. Even excessive chlorination of swimming pools with build-up of free chlorine can be damaging to the skin and eyes. Unfortunately, monitoring of water quality for swimming and other sport and recreational purposes is not as thorough as it should be. Too frequently the presence of medical problems serves notice that something is wrong, e.g., the detection of parasites in the body following use of an inland bay in Florida for water skiing and swimming. While monitoring water quality is usually the duty of the state or local department of health, their checking is periodic and may not necessarily cover the problem. Thus, physicians, trainers, coaches, and the athletes themselves should be ever observant for any sign of deterioration in water quality. The mere presence of particulate matter in the water may indicate that further checking is necessary.

V. AIR QUALITY

A. Poorly Ventilated Spaces

Those involved with athletic programs usually have some control over indoor ambient environments, particularly temperature and perhaps humidity control. Air turnover within the auditorium should equal or exceed 30 cfm of total air flow per person with 15 cfm of filtered outdoor air. This will provide eight air changes per hour. Smoking should be prohibited because of the degradation in air quality that smoke produces. Air temperature should be programmed so that the combination of heating, air-conditioning, and ventilation maintains air temperature in the lower portion of the thermal neutral zone, i.e., about 20° to 23.3°C (68° to 74°F). Thus, before the crowd arrives the temperature should be on the cool side, for the combined heat elimination of the crowd and participants will raise air temperature. Similarly, humidity will rise in a crowded auditorium because of the water vapor eliminated by those present, and humidity should also be kept low before the crowd arrives. If air quality is poor in the neighborhood, the intake air for the building should be improved by filtration or other processing if possible. Nothing detracts from an indoor sporting event more than poor air quality.

B. Crowding

Crowding produced by inadequate seat size and seating arrangements detracts from the event. The spectators are uncomfortable, and in an effort to relieve crowding, infringement on the competitor's space may occur. Such infringement can lead to accidents. In addition, crowding increases the heat and humidity load because of the heat and water vapor produced by the extra people present. Thus, environmental control systems can be overwhelmed and air quality deteriorate.

C. Odors

Odors pose a special problem and are extremely hard to control. Overcrowding leads to an odor problem in poorly ventilated spaces. Odors brought in from outside in the intake air can be removed by selective filtration, but the expense involved may be great. Adding a disguising odor may only complicate the problem. Recirculated air should also be filtered to reduce crowd odor and dust. The filters should have an air cleaning efficiency of at least 80%.

D. Air Pollutants

Several air pollutants probably have a negative influence on the performance of athletes, but only limited and relatively inconclusive studies have been conducted to date. Experimentation is difficult because of the inadvisability of exposing volunteer athletes intentionally to air pollutants. Nevertheless, it is clear that the burden of pollutants gaining access to the body through the lungs is dependent on the metabolic rate. The higher the metabolism, the greater the pulmonary ventilation, and the greater the delivery of pollutants to the airways. Fortunately, the cilia in the airways can clear many of the particulate pollutants if the cilia are not overwhelmed. Most gases and vapors bypass the cilia and reach the alveoli where transfer can occur across the alveolar membranes to the blood. Whenever possible, competition should be scheduled where air pollution is low or at hours when the concentration is the lowest possible if polluted air conditions can not be avoided. Some states, such as California, have already initiated steps to set air quality standards for competition, but setting such standards still leaves practice and training condition advice and regulation in the hands of the team physician, trainers, and coaches.

In addition to the environmental agents reaching their site of action through the lungs, agents can also proceed through other membranes that separate vital areas from the external chemical environment. These membranes include the skin and the epithelium of the alimentary canal. Once a substance has penetrated an external membrane, it enters the circulation and is carried throughout the body as a freely diffusible molecule or as a molecule reversibly bound to proteins, chylomicrons, or formed elements such as red or white blood cells. Other membrane barriers are also encountered in the body by the agent. These barriers are protective in that they prolong the exposure of the agent to sites of metabolic destruction and excretion. The state of ionization, the size, lipid solubility, and type of binding to other compounds all influence the rate and direction of movement of the agent or its derivative. Although there is some understanding of how many substances are absorbed, what their fate may be, and what effects they produce, there are wide gaps in our knowledge when it comes to some classes of environmental agents such as herbicides, insecticides, organic ions, heavy metals, bacterial toxins, and other macromolecules. Very little information is available about changes in performance capabilities upon exposure to and absorption of these agents. Suffice it to say that avoidance and caution should be observed whenever possible. At the present time there is also little evidence of physiological adaptation to air pollutants, although such adaptation undoubtedly exists. Such adaptation would not necessarily be of benefit to the athlete.

VI. NOISE

Noise is a complex factor in athletics, for crowd cheering and applause can stimulate the athlete to peak effort, while an inappropriate sound can ruin his concentration. A golfer or tennis player is particularly vulnerable. In general, nonassociated noise such as ground or air traffic and uncontrolled irrelevant crowd noise detracts from concentration on the event underway. It has been shown that a sudden loud noise can facilitate a maximal muscular contraction or body effort. Karate and weight lifters frequently use a self-generated noise to this end.

VII. OUTDOOR FACILITIES

Insufficient attention is frequently paid to environmental variables when planning outdoor facilities. The best available environmental consultation should be sought to best cope with air movement and direction, temperature, humidity, solar radiation, air pollution, and proximity to other structures and services such as parking.

VIII. GRAVITY

The influences of differences in gravity with variations in longitude, latitude, and altitude, and the lessening of air density with higher altitude may be important in altering performance. Usually, intraindividual or biological variability is sufficiently large to obscure the small competitive advantage the athlete would have from lessened air density and decreased gravitational force. Theoretically, shot put and long jump world records could be set at the highest possible terrestrial altitude where other competitive conditions are favorable. The setting of the astounding World's long jump record in the Mexico Olympics is hardly proof of this contention, for the shot put record was not broken, nor could the long jumper subsequently repeat (or even closely approximate) his extraordinary performance. The combined effects of decreased air density and resistance (increased take-off speed) and lessened gravitational force combined could have made no more than about a 1% or a 4 inch contribution to the long jump record, yet the record was broken by approximately two feet (see also Chapter 4).

IX. ARTIFICIAL PLAYING SURFACES

The current popularity of both indoor and outdoor artificial playing surfaces including turf has had an important impact on athletics. Although use of these surfaces has produced no significant decrease in athletic injuries, the form of some of the injuries has changed, e.g., the incidence of skin brush burns, skin stripping, and abrasions has increased in football players using artificial turf.

There are many advantages provided by the artificial surfaces. For the most part, the surface is close to an all-weather one; footing is good, wear resistance is excellent, and boundary lines can be permanently marked. The surface stays quite clean or is easily cleaned with sweepers or vacuum cleaners, and other maintenance is minimal with proper installation until the surface is well worn and needs to be replaced.

At least one disadvantage has been found when artificial turf is used outdoors. It is hot when exposed to solar radiation and warm temperatures. Grass shades the soil, and the grass is cooled via evaporation of water from leaf surfaces, which also tends to cool the ground. The use of artificial turf renews the concern about heat injury because of its potential for creating a very warm to hot playing environment. Additional heat is gained by the athlete playing on artificial turf as compared to grass turf in three ways: (1) radiation from the artificial turf because it tends to be warmer on sunny days than skin temperature, (2) an increase in air temperature up to at least the 4-foot level, and (3) transfer of heat from the turf through the soles of the feet (or other portion of the body in contact with the turf) to the body core. This relative heat gain leads to greater physiological heat strain. Thus, guidelines for practice and competition on artificial turf should take into account the potential for greater heat stress.

In the medically well-managed players in professional sports and in college, the risk of additional heat injury when using artificial turf is small. Even so, team physicians and coaches would be ill-advised to schedule all initial practice sessions on artificial turf in hot weather until the athletes are at least partially heat acclimatized. Of greater concern is the use of artificial turf by poorly managed interscholastic athletes. Heat injury is most pronounced in this group, and the added heat stress induced by artificial turf makes medical management of high school athletes a critical matter.

X. SPECIAL FACILITIES FREQUENTED BY ATHLETES

A. Locker Rooms

Poorly constructed and maintained locker rooms can be a source of injury and a source of disease transmission. Properly constructed locker rooms are well ventilated, have low humidity, can easily be kept clean, have no protruding handles or sharp corners, and provide athletes room to move around freely on nonslip surfaces. Lockers should be well ventilated so that equipment can be dried thoroughly and dirty or suspect clothing and equipment removed by trainers and managers. The team physician should check the locker room frequently to make sure that it is maintained in the best possible condition. This checking should include floors, benches, lockers, walls, ventilators, etc. Nonsanitary conditions should be remedied immediately. Unfortunately, this checking is not always done, and needless skin infections and other problems arise.

B. Shower Rooms

For some reason or other, most shower rooms are found wanting from an environmental point of view. They are usually poorly ventilated and dehumidified. They seldom dry thoroughly between major periods of use. The floors are usually slippery and soap films prevalent; plumbing fixtures and projections are prominent, and prevention against a flow of scalding water is frequently absent. A well-planned and operating shower room is a pleasure to use, but many athletes are deprived this experience.

An additional feature seldom provided is a well-drained drying room between the locker and shower rooms. Such a room serves the useful function of keeping the locker room much dryer and the shower room less crowded. The floor and walls of the shower and drying rooms should be washed with an antiseptic solution at least once per week to inhibit development and growth of colonies of microorganisms.

C. Weight and Wrestling Rooms

Both of these rooms, plus the tumbling area for gymnastics, commonly have floors covered with plastic coated mats. The surfaces of these mats must be kept clean, and regular cleaning is the only answer. Antiseptic solutions that are noninjurious to the plastic are preferred. Exercising bodies secreting sebum and sweat provide an excellent culture medium on the surface of the mats for the growth of a variety of organisms. Both of these rooms should also be well ventilated and dehumidified. The wrestling room, in particular, should have dehumidification equipment. Warm moist conditions favor the growth of microorganisms and make the cleaning job difficult. Similarly, the wrestlers and weight lifters will sweat considerably more in a hot humid environment.

It is amazing that more injuries do not occur in weight and exercise rooms, for lifters of all degrees of skill and sophistication use these rooms, and supervision is seldom adequate. Nevertheless, the athletic team physician should check the weight room and the special exercise equipment to insure that hazardous equipment is removed and an atmosphere conducive to safety exists.

A common item of clothing worn in these rooms is the rubberized sweat suit. Other than for utilization for a brief warm-up of from 2 to 15 minutes to raise muscle and body temperature, there appears to be little value in using the rubberized suit. The suit simply serves as a container, trapping most of the water vapor lost by evaporation of sweat. When the air within the suit becomes saturated, sweat can no longer evaporate but is absorbed by other clothing worn or forms puddles that are either contained within the suit or drip out. If exercise continues, skin and body temperatures rise. Only extra water is lost from the body when the rubberized suit is worn. This water is replaced later when food and drink are taken. Thus, the suit serves no functional purpose in athletics other than to initiate a more rapid warm-up. If the rubberized suit is used at all, the suit should be removed following the brief warm-up, and the activity continued in the usual athletic clothing. The thoroughly wetted skin produced by using the suit also favors development of skin infections.

D. Steam Baths and Saunas

The contention has been made that steam baths and saunas, as well as hot baths, do little more than stimulate sweating and provide a form of peripheral vascular exercise. Use of warm baths or hot rooms is a well accepted practice by many cultures throughout the world, usually as a means of bathing and a device for stimulation of social interchange. There is little doubt that the hot, wet steam bath and the hot, dry sauna produce maximal cutaneous vasodilation and high rates of sweating. The vasodilation is reversed by vasoconstriction when a cold shower is taken or the body is exposed to a cold environment following the hot exposure. The cutaneous vasodilation vasoconstriction maneuver is responsible for the comment about peripheral vascular exercise. The dangers for the uninitiated are two: (1) the possibility of heat injury, and (2) postexposure collapse due to orthostatic hypotension brought about by pooling of blood in the lower extremities.

The value of steam baths or sauna in athletics is questionable. Normally shower rooms are available to the athlete so that he can keep himself clean, and he need not use the steam bath unless culturally inclined to do so.

A measure of heat acclimatization can be gained and retained through regular use, but exercise in warm environments is more effective. An unexplained sense of mild fatigue and complete relaxation occurs in many who take a steam bath or sauna. This method of relaxation inducement might be valuable to the athlete who has a difficult time "winding down," but there are also other means of inducing relaxation.

XI. ENVIRONMENTAL STRESS AND THE STATE OF THE BODY

A. Adaptation and Acclimatization

In athletics one might arbitrarily view the process of adaptation as referring to any property of the body which facilitates physiological activity leading to enhancement of performance. Acclimation refers to those compensatory changes which occur in athletes under controlled coaching or laboratory conditions where only one environmental variable is altered. Since acclimation of an athlete can almost never happen, acclimatization is a more useful term for it refers to the adaptive changes which occur under natural conditions when multiple factors vary, such as coaches, team associations, conditioning, weather, competitive seasons, etc. Thus, the study of athletes under their usual operating conditions entails the study of their adaptation and acclimatization. The genotype sets the framework within which the environmentally induced variation can occur. A major task remains to separate the causes of variability among athletes, i.e., that genetically or environmentally induced.

B. Conditioning and Training

Two of the most potent environmental factors leading to improvement in the athlete's performance are physical conditioning and training. Physical conditioning refers to the general enhancement of speed, strength, flexibility, and endurance, whereas training refers to the use of education and practice to improve athletic skill. Conditioning and training in the hands of a good coach and an intelligent athlete are synergistic—each complementing the other. It is the responsibility of the team physician to see that conditioning and training are conducted in a safe way within physiological and psychological limits. A well-conditioned athlete is usually better able to resist and adapt to other environmental stresses than his less well-conditioned colleague. Conditioning and training to be most effective should not be a seasonal affair, but a year-round commitment.

C. Nutrient and Fluid Balance

An athlete cannot adapt to subnormal nutrition or fluid balance, although many athletes try to do so, notably wrestlers. Adequate chemical energy in the form of food must regularly be ingested to sustain conditioning and training regimens plus competition. Similarly, fluid balance must be maintained, and this can only be accomplished if fluid intake is adequate. Daily or at least weekly weight records plus regular inquiries about the athlete's nutrition are immensely helpful in evaluating an athlete's status. A well-run training table helps maintain adequate nutrition and educates the athlete as to the importance of proper food and drink in the management of his bodily needs. Other factors including illness, emotional problems, use of drugs, lack of sleep, etc., can influence the athlete's nutritional status and his fitness for competition.

D. Individual Differences

Athletes with a wide range of body types and builds have distinguished themselves on the playing field. In few sports are athletes of different body size separated except in boxing and wrestling. Thus, if the athlete is sufficiently well-conditioned and has the requisite skill and desire, he can successfully compete. Genetic endowment also shows up in other ways than in body type, build, and size. The capacity for conditioning, neuromuscular coordination, the capacity for speed and strength development, flexibility, intelligence, dedication, and many other characteristics serve to differentiate a given athlete from his peers.

Both genetic and environmental components interact in the development of the successful athlete. For example, there are developmental as well as other individual differences in sweating. The number of functioning sweat glands per unit area of skin surface appears to be established at birth. If the youngster is exposed to a hot environment at a very early age the number of sweat glands can increase, and his body is subsequently better able to withstand heat stress. The sweat glands that are present can elaborate more or less sweat depending on the state of acclimatization to heat. If the person adds excess fat and hence weight and skin surface area, the glands are spread farther apart and the evaporative heat loss mechanism compromised. There is no evidence for difference in genetic endowment of functional sweat glands, but it would be surprising if such differences did not exist.

E. Cross-Adaptation

Either continuous or intermittent exposure to a given environmental variable may lead to a gain or loss of tolerance to other environmental variables. This concept is known as cross-adaptation. Thus, there is cross-adaptation between physical conditioning and heat acclimatization. There also may be cross-adaptation between physical conditioning and exposure to hypoxia.

Because the athlete lives, trains, and competes in a complex environment, it is not always possible to describe the cross-adaptation. As a general principle several adaptations and cross-adaptations can coexist, and a negative cross-adaptation need not necessarily cancel a positive cross-adaptation or an adaptation. The presence of multiple stressors may tend to lower both the physiological and psychological resistance of the body and thus reduce performance. Of interest to the athletic physician is the fact that environmental adaptation and some drugs may elicit a cross-adaptation. Physical conditioning may change effective therapeutic drug dosage, but this type of interaction has not been adequately studied.

F. Biorhythms

A variety of biorhythms have been identified in response to geophysical cycles, and these may be termed tidal, diurnal, lunar, and seasonal. The environmental periodicity apparently acts as a synchronizer for a self-sustained oscillation within the organism. The dark–light cycle is a potent synchronizer. There is probably no organ or function that does not show rhythmicity. The body is a different psychological, physiological, biochemical, and physical system at each hour of the day. Thus, exercise will have different effects upon the athlete depending on where he is on his circadian map. This temporal ordering is probably a necessary prerequisite for a healthy state. The drift among presumably coordinated rhythms may dissociate functions and inhibit performance. The question of when is the right time for competition is a pertinent one. Out-of-phase stress may counteract adaptation, for the existence of adaptive cycles within the athlete's body means that he is programmed to do his thing at the right time. He is prepared in advance for the environmental circumstances to ensue. Thus, an added stress can interact with his otherwise normal activity at the wrong time. A changing environment provides the synchronizer, but synchronization, to be adaptive, means regularity. Any physiological characterization of stresses must consider the temporal organization of the environment and the host organism. Little research has been done in this area, and therefore, little attention to these important considerations has been given in the management of athletes. Conditioning and training regimens and competition is frequently based on convenience, as is scheduling of competitive events. It would be unwise, however, to suggest that our common arrangement of living and working habits is out of phase with our biorhythms. The athlete who trains and competes in the afternoon may well be the beneficiary of near optimal biorhythmicity.

G. Concluding Remarks

Consideration of the above leads to the view that the environmental impact on the organism is indeed complex (see Figs. 4 and 5). The athlete must learn to live with those environmental factors he can not control, learn to adapt to and acclimatize to those over which he has control or must live with, and finally, to learn to avoid those factors or combinations of factors suspected to be deleterious, such as air and

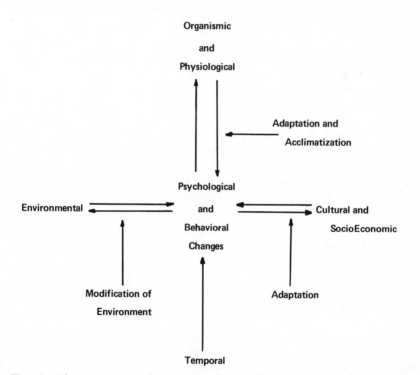

Fig. 4 Schematic pattern of interaction of factors by category in producing physiological, psychological, and behavioral changes. Factors in each category are listed in Fig. 5. It is a tentative list subject to modification with accumulation of additional information through research and literature review.

Organismic and Physiological

Age
Sex
Body Composition
Physical Conditioning and Training
State of Acclimatization
Disability
Disease
Diet — Starvation, Malnutrition
Water Intake — Hypohydration
Metabolic Level
Ability and Skill

Psychological and Behavioral

Environmental

Temperature, Dry Bulb
Humidity — Wet Bulb, Vapor Pressure
Air Movement
Radiation — Infrared, Ultraviolet
Radiation — Ionizing
Light
Sound
Area—Volume, Crowding
Pressure
Gas Mixture
Insulation — Clothing, Buildings, etc.
Housing

Comfort
Dependency — Leadership — Decision Making
Intelligence — Learning
Tolerance
Emotion
Awareness and Sensation — Perception
Accuracy — Efficiency
Attention and Cognition
Anxiety — Apprehension — Well Being
Responsibility — Drive — Incentive
Antagonism — Disruption — Irritability
Enthusiasm — Exhileration
Psychomotor Performance
Fatigue — Lassitude
Personality

Cultural--Socio—Economic

Locale
Customs
Background
Ambitions
Beliefs

Temporal

Exposure Time
Exposure Sequence
Ordering of Tasks
Diurnal — Seasonal
Rhymicity
Transient States
Time Appreciation and Judgement
Time Course of Changes

Fig. 5 Interacting variables affecting the athlete or any other person. Variables in each category can interact with several others in the same or different categories.

water pollution, ionizing radiation, excessive noise, habit forming drugs, alcoholic beverages, and malnutrition.

SELECTED REFERENCES

Adams, T., and Iampietro, P. F. (1968). *In* "Exercise Physiology" (H. B. Falls, ed.), p. 173. Academic Press, New York.

Adolph, E. F. (1956). *Amer. J. Physiol.* **184**, 18.

Balke, B., ed. (1968). "Physiological Aspects of Sports and Physical Fitness." Amer. Coll. Sports Med. and The Athletic Insitute, Chicago, Illinois.

Belding, H. S. (1967). *In* "Thermobiology" (A. H. Rose, ed.). Academic Press, New York.

Bevegard, S., and Shepherd, J. T. (1967). *Physiol. Rev.* 47, 178.

Bullard, R. W., and Rapp, G. M. (1970). *Aerosp. Med.* 41, 1269.

Buskirk, E. R. (1969). *In* "Biomedicine Problems of High Terrestrial Elevations" (A. H. Hegnauer, ed.), p. 204. USARIEM, Natick.

Buskirk, E. R. (1971). *Proc. Symp. ASHRAE Hum. Factors,* 1971, p. 5.

Buskirk, E. R., and Bass, D. E. (1974). *In* "Science and Medicine of Exercise and Sports" (W. R. Johnson and E. R. Buskirk, eds.), 2nd ed. Harper, New York.

Buskirk, E. R., Loomis, J. L., and McLaughlin, E. R. (1971). *NACDA Quart.* 5, 22.

Dautrebande, L. (1962). "Microaerosols." Academic Press, New York.

Dill, D. B., ed. (1964). "Handbook of Physiology," Sect. 4, Williams & Wilkins, Baltimore, Maryland.

Empleton, B. E., (1968). "The New Science of Skin and Scuba Diving." Association Press, New York.

Faulkner, J. A. (1968). *In* "Exercise Physiology" (H. B. Falls, ed.), p. 415–446. Academic Press, New York.

Football Injuries. (1970). Papers Presented at a Workshop. Nat. Acad. Sci., Washington, D.C.

Hardy, J. C. (1967). *In* "Cecil-Loeb Textbook of Medicine" (P. B. Beeson and N. McDermott, eds.). Saunders, Philadelphia, Pennsylvania.

Karvonen, M. J., Friverg, O., Antilla, E. (1955). *Ann. Med. Exp. Biol. Fenn.* 33, 326.

Kollias, J., and Buskirk, E. R. (1973). *In* "Science and Medicine of Exercise and Sports" (W. R. Johnson and E. R. Buskirk, eds.), 2nd ed. Harper, New York (in press).

Lee, D. H. K., and Minard, D., eds. (1970). "Physiology, Environment, and Man." Academic Press, New York.

Leithead, C. S., and Lind, A. R. (1964). "Heat Stress and Heat Disorders." Davis, Philadelphia, Pennsylvania.

Mathews, D. K., and Fox, E. L. (1971). "The Physiological Basis of Physical Education and Athletics." Saunders, Philadelphia, Pennsylvania.

Murphy, R. J., and Ashe, W. F. (1965). *J. Amer. Med. Ass.* 194, 180.

Novich, M., and Taylor, B. (1970). "Training and Conditioning of Athletes." Lea & Febiger, Philadelphia, Pennsylvania.

Rushmer, R. F., and Buettner, K. J. K (1966). *Science* 154, 343.

Weike, W. H., ed. (1964). "The Physiological Effects of High Altitude." Macmillan, New York.

Chapter 11

ROLE OF SKILLS AND RULES IN THE PREVENTION OF SPORTS INJURIES

ALLAN J. RYAN

I. OVERVIEW

Skill in sports practice depends on highly coordinated movements. Many of these movements are inherently dangerous or are rendered

235

so by the circumstances under which they are performed. The unskilled individual is at a greater risk under these circumstances and may endanger others including spectators in certain activities.

Rules of sports and games are developed initially in order to define the nature and limits of competition. Some of these contribute incidentally to safety for the participants. As the result of practice of sports and games, further rules are introduced primarily for the purpose of promoting safety. Coaches, players, and officials have a serious obligation to know the rules thoroughly and to observe them in the spirit as well as according to the letter. Officials may be able to prevent many injuries in situations that are extrinsic as well as intrinsic to play by a careful and impartial enforcement of the rules.

II. THE ROLE OF SPORTS SKILLS IN INJURY PREVENTION

A. The Development of Sports Skills

The development of proficiency in any sports activity, whether the individual is coached or self-taught, depends on the successful interaction of a number of basic abilities or capacities that may be naturally present or acquired by training. A model to illustrate the complex relationships involved is shown in Fig. 1. Strength, cardiorespiratory function, speed of movement, and coordination of movement are conceived of as independent variables with the dependent variables being endurance, whole body movement, power, reaction time, agility, flexibility, and balance.

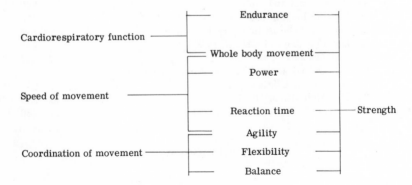

Fig. 1 Interrelationships of basic abilities and capacities required to produce performance skills.

It is possible to influence favorably all of the independent variables by training, although speed of movement appears to be a natural endowment of certain individuals, and the amount which any one individual may improve on his natural speed seems to be much more limited than the development of any other capacity. Since both dependent and independent variables may be improved by training, it becomes especially important to establish what part deficiency in these basic capacities may play in the production of acute and chronic sports injuries.

There are few sports in which all of the dependent and independent variable shown in Fig. 1 are not involved to some extent. It is safe to assume that the greater part any of these variables plays in the activities associated with any particular sport, the greater will be the effect of a deficiency or a misapplication in this quality in the production of injury in that sport. It is possible by analyzing sports carefully to determine for each one which qualities are most demanded and in what order of importance. Such an exhaustive analysis will not be attempted here. Rather, an attempt will be made to assess how the combination of these abilities to produce efficiency may act to prevent injury in certain typical actions common to many sports, leaving the application to a particular sport to be made by those who are interested.

Success in sports is favored by the development of the basic qualities of performance to the point where they may be applied to a maximum degree. The athlete must be able to exercise a control over his application of these qualities, however, which goes beyond the coordination of his efforts. This added quality may best be described in familiar terms as a sense of pace. This implies the ability to discriminate a level of response appropriate to the situation and to vary this level from moment to moment as the situation requires to meet the exigencies of the time and yet to maintain some reserve for the expected duration of the activity.

At the same time the athlete must also maintain a continuing critical appraisal of his situation in order to select the appropriate response from the many responses which he has been trained to make. This might be termed judgment. The exercise of his judgment is facilitated by two factors, anticipation and reflex reaction. Judgment and anticipation come from experience in the particular sport, which indicates the possibility of certain events occurring and, coupled with continuing observation at the moment, selects which occurrence is most probable, initiating a response slightly before the event takes place.

Reflex reaction results from the patterning of activity which is developed by training. The repeated practice of individual sports acts or combinations of these acts which are apt to occur regularly in sequence

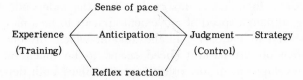

Fig. 2   Interrelationships of skill determinants dependent on central nervous system functions.

allows the individual to respond to a stimulus without having to will the response. Depending on the individual's reaction time, the speed of the response may be so rapid that the individual may not be aware until afterwards that it took place. This ability to "groove" appropriate reactions allows the athlete to progress to the highest level of skill not of a purely physical character, the ability to plan and execute strategy while the action is already in progress.

A model showing the interrelationships of the experience acquired from sports training to the development of sense of pace, anticipation, and reflex reaction, leading to control and allowing the continuous planning and revision of strategy in action is shown in Fig. 2.

B. The Relationship of Skill to Success in Sports

Success in sports depends not only on the development of basic capacities and abilities and directing them in a highly coordinated fashion into skilled performance but also on attitude and good fortune. The role of attitude in producing success or failure as well as its possible role in the production of injury is to be found in Chapter 7.

Good fortune plays a part in every successful sports outcome, no matter what level of skill is required. Generally speaking the part that luck plays is inversely proportional to the degree of skill required by the particular sports activity. In the same way, as the skill of performers increases, fortune plays a lesser role in their competitions.

As a consequence of these considerations, one would expect that, where training had been effective in developing the basic capacities and abilities, where skill was highly developed, and where positive attitudes prevailed among all those engaged in a particular sport, performance would be consistent and that fortune would play a very small part. Where the competitors all fall within the same narrow age range and are engaged in events in which the results can be measured in terms of time elapsed or distance covered the outcomes are predictable with reasonable accuracy if preliminary data on previous performances (form) are available. In a recent Big Ten Swimming Championship, all placings except four in the finals of the swimming events could have been predicted on the basis of the competitors' previous best times for the season.

An individual who manifests basic capacities to an extraordinary degree may be entirely unable to produce a successful performance in any one or a number of sports activities unless he can master the skills involved. The super-heavyweight weight lifting champion of the world could not even take a place in a shot put competition unless he had practiced and learned the skills involved in that event. All skill training is specific and it would only be a coincidence if, without any previous practice, he should make an outstanding throw the first few times he made the attempt. Where refinements of technique can add very little to the effectiveness of basic capacities, however, as in sprinting, an unskilled athlete may be very successful up to a point. If the crouching start is eliminated from a short sprint race, since this is a highly skilled activity, a naturally fast runner might easily defeat a highly trained one.

C. Hazardous Actions in Sports Practice and Competition

All movement of the body or any of its parts invokes a possibility of injury either as the result of the action of the body itself or of its interaction with its environment. The greater the control of the movement the less danger there is of an injury occurring. The internal factors that tend to lessen this control are the speed of the movement, slow reaction time, uncoordinated muscle activity, lack of flexibility, lack of agility, loss of balance, lack of strength, lack of endurance, and loss of concentration. The external factors are persons or objects in the environment and uncontrolled external forces.

Actions of sports are characteristically forceful and vigorous. A tremendous range is involved from the leisurely pace of croquet to the hurtling speed of a racing car. Even within any one sport the variety of activities involved can impose minimum or maximum stresses on the individual from time to time. Since sport involves a testing of the individual against himself or against his environment at a maximum performance level, many of its activities must be viewed in relation to ordinary activities of daily living as manifestly unsafe. It is the development of skill that makes the categorically unsafe activity relatively safe according to the degree of proficiency exhibited.

The performance of a two and one-half, full-twisting forward somersault from a 3-meter diving board is a relatively safe activity for an experienced diver. If he loses his concentration in his approach, mistimes his hurdle, and attempts a midcourse correction to prevent overshooting, form is shattered, the dive is a failure, and the diver may be injured as the result of his improper entry into the water. If he misjudges his distance from the board on an inward dive, he may hit the board in his descent with disastrous results. If he fails to make the proper adjustment to the depth of the pool in his recovery, he may injure himself on the bottom.

Both acute and chronic injuries may occur as the results of the body movement of the individual independent of his environment. In the absence of an inherent weakness in the part affected, the acute injuries rarely occur when the activity is performed in a skilled fashion, unless some environmental circumstance alters the conditions. The skilled halfback in football should be able to run fast and shift his direction quickly to evade pursuers without damage to the meniscus, of his knee. If the turf is wet so that his foot slips as he makes his cut, if the cleats of his shoe hold in the turf a fraction of a second too long, or if he is knocked off balance by a missed tackle, the tear may occur quite easily. The Achilles tendon seldom ruptures in the younger and lighter athlete, but may do so in the older and heavier athlete when its tensile strength is suddenly exceeded by a combination of weight, leverage, and aging of the tendon from previous subclinical strains.

Incoordination of the antagonistic actions of the hip flexor and extensor muscles in the sprinter may result in a tear of the extensor muscles which are normally weaker, the so-called "hamstring pull." Lack of flexibility in the shoulder may result in a tear of the posterior capsule when it is subjected to maximum stress, as in making a tackle. Lack of agility may allow the squash player to collide with his opponent in the court. Loss of balance at a critical moment may cause a gymnast to fall from his apparatus. Lack of endurance may cause a swimmer to drown. Lack of strength may cause a weightlifter to lose his form and dislocate an elbow.

Many sports activities create stresses on the body for which no amount of training or conditioning can compensate. They may do so by requiring an abnormal range of movement or by repeatedly stressing some area an amount close to its maximum ability to resist such a stress or to recover from it. The baseball pitcher in throwing an overhand pitch moves his shoulder and elbow joints through a range of motion which is abnormal for them as it reaches its extremes. At the same time, in throwing a curve ball he puts a strain on the ligamentous attachments of forearm muscles to the internal epicondyle of the humerus, producing a chronic inflammation, which is sometimes known as "pitcher's elbow." At the same time, failure to develop proper skills or periodic failures in technique may cause such chronic conditions to become worse than they might be otherwise or cause flare-ups producing severe disability.

In some sports the contact with other individuals is deliberate since it is a part of the total activity, as in American football. In others it is either semideliberate, as in basketball, or inevitable, as in soccer, where two or more persons are trying to occupy the same space at the same time. In baseball it may be deliberate, as when the catcher blocks the home plate against a base runner, semideliberate as when a runner contacts an infielder on a base path, or accidental, as when two fielders collide in the pursuit of a fly ball. In such potential situations the skilled individual by conscious or involuntary avoidance of his teammate or opponent may be able to prevent serious injury.

In combat sports, injury may arise from personal contact, as in wrestling or boxing, or through a weapon, as in fencing or Kendo. Here the practice of avoidance is an essential skill and takes two forms, which may be designated as defensive and offensive. The defensive aspect involves the abilities to move the threatened part of the body away from the impending blow, to partially avoid, or "slip," the blow so that it is ineffective, or to parry the blow by interposing another less vulnerable or protected part of the body or a weapon to prevent it from reaching its target. The offensive aspect is to press home the attack in such a way that the opponent is on the defensive and less able to land telling blows or holds of his own. Naturally a high premium is placed on skill in the prevention of injury in such sports. A winning boxer may be totally unmarked and the loser severely battered as the result of his inferior skill in avoidance.

Avoidance is a skill based on a fast reaction time, good speed of movement, agility, and balance. Bobby Orr taking the hockey puck up the ice through a swirl of back-checking forwards and waiting defensemen, and somehow arriving in front of the opposing goal without being touched and with the puck still cradled on his stick, exemplifies this art to its highest degree. In ice hockey, as in field hockey, lacrosse, hurling, polo, or in other sports where sticks or rackets are used to propel missiles such as balls or pucks avoidance must become instinctive for players who wish to avoid injury. Protective equipment is being developed increasingly to prevent the unavoidable injury, but its use, unfortunately, tends to lessen the development of avoidance skills and foster an atmosphere of bravado which frequently tests the equipment beyond its capacity to protect.

Speed provides a major hazard to the athlete in any motorized sport which it is difficult for him to control. As speed increases, even the fastest reaction times may be powerless to cope with unexpected events that may occur in the path of the speeding vehicle. Racing automobile speeds are now so high that a driver coming out of a curve on an oval track is actually driving blind for the first section of the straight stretch he is entering. If another car has spun in the track at that point and he has no other signal to warn him, he will be into it before he can actually see it and take diversionary action. In world record speed trials, the driver can bear down or back off on the accelerator and may have some type of brake (usually a parachute) at his disposal. Otherwise he is a victim of any untoward circumstance that may arise during the course of his trial.

Environmental factors that create hazards and may be responsible for injury may or may not be influenced by the skills of the competitors. Very rough and very cold waters have been mastered by skilled marathon swimmers where those of lesser ability have had to give up. Bumpy ice, poorly prepared fields, and splintery floors pose equal hazards to the skilled and the unskilled. Fortune does tend to favor the well-prepared, but human skill and strength are sometimes helpless against implacable natural forces such as gales, electric storms, blizzards, and the like.

Finally, something must be said about the foolhardy athlete who takes unnecessary or unwarranted chances in the face of great danger. They can be divided into three groups: those who are ignorant of what they are getting into; those who know and do not care; and those who know and care but set too great a store in their skills and experience through overconfidence. The first lacks proper instruction, whether this is accidental or deliberate on his part. The second is perhaps driven by complex motives that neither he nor we understand fully. The third finds his archetype in the explorer who seeks to widen the boundaries of human experience by doing what has not been done before.

D. The Occurrence of Injury in the Unskilled

Relatively little has been done so far to document actual rates of occurrence of injury in most sports. Most texts and articles in Sports Medicine deal with the description of typical injuries in sports without reporting injury rates. The few exceptions among sports practiced by large numbers of persons are American football, Little League Baseball, and downhill skiing. It can be expected that little of a definitive nature can be said, therefore, with regard to the relative occurrence of injuries among the unskilled as compared to the skilled in most sports.

There is some evidence to indicate that boys who participate in tackle football beginning in the sixth grade of school suffer less injuries at the eighth and ninth grade levels than those who do not begin until they reach the ninth grade (Robey et al., 1970). High school football players with a history of physical education and tumbling exhibit a significantly lower injury rate than those without this experience (Mc-Carty, 1969). Although 60 to 75% of the injuries in high school football are sustained by varsity players, this appears to be a matter of greater exposure time in practice and games (McClelland, 1965). In college football, sophomores appear to sustain more injuries than juniors or seniors (Moore, 1968). In professional football, rookies are twice as vulnerable to injuries as veterans (King, 1967). Nicholas (1969) points out, however, that rookies make up the largest number of "special team" members and that these players are three times more likely to suffer injury than those who play only on the regular offensive and defensive squads.

Haddon et al. (1962) classified injured and control downhill skiers according to their skills by dividing them into three groups according to their mastery of turning on their skis: (1) snow plow, (2) stem christie, and (3) parallel or wedeln. Skiers' self-ratings as beginner, novice, intermediate, or expert correlated highly with these groups. The injury rate was six times higher in the snow plow than in the parallel turn group. O'Malley (1967) found in a study of ski injuries at Mount Tom, Massachusetts that novice skiers accounted for about two-thirds of all the fractures that were sustained. Spademan (1968) found in a 4-year study of ski injuries at Squaw Valley, California that, when the number of injuries is related to years of skiing experience, there is a substantial reduction after one year of experience. Brody and McAlister (1965) found in a study of the epidemiology of ski injuries in the Anchorage, Alaska area that, although beginning skiers skied less vertical feet per day than the more advanced skiers, they had higher accident rates. Garrick (1971) in the National Ski Safety Research Study (1964–1967) reported that the variables of age, sex, and skiing ability seem to be most closely related to variations in injury rates. He found that the passage from class A (least ability) to class C (most ability) generally results in a decreased injury rate and that this decrease is most pronounced in skiers under 35 and more pronounced in males than in females.

It is quite obvious that the degree of expertise required in order to be able to participate safely in sports varies greatly according to the nature of the sport. The person who is unable to swim, or who can only swim very poorly, may drown if thrown into the water and not rescued. The athlete attempting a giant swing on the high bar with little or no experience will almost certainly fly off and probably be injured. The novice race driver in a race with highly skilled professionals endangers not only his own life but that of others.

Team sports contests where all participants are novices may actually have a low injury occurrence since it is not possible to have a sustained character of play at a high level, where the increased speed of the activity becomes a factor in injury production. In sports in which physical contact of a vigorous nature may take place, however, it is essential that there be classification by abilities as well as by age, height, and/or weight, since the unskilled players will then have a much higher injury rate if they are badly outclassed.

E. Coaching and Learning Skills Correctly

1. The Coach

Although it is required by law that persons teaching in public educational institutions shall possess at least certain minimal educational qualifications and shall be licensed either on the basis of holding a degree or other evidence of such qualification, or by examination, in many places there are no set educational standards that have to be met by coaches in relationship to sports and physical education generally, or to the sport that they are intending to coach specifically. This probably represents to some extent a reflection of the tradition that a sports team was coached by its captain, who was simply a senior member of the team. It gives no assurance, however, that the coach knows the correct skills of his sport or that he knows how to teach them.

Primarily as the result of a concern for the health and safety of the boys and girls committed to the care of coaches in our educational institutions, there is an increasing tendency today in the United States to require certification of coaches. The reason for certification, the problems which may be involved, and recommended standards have been outlined in the publication "Certification of High School Coaches" (Maetozo, 1971). One of the principal problems is that the great expansion of interscholastic and intercollegiate sports activities and the expense of these programs has made it necessary for schools and colleges to hire men and women as coaches who are not trained physical educators. Many of them have never even played the sport they are coaching.

Experience in playing a sport is not of itself a sufficient qualification for a coach. Successful athletes are frequently unable to show anyone else how they do something except by demonstration, since they have developed their skills intuitively without giving thought to the process. Some first class athletes make excellent coaches, but usually because they have a good general sports background and other qualities that help to make a successful coach. Some of the most successful coaches were never outstanding as performers.

2. The Coaching Process

From the standpoint of injury prevention the four essentials in the coaching process are progression, demonstration, repetition, and supervision.

Progression means breaking down the activities of a given sport into teachable elements that may be combined in various ways to produce the fundamental movements required. These are practiced individually and in patterns to reproduce as closely as possible the exact actions of the sport in all of its aspects. All training is specific. It also means that learning progresses from the simpler to the more complex patterns of movement.

Demonstration involves showing the actions desired as they should be performed either by the coach himself or another athlete who has mastered the form required. Live demonstration is supplemented by the use of film to show at natural speed and in slow motion how it is done by the expert, and how the person being taught has done it on a previous occasion. Video tape is particularly useful here since it can be run almost immediately after it has been recorded.

Repetition is essential to the learning of basic skills for any sport. They must become so automatic that they are produced with a minimum of conscious effort. They must be reproduced each time as exactly as possible in accordance with the model. The coach is challenged to keep this necessary repetition from becoming too boring and the execution from becoming careless.

Supervision of practice contributes to the development of skills by allowing a continuous reassessment of progress, the correction of unintentional errors that may creep in as the athlete increases the intensity of his training, the prevention of distraction, and the opportunity for interchange as questions arise in the mind of the athlete.

3. Dangerous Skills

Certain skills may lead to success in sports but they involve unacceptable risks to the athlete and to his opponents. The exercise of these skills may not be expressly forbidden in the rules. Whether such tactics are considered to be ethical by all concerned seems to vary from time to time depending on factors in the sport which are only partially under the control of coach and athlete.

Such a skill in American football is "face blocking and tackling." I categorize this as a single skill since the principle element involved in both is the same, to confront the opponent head-on and, if possible, place the face mask against the numerals on the front of his jersey. What makes this a successful technique, according to the coaches, is that it gives the blocker or tackler the ability to counter easily any effort of the opponent to get to either side of him. What makes it a dangerous technique is that it may place an abnormal strain on the neck. Even more dangerous is the possibility that if not executed with perfect timing the top of the helmet may be driven into the opponent putting an even greater stress on the neck and exposing the brain to injury in spite of the cushioning effect of the helmet.

Face blocking and tackling are perfectly legal in football and are currently considered to be ethical as well as effective techniques. "Spearing," which is the term used to describe hitting the opponent head-on with the helmet, is only illegal if it is done with "malicious intent." It is not considered to be unethical if it develops accidentally, and it is unofficially condoned and even encouraged by some coaches, as long as the player is not found to be using it deliberately by the officials.

The cross-body block is also a dangerous technique for the blocker if not timed and executed so that unprotected areas of the ribs and flank are not exposed to the lower limbs of the opponent. It is a legal block and has always been considered an ethical technique. At the time of this writing an experiment will be made by the NCAA Rules Committee in requiring this block to be made above the level of the knees. It may be very damaging to the knees of the person being blocked, especially if he is hit unexpectedly. This has been the case in the past particularly with the "crack-back" block. This block has now also been made illegal by the Rules committee. An offensive player can no longer move out of the imaginary box which encloses the central line area and then come back into it to block an opponent below waist level.

Additional examples could be cited from other sports. Suffice it to say that a coach teaching or a player practicing such skills must be prepared to take the full consequences for his acts. The possible serious consequences should be known in advance, including being adjudged guilty of unsportsmanlike conduct.

4. The Self-Taught Athlete

Some athletes have learned sports solely through imitation and instinct. If both have been good, they may be highly skilled and relatively safe from an injury due to poor technique. If their model for imitation has not been a good one, then they may have defects in their skills which makes them prone to injury. A pitcher who has learned (incorrectly) to step across his line to the plate may be subject to developing a sore arm. By the time he gets to a coach who can teach him the proper technique it may be very difficult for him to change.

Athletes who are successful in one sport may feel that they can transfer their skills easily to master another sport without having to learn anything new. A dangerous sport in this regard is downhill skiing, where the natural instincts of the athlete trained in another sport may cause him to do the exact opposite from what he should to correct his balance. People will spend hundreds of dollars for clothing and equipment to go skiing and will not spend a few more to take some basic lessons. They frequently end up by spending many more in terms of medical care and time lost from work.

III. THE ROLE OF RULES IN INJURY PREVENTION

A. The Purposes of Rules in Sports and Games

In primitive sports and games rules were developed by common consent and became established by custom. Their initial purpose is to define the nature of the sport. To do this they make specific requirements and set certain limits. They also decide how the winner is to be determined. They are not written down but are passed along by oral tradition and everyone who plays understands them. Changes take place gradually as creative individuals introduce variations, some of which are accepted as rules and become part of the tradition.

Codification begins when someone for historical or other purposes prepares a written description of the game as he has seen it played and heard it discussed by the players. In time this written record is used to recreate the game for those who are not in the direct line of the oral tradition. They may modify it to their own purposes, producing further variations. Competitions between individuals or groups who come from other localities may require consultation to establish common rules which to some extent are local traditions. When competition becomes regular, some rules making and keeping body is appointed to preserve the established traditions in an orderly process.

Somewhere in the course of this procedure, regulations appear which have primarily the purpose of equalizing competition rather than merely defining it or limiting it. These may relate to numbers in group sports, to relative sizes in individual contests, or to creating handicaps in order to account for differences in skill and experience. Implements and objects used in sports are standardized. The appropriate costume may be designated. Judges or officials are provided to interpret and to enforce the rules. Eventually additional rules appear to confirm interpretations that have been made consistently, or to prevent practices that have arisen to the detriment of the game but are not covered by existing rules.

B. The Development of Rules for Safety

Usually, rather late in the evolution of rules, come those that are directed primarily at the problem of preventing or reducing injuries. These rules may be concerned with facilities, environmental circumstances such as weather, personal equipment, and tactics or practices demonstrated to be unsafe.

Coaches and athletes tend to be very conservative with regard to the rules they have learned and played under, and usually demonstrate considerable resistance to changing them. This is particularly true in the case of rules for safety, since these rules frequently produce restrictions in styles of play which are popular and spectacular even though they may be quite dangerous. As a consequence, requests to rulemaking bodies for changes to promote safety should be well documented with a sound theoretical and practical rationale and illustrative cases.

Rules for safety may ban tactics which it has been learned by experience may produce serious injury. The use of a full-nelson hold in wrestling is outlawed because a strong, experienced wrestler may break someone's neck with it. They may require the use of a specific type of protective equipment to safeguard an area that may be endangered in the usual practice of the sport. The football helmet is a good example of equipment that must be worn if the player is to participate. They may provide that a baseball game be called in the event of rain. Control of bat and ball and footing on the slippery field would be greatly hampered under such circumstances. They may require that the blade of a hockey stick be of a certain measurement or curvature and that the tip of the blade be no narrower than a certain distance. The stick is dangerous enough as it is without allowing it to be converted into a lethal weapon. They may specify a certain type of construction and protective covering for the floor of a boxing ring, in order to prevent more severe head injury in a fighter who falls out of control after a stunning punch.

C. Effects of Changes in Sports Techniques on Existing Rules

Those who are responsible for the safety of athletes must be continually on the alert for those changes in the character and style of play which are characteristic of all sports but which may also introduce new elements of danger to the players. Rules previously thought to be adequate for protection become outmoded. A striking example of such a situation occurred in American football where the rules have always permitted blocking from behind within a rectangle based on the line of scrimmage and extending three yards into offensive and defensive zones. The theory was that the dangers of injury to the knee would be much less than in "clipping" in the open field because less impact was involved. The technique of the "crack-back" block, in which an offensive player moved out of the zone and then back into it, altered the situation by introducing the elements of surprise and greater impact.

The introduction of new events into existing sports may require existing rules to be modified or new ones added. The dynamic character of most sports ensures that such events will occur periodically. Many examples are afforded in the present explosive development of auto racing.

Improved technology may require rules changes. The greater heights which can be achieved in the pole vault due to the introduction of the Fiberglas pole have made it necessary to require that the pits be padded with foam rubber rather than sawdust or sand to prevent injury. The change of auto racing fuel from an alcohol-ether-nitro mixture to high-test gasoline has created a greater hazard of fire and explosion, requiring new rules to protect the driver in the way of protective clothing and crash-resistant gas tanks.

D. Who Makes the Rules?

Rules for organized competitive sports are made and revised by national and international governing bodies for the sports concerned. These bodies appoint rules committees who receive suggestions and complaints and adjudicate disputes. Their recommendations for rules changes must be approved by the governing body and ratified by the membership to become effective.

Leagues and conferences in each sport generally adopt the rules of the parent organization which is the national or international sports federation, but may add certain modifications to suit their own purposes but which do not alter the regulation of the sport substantially as far as play is concerned. Local rules may also be established by mutual agreement among the competitors to take into account special problems which may be presented by the facilities or environment existing.

The rules for amateurs and professionals playing in the same sport may vary somewhat, since the rules for professional sports are established by each league for its own use. These differences ordinarily do not disturb the basic character of the sport. There is a tendency for amateur and professional rules to influence each other over a period of time. Special rules may apply to international sports events, such as the Olympic Games, but they tend to follow the rules of the international sports federations very closely.

Rules for many individual sports that are usually conducted informally are established by the governing bodies of the sports for use in competitions but have little or nor effect on the casual practice of the sports. In some cases the governing bodies or safety groups have formulated sets of suggestions or rules as a code for the behavior of the participants. These codes deal with courtesy, sportsmanship, and injury prevention, primarily. There is little power to enforce them except in very closely controlled situations. Such codes, nevertheless, may have great effect as the result of voluntary action.

Where questions of public safety are involved, federal state or local authorities may establish rules that are enforced by patrol and discourage violation by providing fines and jail sentences for violators. Regulations regarding boating in navigable inland and coastal waters, and controlling the use of air space for sports parachuting are examples of such regulatory action.

There is an unfortunate tendency in American sports for rules-making bodies to be dominated by active coaches at the high school and college level. The viewpoints of the athlete, trainer, and physician are seldom represented in these bodies. The coaches view themselves as the only persons qualified to maintain and revise the rules but are notable for their lack of self-criticism and ability to evaluate the games in which they are so involved emotionally and financially in an objective way.

E. Periodic Review and Revision of the Rules

International sports federations, national athletic organizations, private nonprofit sports associations, and collegiate and high school conferences all have rules committees whose functions are to consider requests for changes in rules and make recommendations to the parent body, to conduct studies of the effects of application of existing rules under the changing circumstances of the games and of the times, and to initiate proposals for rules changes based on the observations and experiences of committee members. No consistent pattern can be discerned which is generally applicable to such committees since some tend to be extremely conservative, approving few changes over long periods of time, whereas others are quite active in changing rules almost every year. The number of years for which the sport has had a recognized governing body appears to have some relationship to the rate of rule change, with older organizations changing more slowly, as might be expected.

Outstanding examples of rules committees that are quite sensitive to the need for changes, but are generally conservative in their approach to major revisions, are those of the National Federation in the United States. This organization represents high school federations in the great majority of the states, junior colleges, and many small colleges not members of the two big collegiate federations. Their rules committees in football, basketball, wrestling, swimming, track and field, and baseball annually poll their membership, including coaches and officials, to determine the desirability or necessity of modifying rules, at the same time offering constructive suggestions for consideration in this regard. One of the results of this constant surveillance is that the National Federation leads all other comparable organizations in the introduction and modification of rules that make for safer sports participation.

Federal, state, or municipal bodies that make rules governing sports and recreational activities tend to be responsive to public pressures for changes but are not inclined to be innovative. Their willingness to respond to suggestions and recommendations for changes appears to be inversely proportional to their distance from the person or group seeking the changes.

The United States Ski Association took the unusual step in 1969 of appointing a National Skier's Action Board whose function is to represent "the consumer's voice to the [ski] industry." Composed of leading skiers, ski club officials, and other USSA members from all over the United States, this group has been concerned with safety standards that could be applied locally in the form of regulations and has conducted field tests of some of the ideas suggested at Aspen Highlands. It has invited comment from the skiing public at large, ski area operators, manufacturers of ski equipment, and representatives of ski-related industries. If effective, this mechanism of periodic review and revision of rules in a voluntary association could contribute greatly to ski safety.

IV. THE ROLE OF OFFICIALS IN INJURY PREVENTION

The administration of any but the most informal sports events requires advance planning, preparation, supervision, and frequently certification of the results. The numbers of persons engaged in these duties will vary from one to thousands depending on the nature and scope of the event. The Olympic Games currently require the services of many times the number of officials more than the numbers of athletes. Relatively few of these persons act in positions where they can influence the occurrence of injuries directly, and only a few more may have some indirect influence.

A. Differing Roles of Officials in Sports

When one official takes the entire responsibility for the conduct of a game, he is generally known today as the referee. He has under his surveillance not only the administration of the rules of the game but also the keeping of time, the conduct of players during the action, the conduct of athletes and coaches not participating directly in the action, and the conduct of the spectators. When more than one official is involved, the referee remains the head official (although he is sometimes called the umpire), delegating some of his duties to linesmen, judges, scorers, clerks of the course, timers, and appointees to many other possible duties.

Those officials who have direct control over the conduct of the athletes, such as referees, umpires, field judges, clerks of the course, etc., may by their actions or inactions have great or very little effect on the occurrence of injuries. They have a difficult task of applying the rules and interpreting them, but they are charged also with seeing that the game is played according to the spirit of the rules with due regard to sportsmanship and ethics. The others may influence the outcome of a game by their conduct and their decisions but seldom affect the occurrence of injury.

B. Qualifications of Officials

Since the role of an official is frequently decisive in determining the outcome of a sports contest, and since the outcome is often extremely important to a great number of persons for social, financial, and emotional reasons, it is desirable to have one who is trained as highly as possible in the art of officiating. Since officiating is not usually considered as a full-time career by most persons, full-time study programs are not offered in this field at the college level. Some of the professional sports operate schools for officials which are usually for a relatively short term and lead to a certificate. Isolated courses in officiating are offered at the undergraduate level in most physical education programs.

The typical Official qualifies for his position by home study and then takes an examination for certification. He is ordinarily a person who has been involved in sports or physical education and wishes to supplement his income by officiating. Officiating is only a part-time job for him. He continues at it usually for the love of the sport rather than the income as he gets older.

In professional baseball, basketball, and ice hockey, officials are full-time employees during the season, even though they may have some other business during the offseason. In professional football, the officials are men who work at other jobs during the week and who work mostly because of their interest in the game. In other professional sports, there are mixtures of full-time and part-time officials.

In amateur sports, almost all officials are part-time workers who have other employment. Many are coaches or physical educators. In college sports, undergraduate and graduate students serve as officials for intramural sports contests.

Although professional sports and many college conferences require their officials to undergo periodic reexamination and set certain standards for proficiency which must be met consistently, there is otherwise little attempt to regulate or reeducate officials once they have been certified. Professional football officials keep their skills sharpened by reviewing the films of the games at which they have officiated. This is facilitated by the fact that they work in regular teams that stay together during a season.

A careful review of game films from a high school football conference for one season's play by four qualified observers showed that more than three-quarters of the fouls detected from the films were not called by the game officials. While this might seem to be a serious indictment of the quality of the officiating, it is quite apparent that if all the fouls had been called the games would have become farces. Instant replays on television have shown repeatedly the amazingly high percentage of accurate calls made by officials under difficult circumstances.

Since there are no nationally or generally accepted qualifications for officials outside of professional sports, the quality of officiating tends to vary greatly from one area to another. This leads to difficulty in intersectional contests. More than any other it is probably responsible for officials being accused by players and coaches of teams visiting from other areas of being "homers."

C. The Official as an Observer during Competition

Officials who are working in close contact with athletes on the field, on the court, or in the ring have a responsibility to observe the athletes' mental and physical states during competition. This can be done satisfactorily without unnecessary distraction from the business at hand by a person who is trained to detect the early signs and symptoms of acute illness, exhaustion, and injury. Every official should be required to take at least an elementary course in first aid in order to increase his appreciation of the evidences that an athlete is beginning to weaken and may require assistance.

In the case of mental confusion, often the first sign of injury or illness, the official may be in the best position to detect this, even before the coach or trainer may sense it from the sidelines. By acting promptly to stop play temporarily or remove the player from action, a very serious injury or collapse may be averted.

Since injuries may result from fights between players as well as from the natural consequences of the game the experienced official may prevent the fight from occurring by taking some type of action when he sees trouble beginning between two players. Fights seldom occur, and do not usually amount to anything if they do, when officials maintain a tight control of the game.

D. Pressure on Officials

In an intensively competitive or emotional society, the pressure on the officials increases in direct relationship to the importance of the particular contest. Attacks on officials have been a commonplace for many years in the Latin-American countries. They have, unfortunately, become more numerous and more serious in all countries at the present time. This is one of the problems in trying to find and retain good officials.

The purpose of attacking an official verbally or physically is not to get him to change the decision he has just made and to which you object. No official worth his salt will do this unless it can be quite obviously demonstrated to him that he made a mistake as to a fact; there is really no recall on a decision involving judgment on a blatant foul. The purpose, rather, is to intimidate him so that his future decisions will be made in your favor if any question arises. This could actually mean overlooking foul play, which in turn might lead to serious injury.

Spectators at a prize fight may wish to see it continue, even when one fighter in the eyes of the referee is too disabled to continue safely. Pressure will be exerted here even by the fighter's own corner sometimes to continue a hopeless cause that may terminate in a permanent or even fatal injury for the loser. The referee should seek and be guided by the judgment of the ring physician if he has any question in his mind about the advisability of stopping the bout.

Coaches especially have a serious responsibility to conduct themselves in a restrained and gentlemanly fashion, even when they feel that a decision has gone unfairly against their team. Their failure to do so and, indeed, the deliberate attempts that some make to play to the grandstand and incite the crowd may in the end so disturb the officials' control of the game that unnecessary injuries to athletes on both sides may result. Worse still, a riot may be incited, resulting in injuries to spectators as well.

E. The Authority of Officials

The head official is, or should be, in full control of any sports contest. He signals the start as well as the end, and determines when time shall be called during the play. He is constrained to allow any legal request for "time out," but he must still be asked and signal his acquiescence. Except in a very few instances, he is the only person directly connected with the contest who may stop it at any time that he feels it necessary and may call it off entirely at his discretion.

It has been argued that a properly qualified physician in attendance should be able to stop a contest where there is serious danger to one or more of the contestants. This view has been put forward particularly in boxing, where it is felt that the referee may not always be able to judge correctly the condition of a fighter to continue. In my experience, in the great majority of instances the attending physician has easy access to the head official, and no reasonable request on the part of the physician will be refused by a competent official. In Ohio, a few years ago, a football game was called off at half-time at the instigation of a physician when players were suffering from serious heat exhaustion.

The referee has also the power to call off play if conditions become hazardous to the contestants. Bad weather, especially heavy rain, high winds, and excessive fog or smoke are not infrequent causes of postponements or cancellations in the interests of safety for the contestants as well as the comfort of the spectators. Disturbances among the spectators leading to objects being thrown on the playing surface or persons intruding may cause the officials to cancel the contest or declare a forfeit. Again, safety, as well as the preservation of order, is involved.

The referee has also the power to require a player to leave the game. This may be for reasons of improper behavior but it may also be in the interests of his own safety. He may also refuse to accept a substitute coming on the field if he feels that his presence might endanger himself or others. In certain games he may restrict a player only for a limited time or for the entire match. In the extreme case he may recommend, but cannot enforce, a suspension for an indefinite period of time.

In the interest of safety, the officials are charged with seeing that the facilities, equipment, and wearing apparel of the players, including all items of protective equipment, meet the standards for play and for safety specified by the sponsoring organization and by the rules, insofar as these items are covered by them. The using of illegal equipment, such as a hockey stick with a sharpened tip to the blade or a cast covered by a pad on the forearm, may result in serious injury to the player's opponent. Inspections are usually made by the officials a few minutes before the start of the contest.

In many circumstances that arise in sports, especially in regard to fouls, the official is called upon to judge whether the action was accidental or deliberate. In some cases no penalty may be assessed if the action is inadvertent. Here is where the official must be careful to weigh all factors carefully, and in particular the effect on the safety of the persons involved. If it becomes quickly apparent that deliberate shading of the rules by ignoring the spirit and interpreting very narrowly the letter of the law will not be tolerated, the officials will remain in control of the game, but not otherwise.

Officials who are not in the least hesitant to exercise their authority in small matters of little consequence are sometimes reluctant to act promptly and decisively in the interests of safety. Better training and the complete support of administrators, coaches, and athletes themselves will strengthen their resolution to do what is necessary in the exercise of their unquestioned authority.

REFERENCES

Brody, J. A., and McAlister, R. (1965). *Arch. Environ. Health* **10**, 910–914.

Garrick, J. G. (1971). *Med. Trib.* March 31, 24.

Haddon, W., Ellison, A. E., and Carroll, R. E. (1962). *Pub. Health Rep.* **77**, No. 11, 975–991.

King, J. (1967). *TV Guide* October 21, pp. 7–9.

McCarty, M. J. (1969). *Nat. Fed. Press Serv. Chicago* **29**, 7.

McClelland, M. (1965). *J. Amer. Med. Ass.* **193**, 155.

Maetozo, M. G., ed. (1971). "Certification of High School Coaches. "Amer. Ass. Health, Phys. Educ. and Recreation, Washington, D.C.

Moore, R. J. (1968). *Med. Trib.* February 1, 24.

Nicholas, J. S. (1969). *Med. Trib.* January 30, 15.

O'Malley, R. D. (1967). *In* "Proceedings of a Conference on Winter Sports Injuries," p. 117. Medical Center and University Extension Services, University of Wisconsin, Madison.

Robey, J. M., Blyth, C. S., and Mueller, F. O. (1970). *Med. Trib.* March 22, 22.

Spaceman, R. J. (1968). *J. Amer. Med. Ass.* **203**, 445–450.

Chapter 12

THE IMMEDIATE MANAGEMENT OF
SPORTS INJURIES

FRED L. ALLMAN, JR., and ALLAN J. RYAN

The immediate management of sports injuries entails an evaluation of the injured athlete at or near the site of injury, the proper determination of his playability, and the initiation of treatment when needed.

I. DETERMINATION OF PLAYABILITY

All decisions regarding playability of the injured athlete during a game situation are the sole responsibility of the team physician. Decisions regarding playability of the injured athlete during practice circumstances, in absence of a physician, are the responsibility of the athletic trainer, when one is present, and of the head coach if a trainer or physician is not available. It should be determined whether or not the condition of the athlete is such that he may safely remain in the game or must be immediately removed from the game. Also, if removed immediately from the game, how must he be taken from the field? And, does he need to be immediately evacuated and referred to a hospital or other medical facility? If not immediately evacuated, or even if allowed to continue to play, does he need subsequent referral for follow-up care or consultation?

II. RESPONSIBILITY

Knowledge concerning the responsibilities of the physician, trainer, coach, and administrator as well as certain principles of management and a logical approach to on the field diagnosis are essential prerequisites in order to reach the proper field decision and institute necessary first aid measures.

A. Administrative Responsibilities (School or Other Organization)

1. To appoint qualified medical and paramedical personnel as well as coaches who are knowledgeable concerning not only the game itself

but the medical aspects of the game. A team physician should be selected, his activities coordinated into the school's overall health program, and, when possible, coordinated with the program as recommended by the county medical society.

2. To provide proper equipment for on-site emergency care.

3. To provide an adequately equipped off-site emergency care station for care of athletes whose injuries may not require immediate hospitalization.

4. To have a prearranged plan for obtaining immediate medical consultation and transportation of any injured athlete.

5. In absence of a certified athletic trainer, to appoint and train a member of the school system to assist the athletic department in the capacity as a trainer.

B. Physician's Responsibility

1. The physician should serve as chief of the medical team and must coordinate all efforts of the athletic trainer, coach, school nurse, physical therapist, and all others who might be involved in the health care of the athlete. It is the physician's responsibility to oversee the entire health plan and to provide for immediate and follow-up care of all injuries.

2. To see that the athlete is not unnecessarily deprived of the opportunity to participate if an injury or other clinical condition is not potentially serious and does not interfere with the player's performance.

3. To see that the student's future in athletics and in life is not jeopardized by unwarranted participation in a particular sport or by premature return to competition in any sport after injury or illness.

4. To be sufficiently knowledgeable concerning athletic injuries so that he can make a quick, accurate determination of the type and extent of injury.

5. To be prepared to initiate proper treatment promptly, i.e., establish an airway, assure effective respiratory exchange, and restore or maintain effective circulatory volume.

6. To avoid any procedure or activity that may aggravate an existing injury, i.e., splint all obvious or suspected fractures, and avoid unnecessary movement if spinal cord injury is suspected. In case of open wounds, he should avoid further contamination of the wound.

7. Make prompt referral when necessary, and be sure that follow-up health care is provided.

8. Observe the function or the injured player prior to and upon return to participation.

9. To remain calm and unexcited in all emergency situations.

C. Trainer's Responsibility

1. To be present for immediate evaluation of the injured athlete.

2. To have knowledge of standard first aid measures and techniques.

3. To have knowledge of the proper sequence of events and chain of command in any emergency situation.

4. To be able to relate pertinent information of pre-disposing chronic injury, or other information that may or may not relate to the current injury or catastrophe.

5. To be able to assume the responsibility of determining the playability of the injured athlete following injury in the absence of the physician. In situations where there is any question of the playability, return of activity is withheld until a thorough evaluation by a physician is completed.

6. To supervise and/or assist in the application of protective equipment including strapping and bandaging.

7. To maintain records of all injuries and illnesses.

D. Coach's Responsibility

1. To have a knowledge of serious injuries that may be associated with the sport that he is coaching and the first aid measures necessary to manage these injuries properly.

2. To be knowledgeable and to assist in the proper chain of command that must be established in case of injury or emergency situations, i.e., to know the location and telephone number of the assigned physician, and to know the whereabouts of the trainer at all times.

3. To cooperate with the physician and trainer in making certain that a player does not return to participation until cleared for participation by the physician or trainer.

4. To impress upon each player the necessity of reporting any injury or illness, whether minor or severe, to the trainer or physician immediately.

III. PRINCIPLES OF MANAGEMENT

Following any injury, restrict play of the injured athlete and observe, listen, examine, and then initiate treatment when indicated. Before and following return to play, a functional evaluation is necessary.

A. Restrict Play

Any time that it becomes obvious to the coach, physician, or trainer that a player has been injured, that player should be removed from play.

B. Observe

Initial observations should be made on the spot, and later in a more appropriate area restricted from view of spectators so that all necessary clothing and equipment may be removed. Observe the state of consciousness and the general appearance of the athlete, the color of the skin, the ability to move, the respiratory rate, and the presence of abrasions, lacerations, pain, deformity, or bleeding. If he is unconscious, check the character of the pulse, respiratory rate, pupil size and reaction, presence of blood, especially in the external ear, rhinorrhea or otorrhea, abnormal reflexes, and deformity. Establish a baseline level of consciousness as soon as possible.

C. Listen

If the athlete is conscious allow him to relate the experience of his injury. What is injured? What was the mechanism? Was there contact? Was it a direct or indirect blow? Did he fall or did he twist? What did he hear? Was there immediate disability? Was there a feeling of instability? Has there been any previous injury to the same site? If so, what was the extent of the previous injury? What is the site and nature of the pain?

C. Examine

Note any area of swelling, deformity, or muscle spasm. Palpate for tenderness and crepitus. Check for stability, weakness or dysfunction in the extremities, any sensory defect, and the range of motion. It is necessary to determine the nature as well as the extent of the injury. If after careful evaluation the injury appears to be insignificant, then make a functional evaluation of the injured player. If normal function is present, then the athlete can safely be allowed to return to play. If abnormal function is observed, then further participation should be delayed until a more thorough evaluation or definitive treatment has been concluded. If the injury is significant, then restriction of play should be continued and treatment instituted immediately.

IV. LOGICAL APPROACH TO ON-THE-FIELD DIAGNOSIS AND EARLY TREATMENT

A. Head

An early assessment of the level of consciousness is one of the most important factors in evaluating a head injury. Close, careful observation and evaluation of pupil size, weakness or dysfunction in one or more extremities, radical change in blood pressure, pulse, sensory changes, and respiratory rate are all important considerations. If conscious, the athlete should be carefully questioned to determine orientation to time, place, and substance. These questions should not be routine but instead should offer a challenge to the athlete. The conscious athlete should also be questioned about headache, visual disturbances, dizziness, nausea, memory lapses, as well as any other deviation from normal.

Each head injury should be considered to have possibly a concomitant neck injury, and, after palpating the skull, the cervical spine should also be examined. Rhinorrhea, otorrhea, or blood in the external ear canal suggest a basal skull fracture.

Whenever possible it is important that the force that caused the head injury be known, i.e., a head hit by a golf ball would result in deformation of the skull, a knee striking the head would be likely to produce an acceleration injury of the brain, while a fall to the ground with the head striking it violently would most likely cause a deceleration injury of the brain.

Contusions of the brain are usually associated with the loss of consciousness of more than just a few moments, and individuals suffering such injuries are usually slow to clear mentally. Nausea, vomiting, persistent headache, unsteadiness, or any transient neurological deficit in addition to loss of consciousness are further evidence of severe brain injury. A laceration of the brain may not cause an immediate neurological deficit or unconsciousness, however, and concussions are not always accompanied by unconsciousness. The athlete who has suffered a cerebral concussion or other head injury rendering him unconscious, even if only momentarily, should not be permitted to reenter the game. He should be given several days rest from vigorous activity and no contact for at least one week even if the period of unconsciousness was of brief duration and without any significant sequelae. The complete disappearance of headache, which almost inevitably follows any concussion or contusion of the brain, is a good guide as to the time when a player may return to full activity.

The use of ammonia inhalants, sedatives, and narcotics should be avoided during the immediate postinjury period. If a mouthpiece is present at the time of injury, this should be removed and the airway maintained. Judicious care in handling and transporting an athlete with a head or neck injury is essential. If comatose, the patient should be kept off his back and maintained on his side with proper positioning of head and neck so that the airway is kept patent. All significant head and neck injuries should be transferred under constant supervision as soon as possible to a hospital where further evaluation, including skull and cervical spine X-rays, and periodic reevaluation can be carried out. The level of consciousness should be monitored closely and appropriate measures taken should the patient's condition show signs of deterioration.

B. Neck

Athletes suspected of having a cervical spine injury must be treated with utmost respect. The examining physician must rule out the possibility of fracture and/or dislocation. Any persisting pain around or radiating from the spine requires immediate suspension of the player from play until it is thoroughly understood. Fractures of the neck can, and do, occur without damage to the spinal cord. It is important to examine and handle neck injury patients carefully to prevent such an injury if it has not already occurred. Even in cases with an injury to the spinal cord, prevention of additional spinal cord insult due to additional motion at a fracture or dislocation site is still an important immediate consideration. The examiner should therefore be extremely careful in removing the helmet or in moving the patient.

The state of consciousness, any deformity, and ability to move the extremities should be closely observed. Tenderness, muscle spasm, and stiffness should be noted. The presence of numbness, tingling, burning, or other paresthesias is indicative of injury to the cord.

Lateral flexion injuries of the cervical spine, the so-called "pinched nerve," may produce severe, hot, burning pain in the shoulder and/or extremity. Neurological changes in the upper extremity are common following such injuries with diminished biceps and triceps reflex, decreased sensation, and muscle weakness. These are usually transient in nature with only soreness remaining for any significant period of time. If, following complete evaluation, it can be determined that the injury was a lateral flexion injury and the symptoms subside readily, then the athlete can usually return to competition by using a collar.

If any neck injury is strongly suspected but cannot immediately be diagnosed by standard techniques, the athlete should be protected until further studies can be carried out. Any player who is unconscious on the field must be assumed to have a neck as well as head injury until it can be demonstrated that he probably does not. Only well-trained persons should attempt to move a person suspected of having a serious neck injury. Unconscious patients are usually transported in a semi-prone or side position which helps to keep the airway open and tends to prevent aspiration of fluid into the lungs. The head and neck should be maintained in a properly supported manner and the airway kept patent.

Equipment which should be available on the scene of athletic events for the emergency care of head and neck injuries includes an oral screw, tongue forceps, tongue blades, airway, stretcher, spine board (Figs. 1 and 2), and either a station wagon or readily available ambulance.

C. Spine

Violent contraction of muscles during athletic participation may result in a muscle strain involving any one or more of the spinal muscles. Diagnosis is based upon the mechanism of injury, the character and site of the pain, the localization of point tenderness, and the degree of disability.

Contusions of the spinal muscles may cause severe local pain, spasm, and disability. It is frequently impossible to distinguish them from fractures of the posterior elements of the spine, such as the spinous, interarticular, and transverse processes, unless oblique as well as anterior–posterior and lateral X-ray films are obtained. They should be treated by rest, support, and local application of cold for the first 24 hours.

Fractures involving the spine are usually associated with considerable pain, muscle spasm, and point tenderness. Participation in athletics should be restricted until the full extent of the spinal injury can be ascertained. This will entail X-ray studies including oblique and sometimes bending films, to establish the specific diagnosis of fracture and/or dislocation. Any person with a spinal injury associated with abnormal neurological findings must be moved very carefully, even during the examination, and great care must be exercised in transporting him to a medical facility for further evaluation and treatment.

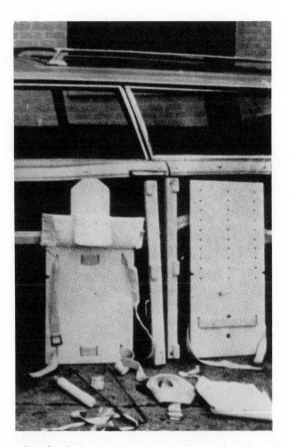

Fig. 1 Spine board which can be easily transported in two pieces and easily assembled by locking the two long struts on the side. Traction accessories are shown in the foreground. The upper portion may be used along for cervical fractures and the patient transported on a conventional stretcher.

Fractures of the transverse processes of the lumbar spine will receive substantial relief of pain from local injection of procaine into the fracture site. These are seldom seriously displaced and do not require special precautions in transportation other than comfortable support.

Subluxations of the spine, especially in the lumbar region, may occur in athletes who are predisposed by the presence of congenital abnormalities such as spina bifida, spondylolysis, and spondylolisthesis. These should be managed initially in the same way as any other acute spinal injury.

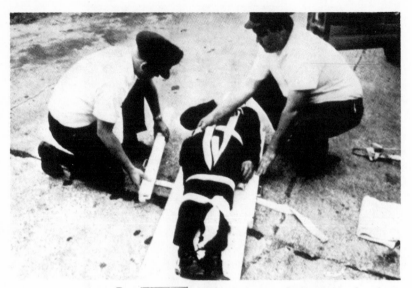

Fig. 2   First aid personnel have secured a patient to the spine board with straps. One strut is locked on and the other is being placed.

D. Chest

Direct blows to the chest may result in contusions, rib fractures, or costochondral separations (sprain). Rib fractures may be complicated by damage to the pleura or lung with resultant subcutaneous emphysema, pneumothorax, or hemothorax. Pneumothorax should be suspected when breathing is shallow and rapid or if the athlete complains of painful shortness of breath. Hyperresonant percussion and absence of breath sounds on auscultation will be noted on the physical examination. The chest should be supported with a rib belt, circular bandaging, or taping until X-rays can be obtained and definitive treatment carried out.

A severe blow to the chest wall may bruise the heart (cardiac contusion) and result in pericardial effusion with cardiac tamponade. Muffled heart sounds, a decreasing pulse pressure, a paradoxical pulse, and increasing venous pressure with engorged neck veins help to confirm the diagnosis. Aspiration of the pericardium through the space between the fourth and fifth ribs on the left may be necessary if the symptoms are rapidly progressive.

Strain may occur to any one of the many muscles that attach to the chest. Overstretching of the muscle or sudden violent exertion is the usual mechanism. Pain and point tenderness are maximum over the involved site. The severity of the disability depends upon the extent of injury. Rest and support by bandaging or with a rib belt is the immediate management.

Chest injuries associated with persistent pain and/or abnormal respiration should be fully evaluated prior to allowing the athlete to return to sports. Athletes with such injuries when associated with tachycardia, a weak, thready pulse, pallor, sweating, cyanosis, or clammy skin should be sent immediately to the hospital on a stretcher and under supervision. The possibility of rupture of the thoracic aorta must always be considered, especially in motor sports.

E. Abdomen and Genitalia

The chief dangers to be considered in injuries to the abdomen are the rupture of a hollow viscus with contamination of the peritoneum and a chemical or bacterial peritonitis and the rupture of a solid viscus with a massive hemorrhage and internal exsanguination. Retroperitoneal hemorrhage may also occur as the result of injury to the mesentery of the intestine, the pancreas, the kidney, and adrenals. Trauma to the pancreas may induce acute pancreatitis without any considerable hemorrhage or extravasation of pancreatic secretions.

The most common injury to the abdomen is "getting the wind knocked out." The sudden and distressing paralysis of respiration is due to a reflex paralysis of the diaphragm from stimulation of the solar plexus which lies deep in the epigastrium. The emergency treatment of this condition is to leave the player alone until his respirations return spontaneously, as they will invariably in a matter of seconds. In the meantime, he should be reassured gently but constantly that he is all right. There is absolutely no need for such commonly employed measures as lifting up the player's legs and flexing the thighs on the hips; in fact these may be dangerous if you don't know the full extent of the athlete's injuries. There is no reason a player should not return to play directly once he has recovered his normal respirations, but he may wish to have a brief respite to pull himself together.

Ruptures of the liver and spleen may result from direct trauma to the abdomen. Signs of peritoneal irritation including pain, distention, nausea, rapid pulse, and fever indicate the possibility of intraperitoneal hemorrhage. These may be followed by increasing pallor and falling blood pressure. Immediate management is to take directly to the hospital by ambulance for X-rays, surgical consultation, transfusion, if necessary, and surgical correction if indicated. The ruptures of the liver can usually be repaired because it has a good capsule. Even small ruptures of the spleen are not ordinarily susceptible to nonoperative management, however, because the spleen has no true capsule and its substance is highly fiable. Unless the injury is very minor, the spleen will have to be removed if proven damaged.

A blow to the pancreas may induce acute pancreatitis, but the onset of severe symptoms usually does not occur until hours later. The immediate management when this condition is recognized is to admit the patient to the hospital for confirmatory tests and treatment. Rupture of the pancreas in sports is very rare and seems to occur chiefly where the pancreas body crosses the vertebral column. It should be treated surgically when recognized.

The signs of retroperitoneal hemorrhage are similar to those of intraperitoneal bleeding. They come on more gradually and often produce pain in the center of the back as well as in the abdominal area. The immediate management is to transport the player on a stretcher to the hospital for further studies and observation. Strong narcotics should not be given for pain before hospitalization since they may obscure the natural development of the particular injury. These injuries may not produce shock until a considerable amount of blood is lost, in contrast to intraperitoneal bleeding. Tenderness should be present in the flank if the kidneys or adrenals are injured. Hemorrhages into the mesentary are ordinarily limited to a relatively small area and are not explored surgically in most cases.

Rupture of a hollow viscus is rare as a sports injury. It occurs most frequently in a loop of distended small intestine but may occur anywhere from the lower esophagus to the rectum just above the peritoneal reflection. Emergency management is to transfer the player directly to a physician or hospital for further diagnostic evaluation and treatment.

The principle sports injury to the male genitalia is contusion of the testis. The immediate management should be the application of a cold pack and elevation of the scrotum on a support, such as can be provided by several towels rolled tightly and placed between the legs. This will minimize hemorrhage and help to shorten disability. If a sizable hemorrhage occurs in spite of this treatment, or if the testis is not seen until some time following the injury, it may be necessary to incise the tunica vaginalis in order to relieve pressure, which may cause atrophy if it persists.

In the female, the vulva may be contused or lacerated as the result of a fall astride some object such as a balance beam or parallel bar. The immediate management should be application of a cold pack and rest to minimize bleeding. Lacerations should be sutured to minimize scarring. The uterus and ovaries are well protected and it is virtually impossible to injure them. Rupture of the vagina has been reported from an inrush of water in a fall from a water ski at high speed. This would require immediate hospitalization and surgical repair.

F. Shoulder

Following an injury to the shoulder, obtain an accurate, careful history of the mechanism that produced the injury. Next, observe the contour of both shoulders with clothing and protective padding removed. Look for any asymmetry or deformity that might be present. Then palpate. Follow the spine of the scapula. Palpate the acromion. Palpate the greater tuberosity and the rotator cuff. Feel for point tenderness or a defect in the rotator cuff. Next, palpate the acromioclavicular joint and then along the shaft of the clavicle. Palpate the sternoclavicular joint and note any prominence or tenderness present at that site. Palpate the inner tubercular groove of the humerus and the lesser tuberosity. Palpate for crepitation. Check the range of motion in the shoulder. Is there pain on abduction? Is there weakness on abduction of the shoulder? Is there any discomfort on rotation or restriction of rotation? Next, check for stability. Is there laxity in the acromioclavicular joint or the sterno-clavicular joint? Is there instability or apprehension on abduction or external rotation of the arm? Finally, check the function of the shoulder by having the athlete perform skillful movement if all other aspects of the evaluation are unremarkable.

1. Fracture of the Clavicle

Fractures of the clavicle are common in many sports. The diagnosis is usually made easy by the presence of pain, deformity, crepitation, and point tenderness at the site of the fracture. First aid consists of application of ice at the site of maximum tenderness and immobilization of the involved shoulder with a sling and swathe bandage. Further participation is restricted until definitive treatment and adequate healing have been concluded.

2. Acromioclavicular Sprains and Contusions

A contusion to the acromioclavicular joint can be diagnosed by the presence of tenderness over the acromioclavicular joint with the absence of any laxity and a history of a direct blow to the joint. Sprains occur as a result of a fall onto the outstretched hand, elbow, or onto the shoulder. Sprains of the acromioclavicular joint are graded according to severity: Grade I is characterized by swelling and tenderness of the acromioclavicular joint but without any laxity; Grade II demonstrates laxity of the acromioclavicular joint but without complete dislocation; and Grade III sprain shows gross laxity in the acromioclavicular joint with displacement of the clavicle out of the acromioclavicular joint. One of the best methods to determine the degree of laxity at the acromio-clavicular joint is to stabilize the arm with one hand while grasping the distal clavicle between the thumb and index finger of the other hand and to move the clavicle forcibly first in an anterior–posterior direc-tion and then in a cephalad–caudad direction. The extent of laxity can also be determined by the use of stress X-rays following removal from the field of play, which is the initial step of the immediate management. The arm and forearm should be supported in a sling until diagnosis is established and definitive treatment given.

3. Glenohumeral Sprain and Dislocation

A history of forcible abduction and external rotation of the arm should lead one to suspect a sprain of the anterior capsule with resultant subluxa-tion or dislocation of the shoulder. In cases where there has been spon-taneous reduction, apprehension will be noted on attempts to abduct and externally rotate the arm while pressure is applied from the posterior aspect of the shoulder, attempting to push the head of the humerus forward away from the glenoid. Frank anterior glenohumeral dislocations usually do not pose any problem of diagnosis because of the deformity that is present, the loss of rotation, and the presence of severe pain. Fortunately, posterior dislocation of the shoulder in athletes is rare. Emergency management should include reduction of any complete dis-location as soon as reasonably possible.

The safest method of reduction for the coach or trainer to attempt if no physician is present or if there may be a delay in getting the athlete to one is to have the player lie face down on a training table with the effected upper extremity hanging down over the side. A weight of 5 to 10 pounds is held in the hand, producing a steady, but not excessive, traction that will almost always reduce the dislocation as muscle spasm gradually relaxes. The physician may want to try the effect of straight traction with the player lying on his back on the table and the arm abducted about 45° from the side of the body. Countertraction may be applied by the physician placing his stockinged foot against the player's chest wall just below the axilla or by an assistant pulling on the same area from the opposite side of the body. The Kocher manoeuver should be avoided by all except the experienced orthopedist.

X-Ray examination of the shoulder should be made in every case of dislocation or subluxation in order to rule out the presence of fractures of the humerus or scapula. The reduction does not have to be delayed until after the X-rays, especially if there will be any great delay in securing them. Increasing muscle spasm and pain in the few hours following dislocation, if it is not reduced, may make a reduction impossible without general anesthesia. Ultimate treatment will depend on the findings of X-ray examination, but the emergency management for either subluxation or dislocation should be to apply cold externally and support the upper extremity with a sling.

4. Sternoclavicular Sprains

Sternoclavicular joint sprains are also classified according to the severity of injury. These injuries are frequently overlooked in the early stages after injury because the pain is frequently felt out on the mid or distal clavicle. The athlete with a sternoclavicular injury characteristically turns his head away from the side of injury, in contrast to the one with acromioclavicular injury who turns it toward the injured side. Palpation over the sternoclavicular joint, however, will indicate an acute area of tenderness, and perhaps a prominence can be observed. Instability can be detected by grasping the proximal clavicle between the thumb and index finger, and forcibly pushing it in an anterior–posterior and then upward direction. This injury usually results from force applied to the lateral aspect of the shoulder. Emergency management requires application of a cold pack, and a sling with immediate referral for X-ray examination.

Retrosternal dislocations may constitute a real emergency that calls for immediate first aid measures. Lateral traction on the arm while pressure is applied to the proximal clavicle will reduce the dislocation if the costoclavicular ligament remains intact. If it does not, open surgical reduction to relieve pressure in the superior mediastinum will usually be necessary.

5. Rotator Cuff Contusions and Strains

Rotator cuff contusions and strains may be identified by the presence of point tenderness over the rotator cuff and by the impaired ability of the athlete to abduct the shoulder normally against resistance. Immediately following complete tears of the rotator cuff, a defect may be palpated prior to the onset of swelling. Management should be to apply a cold pack and a sling and refer for X-ray examination.

Strain of the long head of the biceps tendon will produce tenderness over the long head of the biceps, most easily palpated in the inner tubercular groove. Emergency treatment should include local application of cold, a sling and rest.

G. Elbow

Acute injuries to the elbow during athletic participation usually do not constitute a serious problem in diagnosis, especially as it relates to the ability of the athlete to continue participation, because many of the structures about the elbow can be readily palpated and the extent of injury ascertained. After a careful history has been obtained, the area should be inspected for any deformity or swelling. Next, the area about the elbow should be palpated for any area of tenderness or crepitus. Stability of the collateral ligaments should be checked as well as the range of motion. If all other tests prove to be negative, or if findings are minimal, then the strength of elbow flexion and extension should be determined.

1. Contusion

The increased utilization of artificial playing surfaces has produced an increased frequency of contusions to elbows. The mechanism is a direct blow to the elbow. Diagnosis is made from the history and finding tenderness at the site of the direct blow. Swelling follows frequently, and traumatic olecranon bursitis is a frequent complication that may come on acutely. Less frequently, the ulnar nerve may be contused on the medial side of the elbow and may result in symptoms of varying degrees related to ulnar nerve dysfunction. Management is with immediate cold applications followed by the oral administration of an anti-inflammatory agent.

2. Strain

Strains of the musculotendinous structures about the elbow are especially common in the throwing sports. Most often the pain is on the medial side of the elbow and point tenderness can be elicited over the medial epicondyle or over the flexor-pronator musculotendinous mass. Less frequently, tenderness is located over the lateral epicondyle and along the extensor-supinator musculotendinous mass. Strains may also occur in the triceps muscle at the site of the bony attachment to the olecranon. Immediate treatment is cold application, rest, and oral administration of an antiinflammatory agent.

3. Sprain

Sprains about the elbow are not infrequent in contact sports, especially in football and in wrestling. The most common sprain about the elbow is a hyperextension sprain which is produced by a direct blow to the posterior aspect of the elbow, usually with the weight of the extremity being supported on the hand causing the elbow to hyperextend and the stress being applied to the anterior capsule. Tenderness is often present both anteriorly and posteriorly due to the direct blow hitting on the posterior aspect and due to the secondary damage produced by the stress on the anterior capsule. This is a very painful injury and, if of a significant degree, will exclude the athlete from further participation for a period of 6–8 weeks or more. The lateral ligaments about the elbow may be placed under stress, either abduction or adduction, and when the mechanism of injury is such it is necessary to test them for stability. Sprains about the elbow as in other parts of the body should be treated by early application of ice, a compression bandage in an attempt to limit the amount of swelling, and rest.

4. Fractures and Dislocations

Fractures and dislocations can usually be readily diagnosed by the area of point tenderness, the early appearance of swelling, distortion of the normal relationships of the bony land marks of the elbow, and the significant pain and disability which are present. Crepitus may also be present. Following a dislocation of the elbow, or of a fracture with displacement, it is imperative that the circulation of the forearm distal to the fracture or dislocation should be checked frequently and periodically. The elbow should be appropriately splinted and the patient transferred to a medical facility for definitive care. Reduction by straight downward and forward traction with the shoulder fixed may be necessary as an emergency procedure if circulation is impaired. A cold pack should be applied to minimize swelling.

H. Wrist and Hand

The hand is at risk in nearly all sports. Since its delicate control and skilled function depends on its maintaining its exact mechanical alignment and full range of motion, the correct early management of hand injury is critical. The physician, trainer, coach, and athlete must all be acutely aware of the necessity of the earliest and best emergency measures.

1. Fractures of the Wrist

a. COLLES AND SMITH FRACTURES. The common Colles fracture and the less common Smith fracture should be recognized instantly, X-rayed, reduced, and casted before substantial swelling has occurred. Local anesthesia is usually ideal for the athlete but regional block may be necessary. A fall on the outstretched hand may also produce an avulsion fracture of the tip of the styloid process of the radius rather than either of the above.

b. FRACTURE OF THE NAVICULAR. This injury occurs most often following a fall onto the outstretched hand. There is pain and local tenderness at the base of the thumb and on the radial side of the wrist. Pain may be mild initially but usually increases with use of the hand, especially in radial deviation and palmar flexion. The initial X-ray views of the wrist (anterior–posterior, lateral, oblique, and with the hand in ulnar deviation) may not show the fracture line. If there is any doubt, the wrist should be held in a splint or cast and the X-rays repeated at weekly intervals until all symptoms have ceased or the fracture is shown.

c. FRACTURE OF THE TRIQUETRUM. This causes pain and sometimes clicking in the central area of the wrist on its dorsal surface. Pain in the central area of the wrist may also be produced by damage to the triangular wrist cartilage. Damage to this cartilage is characterized by a "weak" feeling in the wrist and sometimes a click can be heard with motion. Emergency management is application of cold, X-ray examination (including oblique view), and application of a cast.

d. FRACTURE OF THE GREATER MULTANGULAR. This fracture is produced by a force driving the thumb straight back against the wrist. It produces more early pain and disability than the navicular fracture. Early diagnosis by X-ray is especially important in this fracture since early open reduction and pin fixation is usually necessary to maintain normal pain-free function of the thumb.

2. Dislocations of the Wrist

a. RADIOCARPAL DISLOCATIONS. These are very serious injuries which occur only rarely in sports. They may reduce spontaneously or be reduced by the athlete himself so that the history of a serious deformity is very important. These injuries should be managed with immediate application of cold and an air splint and referred directly to an orthopedic surgeon.

b. DISLOCATION OF THE LUNATE BONE. This injury is caused by acute dorsiflexion of the wrist while a force is being exerted against the extensor side of the forearm. A firm tender swelling is palpable under the flexor tendons on the wrist and pain in the distribution of the median nerve may be severe. The wrist is not always locked. Immediate cold application, X-rays, and referral to an orthopedist for closed reduction are indicated.

3. Metacarpal Injuries

These can usually be diagnosed by the point tenderness, swelling, and crepitation that are often present. The treatment of these injuries offers many traps for the nonspecialist. Following initial cold application and elevation to minimize swelling, all should be referred to an orthopedic or hand surgeon.

a. METACARPAL HEAD FRACTURES. These can usually be recognized by the depression or total absence of the normal dorsal prominence of the knuckle. The mechanism is usually striking an object with a closed fist. The necks of the fourth and fifth metacarpals are most frequently broken in this way, as is the shaft or the fifth metacarpal just above the base because the casual and inexperienced fighter hooks his punches instead of punching straight forward.

b. METACARPAL SHAFT FRACTURES. These will frequently be missed unless all bruised and swollen hands are X-rayed immediately. Prevention of swelling is critical for restoration of good hand function.

c. BENNETT'S FRACTURE. This is basically a fracture dislocation at the carpometacarpal joint of the thumb. Pain, swelling, and immediate disability are usually greater than with a navicular fracture. An anatomical reduction of the fractured bone of the metacarpal and of the dislocation, by whatever means secured, are essential to future pain-free normal thumb function.

4. Sprains of the Thumb and Fingers

These are very painful injuries. Dislocations should be reduced by hyperextension of the distal joint and traction before swelling takes place and for relief of pain. This should be accomplished easily and never forced, since a fracture or entrapment of a tendon or ligaments may block reduction by manipulation alone.

a. The proximal interphalangeal joint of the finger is frequently injured in athletics. Disruption of the capsule causes an anterior or posterior subluxation or dislocation. When there is also injury to the collateral ligament, initially deformity may not be present. Because the athlete seldom complains of pain and feels that he is capable of continuing participation, the severity of the injury is often overlooked or minimized. A complete tear of the collateral ligament of the PIP joint can be a very disabling injury with persistent symptoms after injury and resultant stiffness and pain in the PIP joint. If allowed to go untreated, this may result in residual laxity and weakness in that joint with periodic resprains. Tear of the ulnar collateral ligament of the thumb may require surgical repair to prevent disability.

b. The distal interphalangeal joints are the most frequently sprained in the body and the most easily treated ordinarily. If a dislocation has been reduced, X-rays should be taken to identify possible fractures. If the joint is unstable following reduction of a dislocation, surgical repair of the capsule and ligaments will be necessary.

5. Fractures of the Phalanges

The distal phalange does not usually require anything but protection unless there is an avulsion of attachments of tendons or ligaments. In such cases they should be referred to a specialist. The fractures of the middle and proximal phalanges present many problems in management and cannot always be successfully treated by positioning in a plaster cast.

6. Injuries to the Nails and Nail Beds

a. Hematoma beneath the nail should be evacuated immediately by drilling through the center of the nail. This will not only relieve the pain but may prevent loss of the nail.

b. Avulsion of the nail should be completed if it is only partial in order to provide better protection to the nail bed. A dressing of fine mesh vaseline gauze and compression will stop bleeding.

c. Disruption of the nail bed should be treated by anatomical reconstruction of any viable fragments or suture of lacerations to prevent future growth of a distorted nail.

I. Hip

Injuries in the region of the hip are relatively uncommon among athletes. When they do occur they are most commonly related to strains of the musculotendinous unit or to avulsion fractures secondary to muscle pull. The determination of the playability of the athlete following an injury to the hip is determined by the degree of disability present. Athletes with minor contusions, sprains, and strains can usually continue to participate without risk of aggravating the injury, while the more serious, or Grade II and III, sprains and strains as well as severe contusions and fractures should be excluded from further participation until definitive treatment has been performed. The early application of ice to contusions and strains will help to prevent swelling. Those athletes suspected of having fractures or significant musculotendinous injuries about the hip should be protected from weight bearing until the exact nature of the injury is determined.

1. Epiphyseal Avulsions

Tenderness on palpation over the anterior-superior iliac spine associated with pain on flexion suggests a strain of the sartorius muscle with possible avulsion of the anterior-superior spine in the young athlete. Tenderness in the region of the lesser trochanter should lead one to suspect a strain of the iliopsoas with possible avulsion of the lesser trochanter. The mechanism is usually that of forced extension of the flexed thigh. Pain in the gluteal region with tenderness over the ischial epiphysis indicates an injury to the hamstring tendons with possible avulsion of the epiphysis. Following X-ray diagnosis, athletes with these injuries should be referred for surgery.

2. Hip Pointer

Blows over the unprotected or lightly protected iliac crest region produce a painful tender swelling which may be above or below the crest. The injury is very disabling since it usually makes running nearly impossible. Immediate management should include local application of cold packs, rest, and the use of crutches when walking is necessary.

3. Trochanteric Bursitis

The greater trochanter is exposed to bruising, which may result in the development of an acute bursitis. Initial treatment with ice massage and oral antiinflammatory medication may be followed by the local injection of a mixture of procaine and one of the cortisones if pain and disability have not been completely relieved.

4. Groin Pulls

Strain of the iliopsoas tendon occurs in sports when the athlete's thigh is flexed actively on the hip and then suddenly and forcibly extended. Tenderness is usually exquisite below the injured ligament and the athlete resists straightening the thigh. Rest, cold application, and supportive bandaging with the thigh flexed on the hip and externally rotated is the immediate management.

5. Slipped Capital Femoral Epiphysis

In boys and, very rarely girls, between the ages of 12 and 17, pain in the hip and in the knee associated with a limp may come on gradually during the course of sports participation. Physical examination may reveal very little except resistance of the hip to external rotation and pain on compression of the greater trochanter. X-Ray examination will reveal a coxa vara deformity due to sliding upward of the neck and shaft of the femur. Shortening of the extremity may be confirmed by measuring the distance from the lower border of the medial malleolus to the anterior superior iliac spine on both sides or by comparing X-rays of the entire lower extremities made on long films.

The management of this condition is to take the athlete off weight bearing immediately and refer to the orthopedic surgeon for correction of the slip and pin fixation to prevent recurrence before the epiphysis is closed.

J. Thigh

1. Contusion

In contact sports, the most common injury to the thigh is a contusion. This is the result of a direct blow usually to the anterior or anterolateral aspect of the thigh. While many thigh contusions are not serious and do not lead to any prolonged disability, a severe blow to the thigh will often lead to a condition known as myositis ossificans traumatica. It may be 3–4 weeks before evidence of the new bone formation is apparent on X-ray examination, however. Therefore, any athlete who sustains a direct blow to the thigh in which there is disability or inability to flex and extend the knee completely, with or without pain, should be restricted from play and ice applied immediately. A compression bandage should be applied and crutches should be used for walking with no weight bearing. If the contusion is not serious, then function will readily return with early active exercise. Upon full return of function, the athlete may be allowed to return to play.

2. Strain

Strains of the musculature in the thigh are found frequently in track athletes as well as other athletes engaged in running activities. Most commonly the injury is to the hamstring muscles, but may also be seen in the rectus femoris on the front of the thigh. An accurate diagnosis is best made immediately following the injury when a defect may be palpated in the muscle before it is filled with an organizing blood clot. The degree of severity is often indicated by the amount of pain and disability which is present immediately following the injury. Complete rupture, which usually occurs at the musculotendinous junction, requires surgical repair. The athlete who fails to exhibit full function of the hip and knee should not be allowed to continue to participate until further evaluation has been pursued.

Immediate management should be application of cold, compression bandage, and rest with no weight bearing.

3. Fractures

Fractures of the femoral shaft are rare in sports. They are identified by the presence of swelling, deformity, tenderness on palpation over the fracture site, and crepitation on motion as well as significant disability and inability to bear weight. They should be immobilized with splints and the patient transported promptly to the nearest medical facility for definitive care.

K. Knee

Injuries to the knee, considered one of the strongest joints in the body, constitute the most frequent seriously disabling injury in athletics, especially in contact sports. Following an injury to the knee, it is best to bring the athlete to the sideline without permitting him to bear weight on the injured extremity. Once on the sideline, the pants or any other clothing or protective equipment which might interfere with the examination should be removed and a careful examination made of the involved knee. Frequent comparison with the normal knee is very helpful, especially in relation to the general configuration, range of motion, and stability. An accurate diagnosis of the degree of damage is essential before making a determination of playability. The best time for accurate diagnosis of the degree of damage is at the time of injury when muscle spasm is absent, pain is not magnified, and swelling and hemarthrosis have not yet developed.

A vital aid in the diagnosis is an insight into the mechanism of the injury. Listen to the athlete's description of the injury. What is injured? Was there contact? Did he fall or did he twist? What did he hear? Was there a pop or a crack? Was there immediate disability? Was there a feeling of instability? Has there been any previous injury to the same knee? If so, what was the extent of the previous injury? Have there been any chronic symptoms since the previous injury? What is the nature and site of the pain?

Next, observe the knee. Observe the anterior–posterior and lateral alignment. Is there deformity? Is there swelling? Observe the popliteal space for any swelling. Is there muscle spasm? Is there full range of painless motion? Observe the position of the patella. Is it high, pointing lateral, or is it normal?

Then, examine. Palpate for tenderness along the joint line, along the various ligaments, over the pes anserina region, over the patella and the prepatellar bursa, beneath the medial and lateral surface of the patella, along the superior pole of the patella at the quadriceps attachment, along the inferior pole of the patella, and along the patella tendon to the tibial tubercle. Palpate about the fibular head and next to the fibula for any area of tenderness, and the same in the popliteal area. Note the presence of any crepitus.

Next, check the stability of the knee first in forced valgus at 0° flexion, and then in forced valgus at 30° flexion. Next, check in forced varus at 0° flexion and then in forced varus at 30° flexion. Check for hyperextension of the knee. Check for rotary instability with the knee flexed 90° and the leg internally rotated, then in mid position, and lastly in external rotation.

Conventional X-ray examination of the knee in the AP and lateral views help to define bony injuries. The tunnel view is often helpful in finding osteochondral fractures and loose bodies in the joint. The skyline view, taken with the knee against the casette and flexed to 45°, demonstrates the relative height of the femoral condyles, the location of the patella relative to the intercondylar groove, and may show damage to the posterior portion of the patella in cases or recurrent subluxation.

The arthrogram with injection of contrast material, air, or both into the knee joint visualizes the menisci and cruciate ligaments as negative shadows and can be very helpful in making accurate diagnosis of injuries to these structures. Tears in the joint capsule and the collateral ligaments may be identified from leakage of the contrast material outside the joint. Routine use of this procedure in nonemergency situations may help to reduce the number of negative arthrotomies of the knee, although it will still be necessary to operate at times where the arthrogram results are equivocal.

The arthroscope for the knee has been used for only a relatively short time as yet and by only a few physicians. A camera attachment can provide color photographs to supplement the observations of the operator and serve as reference points for subsequent examinations. This valuable tool will undoubtedly see greater use as a supplemental means of diagnosis in sports injuries of the knee in the future.

1. Contusion

Pain and tenderness at the site of a blow usually indicates a contusion, especially when other pathology can be ruled out. These are managed by cold applications and rest.

2. Ligament Injuries

Point tenderness over ligaments and their bony attachments strongly indicates the presence of a sprain. Significant ligamentous injuries are usually associated with swelling or puffiness over the ligament. In cases of severe ligamentous injuries, instability will be present. The medial collateral ligament is usually injured by leverage or angulation produced by forced valgus of the knee. The medial collateral ligament is the ligament most commonly injured in athletics, especially football, due to the frequency of blows to the posterolateral aspect of the knee. Next in frequency of injury is the anterior cruciate ligament. The mechanism of injury to the anterior cruciate is forced rotation in a semiflexed position. This is most often produced by the athlete who suddenly plants his foot and changes his direction. Often the athlete will hear a pop in the knee at the time the cruciate ligament ruptures and he usually will have a feeling of instability. The posterior capsule and posterior cruciate ligament are often injured by the mechanism of hyperextension or by a force directed from anterior–posterior against the tibia with the knee flexed. An injury to the lateral collateral ligament is much less frequent than injuries to the medial collateral ligament and anterior cruciate ligament. It occurs as a result of a rotation force, usually as a result of forceful adduction of the internally rotated knee.

Ligamentous injuries are graded by the degree of severity, the first degree being a mild injury with no instability, the second degree with minimal instability but with slightly increased symptomatology, and the third degree comprising a complete disruption of the ligament with maximal instability. Complete tears of the anterior cruciate ligament may occur as an isolated injury. In such cases, there is usually no demonstrable laxity of the knee, thus making the diagnosis extremely difficult.

Any athlete who is felt to have a ligamentous injury of the knee greater than of the first degree should be withheld from further participation and definitive treatment instituted. Cold should be applied, the joint wrapped for support, and weight bearing not allowed. Athletes with a third degree sprain as indicated by the extreme laxity of the involved ligament require surgery in order to reapproximate the ligament in the most desirable position for solid healing and to prevent chronic disability.

3. Meniscal Injury

The mechanism of injury to a meniscus is any action that disrupts the rotary mechanism within the knee. The medial meniscus is most often injured by any rotary force that causes the femoral condyle to rotate medially while the tibia rotates laterally. The lateral meniscus is usually torn by a rotary force in which the femur rotates externally. Meniscus injuries are characterized by jointline tenderness with the feeling of instability on rotation. Effusion usually occurs but it may not be present in the first moments or hours after the injury occurs. Aspiration of the knee joint should be for diagnosis only unless the effusion is so great that severe pain is present and circulation impaired. Presence of a bloody effusion is indicative ordinarily of severe intraarticular damage. Locking infrequently occurs with the initial injury. Acute meniscal injuries are usually disabling to the athlete and, therefore, continued participation should be restricted until healing or definitive treatment has been concluded.

4. Strains

Extensor mechanism injuries may occur in the quadriceps mechanism proximal to the patella, at the attachment to the patella, at the patellar attachment of the patella tendon, along the course of the patella tendon, or at the tibial atttchment of the patellar tendon. The latter is very common in the preadolescent. Acute tendonitis with swelling, tenderness, pain in extension of the leg or the knee, and sometimes calcification in or beneath the tendon occurs in athletes who jump upwards repeatedly. It can be treated successfully by splitting the tendon and excising the mass of inflammatory tissue and/or calcification found there. Strains may also occur about the knee involving the biceps tendon at or near the fibular attachment or to the hamstring tendons at or near the pes attachment. These are ordinarily controlled by rest and salicylates.

5. Patellar Dislocation and Subluxation

The mechanism is usually one of valgus stress. There is usually spontaneous reduction. The pain, especially in the case of the complete dislocation, is usually quite severe. Physical findings are tenderness along the medial retinaculum adjacent to the patella, rather rapid onset of swelling, and apprehension on lateral displacement of the patella. Occasionally a defect in the retinaculum can be palpated or an avulsed fragment of the patella can be palpated prior to the onset of swelling. Dislocations of the patella in which spontaneous reduction does not occur may be reduced by extending the knee while applying light pressure to the lateral aspect of the patella. Dislocations and subluxations of the patella following reduction are treated by the application of ice, compression, and protection from further injury (sometimes with a plaster knee cylinder) while the retinaculum is allowed to heal. Proper follow-up includes the use of X-ray to rule out the possibility of an avulsed piece of bone.

6. Fractures

The most common fractures about the knee during athletic participation are chondral and osteochondral within the joint and fractures of the distal femoral epiphysis. Those less frequently seen are fractures of the proximal tibial epiphysis, the tibial plateau, and the tibial tubercle. All should be treated immediately by splinting or support and be off weight bearing, with X-ray examination helping to determine the appropriate definitive treatment.

a. Chondral or osteochondral fractures may occur as the result of a direct blow to the patella or to the femoral condyle, but they are more commonly seen as the result of an avulsion from the posteromedial patellar surface or from the lateral femoral condyle as the patella is displaced laterally as the result of valgus stress with the knee slightly flexed. This is associated with the sudden occurrence of severe knee pain with rapid onset of hemarthrosis. There may be an inability to completely extend the knee and there is usually significant pain with weight bearing.

b. Fracture of the distal femoral epiphysis is often mistaken for a ligamentous injury due to the abnormal mobility of the knee on valgus or varus stress. Two diagnostic points are helpful in distinguishing the distal femoral epiphyseal fracture from that of collateral ligament disruption: swelling as associated with a distal femoral epiphyseal fracture is usually above the knee involving the distal thigh as well as the knee while it is infrequent to have swelling in the thigh following ligamentous injuries of the knee and pain and disability are usually much more severe with fractures of the distal femoral epiphysis. This is true even if there is no displacement of the fracture.

7. *Dislocation*

Tibial-femoral dislocation occurs infrequently in athletics, but when it does occur it constitutes a severe injury and all precautions must be taken to assure that if blood supply is impaired it is quickly restored. Spontaneous reduction may occur and the seriousness of the injury may be overlooked in such cases. Numbness, weakness, coldness in the leg, undue pain in the leg or foot, paresthesias, and paralysis should all lead one to suspect that there has been an injury to the popliteal artery. The extremity may be cold, cyanotic, and mottled, with a stocking or variable sensory loss, varying motor loss, and popliteal fullness. The peripheral pulse may be reduced or absent.

The immediate management of the dislocated knee consists of proper splinting, the avoidance of further injury by unnecessary manipulation, and the application of ice, with removal to appropriate medical facility so that prompt reduction may be carried out. It is essential that adequate peripheral circulation be restored and maintained. In case there is any question, the popliteal artery should be exposed, repaired if torn, and explored if intact. Most authorities agree that early open repair of the completely torn ligaments is indicated. Following an injury to the knee in which the blood supply to the leg and foot is questionable, a slightly dependent position of the lower extremity is desirable and external heat should not be applied.

8. General Considerations

Following any injury about the knee in which there is any deformity, crepitus, or instability, athletic activity should be immediately restricted and first aid measures instituted prior to sending the athlete for further evaluation. Only in absence of significant findings, where there is no weakness present, there is a full range of motion, and the athlete has been able to demonstrate to the physician that he has full normal function should he be allowed to return to activity.

L. Leg

1. Contusion

Contusion is very common in the lower leg since in most sports it is exposed to direct blows. The nature and severity of the injury depends upon the site of the direct trauma. Much of the tibia is superficial and therefore has very little protective covering.

a. MUSCLE CONTUSIONS. Direct blows to the posterior aspect of the leg may cause hemorrhage of varying degree but seldom result in myositis ossificans traumatica. If bleeding in the leg is present to any significant degree, then ischemia may result due to increasing pressure in the enclosed space and the limited expansion that may be allowed. Extensive bleeding may cause necrosis of the muscles into the anterior or lateral compartments and even gangrene of the leg. It is extremely important therefore that severe contusions to these areas of the leg be watched closely for an increase of swelling, changes of skin color and temperature, and loss of peripheral pulses. Immediate fasciotomy and evacuation of blood clots will restore circulation.

b. FIBULAR CONTUSIONS. Contusions over the proximal fibula may injure the peroneal nerve. The symptoms will vary according to the extent of injury to the nerve.

2. Muscle Strains

Strains of the muscles and tendons of the leg are frequent in runners and jumpers. The diagnosis of a sprain to a muscle or tendon is based upon the history of the mechanism, the site of point tenderness, and the degree of disability. Management should be directed at rest, ice massage, and the use of oral antiflammatory agents.

3. Shin Splints

This is an injury that expresses itself in the form of painful swelling of the leg muscles, especially the anterior and posterior tibial ones, which may be acute or chronic. It arises from a variety of causes but chiefly prolonged hard running in the untrained or poorly conditioned athlete, hence the English term "fresher legs." Repeated running on very hard surfaces may induce a chronic state. Stretching the muscles forcefully after they have been heated to produce as much relaxation as possible may be helpful. Wearing a shoe with a well-cushioned sole helps to dampen the vibrations if it is necessary for the athlete to continue running or playing on a hard surface.

4. Anterior Compartment Syndrome

Following vigorous exercise, especially in an unconditioned athlete, rapid swelling may occur within the anterior compartment which may lead to early interference with the blood supply and muscle necrosis. Pain, cramping, muscle spasm, paresthesias, and numbness should lead one to suspect anterior compartment syndrome. In such cases the athlete must be kept under close observation so that fasciotomy may be carried out immediately when it becomes indicated. First aid measures consist of ice, compression, and elevation. Further participation in athletics should be withheld until there has been complete restoration of normal vascularity.

5. Epiphysitis of the Tibial Tubercule

Although this may arise gradually from continued strain, it also appears as an acute injury involving the whole epiphysis or only its superficial portion where it is attached to the patellar tendon. A painful swelling develops involving the epiphysis and it becomes very tender to touch. Application of ice and temporary restriction of activity is usually all that is necessary to render the individual asymptomatic. Protective padding should be utilized upon return to activity. Attempts to hasten fixation by insetting a screw through the epiphysis into the tibia should not be made in the child who has not reached full growth since they result in the formation of a back-knee deformity later.

6. Dislocation of the Head of the Fibula

This injury results when a twisting force is applied to the knee, rotating it internally, and at the same time direct force is applied to the head of the fibula, levering it out of the shallow socket in which it lies. The reduction may be accomplished by closed manipulation under anesthesia, but if the joint remains unstable the ligaments may have to be repaired. Particular pains should be taken to determine if the peroneal nerve is injured by testing the athlete's ability to dorsiflex his foot when the reduction has been achieved.

7. Fractures

Isolated fractures of the tibia and fibula occur but are not common in sports. Usually the main concern is restoring the integrity of the tibia, so that, with only a few exceptions, it will be assumed here that both bones are involved when the tibia is fractured. The immediate management, except where it is noted, should be the application of a splint and transportation by stretcher to a facility where X-ray examination can be performed and definitive care given. External application of cold packs, where feasible, and medication for relief of pain should be routine.

a. Tibial plateau fractures must be reduced anatomically and secured by internal fixation in order to prevent chronic deformity and disability.

b. Fracture of the neck of the fibula should always make one think of more serious associated injuries involving the interosseous membrane and bones and ligaments of the ankle.

c. Spiral oblique fractures ordinarily heal well if a good reduction is secured with stable fixation. If this cannot be maintained by the application of a cast, internal fixation is necessary. This also makes early weight bearing, which is desirable, easier and safer.

d. Transverse fractures in the lower third of the tibia may heal very slowly due to relatively poor blood supply. Stable fixation is especially important here to prevent nonunion.

e. Stress fractures may occur in either the tibia or fibula or both. They are usually found in the lower third of each bone and may be single or multiple. They are most frequently confused with shin splints, so that in any case of persistent leg pain X-ray examination should be made. It may be several weeks or more from the onset of symptoms before the first fine break in the cortex of the bone can be seen. As callus forms at the site it may be palpated at the tender spot on the bone. Management is by rest from sports, no cast is required, and ordinary walking is allowed, provided it is not excessive.

M. Ankle

Ankle sprains constitute one of the most frequent injuries in sports. An accurate diagnosis of the degree of damage is essential before making a determination of playability. The best time for accurate assessment of the degree of damage is immediately following injury when muscle spasm is absent, pain is not severe, and swelling and hemarthrosis have not developed.

Following an injury to the ankle, it is best to bring the athlete to the sideline without permitting him to bear weight on the injured extremity. Once on the sideline, shoes, socks, and any tape, wrap, or strapping should be removed and a careful examination made of the injured ankle. Frequent comparisons with the normal ankle are very helpful, especially in relation to general configuration, range of motion, and stability.

When the ankle has been exposed, listen to the athlete's description of the injury. What hurts and where? How did the injury occur? Was there direct contact with another player, the ground or something else? Did he fall, or turn over his ankle? Did he hear a "'pop" or "crack"? Was there immediate disability? Was there a feeling of instability? Has there been any previous injury to the same ankle? If so, what was the extent of the previous injury? Have there been any chronic symptoms since the previous injury? What is the nature and site of the pain?

Next, observe. Is there deformity? Is there swelling or discoloration? Is there muscle spasm? Is there a full range of painless motion? Is the skin intact?

Now, examine. Palpate for tenderness or crepitus. Use one finger tip to ascertain the area of maximum tenderness. Point tenderness over ligaments and their bony attachment strongly indicate the presence of a sprain, while maximum tenderness over bone should alert one to suspect a fracture. Point tenderness over the medial (deltoid) ligament and over the fibula above the joint line should lead one to suspect that there may be a disruption of the ankle mortise and further play should be restricted until a more detailed evaluation can be carried out (including X-rays). Point tenderness over a tendon or its bony attachment suggests a strain. Tendons most often injured about the ankle are the posterior tibial, anterior tibial, and the Achilles. Point tenderness and swelling over lateral malleolus and peroneal tendons suggests peroneal tendon strain or dislocation. Forced eversion with the foot in plantar flexion is the usual mechanism for dislocation of these tendons and reduction may occur spontaneously with little initial swelling. Point tenderness equidistant between the lateral malleolus and base of the fifth metatarsal suggests an avulsion fracture of the anterior process of the calcaneus (seen best on oblique X-ray of the foot).

In the absence of deformity, the active and passive range of motion and stability of the ankle should be compared with that of the opposite ankle. From four to five percent of normal subjects demonstrate an increased talar tilt secondary to relaxation of the fibular collateral ligament without any history of injury, and, therefore, comparison with opposite limb is helpful in determining any abnormal motion. Locking or a catching feeling should lead one to suspect a chondral or osteochondral fracture. Inversion of the dorsiflexed ankle is the usual mechanism. An anterior drawer sign can be demonstrated with complete tear of the anterior talofibular ligament and the anterior joint capsule. If there is any question about the stability of the ankle, these observations should be supplemented by X-ray examination under local or general anesthesia with inversion and eversion stress in the anterior–posterior view and with the foot pulled forward in slight plantar flexion on the lateral view.

The immediate management of all ankle injuries should be to apply cold, compression, and support and to forbid weight bearing. The injection of procaine into or around sprained ligaments for the purpose of allowing immediate weight bearing with or without support is a practice mentioned only to be condemned. Aspiration of a massive bloody effusion may help to relieve pain and allow for more effective support, but it should not be accompanied by the injection of cortisone or any other substance into the joint.

If a diagnosis of sprain without fracture and without complete disruption of the lateral ligaments is established, bandaging of the foot and ankle in midposition with elastic adhesive for compression, followed by elevation as much as possible and no weight bearing for 24 to 48 hours is indicated. At the end of that time, if swelling has past its peak, two courses of treatment are possible. Some prefer a short leg cast if the sprain is moderate to severe, maintaining it for from 4 to 6 weeks and allowing weight bearing. Others tape the ankle in midposition with nonelastic tape, beginning partial weight bearing with crutches and progressing to full weight bearing as soon as the weight can be borne without pain. The average sprain will heal in about 3 weeks if it is kept taped constantly, changing the tape every 3 to 4 days. Athletic trainers prefer to remove the tape daily, or even twice daily, for the purpose of applying contrast or whirlpool baths to the ankle. It is doubtful if either of these treatments facilitates healing, and there is little question that hanging a swollen ankle down in a hot bath without any support increases the venous and lymphatic engorgement, at least temporarily.

Certainly no athlete should be allowed to resume play immediately or on the same day as an ankle appears to have been injured unless he can show a full range of pain-free motion and can stand on his toes, hop, run, and cut sharply without any disability.

1. Complete Disruption of the Collateral Ligaments and Anterior capsule

This amounts to a dislocation of the ankle, even if it does not present itself as such or has spontaneously reduced. Anatomical reduction is essential and must be maintained until adequate healing has occurred.

2. Rupture of the Achilles Tendon

This injury occurs in the very heavy and the older athletes primarily. When the athlete is supported on the toes of one foot, the force exerted on the tendon is a multiple of the ratio of the distance from the point of support on the ball of the foot to the midpoint of the ankle and from the midpoint to the attachment of the tendon to the calcaneus. The heavy, tall athlete with long feet, such as a defensive tackle in professional football, is at the greatest risk. The tendon of the older athlete ruptures as the result of chronic strain and the gradual weakening of the tendon which usually accompanies the aging process.

Rupture of the Achilles tendon should be treated by surgical repair. Advocates of the use of a plaster cast with the foot in plantar flexion have not demonstrated complete rupture conclusively or long-term follow-up in athletes so treated with no recurrence. In fact, it may be better in the long run to treat partial as well as complete rupture by surgical repair.

3. Dislocation of the Peroneal Tendons

Once this injury has occurred there is a strong tendency to recurrence. It is therefore probably best treated initially by repair of the retinaculum even though the initial disability may be somewhat lengthened.

4. Talotibial Exostoses

This chronic condition, which may cause pain and disability when the athlete bears weight on the leg with the foot in dorsiflexion as he drives off it, probably occurs more frequently in athletes than is generally recognized since in most cases it does not cause symptoms. It occurs as the result of repeated impingement of the anterior portion of the talus against the leading edge of the tibia. As the bone builds up on both sides, the contact becomes painful. Although prolonged rest with no weight bearing will relieve the symptoms, cure is usually accomplished only by surgical removal of the exostoses.

5. *Fractures*

a. Fracture of the fibula above the joint line may be accompanied by ruptured tibiofibular and medical collateral ligaments and fracture of the medial malleolus.

b. Fracture of the fibula below the joint line may be accompanied by rupture of the medial collateral ligament and/or fracture of the medial malleolus.

c. Fracture of the medial malleolus may be accompanied by ruptured lateral (including tibiofibular) ligaments and/or fracture of the fibula above the joint line.

d. Bimalleolar fractures with disruption of the mortise may also be accompanied by fractures of the posterior lip of the tibia.

e. Osteochondral fractures on the ankle usually involve the superior surface of the talus, medially or laterally or the inner surface of the fibula. Surgical removal of the bone and cartilage fragments is usually necessary to effect cure. These fractures may be missed if oblique views are not made on X-ray examination of injured ankles.

f. General principles of management of ankle fractures involve chiefly the stability of the ankle joint and maintenance of the mortise. Internal fixation with screws and repair of ruptured ligaments are frequently indicated to restore the integrity of the joint.

N. Foot

The foot is protected in many sports by a shoe, but this does not prevent its being frequently injured as the result of being struck, stepped on, twisted, stubbed, impaled, or otherwise mistreated. The complex structure and mechanism that make it so efficient when normally constituted and uninjured in supporting and transferring body weight to the ground and favoring speed and agility in motion exposes it to a variety of injuries under the stress of sports participation.

All acute injuries to the foot should be managed by elevation, application of cold, and interdiction of weight bearing to minimize swelling and shorten disability. The degree of swelling will usually determine when regular shoes can be worn. Soft slippers or heavy athletic socks may be worn in the meantime for warmth and protection.

1. *Contusions*

The important thing in the management of contusions of the foot is to keep swelling to a minimum. X-rays should be taken routinely to identify possible fractures. On the sole of the foot weight bearing may be painful for a long time if necrosis of subcutaneous fat and fibrous tissue reaction causes the so-called "stone bruise." In such· cases cushioning and padding may be helpful, but prolonged rest may also be necessary.

2. *Strains*

Practically all the tendons entering the foot may be subject to strain depending on the athletic activity involved and the different anatomical peculiarities and modes of weight bearing of the athletes. Strain of the Achilles, anterior tibial, and peroneal tendons are the most common. Treatment involves primarily rest, but restriction of the range of motion stressing the tendon by strapping, the use of a cushioned heel, and the oral administration of an antiinflammatory agent may help.

3. *Sprains*

Any one of the many ligaments that bind the tarsal and metatarsal bones together or that connect the foot to the ankle may be sprained by some type of twisting or compressive force. The management of all of these sprains is quite similar, involving cold, compression, and elevation, at first, followed by support with either adhesive tape or a plaster walking boot depending on the severity of the strain.

a. The cruciform cruciate ligament of the foot and ankle crosses ante-riorly˙from cuboid bone to the medial malleolus and also to the first cuneiform bone creating a Y-shaped structure. Its sprain, which may occur separately or in conjunction with a lateral sprain of the ankle, causes pain, swelling, and tenderness across the instep of the foot. Since it serves mainly to restrain the tendons crossing the anterior aspect of the foot and does not have a weight bearing function it will heal in 7–10 days with adhesive strapping.

b. Sprains of the arch may involve one or several ligaments. Traumatic sprains of this type are more apt to affect those athletes who already have some degree of static sprain due to the configuration of their feet.

c. Sprain of the plantar fascia. This sprain may be very resistant to treatment, requiring a long period of protection from weight bearing, with a strong tendency to recurrence. Pain often attributed to formation of a bony spur on the anterior and plantar surface of the calcaneus is more often due to plantar fascia sprain.

d. Sprain of the intermetatarsal ligaments is seen most commonly in runners early in the season, when they are running on hard surfaces or when they are running very long distances every week. This sprain can be treated very effectively by wrapping adhesive tape in a circular fashion around the foot over the metatarsal heads. The tape should be laid on without tension with the foot at rest so that it does not constrict but prevents spread of the foot as the weight is borne on it.

e. Sprain of the metatarsophalangeal joint of the great toe is considered separately because it is such a disabling condition. The athlete is practically unable to run with it since he cannot push off from this toe. Weight bearing should be forbidden until swelling and tenderness have subsided completely. The toe should then be strapped to the foot in such a way as to prevent it from going into plantar flexion, the motion which causes greatest pain, and the athlete allowed to resume walking. Running should be restricted until walking with taping is pain free. Taping should be continued for the remainder of the season.

f. Sprains of the toes. These are seldom disabling except where the interphalangeal joint of the great toe is involved. They are treated by strapping the sprained toe to the adjacent toe with a small pad of cotton between the toes for comfort and to prevent maceration of the skin.

4. Bursitis

The presence of bursitis in the foot, as elsewhere, is signalized by the presence of sharply localized swelling and tenderness over a bony prominence. Treatment is by cold application, relief of pressure, aspiration, injection of procaine and sometimes corticosteroids, and in resistant cases, excision.

a. Plantar calcaneal bursa. Inflammation of this bursa is sometimes mistaken for plantar fascial strain, "bone spur" or "heel bruise".

b. Retrocalcaneal bursa. This bursa lies between the calcaneus and the most inferior portion of the Achilles tendon. It's inflammation may be mistaken for tendonitis.

c. Bursa under the first metatarsal head. This bursa serves as a gliding surface for the medial seosamoid bone.

5. Ganglion

Ganglia of the feet occur chiefly on the dorsum or lateral aspects of the foot. They may originate from the sheaths of the extensor tendons of the toes or from the peroneal tendon sheaths or from any of the tarsal or tarsometatarsal joints. They usually occur following a specific injury to that area. Aspiration may afford temporary relief, but excision is required for cure with repair of the injured ligament if a joint is involved.

6. Morton's Foot

This is not an injury but the result of having a second metatarsal longer than the first so that a disproportionate amount of weight is borne on this head rather than on the head of the first metatarsal which is stronger and better adapted for this purpose. The characteristic finding is a heavy, tender callus on the sole of the foot over the second metatarsal head and absence of callus over the first metatarsal head. Pain may not have been present until the athlete becomes active in running with the whole of his body weight being thrown forward onto the ball of his foot. Treatment is by placing a felt pad in the shoe under the head of the first metatarsal head so that pressure is removed from the second head.

7. Puncture Wounds of the Sole of the Foot

These wounds are of particular importance because the spike or other sharp object may penetrate the plantar fascia, bringing contamination, and potentially infection, into a closed space where it may cause a serious cellulitis or abscess of the foot. Every puncture wound of the sole of the foot should be opened wide under local anesthesia and explored to its bottom to remove any foreign material which may have been deposited there. Elevation and hot soaks should be carried out for the next few days with no weight bearing even if no active infection is noted when it is first seen. It is one of the few situations where the prophylactic administration of a broad spectrum antibiotic for a traumatic wound can be justified. A booster dose of tetanus toxoid should be administered.

8. Dislocations

Immediate treatment for all dislocations of the foot should be reduction, but in some this reduction will have to be accomplished by open means with internal fixation to prevent chronic subluxation. Only in dislocation of the small toes can sports activity be continued before complete healing has taken place.

a. Dislocation of the talus is a serious injury because it is often associated with a fracture of the talus or other adjacent bones and may lead to a posttraumatic arthritis, but also because interference with the blood supply may result in aseptic necrosis of the talus itself. It requires open reduction.

b. Dislocation between the first and second metatarsals, between the first and second cuneiform bones, and across the foot laterally requires open reduction and internal fixation to prevent chronic painful disability in the foot.

c. Dislocation of the toes is not very disabling except for the great toe where the same principles apply as in the discussion of sprain of this toe above. The small toes can be taped to each other for support following reduction.

9. Fractures

When a fracture has been identified by X-ray examination of the foot, the treatment will almost invariably require the application of a cast, except in the case of the small toes. Weight bearing may be allowed after varying periods of time depending on the nature and location of the fracture. Closed or open reduction with or without internal fixation should precede the cast application.

More time has probably been lost by athletes from effective action because of misguided attempts to treat fractures in the foot without proper reduction and protection with a cast and restriction of weight bearing than would be lost by the same athletes if this treatment had been adopted in the first place. When walking plaster boots are used, they are easily softened and broken and must be replaced frequently. Patience is required of both physician and athlete to see that the necessary time in this protection is not cut short because of the nuisance and inconvenience involved.

a. Talus fractures may result in aseptic necrosis. It is essential to restore the normal relationships of the talus to the ankle mortise and the calcaneus, even if it requires open reduction and prolonged restriction of weight bearing.

b. Calcaneal fractures usually result from falls in which the athlete lands on one or both heels. The normal shape of the bone must be restored almost anatomically to prevent chronic pain and disability. Pin traction may bring about a satisfactory reduction which is followed up by plaster cast immobilization.

c. Cuboid and cuneiform fractures occur only rarely by compression. Avulsion fractures associated with sprains and dislocations are more common. Treatment depends on the ligaments involved and the size and displacement of the avulsion.

d. Metatarsal fractures may occur singly or in combination. The most common single fracture is at the base of the fifth metatarsal which may be pulled off by the strong attachment of the peroneus brevis. Care must be taken to preserve the spaces between the metatarsals in shaft fractures and to restore joint integrity in fractures at the base or head.

e. Stress fractures are usually treated at first as foot sprains or strains. X-Rays may not reveal the fracture at first, but only after several weeks when absorption of bone occurs at the fracture site and soft callus appears. Treatment consists of altered activity and no weight bearing until symptoms subside.

f. Fracture of the great toe. Fractures of the distal phalanx seldom require a cast unless the joint surface is involved. In the proximal phalanx, all fractures should be treated by accurate reduction and adequate immobilization.

g. Fracture of the small toes. These may be treated adequately by strapping to adjacent toes and supporting with some strapping to the forefoot. Avulsion fractures of the toes should be strapped or splinted to prevent the formation of a hammer toe.

V. FIRST AID MEASURES

A. Heart–Lung Resuscitation

If the athlete is unconscious, establish an airway and position properly by tilting the head back. Without an adequate airway, all other efforts at resuscitation will be useless. The airway must be cleared of all foreign material. If not breathing, the lungs should be inflated rapidly, three to five times. Each time the lungs are inflated, a rise in the chest should be observed. The method may be mouth to mouth, mouth to nose, or mouth to airway adjacent to a bag or mask, if these materials are available (Fig. 3). If a carotid pulse is present, continue approximately twelve lung inflations per minute until normal respiration is restored.

If the pulse is absent, then closed cardiac compression is recommended. The pupils may be dilated and the athlete may have a deathlike appearance. He should be lying on a firm surface on his back with the head about 10° below the horizontal plane. One should position oneself at the side of the athlete's shoulder in order to have ready access to mouth and chest. If two people are available, the other should be

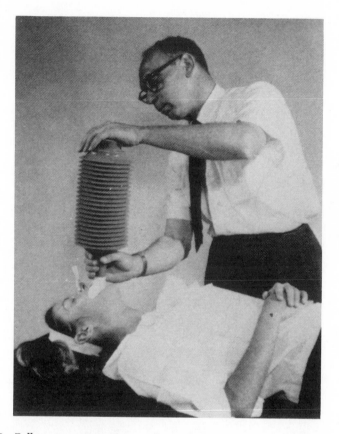

Fig. 3 Bellows-type resuscitator with attached mouthpiece being used to breathe for a patient.

on the opposite side of the athlete (Fig. 4). The heel of one hand is placed on the lower sternum but not on the xyphoid cartilage. The fingers are directed over the ribs. Lean forward so that shoulders are directly over the patient's sternum. Keep the elbows straight and depress the sternum downward, using the weight of the upper body. The downward thrust of the sternum should be approximately 3–5 cm with a moderate thrust or push. Squeezing is not effective. Press for one-half second and then release. Compression is repeated about 50 times per minute.

The lungs should be inflated about every four compressions at this pace. The rhythm should be smooth, even, and uninterrupted. Check the femoral or carotid pulse periodically and also the pupils. Dilation of the pupils often is indicative of insufficient blood supply to the brain.

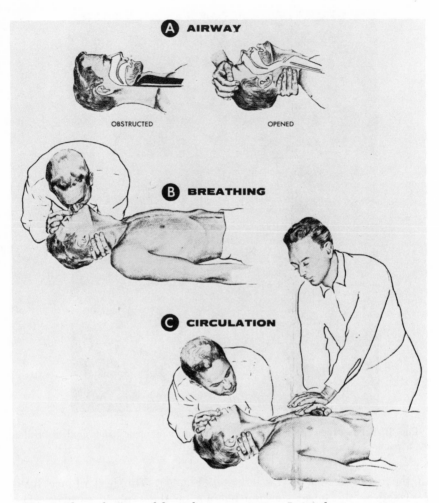

Fig. 4 The techniques of heart–lung resuscitation. In (C) the two operators are shown on the same side of the patient only to make the illustration more clear; ordinarily they would be on opposite sides.

In case of the availability of only one person to administer cardiopulmonary resuscitation, two quick inflations of the lung should be provided for each fifteen compressions of the chest. If there are two operators, then one inflation of the chest should be interposed after every fifth compression of the chest.

Transport the patient to a hospital as soon as possible while continuing cardiopulmonary resuscitation. If an ambulance is available it should contain oxygen equipment and possibly a portable electrocardiograph, defibrillator, and other life-support systems.

B. Shock

Shock may be defined as a state of deficient oxygen supply to various body tissues associated with a decreased return of venous blood to the heart. The types of shock that are most likely to be seen in the athletic environment are traumatic due to fracture or injury of very sensitive body parts, hemorrhagic due to blood loss, neurogenic due to damage of the nervous system, and psychogenic where fainting has occurred. Cardiogenic and anaphylactic shock are much less frequently seen in the athletic environment.

1. Signs and Symptoms of Shock

The face and hands are pale and may be cyanotic. The skin is cold and clammy. Sweating, however, may be profuse. The pulse is weak and rapid. Respiration is irregular and may be shallow, labored, rapid, or gasping. The pupils may dilate. The blood pressure may fall steadily. Nausea, vomiting, restlessness, and anxiety may preceed all other signs.

2. Treatment of Shock

Secure and maintain an airway. Control all obvious bleeding by compression. Elevate the lower extremities slightly if these members are not injured. Splint all known fractures. Avoid rough and extensive handling of patient. Prevent loss of body heat by covering the body but do not overheat the patient. Obtain baseline recordings of blood pressure, pulse, respiration, state of consciousness, and other vital signs and record these indices at five minute intervals. Do not administer liquids by mouth, but, as soon as possible, administer a blood volume expander intravenously and obtain some blood for typing and cross-matching so that transfusions may be given as needed. Do not give narcotic medication for the relief of pain until shock is controlled.

C. Control of Bleeding

Although extensive bleeding is a very infrequent cause of trouble at the time of an athletic injury, the physician, trainer, or coach in attendance must be prepared to control any bleeding which occurs. Bleeding can be external or internal. External bleeding occurs as a result of a laceration, an open fracture, or, occasionally, from a puncture wound.

1. External Bleeding

The best method of controlling external bleeding is by the application of direct pressure using a sterile compress. In cases where direct compression over the bleeding area does not suffice, utilization of pressure points are helpful. The use of the tourniquet should be reserved for those who have had special training in its application and use.

2. Internal Bleeding

Internal bleeding may occur due to blunt trauma to the chest or abdomen especially when it is directed toward the spleen, liver, or kidneys. Signs and symptoms may develop very precipitiously or they may occur over a period of hours or days. When internal bleeding is suspected, one should look for signs and symptoms of shock and treat the shock accordingly. The athlete should be kept without any fluids by mouth in case surgery should be necessary, and oxygen should be administered if necessary. If surgery is not performed, repeated observations of the vital signs and blood indices should be made until the condition is stabilized and danger of further hemorrhage is remote.

D. Splinting and Immobilization

The Committee on Injuries of the American Academy of Orthopaedic Surgeons in the manual "Emergency Care and Transportation of the Sick and Injured" has made the following recommendations concerning splinting:

1. General Rules of Splinting

1. All fractures should be "splinted where they lie." Apply the splint or bandage before moving or transporting the patient.
2. To immobilize an extremity fracture properly, splint the joints both above and below the bone involved in the fracture.
3. To splint a dislocated joint, immobilize the bone above and below the joint. Do not straighten the angle of a dislocated joint.

4. Take care to apply the splint so that it does not interfere with circulation of the extremity.

5. Cover all wounds with a sterile dressing before applying a splint.

6. Apply a gentle continuous pull (traction) to an injured lower extremity while the splint is being applied. Once you have begun to apply traction, do not let go of the extremity until the splint has been properly applied.

7. Pad the splint carefully to prevent pressure points and discomfort to the extremity.

2. Types of Splints

Splints are generally of two types: rigid and traction.

a. A rigid splint is made of stiff material. It is attached along the side, front, or back of the injured extremity. When used correctly, it will prevent motion at the fracture site.

Air splints consist of a double-walled plastic tube. They are applied to the injured limb, then inflated by mouth (never by pump). They provide uniform pressure.

A pillow splint, although not itself rigid, when wrapped around an injured part and bandaged, furnishes considerable support. It may be reinforced by a board or boards.

b. Traction splints are considered rigid and also hold the fracture or dislocation immobile. In addition, the traction splint immobilizes by a steady longitudinal traction pull exerted on the extremity.

3. Precautions in Using Splints

a. AIR SPLINTS. There is a general tendency to inflate air splints with too much pressure. They should be inflated by mouth only. It should be possible to indent the air splint easily with a thumb. Remember to keep checking the air pressure in air splints.

b. TRACTION SPLINTS. The ankle hitch used with a traction splint must not be applied too tightly across the ankle bones, heel cord, or arch of the foot. Be sure to pad these areas. If the ankle hitch is improperly applied, too much pressure will be placed on the skin, cutting off its blood supply, thereby causing great pain and leading to pressure sores.

When placing the upper part of the splint in the groin, be careful not to injure the genitalia or cause pressure in the groin. The pressure should be against the seat bone (ischial tuberosity).

Enough pull must be applied to the limb to hold it in position. Some persons have tried to determine the pull in pounds, but this procedure is too variable. With the proper amount of traction the patient should be reasonably comfortable.

c. BOARD SPLINTS. It is sometimes difficult to obtain adequate immobilization with board splints. Make sure that the splint is long enough, properly padded, and well secured to uninjured parts of the body for support.

VI. TRANSPORTATION OF THE INJURED

Every athletic coach, trainer, and team physician should have a predetermined plan of action in case of injury of a player. Included as part of this plan of action should be the manner and means of transportation of the injured athlete if it should be necessary.

A. Principles concerning Transportation of an Injured Athlete

Avoid being hurried into moving any athlete who is injured. Move the injured athlete only after careful appraisal of his condition. Obtain medical supervision before moving an athlete with a suspected neck or spinal injury. Have readily available a stretcher, a telephone, and a safe means of transporting the injured athlete. At the time the injured player is moved, support the injured part or member. If the injury is to the lower extremity, avoid weight bearing. While en route to the nearest hospital or other medical facility, an airway must be maintained. An attendant should accompany the injured player.

B. Who Requires Transportation?

The following require transportation: an athlete with any serious lower extremity injury, any head or neck injury with loss of consciousness for more than a brief period, any neck injury which is felt to be serious, who is unconscious for any reason or who has experienced numbness and tingling in the extremities, difficult breathing, or any neurological deficit, who has had a fracture or dislocation requiring X-ray examination and urgent treatment, who has had an abdominal injury, a serious eye injury, is hemorrhaging, has had a pneumothorax, has required resuscitation, or is suffering from heat stroke.

VII. NECESSARY EQUIPMENT FOR FIELD EMERGENCIES

In order that adequate care may be provided for the injured athlete, the following items of equipment should be available at or near the sites of organized team sports practices and games:

1. A portable suction apparatus with wide-bore tubing and rigid pharyngeal suction tip

2. A hand operated bag-mask ventilation unit with several varied size masks

3. Oral pharyngeal airways in various sizes

4. Mouth-to-mouth artificial ventilation airways

5. Portable oxygen equipment with adequate tubing and semiopen valveless transparent masks

6. Mouth gags

7. Universal dressings approximately 10 inches × 36 inches compactly folded and packaged in convenient size

8. Sterile gauze pads 4 inches × 4 inches

9. Soft rolls of self-adhering type bandages 6 inches × 5 yards

10. Two rolls of plain adhesive tape 3 inches wide

11. A hinged half-ring lower extremity traction splint with limb support slings, padded ankle hitch and traction strap or some other comparable immobilization device for extremities

12. Two or more padded boards $4\frac{1}{2}$ feet long × 3 inches wide and two or more similar padded boards 3 feet long (a material comparable to four-ply wood) for coaptation splinting of leg or thigh

13. Two or more 15 inch × 3 inch padded wooden splints for fractures of the forearm

14. Uncomplicated inflatable splints

15. Short and long spine boards with accessories

16. Triangular bandages

17. Large size safety pins

18. Bandage scissors

19. Blood pressure manometer with cuff

20. Stethoscope

21. Flashlight

22. Instant cold packs and/or ice

23. Elastic bandages 3 inch × 5 yards

24. Crutches, adjustable in length

25. Stretcher

An ambulance with a driver and attendant should be on duty at the field for all football games.

VIII. PRIORITY OF TREATMENT

Cardiac arrest, airways and breathing difficulties, uncontrolled bleeding, severe head and neck injuries, shock, and open chest or abdominal wounds are considered to have top priority for emergency treatment. Major or multiple fractures, thoracic and lumbar spinal injuries, and unreduced dislocations should have second priority. Uncomplicated fractures, sprains, strains, subluxations, dislocations with spontaneous reduction, and contusions should have the lowest priority for emergency treatment.

Chapter 13

REHABILITATION OF THE INJURED ATHLETE

FRED L. ALLMAN, JR.

I. THE NEED FOR REHABILITATION

In treating athletes, be they football players, basketball players, base-ball players, soccer players, or even those engaged in recreational sports such as skiing, golf, and tennis, no phase of treatment is more important than conditioning and rehabilitation, for the effectiveness of rehabilitation in the recovery period, either postinjury or postsurgically, will usually determine the degree and success of future athletic competition. Kraus (1959) has stated that "Injuries which are sustained during athletic participation are usually produced by circumstances inherent in respective athletic performance, and they are, therefore, characterized by exposure to recurrent identical trauma, making re-injury likely." Yet, in spite of its importance, very few innovations and very few new programs for rehabilitation have been offered since DeLorme (1945) offered the progressive resistive exercise routing during World War II. During this same 30 years, considerable progress has been made in other aspects of sports medicine.

It was only five years later that O'Donoghue (1950) first advocated early surgical repair for torn knee ligaments. Innovations have also been made in protective equipment and playing facilities and the certification of athletic trainers has become a reality. Most important of all, however, has been the development of a greater awareness by coaches and trainers, as well as physicians, of the need for prompt, proper medical care for all injured athletes, and this, of course, includes the need for total rehabilitation following injury. During this last 30 years, there has been an increased participation and emphasis on sports with an increased tempo in these sports. This increased tempo has come at a time when our population as a whole has become less active off the athletic field, and they are, therefore, less well prepared to withstand the stressful forces that frequently produce injury.

II. REASONS FOR INADEQUATE REHABILITATION

There are several reasons for the lack of widespread improvement in reconditioning or rehabilitation in recent years.

1. Most physicians know too little about proper exercise and its beneficial effect.

2. The presence of residual muscular weakness resulting from injury and/or surgery is seldom scientifically evaluated.

3. To much reliance has been placed upon simple restoration of a single muscle (often the quadriceps femoris) and its strength, with little or no attention being directed to other important muscles about the extremity (for example, hip abductor, hip flexor, knee flexor, etc.).

4. Little concern has been given to maintaining flexibility or to the detection and correction of those with too much flexibility.

5. No effort has been made to build local or general body endurance.

6. Bilateral equal muscle balance and antagonistic muscle balance are seldom achieved.

7. Too little time is devoted in an attempt to convert the "neuromuscular idiot" into a "neuromuscular genius."

8. Postural defects often go undetected and therefore contribute to fatigue and muscle imbalance that often results in injury.

9. The physician treating the athlete seldom takes time to supervise the rehabilitation and therefore delegates this responsibility to another person. if this other person is a physical therapist who has devoted most of his professional career to rehabilitating elderly individuals with broken hips or with arthritis, then chances are very strong that he will discharge an athlete as being fully rehabilitated when he can lift 15 to 20 pounds for 10 repetitions with his quadriceps femoris muscle, hardly a safe performance level for any athlete.

10. If the physician supervises the rehabilitation himself, he seldom is specific in the exact exercise prescription. Even the physician who gives the proper exercise prescription seldom evaluates the results functionally, which is really the aim of rehabilitation, that is, *functional return*. Simply to look good is not enough—the athlete must be able to perform well and to perform safely. He must be able to return to normal function.

III. INDICATIONS THAT REHABILITATION FOLLOWING INJURY HAS OFTEN BEEN INADEQUATE

A. All American Game Study

A physical examination was performed on every participant each of the three years that the All American football game sponsored by the American Football Coaches Association was played in Atlanta. These young men were the cream of the college seniors, but each year players were evaluated who had undergone surgery at the conclusion of their regular football seasons and had little or no rehabilitation following the surgery. Many of these young men were scheduled to report for professional training camps only one week following the All American game, and each of them had hopes of being able to make the team. There can be no question, however, that, if any individual reports without adequate conditioning and reconditioning following an injury or surgery, his chances of making the team are greatly diminished, and his chances are greatly increased for sustaining reinjury. If it is true that many of our top quality athletes in the more affluent universities are not adequately rehabilitated following injury, what of the high school boy in a less affluent situation?

B. Induction Center Observations

Orthopedic consultation with inductees at the Armed Forces Induction Center in Atlanta over the past 10 years has revealed numerous high school boys who have sustained serious injuries in high school, yet who have never been exposed to any form of rehabilitation. Many of these youngsters, however, have been released by their physician and allowed to reexpose themselves to further trauma, and many have sustained additional injury.

C. New York Study

A very significant and valuable study has recently been concluded by the New York Public High School Athletic Association (Callahan *et al.,* 1971). Included in the study were over 61,000 varsity high school football players. The most straightforward and clear-cut indication drawn from the data of this survey was that varsity high school football players with a history of previous knee injury were reinjured seriously at a rate some 15 to 17 times greater than the injury rate for players with sound knees. The report further recommended that players suffering a serious knee injury be required to participate in a planned program of rehabilitation under the direction of a physician as a precondition to consideration for further varsity football competition, and that players with a history of previous serious knee injury be carefully and thoroughly examined by a physician at the beginning of each season in order to determine the degree of rehabilitation of the injured knee and ultimate fitness to participate. Implied here, of course, is the need for greater involvement of physicians skilled in all aspects of medical care of athletes, including rehabilitation, in the certification of youngsters for participation in football.

IV. THE GOAL OF REHABILITATION

As mentioned previously, injuries that are sustained during athletic participation are usually produced by circumstances inherent in respective athletic performance and they are therefore characterized by exposure to recurrent identical trauma, making reinjury likely. Too often the physician, trainer, or physical therapist fails to take this point into consideration when supervising rehabilitation. As a result, the end point of treatment is often far short of a safe performance level. In order to achieve a high performance level, the best protection is balanced, bilateral muscular strength as well as antagonistic muscle balance. The goal of treatment must be restoration of function to the greatest possible degree and in the shortest possible time.

A. The SAID Principle

In conditioning or reconditioning for vigorous sports activity following injury, it is necessary to understand the SAID principle (Wallis and Logan, 1964). The letters SAID stand for Specific Adaptation to Imposed Demands. Simply stated, this means that the training program must attempt to adapt the individual to the demands that may be made upon him during athletic performance. Adaptation is specific and refers to the alteration of the structure or function of an organ or part as a result of an altered environment. Function increases with use, and that which we do not use we lose. The intensity, duration, and frequency of activity are all related to the functional capacity that is developed. Unfortunately, today's youth, because of relative inactivity, do not have sufficient exposure to vigorous activity, and are, therefore, poorly adapted to the environment created by certain sports, especially contact sports. The result has been a gradual progressive increase in the frequency and severity of injuries, especially knee injuries, and a very high incidence of reinjury, the reinjury being related not only to poor adaptation over many years, but also to failure in ability to restore normal function following initial injury.

The athlete with ligamentous laxity is far more susceptible to injury than the athlete without such laxity (Klein and Allman, 1971). The stretch effect of a normal ligament is proprioceptive in nature and results in a stimulation to the surrounding musculature that calls the muscle into supportive function of the joint. The muscular action stabilizes the joint and thus defends the ligaments against abnormal stress, if the ligament is stretched or weakened by previous injury. A strong musculature causes the joint to be more firmly bound together and thus reduces abnormal movement. A joint is a torque-transmitting mechanism, and if it is called upon to transmit a force that exceeds its capacity, then damage to the joint or its surrounding soft tissue may occur. In attempting to restore muscle function, therefore, it is important not to overstress the joint beyond its capable range.

B. West Point Survey

A recent survey of previous knee injuries sustained by plebes entering West Point Military Academy (Abbott and Kress, 1969) revealed that 80% of the injuries represented reinjury, the initial injury usually having been sustained in high school. In most cases they had been inadequately treated and poorly rehabilitated, if rehabilitated at all. As a result of this survey, the military academy has instituted a screening program. The cadets are assigned to different sports activities according to their physical capability. Those entering cadets who are found to possess weakness in their thigh muscle strength are not permitted to participate directly in contact sports. A remedial program is provided for them immediately after entrance. As a result of this program, the number of knee injuries has been markedly reduced at the academy.

C. Looseness and Tightness Related Injuries

Nicholas (1970) has presented evidence that specific tests can be conducted on athletes which will determine the degree of looseness and tightness about certain joints, and that this, in turn, is related to the incidence of injury to those joints with a high degree of predictability. This does not agree with the findings of Marshall (1970) and Morehouse (1971).

D. Restoration of Muscle Function

Rehabilitation of the athlete with an injury deals primarily with restoration of muscle function. The effectiveness of rehabilitation in the recovery period, either postinjury or postsurgically, will usually determine the degree and success of future athletic participation. The assurance given the athlete that his muscular strength and functional capacity are at a very high level of supportive quality is both a physiological as well as a psychological necessity in order for him to return to the field of competition. Haphazard, unproven methods of rehabilitation are usually ineffective and fall far short of the desired goal. Practice for the event itself does not make sufficient demands upon all of the physiological systems supporting the performance. The performer must therefore supplement his practice of the event with artificial exercise designed to develop supporting physiological mechanisms to the point that they can make a maximum contribution to the overall effort.

V. INDIVIDUALIZED REHABILITATION

Rehabilitation of the injured athlete must be individualized. No single exercise or piece of apparatus known to science today can be classified as a panacea; likewise, while elaborate and extensive tables and gadgets are available, and frequently desirable, proven methods may be utilized which require little or no special equipment. The disabled must rehabilitate themselves, but they must be given proper guidance and evaluation if they are to succeed.

VI. TYPES OF THERAPEUTIC EXERCISE

Therapeutic exercise is defined as bodily movements prescribed to restore or alter favorably specific functions in an individual following an injury. They may be active or passive. Active exercise is purposeful voluntary motion that is performed by the injured individual himself, with or without resistance, and with or without the aid of gravity. Active exercise may be static, kinetic, or isokinetic. Static exercise is that which is performed without producing joint motion. The muscle being utilized maintains a fixed length, which is an isometric contraction. Kinetic exercise is that which is performed to produce joint movement. The contracting muscle shortens, producing the movement which is an isotonic exercise. Isokinetic exercises are those in which joint motion occurs at a controlled rate (Figs. 1 and 2). Concentric contraction occurs when a muscle is contracted from the extended to the shortened postion. Eccentric contraction occurs when the tensed muscle lengthens. An example of a concentric contraction would be flexion of the elbow in performing a pull-up. An example of an eccentric contraction is that of slowly lowering the body into the extended position from the flexed position after doing a pull-up since the muscle is maintaining tension while ac-

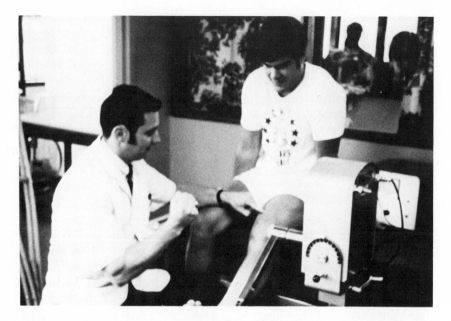

Fig. 1 Subject performing extension of leg on the knee against the self-adjusting resistance of the isokinetic exercise device. The recording device, which produces a graphic record of the force exerted by the subject throughout the range, is seen on the table behind the resistance apparatus. The therapist is encouraging the subject to concentrate on the maximum contraction of the medial head of the quadriceps muscle.

tually lengthening. Passive exercises are those performed for the injured athlete by another person or by a mechanical appliance. Passive exercise is carried out by the application of some external force with minimal participation of the muscle action by the injured athlete. It may be forced or nonforced. The nonforced exercises are those utilized to help maintain normal joint motion and are kept within a painless range of motion, for the most part, while forced passive exercises are those that usually produce movement beyond the limits of the free range of motion and are often associated with some discomfort to the individual.

VII. REHABILITATION AS A TEAM APPROACH

Rehabilitation of the injured athlete should be a team approach involving not only the injured athlete, but also the team physician, trainer,

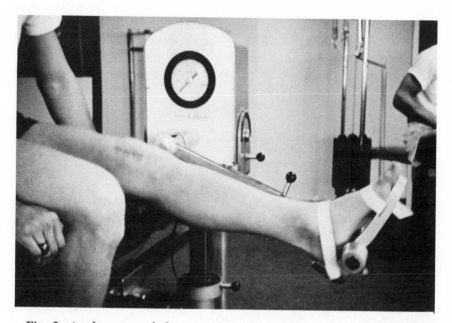

Fig. 2 Another view of the same device for isokinetic exercise seen in Fig. 1. The dial shows the subject and therapist the force in pounds being exerted during the muscle contraction. The subject's leg is in full extension on the knee. The scar on the medial side of the knee indicates previous surgery for the removal of a torn meniscus.

the orthopedic surgeon, and the physical therapist. The injured athlete must rehabilitate himself, but he must be given proper guidance if the rehabilitation program is to succeed. All of the aforementioned individuals are important in making certain that the exercise prescription is formulated properly and carried out correctly.

VIII. IMPORTANT CONSIDERATIONS IN FORMULATING AN EXERCISE PRESCRIPTION

Normal muscle function is restored by a training program. A prescription for a training program must include the exercise to be prescribed, the precautions, the duration and intensity of the exercise, the nature and range of the exercise movement, as well as the rhythm, timing, and proper progression in order to achieve maximum performance in the shortest possible time. The objectives of training are the development of muscle strength and endurance, flexibility, the ability to yield to passive stretch and to relax, and neuromuscular reeducation. In rehabilitating an athlete, the restoration of explosive power is also an essential objective. Explosive power is the ability to release maximum muscular power in the shortest time. Power is the product of speed times strength.

Formulating the Exercise Prescription

1. The Exercise

Three main factors must be considered in prescribing the exercise: the purpose of the exercise; how it is to be administered; and its relationship to other exercises that might be prescribed. Proper selection of an exercise must be based on knowledge of the principles of joint dynamics and of whether the exercise can fulfill its designed purpose. The proper execution of an exercise is very important. Failure to achieve the desired benefits usually indicates poor selection of the exercise. Injury may occur if the exercise is not properly executed.

2. Precautions

The precautions should include care for any existing conditions that might alter the response of the individual to the exercise program. It should be remembered that the exercise must be administered within the limits imposed by the existing status of the individual. The kinetic hazards imposed by the exercise must also be considered. The athlete with chondromalacia of the patella, for example, cannot be placed on the same exercise routine as another athlete with a similar condition but without the chondromalacia. The athlete with chondromalacia of the patella should avoid exercises that include range of motion with weight initially. Even later in the rehabilitation program, when range of motion exercises are added to the routine, it is better to use an isokinetic type of exercise, or an isometric exercise, rather than an isotonic exercise.

3. SAID Principle

It is extremely important in prescribing the exercise that the future plans of the athlete be known. What are his desires for future participation? If it is for a sport such as football, higher performance levels should be sought than for the individual who seeks to play golf, archery, or any one of the other noncontact type sports.

4. Duration

The duration of each exercise period and of the total amount of time required for the program must be considered. The duration may vary from only a few days following a contusion to a period of months following multiple ligamentous injuries which constitute a major disability.

5. Intensity

The intensity will vary according to the extent of the injury for which the exercise prescription is being ordered. For minor injuries, the intensity may be very great initially and of short duration, while, in a more severely injured athlete, the intensity will be very low initially and then, over a period of months, will progress to that of high intensity prior to his being released for further competition. It is the intensity of exercise that regulates growth stimulation in muscle, and growth stimulation relates almost directly to strength gain. Growth stimulation and strength are best produced when the exercise is as hard as possible, yet as brief as possible. Factors which must be considered in the intensity of exercise include the resistance load, the range of motion, to indicate the distance that the load is moved, the speed of movement, and the duration of the activity.

6. Nature of the Movement

The nature of the movement is characterized by its speed, the method of loading as it effects joint dynamics, and whether or not it is performed unilaterally or bilaterally, either simultaneously or alternately. The length of the lever arm, the attachment points of muscles and tendons, and their angles of insertion are important in determining these characteristics.

7. Range of the Movement

The range of movement is determined by the distance the body part covers in exercise. Immediately following injury, or following surgery, an exercise might be prescribed without any movement of the involved joint, whereas, as improvement takes place, the range of movement will be gradually increased. Toward the final stages of rehabilitation, and as soon as possible in the recovery period, the range of motion should

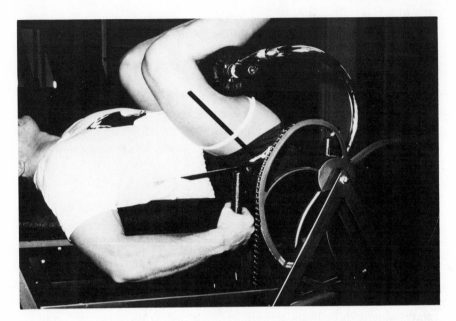

Fig. 3 The subject is lying supine on a Nautilus exercise table with his hips flexed to a maximum degree. A goniometer is attached at his lower ribs and upper thigh to measure the range of motion. This is another type of device designed to provide uniform resistance throughout the range of motion.

be as complete as possible. The best results in restoring full muscle function are achieved when the muscles are contracted throughout the entire range of motion of the joints involved (Figs. 3 and 4).

8. Rhythm

The rhythm relates not only to that which is carried out during each movement but also as it relates to different other movements. In the initial phases of the rehabilitation program, it is important to teach effort–relaxation cycles so that the muscle does not remain in a state of constant tension. As the exercise program progresses, less emphasis needs to be placed on effort–relaxation cycles as they become more or less subconscious. It has been demonstrated that a resting muscle recovers more quickly if it is exposed to a work load of low intensity during the resting period between heavy exertions. Rhythm in the overall exercise scheme is extremely important because it involves utilization of exercises that effect large muscle groups prior to those which effect the small muscle groups. The greater the mass of involved muscles, the

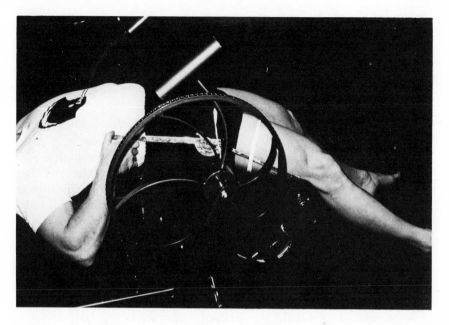

Fig. 4 The subject now has both hips extended to the maximum degree on the Nautilus machine, as indicated by the goniometer.

greater the value of the exercise. For example, in a knee rehabilitation program, it would be far better to have exercises involving the hip extensors work first because of the large muscle group that is involved. Secondly, an exercise such as the half knee bend would be utilized, followed by other more specific exercises, such as knee extension, knee flexion, and, lastly, ankle plantar flexion and dorsiflexion exercises.

9. Timing

Timing relates to exposure with a given exercise as well as the time allowed between each exercise. It relates to the coordination of muscle response, and also the stages of rehabilitation, whether immediately postinjury or late in the rehabilitation program.

10. Progression

Progression in a training program is essential. It relates to range of motion, load, speed, power, and energy expenditure in relationship to each exercise as well as to the total exercise program. An attempt should be made to produce some sign of progress in each exercise session with the development of power potential the ultimate goal. Muscles must be worked to the point of "momentary failure" or "exhaustion" if a high performance level is to be achieved.

11. Neuromuscular Reeducation

Neuromuscular reeducation primarily involves development of a proprioceptive awareness. Correction of posture and the use of passive, active, and resistive movements all seem to be essential to complete proprioceptive response. It becomes very important, therefore, to realize that normal function will in most cases return more quickly to the athlete who is allowed to continue with activities that permit near normal function but do not interfere with the normal healing process.

IX. FUNCTIONAL EVALUATION

As mentioned previously, a functional evaluation is necessary to determine whether or not the athlete is ready to return to normal participation. The functional evaluation should be immediately preceded by an evaluation of girth, strength, and goniometric measurements of all adjacent structures in the involved extremity. Examples of these measurements for both the involved and uninvolved extremity are included in Tables I, II, and III. In addition to the physical evaluation of girth, strength, and range of motion, it is essential to perform certain functional tests.

For the shoulder, a brief functional evaluation would include a dead hang from a chinning bar for two minutes. Some throwing movement should be utilized depending upon the sport in which the individual participates. Punching a bag and jumping rope are other methods of functional evaluation of the shoulder. A somewhat more strenuous evaluation is rope climbing without the aid of the feet, or climbing a peg board.

A functional evaluation of the knee, in addition to the physical determinations of girth, strength, and range of motion, includes a stationary jog, a fast jog, a leaning hop test, a squat, kneeling, and, when carefully administered, the duck waddle. Endurance capabilities can be determined by a mile and one-half run or a jump rope routine for time and speed. Even after the athlete has achieved a safe performance level and is allowed to return to full participation, he should be recalled for periodic reevaluation at appropriate times. It is only through periodic

TABLE I

Shoulder Evaluation Form Completed for Both the Injured and Uninjured Shoulder Which Serves as the Basis for Exercise Prescription in Rehabilitation

	Right	Left
Girth		
Arm	_____	_____
Forearm	_____	_____
Strength		
Hand	_____	_____
Shoulder		
Internal rotation	_____	_____
External rotation	_____	_____
Flexion	_____	_____
Extension	_____	_____
Abduction	_____	_____
Goniometric		
Abduction	_____	_____
Flexion	_____	_____
Internal rotation	_____	_____
External rotation	_____	_____
Extension	_____	_____
Functional evaluation		
Dead hang for endurance, 2 minutes		
Throwing movement		
Punching bag		
Jump rope		

reevaluation that an athlete can maintain a safe performance level. While many will be able to maintain such a performance level with relative ease, others will have to continue with some form of rehabilitation after their return to activity in order to maintain such a high level.

X. SPECIFIC REHABILITATION PROCEDURES

A. Rehabilitation following Shoulder Injuries in Athletes*

1. Rotator Cuff Injuries

a. EARLY REHABILITATION. At this stage the rotator cuff is compromised by its subacute or postsurgical status. The shortness of the cuff muscles and the disproportionate strength of the other musculature

* The program outlined is that used at the Sports Medicine Clinic in Atlanta, Georgia, by William Andrews, R. P. T.

TABLE II

Knee Evaluation Form Completed for Both the Injured
and Uninjured Knee Which Serves as the Basis for
Exercise Prescription in Rehabilitation

	Right	Left
Girth		
Quadriceps		
at _ cm above patella	_____	_____
midpatella	_____	_____
Calf	_____	_____
Strength		
Quadriceps	_____	_____
Hamstrings	_____	_____
Gastroc soleus	_____	_____
Hip flexor	_____	_____
Hip abductor	_____	_____
Hip extensor	_____	_____
Hip adductor	_____	_____
Goniometric		
Extension	_____	_____
Flexion	_____	_____
Functional evaluation		
Stationary jog		
Fast jog		
Leaning hop test		
Squat		
Kneeling		
Duck waddle		
Endurance run, $1\frac{1}{2}$ miles		
Jump rope		

of the pectoral girdle make conventional full range exercise inappropriate, even if active range of motion is possible. The following exercises are indicated:

i. Gripping exercises (Figs. 5 and 6). Gripping a hand dynamometer or tennis ball at several points along the arc from full (pain free) abduction-flexion-external rotation to full adduction-extension-internal rotation. This brings the rotator cuff into synergistic (fixative) contraction, as well as conditioning forearm muscles which have probably atrophied if inactivity has been of long duration.

ii. Codman (pendulum) exercises (Fig. 7). This exercise increases the range of motion while stimulating contraction of the rotator cuff due to the gentle traction applied to the muscle systems.

TABLE III

Ankle Evaluation Form Completed for Both the
Injured and Uninjured Ankle Which Serves
as the Basis for Exercise Prescription in
Rehabilitation

	Right	Left
Girth		
Foot	———	———
Ankle	———	———
Strength		
Plantar flexion	———	———
Dorsiflexion	———	———
Internal rotation	———	———
External rotation	———	———
Goniometric		
Plantar flexion	———	———
Dorsiflexion	———	———
Inversion	———	———
Eversion	———	———

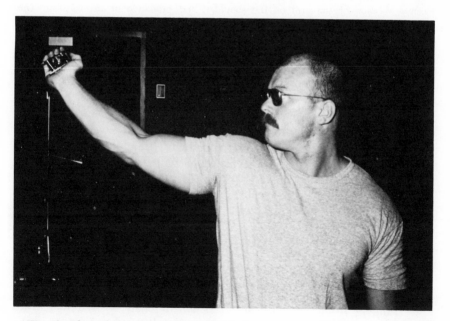

Fig. 5 The subject is gripping a hand dynamometer with the arm abducted, shoulder externally rotated, forearm supinated, and wrist extended.

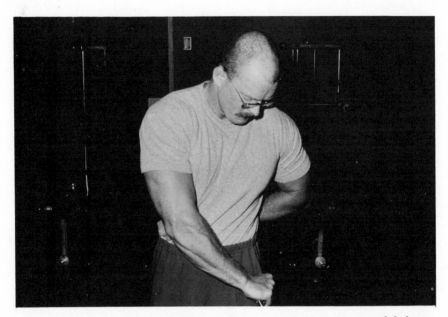

Fig. 6 The subject has continued his compression of the dynamometer while bringing his arm down from the position shown in Fig. 5 to a position of adduction and internal rotation of the arm on the shoulder, and pronation of the forearm. This exercise brings the rotator cuff into a fixative contraction as well as strengthening other muscles of the shoulder, arm, and forearm.

iii. Bench press supports (*Fig. 8*). Lie supine on the bench, holding the barbell in a "locked-out" position. A freely held barbell or dumbbells are preferable to a statically held weight machine since four-way control is stimulated by the free barbell and not by the weight machine. The weight should be only heavy enough to stimulate fixation of the cuff gently. Progression is accomplished by widening the grip gradually from about 20″ to 30″ (to pain tolerance). This increases the external rotation gradually. The weight is also increased gradually.

iv. Deadlift supports (*Fig. 9*). Hold the barbell or corresponding lever of the multistation weight training apparatus with an overhand grip at the front of the thighs. The shoulders are held in a shrug position. Single efforts of 10 seconds are performed. Progression is obtained by widening the grip and increasing weight.

v. Hanging from chinning bar. A bench or chair is used to elevate the body so that the bar can be grasped regardless of a deficient range of motion. The bar is gripped but no effort is made to support full

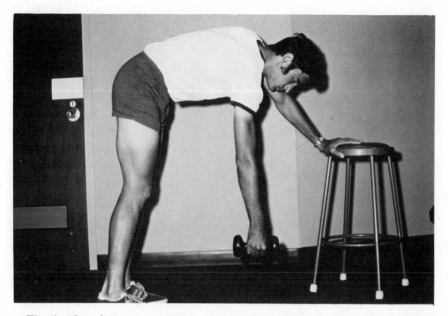

Fig. 7 The subject supports his weight partially with the opposite upper extremity on a stool while he supports a light dumbbell in his hand and moves it gradually into circles of increasing width.

or partial weight until the arms can be painlessly held over the head. The patient merely grips the bar and isometrically sets the latissimus group in a comfortable range. Once full weight bearing is possible, progression is obtained by widening the grip.

b. INTERMEDIATE REHABILITATION. At this stage the rotator cuff should be able to contract fully without pain, but full range is not present, and strength is not yet fully developed. The cuff is, however, adequate to take on conventional shoulder conditioning exercises that will develop strength and further increase range of motion. The following exercises are performed:

i. Light dumbbell circles. This is a progression of the pendulum exercises. Done while standing upright, the dumbbell is directed upward and outward in a rotary manner, and then upward and inward in the opposite manner. These circles progress by widening the excursion of the circle and increasing the weight.

ii. Bench presses. Progressing from supports, the patient gradually adds bending to the movement until a full range bench press is possible.

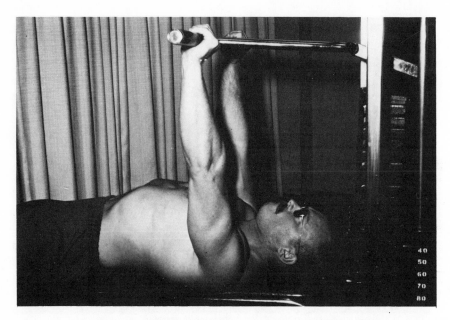

Fig. 8 The subject is supporting with his elbows locked the weight resistance offered by the universal gym in order to strengthen the rotator cuff muscles. His hands, which are now placed as closely as possible to the lever arm, will be gradually moved out in successive exercises to increase the external rotation at the shoulder, and the amount of weight supported will be gradually increased.

More weight is added. Once again, because of the need to support the weight in all directions, freely held weights are preferable to weight machines. Dumbbell bench exercises, or "flyes," while they may present a safety problem, will offer a wider range of motion.

iii. Upright rowing. This is a progression of the deadlift supports, using the same grip, in which the weight is raised to a position high on the chest. Varying the width of hand grips is desirable.

iv. "Lat" machine pull-downs to the rear of neck (Fig. 10). A shoulder-width grip is used at first with later progression to a wider grip. Weight is added until the patient is able to progress to behind the neck pull-ups (only if a minimum of six can be performed).

c. Advanced Rehabilitation. The progress of the intermediate stage has probably left the athlete at near normal development. To develop extra strength of the structures in question, along with increased flexibility, the following program might be utilized:

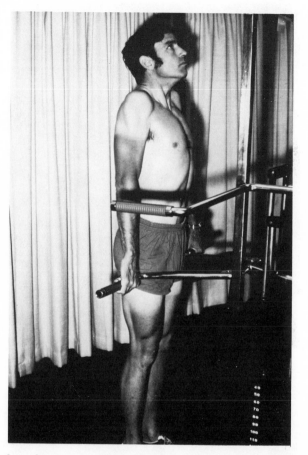

Fig. 9 The subject is supporting weight in the Universal gym by a deadlift as he shrugs his shoulders in order to strengthen the rotator cuff of the shoulder. In progressive exercises he will grip the handles farther out and increase the weight.

i. Alternate dumbbell presses or presses behind the neck.

ii. Dumbbell benches, incline presses, "flyes," or parallel bar dips.

iii. Bent-arm pull-overs.

iv. High pulls with a snatch grip, or repetition "cleans." All of the above are done for strength at a level of weight, repetitions, and number of sets to assure maximum development in accordance with the individual's potential. The exercises are done to the extremes of motion so that flexibility is improved. If properly done in this manner, no specific

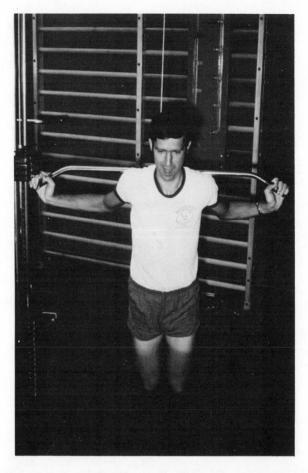

Fig. 10 The subject is pulling down against weight resistance provided by the Universal gym with his hands as widely separated on the bar as possible to strengthen the rotator cuff muscles of the shoulder as well as the latissimus dorsi muscles.

flexibility exercise is needed. To supplement any deficiency, however, the following exercises can be performed:

v. Straight arm pull-overs across the width of a bench, using a progressively wider grip. The weight is kept at a permanently light poundage (30 pounds).

vi. Light dumbbell "flyes" with a medicine ball between the shoulder blades, or elastic cable stretching at pulley weights (Fig. 11). In the latter, the cable is held in back of the shoulders with the palms facing

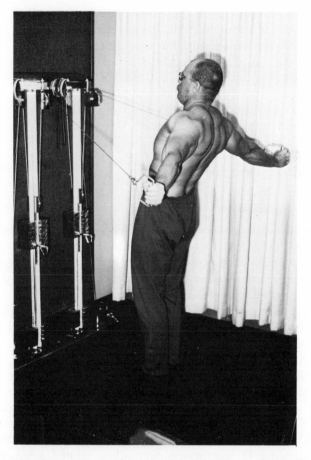

Fig. 11 Advanced exercise for the rotator cuff muscles of the shoulder utilizing pulley weights to create abduction and external rotation of the arm at the shoulder.

forward at shoulder height and the cable is worked forward and backward, stretching the pectoral girdle and rib cage.

B. Glenohumeral Dislocations and Subluxations

All stages of rehabilitation are similar to the rotator cuff with the following exceptions:

1. If surgical intervention has not been instituted to correct the dislocations, no exercise should be done which places the shoulder in a compromised position (abducted and externally rotated). Thus, grips should never be wide, bench work should only be done in the top one-third

of the movement, and presses are best performed in only the lower half of the range. To accomplish this, the use of a "power rack" is beneficial. If unavailable the barbell with the assistance of two spotters is used.

2. The extent of damage to the cuff and surrounding structures may be such that progress is slower, and there is greater atrophy and limitation of range.

3. Special emphasis is given to strengthening the internal rotator (subscapularis muscle).

C. Acromioclavicular Injuries

1. Early Rehabilitation

At the subacute or postoperative stage, pain is often a limiting factor, with associated tightening of all the shoulder musculature (trapezius, pectoral, deltoid, latissimus, etc.) as well as the possibility of tightness and weakness in the adjacent arm muscles. For this reason, the following exercises are used:

a. Light, active range of motion for shoulder flexion, abduction, internal and external rotation, flexion and extension of the elbow, and supination and pronation of the forearm.

b. Light resistive exercise for the trapezius (shrug).

c. Light resistive exercise for the anterior deltoid (upright row).

d. Resistive exercise, to tolerance, for the forearm, biceps, and triceps muscles. All should be done in such a fashion that little or no downward pull is affected at the shoulder (lying or seated rather than standing).

e. Codman (pendulum) exercises are done to increase the tolerance of the shoulder to weight support with a limited range of motion.

2. Intermediate Rehabilitation

Pain should be absent and the range of motion nearly full. The main goal is strengthening the muscular attachments of the trapezius and deltoids in the area of the clavicle and acromion near the acromioclavicular joint. This is done by strengthening the entire deltoid-trapezius group. The following exercises should be done:

a. Dumbbell presses done alternately (emphasis is on the anterior deltoid).

b. Wide grip press behind the neck (emphasis on the lateral deltoid and trapezius).

c. Shoulder shrug (emphasis on the trapezius).

d. Upright row (emphasis on the anterior deltoid and trapezius).

3. Advanced Rehabilitation

Increasing the general muscle bulk in the anterior shoulder area should have a strengthening effect on the acromioclavicular joint. All of the above exercises are appropriate when done intensively with a heavy progression of weight. Also beneficial are all incline presses, all "cleans," snatches, and deadlifts, bench presses, and pull-overs.

D. Injuries Related to the Throwing Sports

The key is prevention. Assuring general fitness of the musculature through adequate strength training is important. More important, however, is the establishment of fluid agonist–antagonist function for each associated movement at the shoulder and elbow. Development of appropriate flexibility and coordination of movement are extremely important, as well as of a proper kinesthetic sense by the athlete. The following general points are important:

1. Full range strength training, mostly with dumbbells. Done to extremes of stretch and with "ballistic" movement to assure the maintenance of quick, fluid reaction in the muscles.

2. Additional stretching movements for the entire shoulder–elbow area.

3. Maintenance of flexibility and fluid motion in the thoracic and lumbar spine. This can have a beneficial effect on the general state of flexibility in the extremities.

4. Thoughtful practice of the throwing skill to establish the most fluid and efficient pattern possible.

5. Always practicing proper warm-up, and not abusing the endurance and recovery capabilities of the structures involved (not throwing too often or too much at one time, or too soon after a lay-off).

E. Rehabilitation following Knee Injuries in Athletes*

1. Injury Classification

It is important to classify injuries by type and extent, since the course of rehabilitation will differ from one type to another. The injury classification and specified therapy routines should not be considered to be inflexible or to limit further detailing or specialization.

* The program outlined is that used at the Sports Medicine Clinic in Atlanta, Georgia, by William Andrews, R. P. T.

a. Single ligament or uncomplicated meniscus injury.

b. Multiple ligament injury or complicated single ligament and/or meniscus injury.

c. Multiple ligament injury associated with other complicating factors, such as a fracture.

d. Chondromalacia of the patella and/or femoral condyle erosion, either alone or in combination with any of the above types.

2. Stages of Rehabilitation

Rehabilitation following knee injury and/or surgery can be divided into five stages: presurgical, immediate postoperative, early intermediate, late intermediate, and advanced.

a. PRESURGICAL STATE. The presurgical stage is usually significant only when elective surgery is to be performed. If a specific diagnosis has not been made, therapeutic exercise may be instituted for purposes of aiding in diagnosis as well as for functional benefits. Therapeutic exercise at this stage is designed to build or maintain strength, while at the same time not to aggravate the existing injury. Thus, the exercise must be, for the most part, not through a full range of motion. Isokinetic exercise is especially desirable during this stage because of its readily controlled, noncompelling nature. The following exercises should be carried out:

i. Quadriceps setting—10-second contractions for 5 minutes each hour while awake.

ii. Straight leg raising—15 nonstop repetitions with the maximum possible resistance each hour while awake (Fig. 12).

iii. Isometric knee extension (at or near full extension—15 repetitions each hour while awake.

iv. Isometric or isokinetic knee flexion—15 repetitions (optional).

v. Hip extension (wall pulley)—20–25 repetitions (optional).

vi. Hip flexion (wall pulley)—20–25 repetitions (optional).

vii. Hip abduction (wall pulley—20–25 repetitions (optional).

viii. Hip abduction (wall pulley)—20–25 repetitions (optional).

The above routine should be performed daily for 10–14 days prior to surgery. In so doing, the preservation of muscle tone and the improved kinesthetic sense will help in preparation for the practice of similar exercises immediately postoperative. Instruction in three-point gait training should also be given during this stage. Touch weight bearing with the injured extremity is allowed; however, while the involved extremity is in the weight bearing phase of gait, the knee is fully extended and

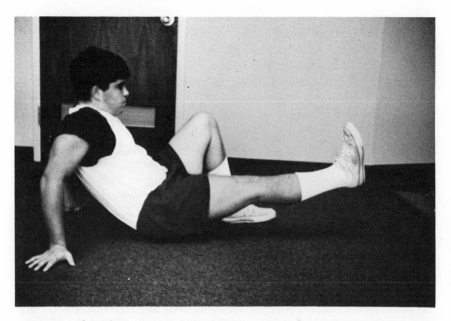

Fig. 12 The subject is raising the lower extremity with the leg fully extended on the knee against the resistance of its own weight. Progression is obtained by adding weight through pulleys or by sand bags.

the quadriceps muscle is "set." Complicated or more serious injuries are usually treated by elective surgery and, therefore, are not included in this stage of therapy, since surgery is most often indicated immediately.

b. IMMEDIATE POSTOPERATIVE OR POSTINJURY STAGE. The optimal time for commencement of therapeutic exercise is approximately 24 hours following surgery or injury. An earlier beginning is often met by an unreceptive and confused patient. Any beginning later than 24 hours must be considered a loss of valuable time. As soon as normal function ceases, atrophy and other debilitating mechanisms begin to occur and serve to delay further return of normal function. Exercises in this stage are similar to those in the presurgical stage, except for those movements that are precluded by the presence of a cast, dressing, or associated immobilization. The following exercises should be carried out:

i. Quadriceps setting—10-second contractions for 5 minutes each hour while awake.

ii. Straight leg raising—10 repetitions each hour while awake with maximum possible resistance.

iii. Isometric hip extension—10-second "presses" onto the bed for 10 repetitions each hour while awake.

iv. Abduction and adduction of the hip—10-second presses against resistance for 10 repetitions each hour while awake.

v. Ankle plantar flexion—10-second presses against resistance for 10 repetitions each hour while awake.

vi. Ambulation. As soon as the patient is able voluntarily to elevate the involved extremity from the bed, he is allowed to ambulate on crutches, using a three-point gait, with touch weight bearing on the involved extremity. The touch weight bearing stimulates proprioceptive receptors that provide the central nervous system with an awareness of body segments (in the involved extremity). Proprioceptive awareness has been shown to be of primary importance in neuromuscular reeducation.

The goals during this stage of rehabilitation are maintenance of muscle mass, strength, and function during the period of time that immobilization is indicated. These exercises should be progressive and continuous during the entire immobilization period. It is important that exercises be prescribed for the entire extremity as well as other major body segments, since bed rest and immobilization deprives all of these segments of normal activity.

The above exercises are recommended for uncomplicated single ligament and meniscectomy cases. More complicated injuries introduce elements of increased instability, increased pain, increased potential for hemorrhage, and the need for more extensive tissue repair. These conditions are, therefore, indications for the most judicious choice of activity and dosage. In most cases, however, given time and proper supervision, the level of activity can approach that of less complicated cases. Careful control of the rate of exercise progression is the key to success, with the obvious testimony of pain and edema serving as primary guidelines. Thus, the following immediate postsurgery, or postinjury routine is usually possible, even with very complicated cases:

vii. Quadriceps setting —10-second sets, for 5 minutes each hour while awake.

viii. Straight leg raising—to tolerance for 30 seconds each hour while awake.

ix. Hip extension (isometric)—to tolerance for 30 seconds each hour while awake.

c. EARLY INTERMEDIATE REHABILITATION. At the end of the immobilization period, the patient proceeds immediately into the early intermediate stage of rehabilitation. This stage is a continuation of the postsurgical stage and the exercises are similar, but with added emphasis on progression. Exercises are also included to increase the active range of motion (ROM). Passive stretching is seldom used, as active ROM exercises usually provide full ROM within a reasonable period of time. In cases in which terminal extension is a problem, the patient is instructed in passive–active exercise to correct this deficit. The following exercises should be carried out:

    i. Straight leg raising—using maximum possible resistance.

    ii. Pulley exercises:

        Hip extension—progressive to 15–20 repetitions.

        Hip flexion—progressive to 15–20 repetitions (Fig. 13).

        Hip abduction—progressive to 15–20 repetitions.

        Hip adduction—progressive to 15–20 repetitions.

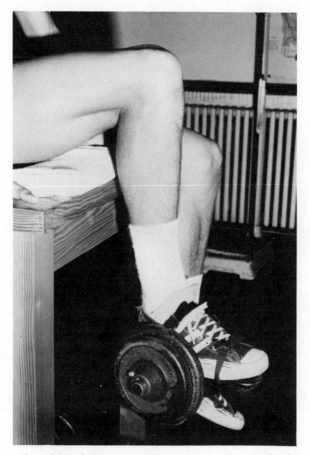

Fig. 13 Unilateral hip flexion against the resistance of a weighted boot following knee surgery.

iii. Knee extension–flexion utilizing isokinetic exercises, beginning with a relatively low speed and gradually increasing the speed.

iv. Ankle plantar flexion—progressive to 15–20 repetitions.

v. Terminal extension exercise (Figs. 14 and 15) ("hurdler's exercise") with the addition of a towel looped over the forefoot for additional stretching of the popliteal area.

The above exercises are done once in a circuit during the first session, two sets at the next, three sets at the next, and never more than three sets subsequently. Progression is consistent and judicious. As soon as a pain-free ROM in excess of 90° is present at the knee with no apparent swelling and no significant pain, the following changes are made:

vi. Leg raises are eliminated.

vii. Isotonic leg extension is added—one leg at a time, alternating legs. Resistance is added progressively, 15–20 repetitions.

viii. Isotonic knee flexion—resistance is added progressively, 15–20 repetitions.

ix. Terminal extension is continued if necessary.

x. Active stretching of the rectus femoris muscle, the hamstring mus-

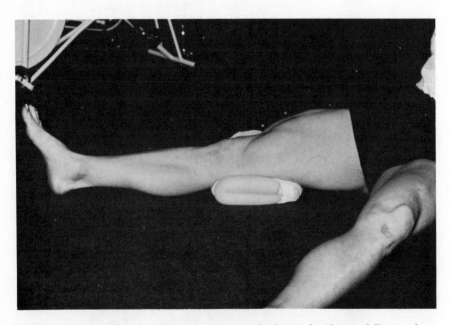

Fig. 14 Terminal extension exercise to stretch the popliteal area following knee surgery. The subject is making an isometric contraction of the thigh and leg muscles against a foam pad placed behind the knee.

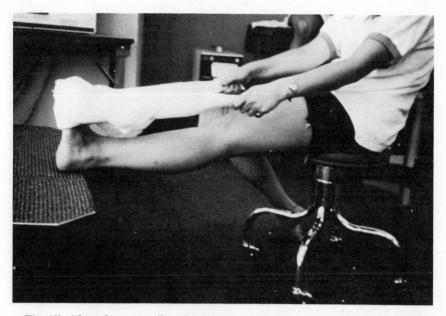

Fig. 15 The subject is pulling his foot into dorsiflexion with a towel while maintaining an isometric contraction of the leg and thigh muscles to stretch the popliteal area.

cles, and the Achilles tendon is initiated at the same time that isotonic exercises are introduced.

xi. Stationary bicycling is added to tolerance, usually 2–4 miles at one sitting, with a resistance based upon the capability of the individual (Fig. 16)

xii. At this stage the leg press is added to tolerance. Resistance is progressive, 20–30 repetitions.

Each of these exercises is performed 2–3 times daily. The rationale at this stage is no longer one of maintenance of function, but is one of building (rebuilding) muscle mass and function. Still, aggressiveness should not gain the upper hand over judicious choice of exercise dosage. Of primary importance at this stage is mobilization and achievement of pain-free flexion and full extension. Secondarily, proper form in the performance of exercise is indicated. Of third importance is the actual amount of resistance used in the exercise, although once motion and proper form have been achieved, the resistance load becomes all-important. More complicated or extensive injury may call for a slower beginning at this stage. By observing the signs of pain and swelling however, as well as following basic precautions as far as the rate of

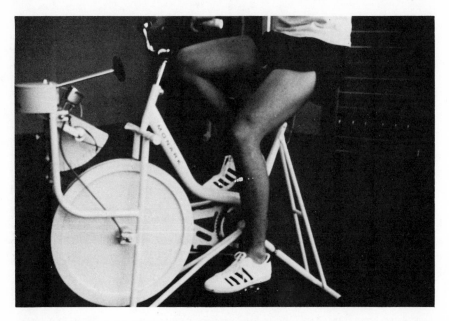

Fig. 16 Subject is riding a Monark bicycle ergometer in order to increase the endurance of his lower extremity muscles. An adjustable electric resistance which can be read directly off a cycle is provided through the weighted fly wheel.

progression is concerned, there is no reason to believe that most such cases cannot eventually progress to the same level of performance as less complicated ones. The difference is one of a slower rate of progress. In many cases of extensive erosion of the joint surfaces either on the patella or the femoral condyle, resistive ROM exercise may be permanently contraindicated. In these cases isokinetic types of exercise usually are helpful.

d. LATE INTERMEDIATE REHABILITATION. The criteria for advancement to this stage are pain-free full range motion of the involved joint, and a strength deficit in the quadriceps group of no more than 25%. The following exercises should be carried out:

i. Leg extension—both legs simultaneously, 15–20 repetitions (Figs. 17 and 18).

ii. Leg flexion—both legs simultaneously, 15–20 repetitions.

iii. Leg press—15–20 repetitions. (Fig. 19).

iv. Stationary bicycle—emphasize high speed and high resistance. Progress with distance up to 5 miles.

v. Running—preferably uphill, or if on the treadmill, with a grade of 5–10%. Progress in distance and speed.

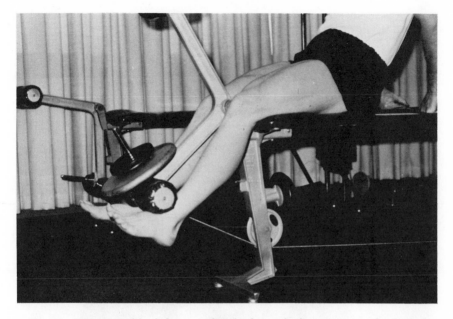

Fig. 17 Extension of both legs simultaneously on the knee against a fixed weight resistance. The subject's legs are in the middle of the range of motion as he leans back to balance the resistance with his body.

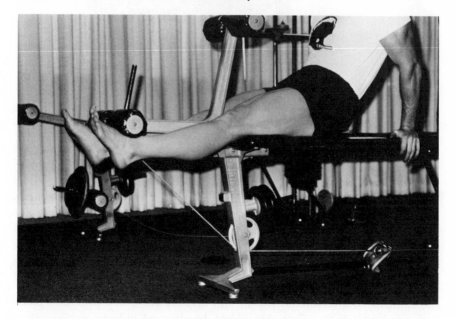

Fig. 18 The same exercise as in Fig. 17, with both legs now in full extension. Progression is obtained by increasing the weight in $2\frac{1}{2}$ to 5 lb. increments.

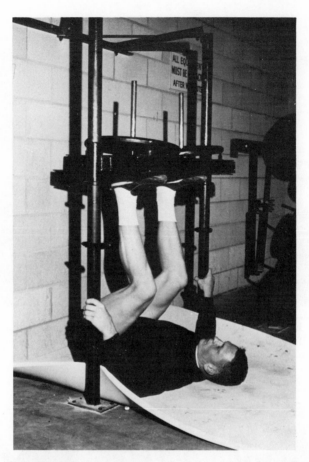

Fig. 19 Late intermediate rehabilitation of the leg and thigh muscles by pressing the lower extremities together into full extension against a weight resistance while lying supine.

At this stage of rehabilitation the rationale becomes less one of therapy and more one of sports conditioning. Sports conditioning centers about a concern for "functional power." Considerations must include resistance, speed of movement, range of movement, and repetitions. By this stage it has been determined whether or not intensive exercise is indicated. If not, then exercise is limited to nonresistive exercise of the isokinetic type, and to non-ROM exercises such as straight leg raises, isometrics at various angles, and full ROM hip and ankle movements.

    e. ADVANCED REHABILITATION. The criteria for entry into this phase of rehabilitation are that the athlete be deemed able to participate in competitive sports, and have no more than 5–10% strength deficit in the quadriceps mechanism. The following exercises are to be carried out:

i. Warm-up using a stationary bicycle or jump rope. Maximum performance, 3–5 minutes duration.

ii. Leg press—to exhaustion, 20–30 repetitions.

iii. Leg extension—to exhaustion, 15–20 repetitions.

iv. Half knee bends—to exhaustion, 15–20 repetitions.

v. Leg curl—to exhaustion, 15–20 repetitions (Fig. 20).

vi. Toe raise—to exhaustion, 25–30 repetitions.

vii. Stationary bicycle—taper off. Moderate resistance for 3–5 minutes duration.

The above exercises should be performed with absolutely no rest between exercises, and, with the exception of the stationary bicycle or jump rope, should be performed in approximately 5 minutes. The central focus of advanced rehabilitation is exactly the same as advanced sports conditioning. Done properly, sports conditioning should simultaneously provide maximum benefit in developing power, endurance, and flexibility.

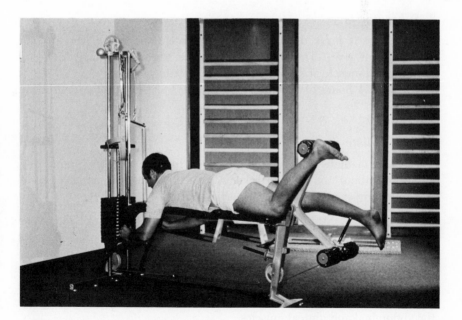

Fig. 20 Advanced rehabilitation of leg and thigh muscles by flexing the leg on the knee in the prone position. The resistance is provided by a pulley weight which is adjustable.

F. Rehabilitation Routines following Sprains and Strains to the Lumbo-sacral Region of the Back

The purpose of these exercises is to improve the mechanics of the back through improved strength, coordination, and elasticity. This is accomplished by developing actively the flexor muscles of the lumbosacral spine and stretching passively the extensor muscles and fasciae. Faulty posture must be corrected, and, once corrected, proper posture must be maintained at all times.

1. Acute Stage

This stage is marked by the presence of pain and muscle spasm, and requires bed rest. Back exercises should not be attempted during this stage. The following exercises should be carried out:

a. Muscle setting of major muscles of the extremities may be performed safely in order to maintain as much strength in the extremities as possible.

b. Deep breathing exercises may also be helpful.

2. Subacute Stage

This stage is marked by the relief of muscle spasm and the absence of significant pain. The following exercises should be carried out:

a. Gluteal muscle and abdominal muscle setting.

b. After 24 hours of the above two exercises, pelvic tilt exercises are initiated.

3. Intermediate Stage

The intermediate stage of rehabilitation for lumbosacral sprains usually starts about the fifth to seventh day following the acute episode. The following exercises should be carried out:

a. ABDOMINAL SETTING AND PELVIC TILT. The knees are bent. The back is flattened against the floor by pulling the abdominal muscles in and up, tilting the pelvis. The lower spine should be completely flat. This exercise must be performed on a rigid surface so that the back can be flattened with certainty. The abdominal and gluteal muscles should be "set" during this exercise. This exercise helps to strengthen the abdominal and gluteal muscles.

* The program outlined is that used at the Sports Medicine Clinic in Atlanta, Georgia, by William Andrews, R. P. T.

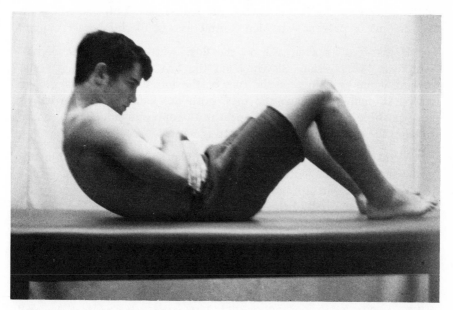

Fig. 21   Lying in the supine position with arms across the lower chest and knees flexed to 45°, the subject raises his head and shoulders from the table by tightening his abdominal muscles. Bending the knees minimizes the contribution of the hip flexor muscles to this exercise.

b. HEAD–SHOULDER CURL. (Fig. 21). Sit-ups often aggravate existing back problems. Therefore, head–shoulder curls should permanently replace sit-ups. From the starting position, with the knees flexed and back flat on the floor, raise the head first, then the shoulders as far as possible, while keeping the small of the back flat. Hold this position in an isometric contraction with the abdominals.

c. KNEE–CHEST. From starting position of the head and shoulder curl, grasp the knees with outstretched hands and pull the knees toward the axilla as far as possible while attempting to push the head between the knees. This exercise passively stretches the erector spinae muscles and the contracted lumbar fasciae and ligaments posterior to the center of gravity at the lumbosacral level. Double leg raises are usually contraindicated in individuals with back problems and therefore should always be avoided.

d. TRUNK FLEXION. Sit on the edge of the chair, slowly drop head and shoulders, and then bend the back so as to attempt to touch the folded elbows to the floor between the feet. Relax. This exercise helps to overcome or prevent extension contractures of the lumbosacral spine.

  e. HAMSTRING STRETCH. Sit on the floor with the legs extended in front in a "V" position. Slowly bend the head, shoulders, and trunk forward while reaching for the toes of the left foot with outstretched fingers. If unable to reach the toes, push the hands along the leg as far as possible. Slowly stretch. Repeat to the opposite side. This exercise stretches the erector spinae and hamstring muscles.

  f. ANTERIOR HIP STRETCH. Assume the squat position, with both hands on the floor, the left foot placed flatly on the floor with the knee fully flexed and the right hip and knee fully extended behind the body with the weight on the ball of the foot and the ankle doriflexed. The forward knee is slightly extended and then flexed repeatedly, thus moving the pelvis up and down, and stretching the anterior portion of the extended hip. This exercise stretches the anterior thigh and hip structures (rectus femoris muscle, fascia lata, and iliofemoral ligament).

  g. BACK FLATTENING AGAINST WALL. Stand with the back to the wall, and heels 6–8 inches from the wall. Flatten the spine against the wall by tilting the hips backward, with the abdomen pulled in and up, the chest up, and the chin in and down. Set the abdominal and gluteal muscles. This exercise helps to strengthen the abdominal and gluteal muscles.

4. Advanced Stage

  This stage is not undertaken until the patient is totally asymptomatic. The goal of this stage is to restore sufficient strength so that the individual may safely participate in athletics, but the weight training program is modified so that it is not likely to aggravate the preexisting back condition. During this stage the exercises that were outlined for the intermediate stage are continued, and in addition endurance activities are progressively added to the program. These include cycling, jumping rope, and running.

D. Weight Training for Persons with Low Back Difficulty

  General notes for this training are as follows:

  1. Avoid lifting unnecessarily heavy weights, but keep repetitions quite high, such as 25–30 for the legs and 12–15 for the upper body.

2. Whenever possible, perform upper body exercises with one arm at a time (press, curl, triceps press, etc.).

3. Whenever possible, perform exercises in a seated position (press, curl, triceps press, etc).

4. Alternate exercises which push down on the spine with those exercises which pull the spine apart (e.g., press alternate with pull-down).

5. Strictly avoid the following:
    a. Sit-ups (do head shoulder curl instead).
    b. Stiff-legged leg raises.
    c. Stiff-legged dead lift or any other dead lift.
    d. Standing overhead presses.
    e. Arch-type bench press (keep feet up on a second bench).
    f. Full squats or heavy leg presses.
    g. Heavy standing curls.
    h. Limit lifts of any type.
    i. Calisthenics such as toe touches (do seated hurdler's stretch instead).
    j. Duck walks and pony back carries.

H. General Conditioning Routine on a Multistation Weight Training Apparatus

(Perform this exercise routine only once daily.)

1. Head–shoulder curl on the abdominal board.
2. Leg extension.
    a. Moderate weight with 25 repetitions with weight on the end, not the weight stack.
    b. Follow within five seconds with the leg press.
3. Leg press.
    a. Moderate weight with 25 repetitions.
    b. Use the closest possible seat position.
    c. Do not pull excessively with the hands but use a restraining belt, if possible, instead of the hands.
    d. Follow within five seconds with the leg curl.
4. Leg curl
    a. 15–20 repetitions.
5. Kneeling behind the neck "lat" pull-down
    a. Use shoulder width grip.
    b. Relax at top of each repetition.
    c. 15–20 repetitions.
6. One arm seated press (alternate arms)
    a. 15–20 repetitions.

7. Head–shoulder curl.
8. Seated pulley curl (alternate arms).
    a. 10–15 repetitions.
    b. Sit on floor with the elbow braced on the inside of the knee.
9. Triceps press-down on "lat" station.
    a. 15 repetitions.
10. Dead hang from chinning bar.
    a. Hang relaxed for 15–30 seconds.
11. Bench press.
    a. Feet supported above floor level.
    b. Keep back flat on bench.
    c. 10–15 repetitions.

REFERENCES

Abbott, H. G., and Kress, J. B. (1969). *Arch. Phys. Med. Rehabil.* **50,** 326–333.

Callahan, W. T., Crowley, F. J., and Hafner, J. K. (1971). "A Statewide Study Designed to Determine Methods of Reducing Injury in Interscholastic Football Competition by Equipment Modification." New York State Public High School Athletic Association, Albany.

DeLorme, T. L. (1945). *J. Bone Joint Surg.* **27,** 645–667.

Klein, K. K., and Allman, F. L., Jr. (1971). "The Knee in Sports," Pemberton Press, Austin, Texas.

Kraus, H. (1959). *Amer. J. Surg.* **98,** 355–362.

Marshall, W. A. (1970). Doctoral Dissertation, University of Wisconsin, Madison, Wisconsin.

Morehouse, C. A. (1971). Read at *Nat. Conf. Med. Aspects Sports, 13th,* New Orleans, Louisiana, Nov. 28.

Nicholas, J. A. (1970). *J. Amer. Med. Ass.* **212,** 2236–2239.

O'Donoghue, D. H. (1950). *J. Bone Joint Surg. Amer. Vol.,* **32,** 721–738.

Wallis, E. L., and Logan, G. A. (1964). "Figure Improvement and Body Conditioning through Exercise." Prentice-Hall, Englewood Cliffs, New Jersey.

Chapter 14

SPECIAL PROBLEMS OF THE FEMALE ATHLETE

CLAYTON L. THOMAS

Even if the day ever dawns in which it will not be needed for fighting the old heavy battles against nature, muscular vigor will still always be needed to furnish the background of sanity, serenity, and cheerfulness to life, to give moral elasticity to our disposition, to round off the wiry edge of our fretfulness and make us good humored and easy of approach.

William James

I. HISTORICAL ASPECTS OF WOMEN'S PARTICIPATION IN ATHLETICS

Examination of artifacts from primitive societies and cultures indicates that mankind has almost always participated in games or play of some sort. Those artifacts do not, however, allow us to determine to what extent women participated. Bloch (1968) states: "Ancient Greece can truly be considered the birthplace of competitive sports as we know them." We also know from Harris' (1964) excellent study that, in the sixth century BC, girls participated in running races and that women of Sparta wrestled. Even this participation was limited to the time of a woman's life prior to marriage. He felt that even though women's life in ancient Greece was quite different from modern women's, the difference has been exaggerated by lack of information. Pericles stated that the greatest glory of a woman is not to be talked about by men, either by praise or blame (Harris, 1964). Because Greek literature deals almost exclusively with the public part of life, we have little opportunity to know whether or not Greek women participated in sports or games at home.

It is of curious interest to note that the ancient Olympic Games were open to all spectators except married women, and that first prize was a woman skilled in domestic arts. Second prize was a pregnant mare.

In all societies in which the ability merely to survive depends upon maximum physical effort of the entire family, there is little reason to expect that either men or women would have the time and energy to participate in athletics. In any case, as leisure time became available, it was the men who were the first to devote time to sports.

This point is well illustrated by examining the history of women's participation in the modern Olympics. They were founded in 1896 by Baron de Coubertin, who was most probably a misogynist. No doubt other forces were in part responsible for the fact that women didn't appear as contestants in the first modern Olympic Games in 1896. Nevertheless, evidence that the founder encouraged women's participation in the Olympics during his tenure as President of the Comité International Olympique is not apparent. Indeed, six women competed in the 1900 Olympics, but none in 1896 and 1904. By 1932, 715 participants (4.1% of all the contestants) were women (Encyclopedia Brittanica, 1964). Contemporarily, representation of girls and women as Olympic contestants has improved, but the record is still dismal. Of the 5,558 athletes at the Tokyo Olympics in 1964, 722 (13%) were women. In Mexico City at the 1968 Olympics, 13.9% of the contestants were women.

Of the 115 countries represented at Mexico City, 57 were represented by men alone. Many of the national teams, though well supplied with men, included only one or two women.

Women will, in the near future, have a greater role in athletics, not only in the present context, but in areas of competition as members of teams composed of men and women. The experience in New York State in 1969 and 1970 (Grover, 1970) has proven that boys and girls can coexist as members of the same team in a noncontact sport, even if it means some boys will lose to better players who happen to be of the opposite sex.

II. BIOLOGICAL FACTORS THAT LED TO SEPARATE MALE–FEMALE SOCIAL ROLES

In all but a very few societies, women have been assigned to, and virtually inextricably bonded to, the role of keeper-of-the-nest. This did, and still, means that, of the two sexes, women have the job with the longest hours, and least pay, even though the greatest security. In primitive societies, childbearing dictated this role. Participation for lengthy intervals in the traditional male endeavors of hunting and fighting was impossible. Even so, in some Amerind groups, though the men killed large game, it was the task of the women to skin the animals and bring them home.

The influence of the male hormone on muscular development is well known. One cannot help but speculate, however, concerning the possible influence of genetic selection working to choose two groups of individuals best suited for the quite different job classifications, i.e., men equipped for strength, speed, and endurance required in hunting and fighting; and women whose job probably required more total energy output, but not expended in short-time intervals. Darlington (1969) has explained how selection can alter one sex without affecting the other.

Through the ages men have found this situation, summarized by the Germans in *Kinder, Küchen, Kirche* (children, kitchen, church) so convenient that they have felt no compulsion to examine either its necessity or fairness. The ethical, economic, and moral validity of this system is being examined in great detail by both the willing and unwilling in what might be termed a revolutionary atmosphere. Women, especially those in the field of athletics, still have a long way to go. Equality of encouragement and opportunity for women's participation in sports is lacking throughout the world and virtually absent even in advanced societies. The winds of change, though slower in eroding the restraints imposed by a male-dominated social system than many think reasonable, are blowing with greater force, over a greater area, and with greater results.

Entrance of females into all-male strongholds, both social and physical, is startling with respect to variety, but not extent. In World War II we became accustomed, in the United States at least, to women working as riveters, as ferry pilots for airplanes, and in virtually all industries previously limited to males. That law, the judiciary, and elected public office did not share equally in those incursions by women could be explained by several factors. Especially important is the length of time required in training or political preparation in order to participate in those fields. The more than three decades since the beginning of World War II, however, has seen no drastic change in representation of women in those professions.

The seemingly absolute barriers continue to fall. We now have women who are jockeys, airline-transport pilots, aircraft-control tower operators, aquanauts, and even training for the Rabbinate. No doubt we will one day have women as astronauts, and increasingly as heads of State. As dramatic as these accomplishments are, or would be, they should be considered in the light of their rarity, and that women are still economically deprived in relation to the planning for their recreational facilities as compared to those for men.

III. CURRENT SOCIAL, ECONOMIC, AND BIOLOGICAL FACTORS THAT ACT TO LIMIT OR INFLUENCE WOMEN'S PARTICIPATION IN ATHLETICS

A. Social Factors

In the Western world, and particularly North America, the social limits on women's participation in sports are rapidly disappearing. Young girls, particularly, have found it possible to compete in almost any sport, and even on teams with boys. So far, this latter type of involvement has been limited almost completely to noncontact sports. A lady has participated as the holder of the ball for place kicks in American professional football.

Traditionally male-only educational institutions have been entered by women. After 222 years, Princeton permitted women to enroll, and, within two years, a girls' eight-oared crew had been formed, and was seeking to schedule races with similar teams at Smith and Wellesley colleges.

The New York State Education Department found that its 16-month-long experimental program of letting girls compete on the same team as boys in golf, tennis, gymnastics, riflery, skiing, swimming, fencing, track, and cross country, was an unqualified success (Grover, 1970). There was no evidence of physical, psychological, or sexual harm to the girls or boys who participated in the experiment.

Even though the social barriers to women in athletics seem to be disappearing, at least in parts of the Western world, there will no doubt be a lag in the number of participants who can be accommodated in sports. This delay will be necessitated by the fact that women have traditionally not been allowed the same share of funds for athletics and recreational equipment. The appearance of girls' teams to utilize sports facilities not previously required by them will have great economic impact on schools, cities, and colleges. As previously pointed out (Thomas, 1970), "If by some miracle, women suddenly began using public and private athletic facilities to even half the extent they are used for men, then the overcrowding would be catastrophic. If women ask their husbands to do domestic chores so that they can participate in recreational activities as often as their husbands now do, men would most probably rebel."

No matter to what extent women become liberated, it is hoped that some will continue to be motivated to continue childbearing and rearing! In the past, this process has required an inordinate length of time, particularly for those who had, by chance or circumstance, large families. In the present context of planned and spaced childbearing, women need not be slaves to the process, and can have time for careers in many fields, including athletics. Motherhood and athletics, as will be discussed later, are not mutually exclusive.

In addition to planning the conception of children, modern girls and women who wish to enjoy sport and physical recreation will need to change other social habits—habits which can be as adverse to freedom of movement and athletic participation as any other single force—such as feeling that social acceptance by peers and society requires hours of personal or purchased grooming. Athletic endeavors at all levels, from playground to the Olympics, are facilitated by the participants being physically unfettered and willing to seek a goal with a certain degree of physical abandon. This cannot be accomplished if an individual is primarily concerned with preserving eyeshadow, false eyelashes, and coiffure with exercising. This is not to suggest that men and women should not be concerned with beauty, but to say that it behooves us to examine the social and economic forces that attempt to deny that physical activity is a basic right and need of all human beings. Fear of perspiring should not have priority over the pursuit of the physical and mental rewards of sports participation. A nice compromise was reached at the Olympic Games in Munich in 1972 when special on the field facilities for primping were provided for women contestants required to go to the winner's stand immediately after concluding their events.

Important to the social aspects of women's participation in sports is the different light in which men and women who excel, or in the latter case even participate, are regarded by society. The young boy who wished to participate in football, softball, or baseball will find a spectrum of national organizations waiting to foster and nurture his interest. There are, however, few counterparts to Little League and other male organizations to administer and supervise team sports for girls. The reasons for this are complex and multiple, but high on the list would be the continued expectation by the Establishment that women's role should not include athletics. Evidence that many young girls, if given the same opportunity and encouragement, will participate in vigorous athletic activity, is available (Brown, 1970; Klemesrud, 1971). Indeed, as Shaffer (1961) has noted, all children have a natural desire to participate in games. Realizing this, it must be assumed that our society has, by marshaling strong negative forces or by persistent neglect, effectively prevented women from realizing their potential in either recreational or competitive sports activities.

B. Economic Factors

No doubt much of what has been presented above as social forces important in preventing or dissuading women from athletic participation can also be ascribed to an economic factor. With rare exceptions, there are no readily apparent sizable economic rewards to institutions, corporations, or individual women which accrue because of women's participation in athletics. In contrast, when a male athlete performs, money is usually involved. Athletic-equipment suppliers, radio and television stations, high school and college stadia—all may be sources of revenue. Many team members at the college level are provided with athletic scholarships. There are many direct and indirect economic gains for individuals or organizations. There is, therefore, minimal economic incentive for a young girl to excel in athletics. She will, even in performing at the championship level, have little opportunity to receive a scholarship to college. Schools and colleges have no compelling incentive to spend money on interscholastic or intercollegiate athletic facilities for women. Such expenditures would increase their indebtedness without immediately providing the opportunity through gate receipts to amortize the costs. Equipment manufacturers are reluctant to attempt to develop women's athletic equipment if redesign costs are involved. The television medium thrives on sporting events that are spectacular enough to attract millions of viewers, and, thus, advertisers to pay the costs of the production. Only rarely are girls' events seen on television. Compare this lack of exposure to that afforded football, baseball, basketball, and ice hockey. As a result, there is rarely an opportunity for women to receive the type of publicity that would create national interest and involvement at the individual or corporate level.

Another economic factor, particularly important to the young housewife and mother who might wish to participate in athletics, is the lack of general availability, as well as the cost, of baby sitters at the time of day when it might be most convenient to exercise. The husband has no such problem. He may come home and leave for the golf course, assured that the children are well cared for by available low-cost labor—his wife!

C. Biological Factors

The biological factors important to women who wish to exercise may be considered under endocrine, biochemical, hematological, and anthropometric classifications.

1. Prepubertal Functional Capacity

Prior to puberty, boys and girls differ very little with respect to their physical work capacity. The study of Åstrand et al. (1963) clearly demonstrates this and the data of Willmore and Sigerseth (1967) confirm it. With respect to age, the maximum work capacity in girls is attained earlier than in boys. There is no reason to believe that these age-related differences in the two sexes beginning at puberty could be attributed to factors other than endocrine.

2. Effects of Menstrual Cycle on Behavior and Sports Performance

In addition to the obvious male–female endocrine differences, the female demonstrates, due to hormonal influences, a cyclic variation in her reproductive physiology which is not, so far as is known, observed in the male. This cycle, which is essential to reproduction, begins at puberty and continues until the menopause. The marked effect of this biological rhythm on women has been reviewed by Southam and Gonzaga (1965). They list the more than 30 different physical, chemical, and systemic changes that have been reported to undergo variation during the phases of the menstrual cycle. A partial summary of their report is included in Table I. It should be noted, however, that the authors state at the end of their review: "It is evident that the ovarian cycle has an effect on many physiologic measurements. Some of the changes presented in this review require further documentation and some of the older observations deserve re-evaluation with modern techniques."

The information in Table I provides some insight into the possibility that variation in a variety of body functions does occur during certain phases of the menstrual cycle. Dalton (1964, 1970) has presented a great deal of information indicating that women's behavior, particularly during the premenstrual portion of the cycle, is severely altered. She has not, however, investigated the effect of premenstrual tension on athletic performance nor has she been concerned with the effect of exercise acting either to mitigate or enforce those potentially negative effects. Investigations of the effect of the menstrual cycle on athletic performance must be considered and evaluated with respect to the possibility of selection bias. This is especially true of studies of world-class athletes. D. Hanley, B. Sebasteanski, and A. Martin (personal communications, 1968) have ascertained that, as would be expected, women on the United States Olympic teams in 1964 and 1968 have won Gold medals and established new World records during all phases of the menstrual cycle, including menstruation itself. This confirms the reports of other investigations of championship performance (Bausenwein, 1960; Zaharieva, 1965; Noack, 1954). To interpret this as being proof that all women can be expected to perform at maximum capacity and ability during all phases of their menstrual cycle would be ridiculous. The factors that determine one's best achievement, be the performer male or female, are multiple, and include much more than physiological variation.

3. Influence of Physical Exercise on Reproductive Function

It is, indeed, valid to attempt to examine the other side of the coin concerning women and athletics, i.e., does exercise interfere with maintenance of general health of women and specifically their reproductive function?

Almost a century ago, Jacobi (1877) wrote: "There is nothing in the nature of menstruation to imply the necessity, or even the desirability, of rest for women whose nutrition is really normal."

TABLE I

Changes during the Menstrual Cycle[a]

Item	Character of change
Temperature	Decreased at time of ovulation then sharp rise to a plateau
Blood Pressure	Arterial pressure lower at midcycle
Respiration	Increased ventilation of lung with decreased arterial CO_2 tension in the luteal phase
Weight	Some women gain in premenstrual period
Red blood cells	Decreased survival time in luteal phase
Leukocytes	Decreased during menstruation and proliferative phase
Eosinophils	Decreased during midcycle
Platelets	Decreased in latter half of cycle
Proteins	No distinct
Carbohydrate metabolism	Tolerance to glucose is less during menstruation; fasting blood sugar is higher during menstruation
Lactic acid	Increased at time of ovulation
Cholesterol	Total serum cholesterol rises following menstruation
Total nonprotein nitrogen	Increased at onset of menstruation
Calcium	Lower in premenstrual phase
Inorganic phosphate and phosphorus	Higher at time of menstruation
Serum magnesium	Decreased to minimum immediately prior to menstruation
Endocrine	Midcycle peak of total urinary gonadotropins
Thyroid	Premenstrual rise in basal metabolic rate during menstruation
Mucus	Arborization of both nasal and cervical mucus during proliferative phase
Cytology	Cornification of epithelial cells of vagina, cervix, mouth, and bladder at time of ovulation and during menstruation
Skin	Darkening of skin premenstrually; increased sebaceous gland activity premenstrually
GI Tract	Increased gastric motility during menstruation
Electroencephalogram (EEG)	Rhythm disturbances at time of menstruation in some women
Equilibrium	No difficulty in response to vestibular stimulation
Mental and physical efficiency	Pedometer-measured activity is greatest during postmenstrual phase; time or speed of movement is not affected
Behavior and emotions	Premenstrual complaints of breast pain and tenderness, abdominal discomfort, back pains, headache, depression, and decreased mental efficiency; insomnia occurred more frequently during the menses; misdemeanors increased

TABLE I (Continued)

Item	Character of change
	among school girls during menstruation; suicides and attempted suicides more frequent in premenstrual and menstrual phases; more crimes committed in those same periods
Premenstrual tension	Protean clinical syndrome which includes physical and emotional components; etiology is obscure; does not occur in anovulatory cycles
Systemic diseases	Certain infectious diseases are more likely to have their onset in the immediate premenstrual period (this is also true for accidents and pancreatitis; diabetic coma more frequent and insulin requirement is increased at time of menses; allergic conditions, including asthma, are worse during the menstrual and premenstrual periods; skin disorders, including eczema and herpes, are worse premenstrually and during the menses; peptic ulcer symptoms are increased during the menstrual period; urinary incontinence becomes worse during the progestational phase of the cycle; epileptic seizures are more common during the premenstrual and menstrual phases, according to some, but others dispute this

[a] Abstracted from Southam and Gonzaga (1965).

Both the short-term and the long-range effect of women's participation in competitive swimming was thoroughly investigated and reported by Åstrand *et al.* (1963). They investigated 30 contemporary Swedish champion girl swimmers and 84 former championship contestants. The latter were called the post-active group. The 30 champion girls had trained by swimming 3.73 to 40.39 miles (6000 to 65,000 meters) per week. The others had averaged 5.59 miles (9000 meters) per week. None of the 30 was injured by that vigorous program. The obstetrical and gynecological history of the post-active swimmers was normal.

Anderson (1965) in a study of synchronized swimmers at North High School in Des Moines, Iowa compared 65 girl swimmers with 138 students whose swimming experiences were minimal. The synchronized swimmers had less difficulty with dysmenorrhea, and it was less severe as compared to the nonswimmers. The author also questioned 111 women who had previously participated in vigorous athletic activity. Their obstetrical and gynecological experiences had been uneventful.

The Pacific Association of the Amateur Athletic Union of the United States (Amateur Athletic Union of the United States, 1960) published a booklet containing data and opinion from virtually all medical and athletic disciplines. They found no evidence that athletic competition has a deleterious effect on girls and women.

Hong and Rahn (1967) have described women who make their living by diving throughout the year:

> The Korean women dive even in winter, when the water temperature is 50 degrees Fahrenheit (but only for short periods under such conditions). For those who choose this occupation, diving is a lifelong profession; they begin to work in shallow water at the age of 11 or 12 and sometimes continue to 65. Childbearing does not interrupt their work; a pregnant diving woman may work up to the day of delivery and nurse her baby afterward between diving shifts. The divers are called ama. At present there are some 30,000 of them living and working along the seacoasts of Korea and Japan. About 11,000 ama dwell on the small, rocky island of Cheju off the southern tip of the Korean peninsula, which is believed to be the area where the diving practice originated. Archaeological remains indicate that the practice began before the fourth century. In times past the main objective of the divers may have been pearls, but today it is solely food. Up to the 17th century the ama of Korea included men as well as women; now they are all women. And in Japan, where many of the ama are male, women nevertheless predominate in the occupation. As we shall see, the female is better suited to this work than the male.

In a personal communication, Doctor S. K. Hong wrote concerning the diving ama: "Some years ago we have made a survey on their menstruation, according to which they engage in usual daily diving work even during menstruation. As far as we learned, they use no particular menstrual protection. Our survey also indicated that their menstrual cycle is quite regular." Social and occupational aspects of the diving ama of Japan have been described and photographed by Maraini (1962) and Marden (1971).

Erdelyi (1961) surveyed 729 Hungarian female athletes and found the incidence of cesarean section was only 50% of a control group. Bausenwein (1960) states that, in events of short duration, women have attained their best personal performance and even established Olympic and World records while menstruating. Yet, without presenting data, she contends that exercise during menstruation causes pelvic congestion, and that strenuous exercise by younger girls may cause irreparable harm to ovarian function.

Javert (1960) has discussed the role of a patient's activities in the occurrence of spontaneous abortion. He quotes Potter as follows: "As well stated by Potter, the packaging of the child in utero is such that the tough skin, muscles, and fascia of the abdominal wall, the thick uterine muscle lined by membrane, and the ammoniotic fluid absorb physical trauma encountered in the daily routine of the mother to protect the growing fetus from ordinary harm." Javert (1960) concluded: ". . . that normal physical and mental activity do not predispose to spontaneous abortion. However, violent physical and mental trauma engendered by unexpected accidents are rare but significant factors in abortion."

There is no evidence that strenuous and vigorous physical activity harms the nongravid uterus. McCloy's (1931) discussion of Paramore's comparing the protection afforded the uterus to that supplied by the water surrounding an egg in a jar provides an easily duplicated model for demonstrating this principle. As long as the egg is not resting against the wall of the container and the container remains intact, it is not possible to break the egg by hitting the jar.

The type and amount of exercise either indicated or permitted during pregnancy is something each patient, in consultation with her doctor, will have to decide. The patient who has been almost completely sedentary prior to her pregnancy might require a somewhat vigorous fitness program. On the other hand, the highly trained athlete might find it advisable to decrease her exercise schedule.

In a study (Ueland *et al.*, 1969) of 11 normal women, cardiac output and pulse rate were found to be elevated during most of the last two trimesters of pregnancy. Stroke volume progressively decreased during the same period. Cardiac output investigated in six patients during light exercise (100 kpm per minute) and in five during moderate exercise (200 kpm per minute). In moderate exercise, there was a progressive decline in circulatory response as pregnancy advanced. This was not attributed by the authors to a change in cardiac function, but to peripheral pooling of blood and obstruction to venous return by the large gravid uterus. Following exercise, cardiovascular function returned to resting levels at the same rate during pregnancy as in the postpartum period. To the extent the results of this study (Ueland *et al.*, 1969) could be applied to well-conditioned subjects, it is not surprising to find that championship-level athletes have competed until a few days prior to onset of labor (Rumpf, 1952) and that there was one Olympic Bronze medalist in swimming competition in the 1952 Games during her pregnancy (Amateur Athletic Union of the United States, 1960).

Noack (1954) investigated 10 women who continued their sports activity after delivery. He reported:

> . . . two retained their physical abilities, and eight clearly increased them. All the women reported that after the birth of a child they had become tougher, more enduring and stronger. It is striking to learn from this survey that everything went smoothly from the obstetrical point of view. The generally

short duration of the delivery indicates that the frequently asserted rigidity of the soft parts (Sellheim) is insignificant. Certainly, the seven ruptures of the perineum are above the normal number. It cannot be excluded that the good activity of the abdominal muscles in the sports-trained woman was a disadvantage for the perineum. In spite of the desire to resume sports, breast feeding was apparently carried out for a normal length of time. It is especially significant and noticeable that six of these women won championships after delivery. We would not be able to find thirteen German Champions, three DDR-Champions, three Berlin Champions and two Silver Medals during the Olympic Games of 1948 in our German sports, if these women had not resumed sports after delivery. We believe that this fact deserves attention in interested sports circles. Naturally, our material is small and selected, but the top performances are objective facts which should give food for thought.

4. Influence of Exercise on Growth and Development of Young Children

It is reasonable to question whether or not a young child, particularly a girl, might be permanently harmed by being allowed to participate in strenuous athletic activity. Establishment of the concept that physical exercise promotes health in children was set back for at least two generations by Beneke's (1879) publication on heart size. His data were misinterpreted by himself, as well as by most of those who read his report. It was generally thought that Beneke's study indicated that in the developing child the growth rate of the heart lagged behind that of the aorta and pulmonary artery. This anatomical myth was believed and quoted extensively. Finally, Karpovich (1937) demonstrated that a fallacy had been perpetuated because Beneke and subsequent authors had failed to compare the *volume* of the heart with the *cross-sectional area* of the aorta and pulmonary artery. Karpovich used Beneke's original data to demonstrate this point. He concluded:

1. Contrary to an established notion, there is no discrepancy between the development of the heart and the cross section of the largest arteries.
2. The heart volume and the cross section areas of the aorta and the pulmonary artery show a close proportionality. It would be of interest to use the heart capacity instead of the volume, but unfortunately there are not enough data available.
3. The ratio of the heart volume to the size of the blood vessel is not decreased at the age of seven. There is a steady gradual increase in this ratio which starts at the end of the first year.
4. Hygienic warning based upon erroneous interpretations should be discarded.

5. The Suitability of Sports for Young Children

We do not have data that would allow a precise and significant statement to be made concerning which sports are suitable for various age groups. Even though it has been customary to prohibit prepubertal girls from competing, there is ample evidence that some girls have competed during and before puberty and have not been harmed by this experience. For example, the average age of the girls who were members of the 1964 United States Olympic swimming team was $15\frac{1}{2}$ and they had been competing for over 5 years (Counsilman, 1965). Obviously, many of the girls on the team had begun to train and compete prior to menarche.

6. The Female Breast in Sports Activity

Whether or not females who have an excess of breast tissue will be at a disadvantage in sports participation is largely determined by the requirements of individual events. Since breast size is determined to some extent by excess body fat, one rarely sees a gymnast with extremely large breasts. Excess breast tissue would, however, be less of an impediment in other sports such as equestrian events, sailing, and weight events. With respect to protecting the breasts from trauma, there is no reason why, with engineering techniques available, that proper protection cannot be provided. Bayne (1968) has described a special protective brassiere. It is possible that clothing which restricts free movement of the thoracic cage would interfere with oxygen consumption. Valsik and Kostkova (1964) reported a statistically significant decrease in oxygen consumption in the 198 18- to 19-year-old students they tested wearing a brassiere as compared to those not wearing one.

7. The Onset of Puberty in Girls

The appearance of puberty approximately two years earlier in the female than the male is well documented. This should, and probably does, give the pubescent girl, of the same chronological, but more advanced maturation age than a boy, an advantage in athletic endeavors requiring skill and strength. This has, however, been little studied. The exact cause of earlier onset of puberty in the girl is not known, but Van Wyk and Grumbach (1968) noted:

> The female skeleton is normally, at all ages, somewhat advanced beyond that of the male, and pubescence likewise occurs earlier in girls than boys. These physiologic differences in timing are frequently exaggerated, since true sexual precocity occurs more commonly in females, whereas a physiologic delay in the onset of adolescence is predominantly a disorder of the male. Although ordinary methods of hormone assay fail to reveal significant sexual differences until the onset of pubescence, ovaries undergo greater enlargement and ex-

hibit far more histologic activity during childhood than do testes; these histologic differences suggest that the prepubescent ovary also has more secretory activity than the infantile testis. Thus, the secretion of small amounts of estrogen throughout the prepubescent years could readily explain both the more rapid skeletal maturation and the earlier onset of pubescence in the female.

8. Biochemical, Endocrine, and Hematological Differences in Men and Women

Tables II and III list some of the endocrine, biochemical, hematological, and urine laboratory tests in which women have been found to be significantly different from men at certain ages. Interpretation of individual tests for women should be made cautiously, particularly if a certain value is closer to the male range than the female. Williams (1956) and others (Elveback *et al.*, 1970; Files *et al.*, 1968) have clearly shown that "normal" is difficult to define. Thus, an individual girl may be found to have a laboratory test value which is quite normal for her, but still quite different from what would be expected from comparing

TABLE II

Certain Physical and Biochemical Differences between Prepubertal and Postpubertal Girls and Boys[a]

Characteristic	Prepubertal		Postpubertal	
	Girls	Boys	Girls	Boys
Height	$<$[b]		$<$	
Weight	$\cong$		$<$	
Strength	$=$		$<$	
Reaction time	$=$		$\cong$	
Earlier onset of puberty	$>$		—	
Body hair	$<$		$<$	
Calcium, serum	$=$		$<$[c]	
Total protein, serum	$=$		$<$[c]	
Albumin, serum	$=$		$<$[c]	
Blood urea nitrogen	$<$		$<$[c]	
Uric acid	$=$		$<$[c]	
Alkaline phosphatase	$=$		$<$[c]	

[a] From Arena (1969), Åstrand *et al.* (1963), and Werner *et al.* (1970). $<$, Less than; $>$, greater than; $=$, equal; $\cong$, approximately equal.

[b] Except ages 12–14.

[c] From Werner *et al.* (1970). These data from a different population are not in complete agreement with those given for these substances in Table III (Castleman, B., and McNeely, B. U., 1970).

TABLE III

Sex Differences in Hematological, Blood and Urine Chemistry Values in Adults[a]

Item	Women	Men
Cholesterol	=	
Calcium	=[b]	
Creatinine phosphokinase	<	
Inorganic phosphate	<	
Total bilirubin	=	
Albumin	=[b]	
Total protein	=[b]	
Uric acid	=[b]	
Blood urea nitrogen	=[b]	
Fasting blood glucose	<	
Acid phosphatase	<	
Alkaline phosphatase	=[b]	
5-Hydroxy indole acetic acid (urine)	<	
Plasma testosterone	<	
Growth hormone	>	
Luteinizing hormone	>	
Erythrocytes	<	
Hematocrit	<	
Hemoglobin	<	
Serum iron	<	
Urine 17-ketosteroid excretion (except prepubertally when it is equal in both sexes)	<	
Urine 17-hydroxy steroid excretion	<	
Basal metabolic rate	<	

[a] From Wintrobe (1967), Castleman, B., and McNeely, B. U. (1970), and Metropolitan Life Insurance Company (1971b).

[b] See footnote to Table II regarding data (Werner *et al.*, 1970) from a different population.

her results with the mean value for a large group of women of a similar age group.

When discussing "normal" values for endocrine, biochemical, and hematological laboratory studies, it is important to define the variable factors such as age, sex, time of day, metabolic, and exercise state when the test was done.

9. Anthropometric and Growth Differences

In discussing body size of adult women, it is of utmost importance to keep in mind the human group to which the individuals belong. This has been thoroughly reviewed by Meredith (1971).

Infant girls are, on the average, very slightly shorter and lighter in weight than boys (Arena, 1969). The heights and weights of children aged 6–11 were obtained from a probability sample of 7417 children selected to represent approximately 24 million noninstitutionalized children in the United States. Height was obtained in stocking feet, and weight was measured in standardized clothing weighing less than two-thirds of a pound. "American boys at age 6 are slightly taller and heavier than the girls; but by age 11 the girls are larger, this holds true for both white and Negro children analyzed separately and together" (Hamill *et al.*, 1970).

Shortly after the onset of puberty in the male, the adolescent boys attain, on the average, greater height and weight than the girls.

From the age of 2 months to 16 years, the overall increase in muscle cell number in the entire body is 14-fold for boys. For girls, during the same period, the increase is approximately 10-fold (Cheek, 1968). The increase in individual muscle-cell size in girls reaches a peak at about age $10\frac{1}{2}$, but in boys the maximum rate of growth of muscle-cell size begins at $10\frac{1}{2}$ and may continue to age 25. Until the onset of puberty, however, the strength of boys and girls of the same biological age is quite similar (Cheek, 1968). Cheek (1968) is unable to explain the difference in cell growth between girls and boys. He speculates it could be due to androgens, growth hormone, or the influence of exercise. He points out that in rats exercise has been shown to increase the DNA and protein content of muscles.

Rauh and Schumsky (1968) report that for children from age 5 to 17, the average percent of body fat is greater in the female, except for the age period of approximately 7 to 10, reaches a peak in boys at age 11, but, after decreasing in the female for ages 5 through 7, increases continually through age 17. The implication of this is, of course, obvious. In swimming, girls would, at certain ages, be relatively more buoyant than boys. This advantage has to be considered in light of the buoyancy being gained at the expense of relatively less lean body mass and, therefore, less muscle mass. Even though contemporary champion girl swimmers beat the World and Olympic records of men several decades ago, they do not equal the record times of contemporary males. Thus, the advantage girls gain over boys in aquatics, because of greater buoyancy, is not sufficient to overcome their absolute deficit in muscle mass. In nonaquatic sports, the increased fat percentage in girls serves to place them at a disadvantage when competing against boys.

In summary, girls are, except for a short period in their earlier life, shorter, lighter, and possess a greater percentage of body fat and a fewer number of muscle cells than boys.

IV. SPECIFIC PROBLEMS OF WOMEN ATHLETES

A. Iron Metabolism and Requirements

Until puberty, the daily intake of iron required for boys and girls is the same. Once the menstrual cycle begins, however, girls require, on the average, twice the daily iron intake of boys. Because of the wide variation in the amount of blood loss during menstruation, some girls may require from three to four times as much iron as the average male (Wintrobe, 1967). All persons concerned with the health of young girls—parents, the individuals themselves, coaches, physicians, and nurses—should be aware of the absolute necessity of an adequate diet, including sufficient iron intake to compensate for iron losses, in maintaining an optimum state of health in postpubertal girls, especially those who wish to participate in athletics.

C. E. C. Harris (1971) stated that during puberty neither boys nor girls should be allowed to be blood donors; and even as adults, women should give blood no more than twice yearly.

In general, women who use an intrauterine contraceptive device (IUD) should be aware that they will lose more blood each menstrual period (Guttorm, 1971; Hefnawi *et al.*, 1970). This means that persons using an IUD have an even greater requirement for dietary or supplemental iron.

B. Injuries and Protective Equipment

With few exceptions, athletes of either sex experience the same kind of injury when they participate in the same sport. The risk of injury and severity of injury might be quite different, though. Except for downhill skiing, this has been little studied. In several reports (Haddon *et al.*, 1964; Ellison, 1970), women have been found to have a much greater chance of experiencing injury while skiing than men. The principal factors appeared to be less strength, less skill, and, in the case of fractures, less bone density.

The experience of women with respect to accidents while skiing as compared to the accident rate in men is a reversal of the usual trend. In almost all other situations involving accidents, women have a much lower rate than men (Metropolitan Life Insurance Company, 1971a; Bergner *et al.*, 1971; Sklar and Downs, 1968).

Women who water ski, when they capsize in a leg-spread position while moving forward or gaining momentum at the beginning of skiing while their pelvis is submerged, have the risk of forcing water into the reproductive tract. The water can produce such force as to gain entrance into the peritoneal cavity either by rupturing the vaginal wall or by traveling via the uterus and fallopian tubes. This has been reported to cause inflammation of the peritoneal cavity (Pfanner, 1964; Ellsworth *et al.*, 1969). The same circumstances that will produce this type of injury may also damage the rectum due to forceful entry of water through the anal orifice. Occasionally in sports a girl will experience trauma to the vulval area with resultant hematoma formation. These types of injuries suggest that girls and women who participate in water skiing and in sports that may injure the vulvae should wear clothing designed to provide perineal protection.

Breast tissue is liable to injury in both contact and noncontact sports. The use of specially designed and fitted protective brassieres, previously mentioned, should be encouraged.

C. Advisability of Athletic Activity during Menstruation

The fact that about one of each seven girls and women of menstrual age would, if not pregnant, be menstruating on any given day provides sufficient information to establish the virtual impossibility of scheduling team amd competitive athletic events in such a way as to be certain none of the contestants was menstruating. Nevertheless, ridiculous regulations designed to prohibit women from participating in athletics during the menstrual period have been established. At one coeducational college I was told by the chairman of the women's physical education department that girls were not allowed to swim during menstruation. One of the younger instructors in her department told me that most students were not aware of the regulation, and those who were ignored it for the most part. At one girls' college the practice was, at one time, to ask that young women not swim while menstruating. This prohibition did not apply to lifeguards. It is suggested that the reader might wish to calculate the number of female lifeguards required to staff a pool to be assured that none would ever be on duty during their menstrual cycle!

Whether or not a girl exercises during all phases of the menstrual cycle should be her personal decision. She should certainly not be forced to participate, nor should she be prevented from so doing, even if the activity includes swimming. This latter statement immediately raises questions concerning the type of menstrual protection to be used, normal bacteriology of swimming pools, and whether or not pool water will flow in and out of the vagina.

The work of Robinton and Mood (1966) utilizing a tank in which young women swam at various times during their menstrual cycle, using either tampons or no form of menstrual protection, is of interest. In their summary they state in part:

> Five healthy young women swam in untreated water of known bacterial quality under a variety of hygienic conditions. Evidence based on bacteriological examination of water samples leads to the following conclusions:
>   1. There is a marked variation in the number and types of bacteria shed by a bather while swimming and the variations do not seem to be correlated to the differences in personal hygiene or the menstrual period . . .

In a review article, Marples (1969) reported that a gram of tissue scraped from the skin contained as many as 530,000,000,000 bacteria. This is quite close to the median figure of the number of bacteria and fungi found in a gram of fertile soil.

Just as no girl should be forced to or prohibited from exercising during all phases of her menstrual cycle, she should not be forced to use a particular form of menstrual protection. It is pointed out, however, that physically active girls, particularly ballet dancers, used homemade tampons long before they became commercially available. Indeed, the examples these young women provided physicians led to the commercial production of tampons.

Women who participate in track and field events have found perineal pads to be hot, uncomfortable, and cumbersome. The use of that form of menstrual protection while swimming is, of course, impractical and would, if attempted, provide no protection. Those who participate in aquatic sports, whether as members of a synchronized swimming team, recreationally, or as competitive swimmers and divers, consider tampons to be the menstrual protection method of choice.

The work of Siegel (1960), as well as the earlier work of Haselhorst (1949), has demonstrated the ability of the vagina to exclude water even when tested almost immediately following childbirth. Thus the possibility of the contamination of the pool by water entering and leaving the vagina is nil. Even if it were possible, the normal vaginal and menstrual fluid do not contain pathogenic organisms. Quantitatively and qualitatively, the skin, nasal, and oral cavities represent a greater source of potentially pathogenic organisms than the vagina.

D. Influence of Sexual Activity on Women's Performance

This subject has not been investigated in women. Johnson (1968) found that sexual activity had no effect on the muscular performance of men. It should be mentioned that there are no investigations on the effect of sexual activity on the psychological attitudes of athletes of either sex. Coitus has been reported to represent submaximal work (Boas and Goldschmidt, 1932). The current feeling, despite Tissot's work (Editorial, 1969), is that masturbatory activity is not harmful. It is worth noting, however, that there are no studies which indicate that masturbation has a beneficial effect on athletic performance!

E. Dysmenorrhea

Some women, in the absence of pelvic or other organic disease, will, upon questioning, indicate that they experience pain and discomfort at the time of menstruation. This poorly understood symptom complex, called primary dysmenorrhea, occurs only if ovulation precedes the menstrual flow. Clitheroe (1964) found that its frequency, as reported by various authors, ranged from 3% to 90% of women of childbearing age. He believes the wide range was due to the varying definition of the term dysmenorrhea.

The symptoms experienced include some or all of the following: lower abdominal cramps, backache, feeling of fullness in the abdomen, headache, and, rarely, nausea and vomiting.

Because of the subjective nature of the symptoms, with the exception of nausea and vomiting, evaluation by an observer of the severity of the illness, or indeed of its presence, is difficult if it is possible. This feature is a principle reason why the disease has remained so poorly understood and defined.

It is important to note, as D. V. Harris (1971) has done, that the interviewer interjects a group of variables, each of which may have an important influence on responses provided. Also, Bukowski (1968) has pointed out that individuals who are warned in advance that they will be subsequently questioned concerning symptoms will provide a greater number of responses than persons not forewarned.

Dysmenorrhea may severely handicap the woman who wishes to exercise. On the other hand, there is evidence that persons with this condition experience relief from therapeutic exercise programs (Clow, 1932; Golub et al., 1958; Billig, 1943).

In addition to exercise therapy, dysmenorrhea may be effectively treated by preventing ovulation. This can be done by administering the progestational antifertility agents in a dose sufficient to prevent ovulation. Symptomatic therapy, including aspirin and the application of heat to the abdomen, is also beneficial.

Hysteria has been reported to be contagious (Ebrahim, 1968). There are no data to support my suspicion that dysmenorrhea also may be contagious.

F. Sexual Identification of Athletes

The cells of the genetic female contain 22 pairs of chromosomes plus two X chromosomes. The male has the same number of paired chromosomes, but an X and Y chromosome. In the cells of a genetic female, the X chromosomes appear as dark staining masses of chromatin at the inside edge of the nuclear membrane. This material, called the Barr body, is present in 20% to 50% of her cells. It is not present in the nucleus of cells from normal males. Establishing its presence is useful in defining the genetic sex of an individual. Anatomical and secondary sexual characteristics (phenotype) of an individual may not be in agreement with the genetic sex. Thus, a genetic male may appear to be a female. If this person were to compete as a female, an unfair advantage over the female competitors might be gained because of the effect of the male hormone in producing greater strength and muscle mass. It is for this reason that the apparent female, who is a genetic male or a male masquerading as a female (transvestite), should not be allowed to compete against women.

There are several types of genetic abnormalities that make it possible for a true male to appear to be an anatomic female or a true female to appear to be an anatomic male, but not very many of these allow normal growth and development to an extent that would permit the person to compete in athletics.

A genetic female may develop an adrenal tumor that produces excess male hormones and subsequent changes in the secondary sex characteristics such as hair growth, voice, and breast tissue. Even though this person might be mistaken for a male by the casual observer, she is actually a female. Occasionally a true genetic male will develop an abnormality of the testicle which will cause excess secretion of female hormones. This person might very well appear to be female, but would be a genetic male.

G. Menstrual Synchrony

Previously, in this chapter, I have indicated that a nonpregnant woman in the menstrual age has approximately a one in seven chance of being in the menstrual phase of her cycle on any given date. It would be statistically reasonable to assume that this would apply to each member of a girls team. Evidence that this may not be entirely true has been presented by McClintock (1971). She reports that women living together in a college dormitory as roommates or close friends tend to develop synchronization of their menstrual periods. If this influence held true for athletes who were members of the same team, the chance of any individual being in the menstrual phase of her menstrual cycle on a given day would still be one in seven, but it could be that the menstrual phase of the entire team would be clustered in a portion of the month rather than by chance throughout the entire month.

H. Drugs

1. Anabolic Steroids

The use of male hormones, in the form of anabolic steroids, may facilitate the increase of muscle mass. It is not known whether this increase would exceed that which could be attained by normal training methods. It is important to note, however, that no coach, athlete, trainer, physician, or parent should permit a woman of any age to use male hormones in the hope that her effectiveness as an athlete would be enhanced. The possibility of damage to the individual is considerable. This is particularly true when anabolic steroids are given to the female athlete who has not attained her full growth. When given before or during puberty, these medicines may prematurely stop the growth of long bones. The individual so treated would not attain her full height.

2. Birth Control Pills

For more than a decade, various combinations of estrogenic substances and synthetic progestational agents have been available for the prevention of conception. Whether or not these hormones have the potential for enhancing or interfering with the quality of an individual's performance by altering her strength, coordination, timing, endurance, emotional stability, or metabolism is not known. The effect of these powerful hormonal substances on athletes is also unknown. Morris and Udry (1969) compared the pedometer-measured activity of eight women taking birth control pills with 26 who did not. The former walked an average of 4.17 miles (6711 meters) and the latter 4.86 miles (7821 meters) each day. These differences were statistically significant. The authors pointed out, however, that, until a prospective study of women before and after taking the pills is done, their data will have to be regarded as presumptive evidence that the use of various hormone agents as contraceptives causes women to be less physically active.

The various metabolic effects of contraceptive steroids have been thoroughly discussed in the volume edited by Salhanick et al. (1969). It would be somewhat surprising to find that these hormones did not alter performance. It is important to bear in mind that there are a variety of combinations of hormonal antifertility agents available and they are not identical in their composition. If these drugs are prescribed for athletes, they should be given only those preparations containing no more than 50 μg of estrogen. The reason for this is that the use of formulations limited to that amount of estrogen causes fewer side effects than those preparations containing larger amounts (Editorial, 1970a,b; Inman et al., 1970).

V. FUTURE PROSPECTS FOR WOMEN'S PARTICIPATION IN ATHLETICS

The future is patently unpredictable and persons who ignore this reality are usually sorry, but some indirect predictions and comments are possible. Whatever the future holds for women, it will be directly proportional to the interest or, conversely, the apathy of all of us, but particularly women themselves. Wyrick (1971) has pointed out the little interest investigators have in using women as subjects in studies of physical education. It is almost as if there were a cultural or professional taboo against designing a research study involving women. Until this condition is altered, we will continue to be penalized by lack of information concerning half of the human race.

It is essential that men learn more about women. Tiger (1970) stated:

> It is curiously anomalous that while young males may be taught about the tax system, about the value of exercise, or about the poetry of Browning, they are unlikely to receive systematic knowledge about the specialized patterns of behavior of members of the sex with whom the great majority will spend a good deal of their adult lives. More realistic and analytic treatment of the different typical careers and life-chances of males and females might alleviate what appears to be frequent disharmony between what many females expect about their working and married lives and the extent to which communities help to meet these expectations. In particular, some objective discussion of the anti-female tradition and the nature of male exclusion of females from various male groups could simplify or clarify the problems women may feel who seek careers in predominantly male organizations.

The image of the female athlete and the risks she takes by winning when in competition with a man has been discussed by D. V. Harris (1971) who feels that many women take the easy route, that is, they avoid all participation in athletics. The deprecation of female athletes by themselves and their peers of both sexes is a powerful force that will have to be attenuated, if not abolished, before women are allowed to and indeed allow themselves the opportunity to realize their full potential in sports endeavors.

Finally, we must never lose sight of the biological fact that each sex is responsible for half of human genetic material. This being true, if we all continue to tolerate a system that places women in an impoverished milieu with respect to allowing them to participate in vigorous physical activities, then we must be prepared to accept depreciation of our most valuable asset—the *sine qua non* for a vigorous, healthy, productive, genetic substrate—human beings with sound minds and sound bodies.

REFERENCES

Amateur Athletic Union of the United States. (1969). "Study of the Effect of Athletic Competition on Girls and Women." Pacific Association of the Amateur Athletic Union of the United States, San Francisco, California.

Anderson, T. W. (1965). *J. Health Phys. Educ. Recreation* 36, 66–68.

Arena, J. M., ed. (1969). "Davison's Compleat Pediatrician." Lea & Febiger, Philadelphia, Pennsylvania.

Åstrand, P.-O., Engstrom, L., Eriksson, B. O., Karlberg, P., Nylander, I., Saltin, B., and Thoren, C. (1963). *Acta Paediat. Scand., Suppl.* 147.

Bausenwein, I. (1960). *Sportaerztl. Praxis* 3, 12–19.

Bayne, J. D. (1968). *J. Sports Med. Phys. Fitness* 8, 34–35.

Beneke, F. W. (1879). "Uber das Volumen des Herzens und die Weite der Arteria pulmonalis und Aorta ascendens in den verschiedenen Lebensaltern." V. Theodor Kay, Marburg, Germany.

Bergner, L., Mayer, S., and Harris, D. (1971). *Amer. J. Pub. Health* 61, 90–96.

Billig, H. E., Jr. (1943). *Arch. Surg.* (*Chicago*) 46, 611–613.

Bloch, R. (1968). *Sci. Amer.* 219, 78–85.

Boas, E. P., and Goldschmidt, E. F. (1932). "The Heart Rate." Thomas, Springfield, Illinois.

Brown, H. C. (1970). *Proc. Nat. Conf. Med. Aspects Sports, 12th, 1970.*

Bukowski, Z. (1968). *Pol. Tyg. Lek.* 23, 1238–1241; abstracted in *Hum. Reprod.* 2, 1 (1969).

Castleman, B., and McNeely, B. U., eds. (1970). *N. Engl. J. Med.* 283, 1276–1285.

Cheek, D. B. (1968). *In* "Human Growth," (D. B. Cheek, ed.), pp. 337–351. Saunders, Philadelphia, Pennsylvania.

Clitheroe, H. J. (1964). *Obstet. Gynecol. Surv.* 19, 649–659.

Clow, A. E. S. (1932). *Brit. Med. J.* 1, 4–5.

Counsilman, J. E. (1965). *Proc. Nat. Conf. Med. Aspects Sports, 6th, 1964* pp. 19–23.

372   *Clayton L. Thomas*

Dalton, K. (1964). "The Premenstrual Syndrome." Heinemann, London.
Dalton, K. (1970). *Brit. Med. J.* 2, 27–28.
Darlington, C. D. (1969). "The Evolution of Man and Society." Simon & Schuster, New York.
Ebrahim, G. J. (1968). *Clin. Pediat.* 7, 437–438.
Editorial. (1969). *J. Amer. Med. Ass.* 209, 1083.
Editorial. (1970a). *Brit. Med. J.* 2, 189–190.
Editorial. (1970b). *Brit. Med. J.* 2, 231–232.
Ellison, A. E. (1970). *Proc. Nat. Conf. Med. Aspects Sports, 12th, 1970.*
Ellsworth, H. S., de Vries, K. L., McQuarrie, H. G., and Harris, J. W. (1969). *J. Sports Med.* 9, 107–109.
Elveback, L. R., Guillier, C. L., and Keating, F. R. (1970). *J. Amer. Med. Ass.* 211, 69–76.
Encyclopedia Britannica. (1964). Vol. 16, p. 782. William Benton, Publisher, Chicago, Illinois.
Erdelyi, G. J. (1961). *Proc. Nat. Conf. Med. Aspects Sports, 2nd, 1961* pp. 59–63.
Files, J. B., Van Peenen, H. J., and Lindberg, D. A. B. (1968). *J. Amer. Med. Ass.* 205, 94–98.
Golub, L. J., Lang, W. R., Menaduke, H., and Brown, J. O. (1958). *Amer. J. Obstet. Gynecol.* 76, 670–674.
Grover, G. H. (1970). *Nat. Conf. Med. Aspects Sports, 12th, 1970.*
Guttorm, E. (1971). *Acta Obstet. Gynecol. Scand.* 50, 9–16.
Haddon, W., Jr., Ellison, A. E., and Carroll, R. E. (1964). *In* "Accident Research" (W. M. Hazzon, Jr., E. A. Suchman, and D. Klein, eds.), pp. 559–612. Harper, New York.
Hamill, P. V. V., Johnson, F. E., and Grams, W. (1970). "Height and Weight of Children," Pub. Health Serv. Publ. No. 1000, Ser. 11, No. 104. U.S. Dept. of Health, Education, and Welfare, Health Services and Mental Health Administration, Rockville, Maryland.
Harris, C. E. C. (1971). *Can. Med. Ass. J.* 104, 767.
Harris, D. V. (1971). *In* "DGWS Research Reports: Women in Sports" (D. V. Harris, ed.) pp. 1–4. Amer. Ass. Health, Phys. Educ., and Recreation, Washington, D.C.
Harris, H. A. (1964). "Greek Athletes and Athletics." Hutchinson, London.
Harris, S. L. (1971). *Family Coordinator* 20, 149–150.
Haselhorst, G. (1949). *Aerztl. Wochenschr.* 4, 746–748.
Hefnawi, F., Younis, N., Zaki, K., and Mekkawi, T. (1970). *Egypt. Population Family Planning Rev.* 3, 1–4.
Hong, S. K., and Rahn, H. (1967). *Sci. Amer.* 216, 34–43.
Inman, W. H. W., Vessey, M. P., Westerholm, B., and Engelund, A. (1970). *Brit. Med. J.* 2, 203–209.
Jacobi, M. (1877). "The Question of Rest for Women During Menstruation." Putnam, New York.
Javert, C. T. (1960). *Fert. Steril.* 11, 550–558.
Johnson, W. R. (1968). *J. Sex Res.* 4, 247–248.
Karpovich, P. V. (1937). *Res. Quart.* 3, 33–37.
Klemesrud, J. (1971). *N.Y. Times* CXX, No. 41, 324.
McClintock, M. K. (1971). *Nature (London)* 229, 244–245.
McCloy, C. H. (1931). *Arbeitphysiologie* 5, 100–111.
Maraini, F. (1962). "The Island of the Fisherwomen." Harcourt, New York.

Marden, L. (1971). *Nat. Geog. Mag.* **140**, 122–135.

Marples, M. J. (1969). *Sci. Amer.* **220**, 108–115.

Meredith, H. V. (1971). *Amer. J. Phys. Anthropol.* **34**, 89–132.

Metropolitan Life Insurance Company. (1971a). *Statist. Bull.* **52**, 3–7.

Metropolitan Life Insurance Company. (1971b). *Statist. Bull.* **52**, 8–10.

Morris, N., and Udry, J. R. (1969). *Amer. J. Obstet. Gynecol.* **104**, 1012–1014.

Noack, H. (1954). *Deut. Med. Wochenschr.* **79**, 1523–1525.

Pfanner, D. (1964). *Med. J. Aust.* **1**, 320.

Rauh, J. L., and Schumsky, D. A. (1968). *In* "Human Growth" (D. B. Cheek, ed.), pp. 242–252. Lea & Febiger, Philadelphia, Pennsylvania.

Robinton, E. D., and Mood, E. W. (1966). *J. Hyg.* **64**, 489–499.

Rumpf, E. (1952). *Zentralbl. Gynaekol.* **74**, 870.

Salhanick, H. A., Kipnis, D. M., and Vande Wiele, R. L., eds. (1969). "Metabolic Effects of Gonadal Hormones and Contraceptive Steroids." Plenum, New York.

Shaffer, T. E. (1961). *Proc. Nat. Conf. Med. Aspects Sports, 2nd, 1960,* pp. 48–49.

Siegel, P. (1960). *Obstet. Gynecol.* **15**, 660–661.

Sklar, H. S., and Downs, E. F. (1968). *Clin. Pediat.* **7**, 220–225.

Southam, A. L., and Gonzaga, F. P. (1965). *Amer. J. Obstet. Gynecol.* **91**, 142–165.

Thomas, C. L. (1970). *P. Med. J.* **73**, 50–55.

Tiger, L. (1970). "Men in Groups." Vintage Books, New York.

Ueland, K., Novy, M. J., Peterson, E. N., and Metcalfe, J. (1969). *Amer. J. Obstet. Gynecol.* **104**, 856–863.

Valsik, J. A., and Kostkova, E. (1964). *Aerztl. Jugendkunde* **55**, 399–400.

Van Wyk, J. J., and Grumbach, M. M. (1968). *In* "Textbook of Endocrinology" (R. H. Williams, ed.), pp. 559–560. Saunders, Philadelphia, Pennsylvania.

Werner, M., Tolls, R. E., Hultin, J. V., and Mellecker, J. (1970). *Z. Klin. Chem. Klin. Biochem.* **8**, 105–115.

Williams, R. J. (1956). "Biochemical Individuality." Wiley, New York.

Wilmore, J. H., and Sigerseth, P. O. (1967). *J. Appl. Physiol.* **22**, 923–928.

Wintrobe, M. M. (1967). "Clinical Hematology." Lea & Febiger, Philadelphia, Pennsylvania.

Wyrick, W. (1971). *In* "DGWS Research Report: Women in Sports" (D. V. Harris, ed.), pp. 15–20. Amer. Ass. Health, Phys. Educ., and Recreation, Washington, D.C.

Zaharieva, E. (1965). *J. Sports Med.* **5**, 215–219.

Chapter 15

NONTRAUMATIC MEDICAL PROBLEMS

ALLAN J. RYAN

I. INTRODUCTION

The physician who only sees and treats athletes very occasionally, or the orthopedic physician, may imagine that most of their problems result from injuries. The sports physician who sees them daily knows that 75% of their medical problems are nontraumatic in origin. Since these problems may include the entire spectrum of disease, if athletes of all ages are to be considered, there will be no attempt made here to write a complete textbook of medicine. Instead, I should like to focus on those problems that seem to be particularly common in young athletes, and that may be to some extent related to their competition, either in their origin or because they may be aggravated by it.

The control of environmental problems is dealt with in Chapter 10; therefore, in this section I will not discuss etiology or prevention to any extent but mainly treatment. Those problems which are peculiar to the female athlete are discussed in Chapter 14 and will, therefore, not be covered again here.

Many of these problems should not be disabling to the athlete if they can be recognized and treated promptly. This is one of the main advantages of having a physician closely associated with sports teams. If left to themselves, athletes are inclined to ignore or put up with such illness until it reaches an advanced stage, so that they may have already lost their effectiveness before they are driven to the physician, and then have a disproportionately long disability before they recover. Paradoxically, the team physician's real value to the team may be overlooked, since by acting promptly he keeps everyone well, or so nearly so that they can keep active, and it looks as if what he is doing is really very simple.

II. INFECTIOUS DISEASES

A. Skin Infections

1. Folliculitis

These range from the simple pimple, or furuncle, which is isolated or multiple, to the coalescence of a group of furuncles producing the carbuncle. They are a particular menace to the athlete because when

his skin is soaked with sweat and he rubs one with his hands or his clothing, the organisms have a means of spreading to establish new sites of
infection. By personal contact, and through clothing, equipment, or
lockers that become contaminated, these infections can spread rapidly
through a team.

In the majority of cases the offending organism is a staphylococcus.
The hemolytic *Staphylococcus aureus*, particularly the so-called "coagu-
lase-positive" strains, are difficult to eradicate from the individual and
appear to be highly contagious.

Prompt and vigorous treatment of all folliculitis is indicated in the
athlete, with unroofing of all "white-heads," drainage of small abscesses,
local application of antibiotic ointments, hot soaks, if necessary to local-
ize the infection, and systemic administration of antibiotics if more than
one lesion is identified. This administration may have to continue for
several weeks or even months in very resistant cases.

2. Acne

It seems hardly necessary to point out that acne is associated with
excessive secretions of sebum, and that the papular to pustular lesions
that result appear to be associated with secondary infection by a species
of corynebacterium that is commonly found on the skin, and that can
be well controlled in most cases by the regular oral administration of
a daily dose of tetracycline. Diets rich in carbohydrates and fats have
been pretty well absolved of any responsibility for this condition.

For an athlete, acne can be a serious problem, since he may actually
become disabled from secondary infection. The vigorous physical activity
of sports seems to increase sebum secretion, probably through some
endocrine mechanism. The heat and perspiration of exercise aggravate
existing acne unmercifully.

Every athlete known to have acne or a strong tendency to it should
be maintained on tetracycline from the start of his season and instructed
in proper skin cleanliness and care. If any lesions do become pustular
under this regime, which is unlikely if it is carefully followed, they
should be drained promptly through a very small incision to minimize
scarring.

3. Herpes Infections

The cold sore of the lip is more annoying than disabling to most
people. When it spreads to other skin on the face or to other parts
of the body, as it may in wrestlers particularly, it can be a hazard
not only to the person who has it but those with whom he comes into

intimate contact. Such an infection can spread rapidly through a wrestling team.

The virus can apparently be inactivated by heat, and exposure to the heat of a hair dryer has been used effectively. Felber (1971) has found that the virus can be apparently killed by a photosensitivity reaction after its location on the skin has been treated with neutral red or proflavine.

Herpes zoster (shingles) can be very painful, even long after the characteristic line of vesicles has dried up and disappeared. No consistently effective treatment has been found for this condition. Its chief importance in the athlete lies in the ability to distinguish it from other pain provoking conditions in the stage before the vesicles appear. When they are present, efforts should be directed at avoiding secondary infection. Oral administration of thiamine or vitamin B complex may be of some value of mitigating the pain.

4. Warts

The verruca vulgaris is apparently caused by a virus, which has been isolated but for which no vaccine has ever been prepared. It is difficult to eradicate by any means because of its strong tendency to recur and to spread to other areas. The type of juvenile warts which occur in crops, chiefly on the fingers, will ultimately disappear. The waiting time averages about two years, unfortunately.

Athletes do not want to wait for the wart to disappear since it may be causing destruction of a fingernail or bleeding as the result of being partially rubbed off. The method of removal which seems to produce the least scarring and lowest recurrence rate is the use of liquid nitrogen. More than one application is usually necessary.

Plantar warts are usually sensitive to pressure and have to be removed once they reach any considerable size. If they occur over a bony prominence, such as a metartarsal head, there is a great tendency to recurrence.

5. Fungus Infections

Athlete's foot is caused by an organism that has a universal distribution and whose growth on human skin is favored by warmth, moisture, and breaks in the skin surface. It is not highly contagious, but tends to occur among members of a sports team when they are subject to similar conditions. The occurrence is ordinarily greatest during the early part of a sports season and lowest toward the end, indicating that the general state of conditioning may be a factor in resistance.

Undecylenic acid, triacetin, and tolnaftate are all effective in eradicating the fungus. Neglected cases may develop secondary infections causing cellulitis and lymphangitis. These have to be treated with soaks, elevation, and systemic administration of antibiotics. The use of medicated foot powder and care in keeping the feet clean and dry help to prevent recurrences. Chronic infection of the toenails will respond to the oral administration of griseofulvin.

Tinea cruris (jock itch) is a fairly common and disabling fungus infection involving the groin area, perineum, and, on some occasions, the scrotum. Tolnaftate is quite effective, but in more severe cases it may be necessary to use griseofulvin by mouth as well.

6. Arthropod Infestations

Scabies appears characteristically in the finger webs, the anterior surface of the wrist, the axillary folds, the umbilicus, the skin of the lower back, and on the glans penis. It can be identified with a magnifying glass by the burrows which can be found in the affected areas. Scraping with a scalpel and placing the material with a drop of potassium hydroxide on a glass slide will alow identification of the ova or female parasite under the microscope. Benzyl benzoate, crotamiton, and gamma benzene hexachloride lotions are all effective in clearing the infestation.

Pediculosis pubis is caused by a louse with a predilection for the pubic hair. It is transmitted usually by sexual contact. The eyebrows or eyelashes may become involved. A positive diagnosis is made by finding the nits on the hair. The same lotions used for scabies are effective in ending the infestation.

7. Infected Wounds

Any wound of the skin which is badly contaminated, as well as any which appears to be infected, should, of course, be left open and treated locally with antibiotic soaks or ointment. Secondary closure with or without drainage may be possible at a later date and with the systemic administration of antibiotics.

B. Eye Infections

1. Conjunctivitis

This is quite a common infection in athletes due to the fact that, when perspiring, they tend to rub the sweat from their eyes with fingers that are not always clean. It may also occur secondary to the incurrence of small foreign bodies, especially dust and dirt from playing surfaces.

Treatment should be prompt with the administration of an appropriate antibiotic ointment to the eye three times daily. Although the ointments that also contain a corticosteroid will reduce inflammation more rapidly, there is some danger to the eye from the indiscriminate use of these agents locally, and they are better avoided unless recommended specifically by an ophthalmologist.

2. Stye (Hordeolum)

These infections of small glands just beneath the surface of the palpebral conjunctiva can be very painful and disabling. If they do not respond quickly to the local use of an antibiotic ointment, the patient should be referred to an ophthalmologist for possible incision and drainage.

C. Ear Infections

1. Swimmer's Ear

This is not an infection to begin with, but is often secondarily infected by the time it is first seen by the physician. It is an eczema of the ear canal caused by retention of water in the ear following bathing, showering, or swimming. The most common secondary invader is *Pseudomonas aeruginosa*. It can be an extremely painful condition.

This condition can be entirely prevented by having the susceptible individual instill three drops of glycerin into each ear canal after bathing and swimming and hold it in with a little cotton for an hour. The glycerin takes up the water and the cotton the glycerin. When secondary infection has occurred, drops containing a mixture of colistin and neomycin sulfate are usually effectual.

2. Middle Ear Infections

These are no more common in athletes than in the general population. They result typically from infected material being forced through the Eustachian tube into the middle ear. Swimmers and divers are more exposed to these infections but will not get them if upper respiratory infections are treated promptly and efficiently.

Although the acute otitis is more painful, it is more easily resolved than the chronic catarrhal variety that requires repeated drainage. The administration of antibiotics orally or systemically is necessary to clear the acute infections, but is relatively ineffective in the chronic catarrhal form.

D. Respiratory Infections

1. Common Cold

The chief importance of a cold to the athlete is that it may initiate a more serious secondary infection. The inconvenience and impairment of breathing due to a stuffed nose can usually be well controlled with an oral antihistamine and decongestant. Repeated use of nasal sprays may aggravate rather than alleviate the problem.

There is no known reliable method of preventing colds. Athletes who are overly fatigued and not properly conditioned seem to be more susceptible to catching a cold. Vitamins do not have any value as cold preventatives. If a cold lasts more than a week, you may be suspicious that a secondary infection has occurred in the sinuses.

2. Sinus Infection

This is a much more common condition than most people imagine and is a major cause of chronic partial disability in athletes. Most cases of sore throat with cough and sputum production in young persons are secondary to infected sinus drip coming down the back of the throat. Posterior cervical lymph nodes may be enlarged and tender. Two red streaks are seen running down the posterior pharynx, one on each side. Frontal headache is almost always present and may be very severe.

It is foolish to temporize with these infections. Antibiotics are indicated and should be given as long as necessary to clear the infection. The infections are usually mixed but will be sensitive in most cases to penicillin or erythromycin. With either of these, an analgesic–decongestant tablet should be given for relief of headache and stuffiness. The tremendous reduction in cases of bronchiectasis in young persons today is due to earlier use of antibiotics for these infections.

Once temperature has returned to normal and headache is controlled, players may return to practice but should continue their medication until the infection is eradicated. Swimmers may have to stay out of the water a few days longer.

3. Sore Throat

This may be a symptom of sinus infection, but in some cases the throat infection is primary, usually due to a streptococcus. Penicillin is the mainstay of treatment. Even though it is encountered rarely today, diphtheria should always be remembered as a cause of sore throat. Mononucleosis and measles are more common causes.

4. Bronchitis

This is usually secondary to an infection in the sinuses in its acute form. Chronic bronchitis is frequently associated with asthma in younger individuals. Sputum cultures may not reveal organisms of any apparently great significance. Antibiotics should be administered in acute cases according to the sensitivity of the organisms involved.

5. Influenza

There are many strains of influenza, and their behavior is almost as various as their numbers. People of athletic age are seldom seriously affected by it but may be disabled for a week or more. Multivalent vaccines are prepared every year to include the major strains that have been isolated during the preceding year. It is worthwhile to immunize athletes with this vaccine before the start of their seasons.

6. Pneumonia

a. LOBAR PNEUMONIA. This is no longer the threat to life for young people that it used to be. Many factors may be responsible for the change, but one of the most important is the effectiveness of antibiotics against it. Complications are minimal and recovery is usually rapid.

Localized areas of consolidation with hemorrhage may be due to contusion of the lung in athletes. This could be classified as a traumatic pneumonia. It is usually accompanied by some elevation of temperature and secondary infection may occur. It is therefore prudent to treat it with antibiotics from the outset rather than awaiting such a result.

b. VIRAL PNEUMONIA. This is characterized by a subacute course, by cough, and moderate fever. Positive physical signs are not often elicited, and the diagnosis is usually made by viewing a chest X-ray. The course is apt to be prolonged. Although in theory broad-spectrum antibiotics should not be effective, in practice they seem to be helpful in speeding resolution.

E. Cardiovascular Infections

1. Rheumatic Heart Disease

The occurrence of this serious condition seems to have been reduced substantially since the advent of penicillin for the treatment of severe upper respiratory infections in children and young adults. The exact etiology is still in doubt in spite of the many years of study and research which have been expended on it. The streptococcus in some form appears to be related in some way to its origin and recurrence.

There is no question that anyone suffering from this condition in the acute or subacute phase should not participate in sports activity. The problem arises in those who have had the disease and recovered. Some young persons with a definite history have no heart murmur, no functional deficit, and questionable evidence of change in the electrocardiogram, usually a moderate prolongation of the PR interval.

The decision with regard to participation should be made on an individual basis. Some young persons who have frank evidence of valvular disease but no functional deficit are capable with a reasonable degree of safety of very vigorous activity (Feinstein *et al.*, 1962). Some who do not have an organic murmur and with minimal evidence of myocardial damage are capable of only very light activity.

Recurrence should be treated promptly with complete rest, antibiotics, and corticosteroids, if indicated.

F. Gastrointestinal Infections

1. Intestinal Grippe

This is perhaps as good as any name for a condition characterized by acute onset of fever, nausea, vomiting, abdominal cramps, and diarrhea. Not all of these symptoms are invariably present or in that order. High fever may be present in the first 6 to 12 hours and then disappear spontaneously. Fever usually comes down with the onset of diarrhea. Weakness and generalized aching pains, particularly during the period of fever, are common. A feeling of unusual fatigue may last for some days after other symptoms have disappeared.

The nature of the condition and its course, which is uninfluenced by the administration of antibiotics, suggests that it is due to a virus, possibly to several different viruses. There is no lasting immunity because attacks may occur every year or more frequently. The feeling of weakness and fatigue appears to be due to involvement of the liver, since liver function studies frequently show significant changes.

Treatment should be by rest, restoration of fluid balance, and antidiarrhetics, which may be administered orally as soon as nausea and vomiting cease. If a low fever and intestinal symptoms persist after 48 hours, it may be advisable to give a saline cathartic such as citrate of magnesia. This appears to flush the virus out of the intestines and may result in a rapid recovery following catharsis.

The infection appears to be mildly contagious and may spread through a whole team in short order. The incubation period is unknown and attempts to isolate affected individuals as a means of preventing its spread are generally ineffective.

2. Food Poisoning

The common pathogen is the staphylococcus, which multiplies readily in foods prepared in advance and not kept adequately refrigerated. It is justly feared by coaches whose teams travel and eat together in restaurants in which they have no control over the conditions of food preparation or conservation.

Antibiotics and restoration of fluid balance are the mainstays of treatment. Gastric lavage is generally ineffective because the contaminated food has usually passed through the stomach before symptoms are apparent.

3. Diarrhea of Travelers

In spite of many attempts to identify the causative agent of this common affliction, its etiology has not been conclusively demonstrated. A recent study of its occurrence in British soldiers in Aden (Rowe *et al.*, 1970) suggests the reason for this difficulty. Rather than being due to some hitherto unidentified organism, it may be due to certain strains of *Escherichia coli* to which the local population has developed an immunity but which are pathogenic to those who have not been exposed.

The British have used a combination of streptomycin and triple sulfonamides quite effectively for prophylaxis. Because of the dangers of toxic reactions to streptomycin, even when given orally, it is probably wiser to use a poorly absorbed sulfonamide such as sulfathalidine. When given in doses of 1.0 gm twice daily, it is quite effective as a prophylactic and will not exert any unfavorable effect on sports performance (Nicholas *et. al.*, 1968).

4. Hepatitis

The occurrence of this condition in athletes, usually due to a viral infection, is fortunately rare. When is does occur, it requires immediate and sometimes prolonged complete bed rest. In the more severe cases, the administration of corticosteroids and liver extract may be necessary as supportive measures. Return to sports activity depends on the return of liver function tests to normal values.

G. Genitourinary Infections

1. Urethritis

Gonococcal urethritis is the most common genitourinary infection in athletes. Current recommendations call for large doses of penicillin (1.0 gm) to be given intramuscularly to males and twice this amount to females. Resistant cases and those who are sensitive to penicillin are treated with doxycycline orally.

Mycoplasmal urethritis is being identified more frequently at present. The secretion is light and glairy, as opposed to the thick white discharge of gonococcal infection. It is also transmitted by sexual contact. It responds very well to tetracycline administered orally in a dose of 250 mg four times daily for 10 days.

An occasional case of urethritis and prostatitis will be due to a staphylococcal or streptococcal infection. These respond well to the administration of the appropriate antibiotics.

2. Cystitis

This is unusual as an isolated phenomenon in male athletes but is more common in females. One should always suspect some associated anomaly or infection in the upper genitourinary tract. Although these infections respond well to antibiotics, the rate of recurrence is high until the underlying cause is corrected.

3. Prostatitis

When this condition involves the seminal vesicle on the right side, it may be mistaken for acute appendicitis. The organism is usually a staphylococcus or a streptococcus. It is best treated by the systemic administration of antibiotics and prostatic massage.

4. Pyelitis

Just as it is more common in females generally, pyelitis is more common in girl athletes. The basis is usually some congenital anomaly involving the ureter or kidneys. Although it responds well to the administration of the appropriate antibiotic, the rate of recurrence is high. Surgical correction of the anomaly is often necessary.

5. Proteinuria

Although not usually associated with acute infection, except in the case of acute or subacute nephritis, proteinuria may be a puzzling and difficult sign. According to Robinson (1971), three major patterns of proteinuria not specifically connected with nephritis may be identified: (1) persistent or "constant" proteinuria during both recumbent and upright postures; (2) transient "orthostatic" proteinuria that is inconstant from day to day; and (3) "fixed" orthostatic proteinuria that is demonstrable constantly on separate days. The distinctions between the three groups are not sharp. Although about half of the patients with "fixed" proteinuria show pathological changes in the kidney tissue on microscopic examination, their 10-year outlook for good kidney function is very good and their eventual fate at the moment is uncertain. There does not appear to be any reason to exclude persons with either of these three types of proteinuria from sports participation.

H. Systemic Infections

1. Mononucleosis

This ubiquitous condition is more feared, and probably with less reason, than any other common infectious disease. Even without the benefit of any specific therapy, the mortality rate has been virtually zero. Less than 0.1% of all persons afflicted with it develop serious complications of hepatitis or encephalitis. Most people have it, and develop the lifelong immunity that goes with it, without ever being aware of it. This is why it appears to be characteristically a disease of young persons.

The chief danger arises from overtreating it. Those persons who are put to bed for extended periods and kept quiet for even longer times take months to recover from the effects of the enforced inactivity. The one complication to be feared is rupture of the enlarged spleen. For this reason, young athletes who develop it are kept out of vigorous sports activities until spleen size has returned to normal, usually about 4 weeks after onset. It is much safer to determine spleen size by a single supine X-ray film of the abdomen than by palpation. Bed rest is prescribed only during the acute febrile stage, and then normal activities, other than heavy work or vigorous sport, are immediately resumed.

2. Septicemia

Fortunately, since the advent of antibiotics this is a rare condition today. When it does occur, it is important to identify the responsible organism by blood culture, find the original point of infection and treat it vigorously, and administer the appropriate antibiotic in adequate doses.

3. Tuberculosis

The great success that we have enjoyed in the United States in the past 75 years in reducing tuberculosis from the position of number one killer of young persons to a place far down on the list has led many people to assume that it is under complete control, like smallpox, and not any longer a source of concern. Our complacency in this regard has caused a slackening of vigilance which has prevented our control measures from being more effective. Every year cases of tuberculosis are picked up in athletes, some of them very prominent and successful in amateur and professional sports.

The keystones to control remain early detection by skin testing and chest X-rays and early treatment by one or more of the several drugs now shown to be effective against the tubercle bacillus. The newest of these, Rifampin, may be the best yet. The availability of effective drugs has greatly shortened the time of treatment and practically eliminated the need for thoracoplasty. Within a year following treatment, most young persons who have contracted tuberculosis should be able to return to normal sports activity.

4. Syphilis

The advent of penicillin has given us a false sense of security regarding venereal disease generally and syphilis in particular. It is still widespread and escaping former control in many areas because it has been impossible for public health measures to keep up with the radical change in attitudes towards sexual activity and the rapid mobility of young persons today.

Prompt recognition and treatment with adequate doses of penicillin, isolation of infected persons until they are noninfectious, and treatment of contacts are the necessary bases for control of venereal disease. These desiderata are not being sufficiently realized at the present time. Professional athletes, because of their promiscuous attitudes when away from home, are important as spreaders and victims of these diseases.

III. ALLERGIC AND TOXIC MANIFESTATIONS

A. Seasonal Rhinitis, Sinusitis, and Tracheobronchitis

Sensitivity to pollens and other airborne allergens, such as the spores of fungi and other substances contained in dust particles, produces a high occurrence of rhinitis and related problems in young people, especially in urban environments. This frequently sets the stage for secondary sinus infections, wihich in turn cause sore throats, tracheobronchitis, and even pneumonia.

Young athletes who are subject to this cycle of problems may be kept well in most instances by keeping them on regular doses of antihistamines during the seasons in which they are susceptible. When secondary infections occur, they should be treated promptly with the appropriate antibiotic to reduce morbidity and shorten disability.

Inoculations with the responsible allergens to produce immunity may be very successful in some persons and unsuccessful in others for reasons that are not entirely clear. The disadvantage is that the testing is sometimes prolonged and expensive, and the desensitizing doses may have to be repeated over a long period of time. Corticosteroids should be used sparingly in young persons to control problems of this sort unless they are unresponsive to the other conventional methods. In athletes, particularly, they may be dangerous because of a tendency to produce osteoporosis following prolonged administration.

B. Contact Dermatitis

The multiplication of synthetic substances has given us almost limitless opportunities today for the development of sensitivities. Many of these substances are used in the manufacture of uniforms and protective equipment for athletes. The appearance of any localized and persistent skin rash, particularly one that follows the outline of any piece of equipment that the athlete wears, should be viewed as a probable manifestation of sensitivity until proven otherwise. Removal of the offending equipment and local treatment with corticosteroids will usually clear the problem up quickly.

Tincture of benzoin is used as a tape adherent, or is contained in some commercial tape adherents. It is a potent sensitizer and should be avoided in sports since effective adherents are available which do not contain it. Many cases of sensitivity which have been attributed to adhesive should probably be credited to benzoin instead. Adhesive tapes today are relatively nonallergenic, and some cloth-backed tapes that are even less sensitizing are available.

The athlete's street clothes may be the source of sensitization. Substances that are used to give clothing the appearance of being permanently pressed can be allergens and should be suspected particularly when they have been recently purchased. Even some of the cream bases that are used as vehicles for corticosteroid preparations for use on the skin may be sensitizing, setting up a vicious cycle in which the treatment makes the rash worse.

C. Drug Sensitivity

It is well to remember that in certain individuals almost any drug may produce almost any type of reaction. These reactions may be either local or systemic. When an individual taking any medication experiences any unusual symptoms or manifests some external sign that cannot be related to the condition for which he is taking the medication, it should be stopped and the signs or symptoms treated appropriately.

Among drugs that are commonly used, aspirin probably causes more unfavorable reactions than any other. These may range from simple gastric distress to abnormal bleeding tendency and even to anaphylactic shock. Every athlete should be asked about any known sensitivities at the time of his annual physical examination. Penicillin reactions are among the most commonly identified because the usual rash is quite troublesome and often difficult to clear up if the penicillin was being given parenterally in a long-acting form. Fatal anaphylactic reactions have occurred with the administration of penicillin parenterally to a sensitized individual. Since parental administration also seems to increase the occurrence of sensitization, it is better on all counts to give it orally when it is possible.

Sensitivity to vitamin B complex following parental administration is not well known, but is common, although often unrecognized. The premonitory symptom is a feeling of faintness following an intramuscular injection. Fatal anaphylaxis has recurred following parenteral administration to sensitized persons. For these reasons it is inadvisable to give athletes intramuscular injections of B complex vitamins unless there is an absolute indication for it, and no way the vitamin can be given to be effective by the oral route.

D. Sunburn

This may be classified as a toxic reaction to uncontrolled exposure to ultraviolet light. Protection of the skin against burning is dependent in great measure on the presence of melanin pigment and its multiplication in the skin (tanning). Persons who "tan" well may avoid sunburn by beginning with short exposures to the sun and gradually increasing the length of time. Although they thus avoid the burning reaction, their skins are subjected to the chronic effects of ultraviolet exposure that brings about premature aging of the skin.

Light-skinned persons, particularly those of Celtic and Scandinavian origin, never tan, and will be repeatedly burned if they do not protect their skins. Sunscreening agents are available which help to protect the skin if other reasonable precautions regarding exposure are taken. The most effective are the preparations in an alcoholic vehicle that penetrate the skin and are not washed off by perspiration or swimming.

Athletes should be cautioned against sunbathing, especially on competition days, because of the danger of burning and the enervating effect of lying exposed to the warm sun for extended periods.

IV. ENVIRONMENTAL STRESS

A. Altitude Sickness

Symptoms of altitude sickness may appear at elevations of only 4500 feet. At 7500 feet they are common, and at 10,000 feet are felt by almost everyone during the first week of acclimation. They include headache, anorexia, fatigue, and vague muscle aches. In most persons they are completely gone after the first week. They are apt to be more severe in very young and very old individuals. No specific therapy other than rest, a light diet, and an analgesic is required.

In persons who are more seriously affected and in higher altitudes,

15,000 to 29,000 feet, altitude sickness may become subacute or chronic. In this case the person should return as rapidly as possible to sea level.

Pulmonary edema occurs in some individuals as the result of prolonged (days) exposure to high altitutde. It is most apt to occur in those who are lifted suddenly to a high altitude, and least apt to occur in experienced climbers who make their way up slowly in stages. It should be treated by the administration of oxygen and immediate evacuation to lower levels. Delay in this procedure, based on the assumption that the condition was pneumonia, has often proved fatal.

B. Heat Cramps, Exhaustion, and Stroke

1. Heat Cramps

Due to excessive salt loss under conditions of high ambient temperature, heat cramps may be prevented effectively by loading the system with salt before exposure. They should be treated promptly by the administration of salt solution by mouth, or, if necessary, by infusion. Massage of muscles affected by heat cramp only aggravates the pain. Relief is quick when salt balance has been restored.

2. Heat Exhaustion

This is primarily due to loss of body water with resultant decrease in venous return to the heart and collapse. Peripheral vasodilation and pooling of blood in the lower extremities due to long standing also contribute to this condition. It may be prevented by provision of adequate fluids without restriction before, during, and after practice and the maintenance of salt balance.

3. Heat Stroke

Failure of the body to be able to dissipate heat at a rate faster than it is storing it due to the ambient temperature and humidity and continuing high rate of heat production and absorption is responsible for heat stroke. The critical period comes when sweating ceases, due to the onset of hydromeiosis, and the body loses its chief cooling mechanism.

It can be prevented by loading the body adequately with salt and water and keeping its surface as dry as possible by preventing sweat from standing on the skin. Once heat stroke occurs, resuscitative measures must begin promptly, since the temperature will rise rapidly to levels (108–115°F) where permanent damage to the central nervous system and/or death may result. Treatment involves rapid cooling of the body with ice or a refrigeration blanket, administration of promazine parenterally, restoration of fluid and electrolyte balance, and digitalization to support the heart.

C. Hypothermia and Frostbite

Prolonged exposure of the human body to very cold temperatures without adequate protection will produce hypothermia and, if not counteracted by rewarming, death. The relative humidity of the air is a negligible factor, but, if clothing is wet through, or if the individual is in the water, hypothermia will come on rapidly. The effect of air movement is of paramount importance. The relationship between speed of air movement and air temperature can be seen in charts of the so-called "wind chill" effect. Frostbite results from cooling of the skin and subcutaneous tissues to the point where the circulation becomes virtually zero. If not rapidly corrected, the skin loses its viability.

Prevention of hypothermia depends on wearing clothing that insulates the body against the cold by reducing heat loss and preventing penetration of wind and water. Prevention of frostbite is favored by keeping exposed areas of skin covered, reducing local heat loss and preserving local circulation by avoiding constricting types of clothing.

The proper treatment for hypothermia is rapid rewarming. This should begin at the scene of exposure and continued until the individual's core temperature returns to normal. One must be careful in rewarming not to use temperatures that will damage skin whose temperature may already be critically low. The same treatment is applicable to frostbite. The oral administration of anticoagulants and vasodilators may also be very helpful.

D. Motion Sickness

Travel in cars, buses, or trains and on the water and in the air will produce motion sickness in some individuals invariably, and in others depending on the particular circumstances. It is almost entirely preventable by using drugs that prevent vertigo prophylactically. Meclizine seems to be most reliable at present with dramamine second. The main disadvantage of these drugs is that they also induce some drowsiness. For this reason they should not be given within six hours before a contest if possible.

E. Underwater Problems

The medical problems that relate to underwater diving and swimming are due to the fact that air is compressible and water is not. The soft tissues of the body are intermediate in their compressibility. Whether the diver is breath-holding or with scuba, the problems are the same with only minor differences.

1. Squeezes

If air is prevented from entering freely any of the air-containing spaces of the body, a relative vacuum develops which will disturb or rupture the lining of such a space. Pain and bleeding into the sinuses, bleeding in the middle ear with rupture of the tympanic membrane, bleeding into the lung, and conjunctival hemorrhage from failing to breathe into the face mask while descending are all examples of such a mechanism. Gas in the intestinal tract and air under dental fillings may also expand painfully during descent.

Prevention of squeeze involves avoiding diving when colds or other conditions impair free exchange during descent, and not holding the breath during descent, but allowing pressures to be equalized gradually. All these squeezes tend to correct themselves spontaneously, but repeated barotrauma may cause permanent hearing loss.

2. Gas Problems at Depth

a. NITROGEN NARCOSIS. At pressures as low as 1.6 atmospheres, the first symptoms of intoxication from nitrogen may be experienced. At 4 atmospheres, most divers suffer from some loss of judgment, and at 125 feet euphoria is usually present. At 200 feet and below, there is serious danger of death due to loss of consciousness or irrational acts such as removing the face mask and mouthpiece.

Prevention is by limiting sports dives to 125 feet and returning quickly to shallower depths if euphoria begins. Neon is less narcotic than nitrogen but somewhat more so than helium. Helium is well tolerated to about 35 atmospheres but causes an unfortunate distortion of speech. The accumulation of carbon dioxide seems to be an important factor in narcosis with any inert gas.

b. OXYGEN POISONING. Pure oxygen may cause convulsions and unconsciousness at 2 atmospheres pressure in a closed circuit system. It is treated by lowering the oxygen tension.

c. CARBON DIOXIDE POISONING. Symptoms appear when the partial pressure gives a concentration of 1%, and will cause unconsciousness at or before a concentration of 10%. In closed circuit scuba, this is due to failure of carbon dioxide absorbent, and in open circuit to accumulation in the face mask.

d. ANOXIA. This may occur on ascending when overbreathing before descending has blown off so much carbon dioxide that the stimulus to breathing is temporarily lost. This is the cause of "shallow-water blackout."

e. AIR CONTAMINATION. When a diver is using compressed air as his supply, the air may have been contaminated during its compression with oil droplets, carbon monoxide, or pathogenic bacteria. If the air was very humid at the time of compression, the diver may get a mouthful of water with his first breath, start to choke, and then panic. A concentration of 0.1% carbon monoxide at sea level may cause poisoning at depth. The remedy is to have a reliable source of supply in which the air is certified to be pure.

3. Problems of Decompression

a. BENDS. Decompression sickness is caused by the formation of nitrogen bubbles in body tissues. Being inert, the amount of nitrogen absorbed into the body through the blood is directly related to the depth underwater reached and the time spent there. The critical ratio that causes the formation of large bubbles in the blood and tissues is reached when the partial pressure due to nitrogen in the tissue is twice that in the atmosphere. This ratio can be achieved when a diver ascends rapidly from a depth of 33 feet or more. On dives to 600 feet, bends may appear as low as 350 feet beneath the surface.

Prevention involves using the greatest care in observing decompression times, avoiding repetitive dives within 12 hours, and avoiding flying shortly after scuba diving.

Treatment requires recompression in a pressure chamber, usually to pressures equivalent to a depth of 100 to 155 feet, and then very slow decompression under medical supervision. It has been recently demonstrated that serious plasma losses may occur in deep diving and that the effectiveness of recompression and gradual decompression may be greatly enhanced by plasma infusions to restore normal blood volume and rate of flow.

b. AIR EMBOLISM. Failure to breathe out steadily during ascent may result in internal rupture of the lungs allowing air emboli to form in the pulmonary artery, or in rupture into the mediastinum or pleura with air passing into both spaces. In the upright diver, the emboli frequently enter the brain with a fatal result. Rapid ascents from depths as shallow as 10 feet may cause this phenomenon. Treatment is supportive with administration of oxygen.

V. NEUROLOGICAL AND EMOTIONAL PROBLEMS

A. Epilepsy

1. Grand Mal

The classic seizure with aura, loss of consciousness, and clonic and tonic muscle spasms followed by sleep, whether due to antecedent trauma or an undertermined cause, requires careful management in the athlete, but should not disqualify him from any sports except those in which there is a high frequency of head injuries. The athlete who has such a condition and has been careless about taking his medicine may become motivated to be more regular if he knows that his ability to participate in sports depends on this.

2. Petit Mal

Although this type of epilepsy produces less alarming attacks, it may be much more difficult to control with medication. In the presence of effective control by medication, there should be no reason for barring a person from sports competition.

B. Cerebral Hemorrhage

Spontaneous cerebral hemorrhage, due to an aneurysm of a cerebral artery, or sometimes to an unknown cause, is not uncommon in young persons. There is no way to predict its occurrence, and the bleeding may cause death before resuscitative measures can be brought to play.

Depending on the area of the brain affected, hemiplegia and/or speech loss may occur.

Treatment is chiefly symptomatic and supportive. In patients who survive the initial hemorrhage, an aneurysm may be detected by an arteriogram. A definitive surgical approach towards these aneurysms is now possible and should probably be attempted if the location is reasonably accessible.

C. Psychoneurosis

The definition and limitations of this term depend on what school of psychiatric thought one subscribes to. Classically it is supposed to differentiate mental disorders that are less serious in their effect on the total personality of the individual, allowing a reasonably normal life and not requiring close supervision or institutionalization. Phobias are an example of a psychoneurotic state in which the individual can carry on a normal life with the exception of a particular fear that only affects his personality overtly when he is confronted with it. Paradoxically, although psychoneurosis by definition should be more curable than the psychosis, it is practically impossible to cure a phobia by any form of treatment.

The athlete who is apparently suffering from some type of mental or emotional disorder should be counseled by the team physician, who must then act on his assessment of the situation, and either decide to treat the patient himself or refer him to a psychologist or psychiatrist. Tranquilizing drugs may play some role in the treatment but their use should not take the place of a thorough inquiry into the roots of the problem and help to the patient in working out possible solutions.

D. Psychosis

These were called "organic" for many years because it was thought that they arise from some chemical or biological disorder and are grounded in physical causes, in contrast to the psychoneurosis which appeared to be largely an emotional problem. Although the graduations between the two main disorders considered under this classification, schizophrenia and manic-depressive psychosis, may create subvarieties of mental disease, the chief value of making the distinction lies in the possibility of predicting the result. The prognosis for recovery from schizophrenia appears to be somewhat better than that for manic-depressive psychosis.

Treatment has ranged all the way from drug and shock therapy to psychoanalysis. No one can say categorically whether one treatment or another would be more successful for all people. It should be individualized, and the physician should stand ready to change it as indicated.

VI. MISCELLANEOUS PROBLEMS

A. Spontaneous Pneumothorax

This condition occurs in young persons who clinically may not be found to have any demonstrable lesion in the lung. Lichter and Gwynne (1971) have found, in operating on 20 young persons for a persistent air leak or recurrent pneumothorax, a small area of fibrosis at the apex of the lung surmounted by a thin-walled bullous cyst or cysts. The remainder of the lung in each case appeared normal. All were treated by wedge resection with no recurrence. The origin appears to be congenital and connected with defects in blood supply and aeration of this portion of the lung in tall, thin individuals. Basketball players, among all athletes, as a group fit this description best.

With a small amount of air in the chest, it is not necessary to aspirate it and the partial collapse seems to favor healing of the cyst. The air is eventually absorbed with complete reexpansion of the lung. With a large amount of air, aspiration is indicated for relief of breathing and to correct any mediastinal shift. With a persistent leak, underwater drainage through an intercostal catheter is the primary treatment of choice. In the event that the lung does not reexpand, thoracotomy and wedge resection is indicated. Surgery is also indicated for a recurrence.

Sports activity should be restricted following nonsurgical management until healing of the lung has occurred, which may be 6–8 weeks.

B. Excessive Perspiration

This may be a critical problem for athletes, particularly as a precipitating cause of athlete's foot. The reasons for its occurrence in otherwise healthy individuals are not known.

Sympathectomy has not been successful as a treatment for this condition. Mild sedation with tranquilizing drugs appears to work better than anything else. Keeping the body clean and using a germicidal soap helps to control unpleasant body odor.

C. Back Problems

An entire chapter, or perhaps a book, could be written on this topic. Only a few general principles will be referred to here.

The first is that "muscle spasm" is not a diagnosis of a back disorder but a symptom or sign of many different disorders. The second is that ordinarily there is little or no motion at the sacroiliac joint and that a diagnosis of sacroiliac strain is not a viable one. The third is that most acute low back strains seen in athletes have a structural origin, most of which are congenital in nature.

The formation of the lumbar and sacral spines is apparently so complex that many errors appear in its development in the infant and child. These defects, unless of a major nature, are not usually productive of symptoms in early life. As the individual matures, the lower part of the spine has to bear a greater weight, and as the result of increased activity the supporting ligaments are stretched. When this happens the spine begins to slip and then, under some acute stress, as in lifting or twisting, the tolerance of that portion is exceeded, nerve root traction or pressure is exerted, and pain begins.

The best treatment for any acute low back pain is rest, lying in the lateral position with the knees drawn up toward the abdomen. Muscle relaxants are of limited value. Medication for relief of pain is more effective. Rest should continue until the pain is gone, and then activity should be resumed very gradually.

The person who has recurrent or persistent low back pain following this type of management usually needs to have a support in the form of a lumbosacral belt and to wear it all times when up and about. Spinal fusion should only be considered as a last resort, except in the case of a severe spondylolisthesis where it should be a treatment of choice.

D. Foot Problems

There are really only two major sources of foot problems: those that are due to congenital deformities; and those that arise from the fact that shoe lasts come in standard sizes and feet do not. Athletes suffer from these problems to roughly the same extent that the remainder of the population does, except that an element of self-selection tends to eliminate a certain percentage of those with the more severe congenital deformities. Because of their greater intensity of movement, athletes also suffer more commonly from blisters.

1. Blisters

Friction produces blisters, but particularly the friction developed by movement in a rotary plane. The premonitory sign of a blister on the sole of the foot is the appearance of redness and tenderness of the skin, a so-called "hot spot." If this is treated promptly with the application of ice and covering with adhesive tape, the formation of a blister may be prevented.

Once the blister has formed, the roof should not be removed unless it has ruptured spontaneously. Premature removal of the roof prolongs pain and disability. Instead, the fluid should be aspirated, or otherwise evacuated from the blister, and the roof preserved by taping or the use of some substance which will make it adherent to the underlying skin. Aspiration should be performed with a fine gauge needle through intact skin outside of the blistered area. The fluid may be evacuated by making a curved incision along one border of the blister, and then using tape adherent or a jelly such as Xylocaine viscous under the roof to cause adherence and covering the roof with tape.

When a blister has ruptured spontaneously, the space between the roof and skin has already been contaminated and care must be exercised not to seal infection inside the blister. The whole roof does not have to be removed but a wide area should be excised including all loose portions that cannot be used effectively for protection. The remaining portion of the roof may then be taped but should not be sealed.

The prevention of blisters depends on minimizing the unfavorable effects of friction. This means fitting shoes properly, wearing socks that fit properly and stay up on the foot to avoid wrinkling, using insoles that are made in such a way that they do not bind the sole of the foot in rotary movements, and lubricating the sole of the foot before practice. For the latter purpose, a thin coating of mineral oil is very effective. The use of tape adherent covered with powder is apt to be dangerous since heavy perspiration causes the powder to aggregate in small lumps and the sole becomes sticky and will not move freely against the insole.

2. Congenital Problems

Flatfoot is one of the most serious of these problems seen in athletes. The complete absence of the normal longitudinal and transverse arches is very difficult to compensate for with any type of support which will still allow freedom of the foot to run. The use of adhesive strapping is of limited value. If an athlete with this problem is willing to suffer the painful effects of long hours of running and standing on these feet, he may be quite successful in spite of them.

A more common problem, and one frequently confused with flatfoot is pronation of the foot. This is due primarily to the axis of weight bearing coming down inside of the center of the foot. It can be corrected by the use of arch supports and sometimes a slight lift on the inner side of the sole of the shoe. Exercises to strengthen the muscles that support the inner longitudinal arch are very beneficial.

The condition of the second metatarsal being longer than the first (also called Morton's foot) produces a heavy callus over the second metatarsal head rather than the first, and produces pain on running and long standing. This can be compensated for by placing a pad in the sole of the shoe under the head of the first metatarsal, making this more prominent and shifting the weight toward it. Removal of the second metatarsal head is generally not successful in relieving the pain, and weight may then be transferred to the third metatarsal head.

The keel-shaped foot is fortunately rare but sometimes seen in athletes. By careful application of felt pads to the sole of the foot medially and laterally, the pressure may be kept off the center of the foot so that relatively pain-free competition may be possible. Clubfoot, even with surgical correction, is not usually consistent with sports performance.

3. Problems Generated by Shoes

Calluses and bunions due to improperly fitting shoes have to be treated by removing the source of pressure and irritation. A tendency to hallux valgus which might not otherwise become symptomatic is often exaggerated by wearing shoes that do not allow enough room for the metatarsal heads and toes to lie naturally. Hammer toes with resultant painful calluses may also be caused by ill-fitting shoes.

If the source of pressure is removed, the conditions may correct themselves spontaneously. If it is not removed, no amount of surgical excision or planning down will correct the lesions. Heavy calluses in normal weight bearing areas can be prevented from cracking and splitting the underlying skin by being cut down or filed down regularly.

E. Heart Problems

1. Rheumatic Heart Disease

Many boys and girls who have had rheumatic heart disease have recovered with apparently minimal valvular and myocardial damage and are able to participate safely and effectively in sports. Each case must be evaluated individually. If the decision has been made to allow sports participation, and to what extent, vigilance should not cease at that point.

Every precaution must be taken against possible recurrence, including the prophylactic use of penicillin during the high risk season. The electrocardiogram should be monitored before and after each sports season, and more frequently if indicated by the appearance of any symptoms, particularly any precordial distress. X-Ray examination of the chest for heart size should be repeated annually.

Generally speaking, asymptomatic children who have had rheumatic heart disease and are allowed unrestricted physical activity do just as well over a 20-year period as those who are restricted, and they have 25% less incidence of adverse psychosocial reactions (Feinstein et al. 1962).

Individuals who have had reconstructive surgery for valvular disease of the heart are a special risk category. Several fatalities have been recorded in individuals who were allowed to play basketball after surgery for heart disease. It would seem advisable not to allow these persons to participate in sports in which very vigorous activity and great endurance are required.

2. Congenital Heart Disease

The great majority of young persons who have congenital heart disease, with or without surgical correction, will not present themselves for sports participation. The exceptions might be those with small intraauricular or intraventricular septal defects who have no cyanosis or functional deficit, and those who have had surgical ligation of a patent ductus arteriosus. The management of these individuals as athletes should follow the same plan as for those who have had rheumatic heart disease, with the exception of the prophylactic use of penicillin.

3. Coronary Heart Disease

Young persons may suffer from coronary artery disease. Since the initial occlusion in a young individual is frequently fatal, there may be no previous warning of the condition. The occurrence of precordial pain, with any of the usual types of radiation, should be carefully investigated with electrocardiograms taken before and during exercise. Positive identification of coronary disease should lead to a therapeutic exercise program rather than sports participation.

4. Irregularities of Rate and Rhythm

As the result of recording 1219 electrocardiograms of high school and college athletes and observing their tolerance for sports, Rose (1969) has offered the following conclusions.

> Based on current knowledge, Wolff-Parkinson-White syndrome without a history of paroxysmal arrhythmia is acceptable for strenuous sports; acquired bundle-branch block, right or left, should be suspected and thoroughly investigated; nodal rhythm and other second-degree block aggravated by exercise is cause for rejection, as is myocardial ischemia and active myocarditis, but not isolated T-wave changes.

According to Hyman (1965), sinus arrhythmia is the chief cause of irregular heart activity in young persons and is normal up to age 35. Premature beats are next most common, and are often associated with air swallowing and other benign upper gastrointestinal conditions. Neither of these should prevent indulgence in sports. Paroxysmal atrial flutter and/or fibrillation is potentially more serious but is not an uncommon finding in competitive athletes. Complete heart block of congenital origin should not contraindicate vigorous athletic activity.

F. Anemia

1. Iron Deficiency Anemia

This fairly common anemia in young athletes is usually due to taking a diet deficient in iron. In girls it may indicate heavy losses of iron during menstrual periods. Since aspirin is taken commonly by athletes for bumps and bruises, it should be remembered that it may cause a secondary anemia through regular loss of microscopic quantities of blood from subacute gastritis.

Treatment is to supply iron by mouth until the red cell count and hemoglobin levels are restored to normal.

2. Sicklemia

The increased participation of Negroes in sports has brought many of them with the sickle-cell trait and some with frank sicklemia under observation. The former are not usually anemic, but the latter usually are, due to the periodic crises in which the sickled cells are destroyed. The use of multiple transfusions for the victim of sicklemia appears to improve his prognosis. Recently there have been reports of improvement following treatment with urea in invert sugar (Nalbandian, 1971).

There is a danger of splenic infarction in persons with sickle cell trait who ascend rapidly to altitudes as low as 6000 feet (Doenges *et al.*, 1954; Cooley *et al.*, 1954; Conn, 1954). This should be kept in mind, since many sports teams travel by air today and compete at altitudes as high as 7500 feet.

G. Diabetes

The young diabetic who can be well controlled by diet and insulin or other medication can participate actively in sports without unfavorably affecting his prognosis. He or she is much more apt to be conscientious in control measures if sports participation depends on keeping sugar free. The so-called "brittle" diabetic who is difficult to control may still participate in physical activity and sports but requires closer supervision.

Two major precautions are necessary for the diabetic athlete: to treat even minor infections as major problems; and to remember that physical activity decreases insulin requirements and to be prepared to treat hypoglycemic shock with sugar if the need arises.

REFERENCES

Conn, H. O. (1954). *N. Engl. J. Med.* **251**, 417–420.
Cooley, J. C., Peterson, W. L., Engel, C E., and Jernigan, J. P. (1954). *J. Amer. Med. Ass.* **154**, 111–113.
Doenges, J. P., Smith, E. W., Wise, S. P., III, and Breitenbucher, R. B. (1954). *J. Amer. Med. Ass.* **156**, 955–956.
Feinstein, A. R., Taube, H., Cavalier, R., Schultz, S. C., and Kryle, L. (1962). *J. Amer. Med. Ass.* **180**, 1028–1031.
Felber, T. D., Smith, E. B., Knox, J. M., Wallis, C., and Melnick, J. L. (1971). *Sci. Assembly, AMA Sect. Dermatol. 1971.*
Hyman, A. S. (1965). *Proc. Nat. Conf. Med. Aspects Sports, 7th 1965* pp. 36–40.
Lichter, I., and Gwynne, J. F. (1971). *Thorax* **26**, 409–417.
Nalbandian, R. M. (1971). *N. Engl. J. Med.* **285**, 408.
Nicholas, W. C., Kollias, J., Buskirk, E. R., and Tershak, M. J. (1968). *J. Amer. Med. Ass.* **205**, 757–761.
Robinson, R. R. (1971). "The Kidney," Vol. 4, p. 3, Nat. Kidney Found., New York.
Rose, K. D. (1969). *J. Amer. Med. Ass.* **208**, 2319–2324.
Rowe, B., Taylor, J., and Bettelheim, K. A. (1970). *Lancet* **1**, 1–5.

PART III

SPECIAL PHYSICAL EDUCATION

Chapter 16

THE PURPOSES OF PHYSICAL EDUCATION

ANN JEWETT

I. DEFINITION OF PHYSICAL EDUCATION

Voluntary movement is a significant function of man. Thus, the education essential to each individual person includes learnings concerned with how human movement functions in his experience and in achieving common human goals. Physical education has long been recognized as the school subject using games, sports, dance, gymnastics, and other movement activities as media for learning. More recently, physical education has been viewed as the series of school programs concerned with the development and utilization of the individual's movement potential. Currently, physical educators attempting to realize the full potential of this area of human experience are seeking to extend concepts of physical education to the needs of learners of all ages in both school and noninstitutional contexts. Physical education is increasingly viewed as personalized, self-directed learning, using selected movement learning media to achieve individual human goals. A physical education program is now defined as a sequence of experiences in which an individual *learns to move* as he *moves to learn*. This definition, developed to clarify the role of physical education in society generally, is equally appropriate to the planning of special physical education programs for handicapped persons.

II. FUNCTIONS OF HUMAN MOVEMENT

Human beings of all ages have the same fundamental purposes for moving. The child needs movement learnings that will function meaningfully in his real world; the youth needs physical education that will aid him in becoming a fully functioning adult; the adult needs movement activities that will permit continuing self-actualization and more nearly complete individual–environment integration. Physical education experiences fulfill the same key purposes for apparently healthy persons of all ages; movement learnings are needed by handicapped persons to serve the same significant functions. Man *learns to move* to achieve these human purposes. Every individual person shares the following human movement goals:

> *Man Master of Himself:* Man moves to fulfill his human developmental potential.
> *Man in Space:* Man moves to adapt to and control his physical environment.
> *Man in a Social World:* Man moves to relate to others.

A. Man as a Developing Organism

The unity of man cannot be overemphasized. Ever since the fallacy of the old mind–body dichotomy was first recognized, educators have been trying to organize school programs so as to focus on the development of fully functioning, integrated individuals. Acknowledging the primacy of this concept, it is, however, not inappropriate to conceptualize complementary physiological and psychological purposes of human movement in fulfilling the individual's developmental potential.

1. Physiological Efficiency

Man moves to improve or maintain his functional capabilities. Physical education has frequently put its major emphasis on circulorespiratory efficiency as a key aspect of physical fitness. Physical activity programs can be designed to achieve maximum training effects by placing appropriate demands for the processing of oxygen on heart, lungs, and the vascular system. Exercise programs are individually prescribed and progressively increased according to aerobic capacity and current level of conditioning. The educator's responsibility includes encouragement of positive attitudes toward maintenance of optimum levels of physiological efficiency as well as provision of factual information and techniques useful in planning and conducting personal exercise programs.

Man moves to increase and maintain his range and effectiveness of motion. Goals in the area of mechanical efficiency include joint flexibility, functional body alignment, and appropriate applications of force to achieve the most effective body leverage. Physical education is properly concerned with the development of efficient body mechanics in daily life and work tasks as well as in sports, games, and other recreational activities.

Neuromuscular efficiency is also an important capability to maintain and improve. Muscular strength and endurance, power, balance, agility, and basic neuromuscular coordination are all important to physiological functioning. These components of fitness should all receive appropriate emphasis in physical education programs.

2. Psychic Equilibrium

Man moves to achieve personal integration. Physical education can play an important role in the growth of self-actualizing persons if its potential in this area is fully realized. Most young children experience genuine pleasure in strenuous physical activity, but the pure joy of movement is lost to many individuals during adolescence. Good physical education programs are planned so as to maintain pleasurable sensations in movement for individuals of all ages and abilities and to maximize personal opportunities for finding peak experiences in human motion.

Self-knowledge basic to self-appreciation and self-actualization can be enhanced through participation in varied movement activities. Movement exploration enriches any child's perceptual field. The adaptation and refinement of basic movement patterns and creation of unique movement designs or combinations permits the individual to determine what he, as a functioning organism, is capable of doing and becoming. Successful learning may increase his self-appreciation as he extends his own physical capabilities beyond limits he had previously accepted.

Physical education may also contribute to individual psychic equilibrium by providing opportunities to release tensions and frustrations precipitated by the common pressures of modern living or by unique personal difficulties in launching oneself fully into the stream of life. The range of movement activities through which different individuals experience such catharsis is almost endless. Conditioning exercises, running, cycling, dance, skating, sailing, handball, tennis, golf, casting, wrestling, karate, volleyball, and softball are examples.

A wide spectrum of movement activities offers the challenge to any person to test his prowess and courage through physical activity. The specific movement forms which constitute challenge vary with age, interest, and physical capability. Popular challenges include skiing, sailing, surfing, riding, mountain climbing, sky diving, scuba, and gymnastics.

B. Man Interacting with His Natural Environment

Human ecology dictates a dynamic interaction between man and his environment. This interaction permeates all aspects of living. Man learns to move in order to adapt to and control his physical environment. His movements, both as an individual and as a member of a large population, modify the environment. In learning to move within his environment, he needs varied and sequential experiences in spatial orientation and object manipulation.

1. Spatial Orientation

Man moves to relate himself in three-dimensional space. His earliest experiences in physical activity develop his conception of his body and how it moves in space. Physical education encompasses concepts of relationships of different body parts, body shapes, directions, pathways, levels, and range of movement.

Man learns to move in order to propel or project himself from one place to another in a variety of settings. Beginning with the simplest forms of human locomotion, he ultimately learns complicated step patterns, skilled variations of basic locomotor patterns, modifications required for locomotion on different surfaces, and complex forms of body propulsion and projection in aquatics, gymnastics, dance, skiing, skating, rock climbing, and track and field. Such skills can be learned or utilized in physical education class, recreational sport, work, or survival contexts.

Man also moves to regulate his body position in relation to stationary and moving objects and persons in the environment. He learns to dodge, to stop and start moving in accordance with boundaries and hazards, to adjust his movements to those of other persons with whom he is cooperating or competing, and to modify his movements for effective interception or pursuit of moving objects.

2. Object Manipulation

Man moves to give impetus to and to absorb the force of objects. Physical education includes experience in lifting, carrying, pushing, and pulling. It provides instruction in effective techniques for supporting, resisting, or transporting the weight of another person's body in rescue, self-defense, or sport activities such as water safety, judo, wrestling, football, ice hockey, hand-to-hand balancing, stunts, and pyramid building.

Many sports and games commonly used in physical education programs require proficiency in various skills of object projection and reception. Children learn throwing, catching, and striking skills in moving with balls, hoops, wands, bats, paddles, bean bags, frisbies, and quoits. Youth enjoy the challenge of seeking increased speed and accuracy in object projection and reception activities, as well as the social satisfactions of group interaction, in many sport and recreational activities. Almost all the team and dual sports provide such learning opportunities. In the lifetime sports selected by many adults, the major skill emphasis is object projection. Golf, archery, handball, bowling, billiards, shuffleboard, badminton, softball, and casting are examples.

C. Man Interacting in a Social World

Man is gregarious by nature. He must therefore learn to live and work with other persons. Physical education aims to contribute to this goal by providing opportunities for learning movement skills through which the individual can relate to others and by using movement activities as media for intergroup understanding. The social purposes of physical education include communication, group interaction, and cultural involvement.

1. Communication

Man moves to share ideas and feelings with others. Communication is a fundamental human activity. Although schooling has consistently emphasized verbal language skills, words do not represent the only means of human communication. Nonverbal communication is also significant in human interaction. Movement is an important medium for sharing personal meaning.

Physical education provides opportunities to develop skill in expressing one's uniqueness in the movement dialogue that is inherent in daily living. It also offers potential learnings in self-expression through such particular movement forms as dance, water ballet, gymnastic routines, and other movement media selected to convey individual ideas and feelings.

Program opportunities in human movement are concerned with the use of gesture and movement style to clarify verbal communication. In addition, movement can be designed to enhance the meaning or increase the impact of other nonverbal communicative forms—music, graphic arts, and various audio-visual media. On the other hand, human movements can be consciously controlled to mask or divert attention from feelings the individual perfers not to share or to obscure his true intent, as with postural styles associated with poise and self-confidence, or in deceptive game strategies intended to throw the opponent off balance or to catch him off guard.

2. *Group Interaction*

Man moves to function in harmony with others. Sport has frequently been viewed as society in microcosm. One of the functions often attributed to educational programs in human movement is guided experience in group interaction. The individual can learn to understand, appreciate, and participate in teamwork as he accepts rules, regulations, and the authority of officials, and shares in achieving common goals in the team play of children's games or adult forms of team sport. He can develop skills of teamwork as he cooperates with a tennis opponent or a golf partner for satisfying recreation, or as he masters the specialized role of a particular position on a basketball or softball team.

Competition characterizes man's movement activities from the simple races, tag games, stunts, and combatives of children to Olympic contests among the world's outstanding athletes. It is normal in most Western societies to vie for individual or group goals. Competition may be directed toward individual excellence in achieving progressively higher levels of performance or toward superior group performance in team competition. Sound competition experiences in educational programs emphasize excellence in performance in contrast to conflict requiring degradation of opponents. The development of leadership abilities in movement activities is associated with the need for motivating and influencing individual group members to achieve team unity and to focus competition upon the striving for excellence of performance.

3. Cultural Involvement

Man moves to take part in movement activities that constitute an important part of his society. Sport and dance are cultural universals. The popularity of specific activites varies cross-culturally, but participation is a phenomenon that exists in all societies. A major role of physical education in school programs is derived from man's desire for participation in the movement activities of his society.

Another aspect of cultural involvement is the understanding and appreciation of sports and expressive movement forms as a spectator or audience participant. Such appreciation is extended to the movement activities of other cultures as well as to those of one's own culture which are not especially enjoyed as a primary participant. The role of sport, dance, and unique physical activities in preserving the cultural heritage of a particular ethnic group is another appropriate concern of physical education.

III. SELF-ACTUALIZATION THROUGH MOVEMENT

Physical education has been defined as a sequence of experiences in which an individual learns to move as he moves to learn. Man learns to move in order to achieve the three key human purposes of individual development, coping with the environment, and social interaction. He *moves to learn* more about himself interacting in the world in which he lives. This goal is variously expressed as independent maturity, full human functioning, or self-actualization. Moving to learn shifts the learning focus from task or product to process.

A. Processes of Human Movement

Movement processes represent one large segment of human behavior. Process learnings are, therefore, essential physical education outcomes. Important learning opportunities include those concerned with the processes by which an individual learns to facilitate, extend, and utilize fully his unique movement capabilities.

Movement processes can be categorized in three major classifications: (1) generic movement, or movement operations that facilitate the development of human movement patterns; (2) ordinative movement, defined as meeting the requirements of specific movement tasks through processes of organizing, performing, and refining movement patterns and skills; and (3) creative movement, or processes of inventing or creating skillful movements that will serve the unique purposes of the learner. Mastery of these different types of movement operations or processes extends the potential channels for individual self-actualization. It is for this reason that physical education is concerned with the learning of human movement processes.

B. Designing Human Movement Learning Environments

The key concepts in the field of human movement are (1) those related to the functions of movement in prolonging and enriching the quality of life, which define the scope of the curriculum in physical education, and (2) those concerned with the processes of self-actualization through movement, which provide a basis for sequencing potential learning experiences in physical education. Purposes and processes of human movement provide an action-oriented framework for designing learning environments that focus on the individual learning to move as he moves to learn.

Learning of movement processes is combined with the learning of key purpose concepts as teachers develop instructional objectives, using elements of human movement as the content focus and movement processes to identify the level toward which instruction is directed. This procedure can be used to generate educational objectives for individual learners and for instructional groups in any learning environment, utilizing a wide variety of learning media encompassing traditional and popular games, stunts, sports and dance activities, innovative movement education challenges, and unfamiliar but potentially satisfying physical recreation opportunities.

Curricular planning in physical education is concerned with the role of movement in developing a healthy self-concept. The individual's personal body image, his knowledge of his movement abilities, his feelings about how well he moves, and his estimate of his movement capabilities and potential movement skill all contribute to this self-concept. A primary focus of the physical education curriculum is the growth of the self-actualizing individual who strives to enrich the quality of life by seeking functional fitness in terms of his personal goals, individual abilities, and unique capacities. Physical education encourages him to build physical recreation into his personal life style by helping him to select appropriate forms of physical recreation, to learn skills that increase his satisfactions in physical recreation, and to understand how to plan and modify his personal physical recreation programs throughout life.

IV. SUMMARY

Physical education serves three key human purposes. Its overall purposes are highly individualized and personalized as each participant seeks to fulfill his human developmental potential, to adapt to and control his environment through movement, and to relate to others through movement activities. Physical education seeks the development of self-actualizing individuals by providing human movement process skills, by offering unique opportunities for creating healthy self-concepts, by designing many alternatives for experiencing functional fitness, and by encouraging satisfying physical recreation in determining personal life styles. Physical education experiences in which man learns to move as he moves to learn vary with each human being, regardless of his unique abilities, and are as vital in achieving self-actualization to the handicapped person as to the apparently healthy. Every physical education program should be special to the person for whom it is designed.

SELECTED REFERENCES

American Association for Health, Physical Education and Recreation (1965). "This Is Physical Education." The Association, Washington, D.C.

Brown, C. and Cassidy, R. (1963). "Theory in Physical Education—A Guide to Program Change." Lea & Febiger, Philadelphia, Pennsylvania.

Jewett, A. E., Jones, L. S., Luneke, S. M., and Robinson, S. M. (1971). "Educational Change Through a Taxonomy for Writing Physical Education Objectives," Quest 15, 32–38.

Mackenzie, M. M. (1969). "Toward a New Curriculum in Physical Education." McGraw-Hill, New York.

Nixon, J. E., and Jewett, A. E. (1974). "An Introduction to Physical Education." Saunders, Philadelphia, Pennsylvania.

Oberteuffer, D., and Ulrich, C. (1970). "Physical Education," Harper, New York.

Chapter 17

EXAMINING THE DISABLED INDIVIDUAL

ALLAN J. RYAN

417

I. CRITERIA FOR INCLUSION IN AN ADAPTED
PHYSICAL EDUCATION PROGRAM

Since the purposes of an adapted physical education program include goals of a physiological, psychological, and therapeutic nature as well as educational, it is desirable to include every student who does not qualify for inclusion in the regular instructional program if possible. In any school program, there will be relatively few students who cannot participate in such a program provided that it can be organized to meet the needs of individuals. At the same time there are in many schools and colleges boys and girls and young men and young women who are participating in regular programs who would benefit far more from the adapted program.

The following criteria are offered as a basis for deciding who should and who should not be included in an adapted program. They are certainly not absolute, since the conditions described can be present to such a slight degree that they do not handicap the individual in any sense as far as physical activity is concerned, or to such an extreme degree that no suitable exercise program can or should be prescribed. They are not all-inclusive, since it would take a textbook of general medicine to describe all the possible conditions which could be included. Four broad areas, i.e., mental and emotional handicaps, physical handicaps, physical immaturity, and obesity, are laid out, and representative examples of specific conditions described as models for making decisions in related states.

A. Mental or Emotional Handicaps

One of the difficulties in discussing the management of persons suffering from mental and emotional disorders is that there is as little agreement among psychologists and psychiatrists regarding classification (on an etiological or any other basis) as there is regarding therapy. I make no brief for subdividing persons with such problems into the five groups of unstable personality, psychoneurosis, psychosis, homosexuality, and mental retardation, other than that those who appear to me to fall into these groups seem to have certain things in common which indicate particular types of management in a physical education program.

It should also be understood that there is no implication that programs of special physical education should be restricted to schools and colleges. They may be a highly desirable means of education for persons who are not approachable by academic education in the ordinary sense, such as severe psychotics or mentally retarded persons. For the institutionalized or otherwise segregated individual, such a program may be a significant means of socialization.

1. Unstable Personality

The individual given to explosive emotional outbursts or severe depression, but who otherwise makes a good adjustment to his environment, would fall into this category. A tendency to irrational behavior, purposeless lying, or unexplained absences might also classify persons in this category. It could be expected that a relatively larger proportion of these people might be drug users.

Persons with this type of problem cannot be handled easily in a large group. They tend to disrupt it and may even destroy it. On an individual or small group basis they are ordinarily easily approachable and may even prove to be extremely cooperative. They manifest a high injury rate unless closely supervised because of the tendency to impulsive action.

2. Psychoneurosis

A major difference between this group and the psychotics is that they have for the most part maintained their contact with reality and have some insight into their problems, even they may not be able to do anything to correct them without help. Neurasthenia, the milder anxiety states, and obsessive–compulsive neuroses are typical examples of this group of syndromes.

The psychoneurotic may shun and fear physical education activities because he feels that exercise in any vigorous form may be somehow harmful physically or mentally to him. Fears of bacterial contamination, of water, and even of associating with others cause them to seek to be excused from regular programs. On an individual basis, with considerable reassurance, they frequently prove to be good candidates for physical education, and may become very strongly attached to suitable continuing activities when they leave the program.

3. Psychosis

Persons suffering from a true psychosis of a so-called "organic" type, such as schizophrenia, are seldom found in educational institutions except in the recovery phase following therapy. They may be quite strong physically and capable of very vigorous activity, but in most instances will require careful personal supervision. A tendency to violent reaction may make them dangerous to themselves as well as others.

Institutionalized patients with psychoses may be good candidates for adapted physical education. Even the most withdrawn may find recreation in participation if given the opportunity. Although there is so far little solid evidence to support it, recreational exercise appears to be therapeutic for these patients.

4. Homosexuality

There are undoubtedly covert and latent homosexuals participating in regular physical education programs. Those who are professed, however, usually request excuse from regular physical education programs with members of the same sex or even in coeducational classes. Some overt homosexuals may present a threat to the heterosexual members of a regular class, particularly at the high school level. Sometimes their confusion or ambivalence regarding their sexual identity carries over into areas of sports and physical education where they are extremely uncertain as to what their roles should be.

An individual dressing facility is necessary if a homosexual with an emotional problem is going to be safely included in an adapted program. The type of individual attention and reeducation toward physical activity which is best given in the adapted program is best suited to their needs.

5. Mental Retardation

The physical education of the retarded person has become almost as specialized as his general education. It appears to offer significant gains to the process of his education as a whole. Remarkable achievements in simple individual sports activities are possible for retarded young people, as demonstrated by the Special Olympics for the Handicapped which were started in the United States in 1968.

There is some question as to whether the mentally retarded do better when segregated in small groups for adapted physical education or when paired one to one with children of normal intelligence. Both such groupings are possible in an adapted program, and might be started simultaneously or asynchronously.

B. Physical Handicap

Many physical handicaps are of such slight significance that the possessors may participate in a regular physical education program without any difficulty. The attitude of each person toward his handicap varies so much, however, that it becomes the decisive factor frequently in deciding whether that individual will enter the regular or the adapted program. Although some conditions are only temporarily handicapping, the exigencies of scheduling physical education programs may be such that the possessor may have to take his course before he is completely recovered. In such a case, he is better off in the adapted program, which may also have a therapeutic aspect for him.

1. Acute Illness

The typical common acute illness is an upper respiratory infection, which has ordinarily a brief and not very severe course. On the other hand, a more severe illness such as acute rheumatic fever, acute nephritis, or acute hepatitis may leave an individual in a weakened state for a prolonged period after the critical phase of the illness has subsided. In such cases, where the time factor will not allow a more complete recovery to occur, an adapted program would be suitable. In an acute infectious disease such as hematogenous-type tuberculosis of the lung, the advent of chemotherapy has changed the picture for the patient from complete rest to modified physical activity, a state suitable for an adapted program.

There is not any rationale at present for recommending or requiring physical education for young persons with acute leukemia, in spite of the relatively long-term survivals now recorded with combined chemotherapy.

2. Chronic Illness

The presence of a chronic illness that is under some kind of control should not necessarily prevent a person from participating in a regular, let alone an adapted, physical education program. Many diabetics who are well-controlled with diet and medication are active in sports competition and can easily take a full program of physical education. Others whose condition is under poor control, the so-called "brittle" diabetics, are better off in the close supervision of the adapted program. Many chronic illnesses, however, are sufficiently debilitating that a full program of exercise is not possible, or might create physical problems, such as in rheumatoid arthritis, which would make such a program undesirable.

The question of whether any person with a chronic illness should be included in an adapted program can only be answered by considering the following problems: (1) Is the degree of debility so slight that it would not be aggravated by a full program? (2) Is the degree of debility or handicap of a nature or extent that would permit any type of adapted program? (3) Would any harm result to the person's present condition as the result of participation regularly in a modified program? When these questions are carefully answered, it will become apparent that there are very few persons suffering from a chronic illness who cannot participate in some form of adapted physical education program.

3. Congenital Defect

Significant defects that might preclude participation in regular physical education programs would include those involving the special senses, heart, extremities, and genetic disorders producing characteristic complex syndromes.

a. SPECIAL SENSES. Congenital deafness is always complicated by difficulty in speaking. The problem of effective communication between teacher and student may make it imperative to handle this problem in an adapted setting. Blindness naturally requires special teaching in physical education and working in small groups under very close supervision.

b. CONGENITAL HEART DEFECTS. Those persons whose defects do not cause either a reduced functional capacity or a high resting blood pressure may participate in regular programs, either with or without surgical correction of their abnormalities. Small septal defects, ligated patent ductus arteriosus, and slight pulmonic stenosis would fall in this category. The others should be placed in an adapted program following surgery, if it is indicated, or without surgery if it is not recommended.

c. DEFECTS OF THE EXTREMITIES. These are usually the result of intrauterine amputations but may also result from toxic states produced by the use of drugs during pregnancy. The problems of inclusion in an adapted program depend on the extent of the defects and their number. The presence of extra digits can produce a handicap if not treated surgically.

d. COMPLEX GENETIC DISORDERS. Turner's syndrome and Marfan's syndrome are examples of conditions that might allow normal participation in activities of daily living but require special consideration in physical education. The tendency for persons with Marfan's syndrome to die suddenly from heart attacks in early life poses a serious question as to whether persons suffering from such a condition should be allowed to participate in physical education at all. The decision to include him in an adapted program should probably be reached on the basis of his apparent interest and desire in being able to participate in some type of activity program. It is probably not going to shorten his life to do so, but the hazard of dying suddenly, perhaps shortly after having been engaged in some physical activity should be understood by his parents and himself.

4. Musculoskeletal Problems

These may be related to genetic defects, disease or injury. Many in all three categories are not completely correctable, although some may be compensated for to some extent.

a. HEREDITARY MUSCULAR WEAKNESS. These conditions are not usually compatible with vigorous physical activity of any kind. In some cases of muscular dystrophy which are delayed in developing, there may be considerable potential for physical activity in the early years. These persons might participate with benefit in an adapted program.

b. NEUROMUSCULAR DISEASE STATES. Cerebral palsy provides an example of a state in which many persons may participate in and benefit from adapted physical education. In those conditions that are of a rapidly progressive and inevitably fatal character, such as amyotrophic lateral sclerosis, there is no point in involving the patient in an activity program. In the case of multiple sclerosis, some young persons in whom the disease appears to be following a very slow course may benefit from some supervised and controlled physical activity.

c. MUSCULOSKELETAL INJURIES. This group makes up one of the largest among those persons who might be considered for inclusion in an adapted program. Some of these problems may be acute, others subacute, and still others chronic. The acute problems are usually best handled by continuation of the necessary rehabilitative treatment, after which a regular program of physical education may be taken, providing there is no serious residual defect.

The subacute and chronic problems that are handicapping are chiefly those affecting the ligamentous origins and tendinous insertions of muscles, the ligaments and capsules of joints, and the bones themselves. Inflammations of origins and insertions, shortening and thickening of muscles due to proliferation of fibrous connective tissue with or without calcium deposition, excessive laxity or contraction of joint capsules, chronic bursitis, muscular atrophy, injuries to joint cartilage with or without formation of loose bodies, synovitis, chronic epiphysitis, delayed fracture healing, fibrous union, and osteochondritis are typical problems. These are most apt to produce partial or complete disability when they affect the spine and the lower extremities.

In deciding whether the affected person should be included in the adapted program, the physician must take into consideration not only the apparent functional capacity but the potential for aggravation of the existing condition. The complete rehabilitation of any permanently handicapped individual may depend as much on his ability to move safely and effectively as on any other factor. Where surgical procedures are anticipated in the individual's rehabilitation program, the adapted program may be of great assistance in preparing him physically for the surgery and speeding his recovery.

d. CONGENITAL LAXITY OF THE JOINTS. These individuals can usually be easily identified by the hyperextensibility of their finger joints. In the extreme degree, this condition may produce repeated subluxations of the shoulders and increased susceptibility to ankle and knee sprains. Those with lesser degrees of involvement should be assigned to adapted programs for their own protection; those with major degrees are better excluded from any vigorous activity program since there is really no way they can learn to move safely and effectively.

e. CONGENITAL DEFECTS OF THE SPINE. Although many physicians, including radiologists, attach little significance to the finding of spina bifida of the first sacral segment, lumbarization of this segment, and sacralization of the fifth lumbar vertebra, these findings appear consistently in patients complaining of recurring and disabling low back pain, and relatively infrequently in those who are asymptomatic. Back pain usually begins after some acute back strain in the early or late teens and then gradually becomes persistent. Loss of firm support from the spinous ligaments is usually responsible for the change. These persons have to learn to live with weak backs and how to protect them. They should be included in an adapted program.

5. Amputations

The amputee with a functioning prosthesis may be easily able to participate in a regular physical education. Some are embarrassed, however, by the presentation of their deformity to a class en masse and are therefore better handled in the more intimate setting of the adapted program. Upper extremity amputees without a prosthesis may also be able to function in a regular program, and prefer it frequently. Bilateral lower extremity amputees probably belong in the adapted program also.

Instruction in physical activities is an important part in the rehabilitation of the recent amputee. He should learn not only what things he can still do but also new ways of doing things that he was able to do before. Skiing on a single ski, once the technique has been mastered, is actually as easy as on two skis, and somewhat safer.

6. Blindness

Many of the nearly blind as well as the completely blind belong in the adapted program. There is no exact limit of visual acuity which can be used as a standard for determining the separation point. It is strictly an individual matter. Persons with severe myopia should probably be in a restricted program because of the dangers of retinal detachment occurring in vigorous activity.

7. Postsurgical Status

Although for most of the common surgical procedures the recovery period is relatively short and a regular program may be undertaken after a period of a few months, some procedures may impose a more lasting or permanent handicap on the individual. The treatment of a hip fracture by surgical pinning may result in shortening of the affected lower extremity, for example. Surgical repair of extensive or complicated ligamentous injuries to the knee does not always result in a stable knee. Creation of an ileostomy or colostomy causes special problems for the individual.

The desirable situation for the postsurgical patient is to include him in an adapted program if his functional recovery is not estimated to be complete eventually, as soon as his wounds are healed, nutrition restored, and other necessary rehabilitative measures, such as physical therapy, completed. The activity itself may then be able to play a significant role in completing his recovery.

C. Physical Immaturity

Functional capacity in terms of cardiovascular and pulmonary efficiency increases steadily during the early years of life and reaches a peak of efficiency in proportion to body weight before the individual develops much in the way of overall strength. Strength development is minimal until the age of puberty but then increases rapidly. It is roughly proportional to height in the untrained individual. The effects of delayed or arrested maturation are felt therefore more in connection with strength than endurance.

1. Delayed Maturation

A state of constitutional delay of normal growth which seems to be associated with a failure of the usual growth spurt at puberty has been recognized for some time but is still not clearly understood. Maturation is not complete until the late twenties at which time the epiphyses finally close. Individuals with this condition belong in adapted physical education where they can be given programs suitable to their degree of development rather than their constitutional age.

2. Endocrine Disorders

Failure of the thyroid and/or pituitary glands to function normally will result in a delay in reaching maturity. Normal physical growth may never be attained, even with treatment. Those who are suffering from pituitary deficiency will grow steadily, but at about half the normal rate. Epiphyseal closure occurs at the usual time. Strength develops proportionately to size. Some endocrine dysfunctions produce asymmetrical types of growth. Dyschondroplastic dwarfs have normal trunk and head size but short extremities. Persons suffering from these disorders should be included in adapted programs primarily because of their small stature and self-consciousness.

3. Primordial Dwarfism

This is a term that merely illustrates our ignorance of why certain individuals develop symmetrically but never reach any considerable height when fully grown. These persons have to be included in adapted physical education programs because their extremely small size makes it impossible for them to participate effectively in regular programs.

D. Obesity

This is properly defined as an excess percentage of body fat. This percentage can be determined by underwater weighing or skin fold thickness measurements. There is no arbitrary point at which a person may be considered too obese to participate in a regular program. The decision should be based on the person's ability to move well and without unusual effort, previous experience in physical activity, sensitivity with regard to personal appearance, and attitude toward exercise generally.

II. EVALUATION OF THE HANDICAPPED INDIVIDUAL

A. History

A good history of the origin of the handicapping condition and of its progress to date, including treatment, provides a sound basis for the remaining portion of the evaluation. The history may not only explain present findings that would otherwise be puzzling, but helps to reveal the patient's psychic reaction to his condition. If any surgical procedures have been performed, it is important to know exactly what they were and what was found. If medication has been given or is being taken currently, this should also be recorded accurately.

Since handicaps are frequently multiple in the same individual, it is important to know about any other significant conditions that may not be directly related to the condition that offers the chief presenting complaint. Accompanying and previously untreated conditions may require treatment adjunctively to the adapted physical education program.

The duration of the major complaint is of especial significance since it will indicate whether it is acute or chronic, but also gives some indication of whether the prognosis for recovery is good or not. If it appears to be poor, then a greater emphasis must be put on learning to compensate for it over an indefinite period through adapted ways of moving. Close questioning is sometimes needed to establish the duration, since there is a tendency to forget events that may not have seemed of great significance at the time of their occurrence.

B. Physical Examination

The examination to determine whether an individual should be included in an adapted program may be considered from two standpoints: as one of a series of examinations made on all individuals who present themselves as candidates for a physical education program; and as a special examination conducted after it has already been determined that the individual is not acceptable for the regular program.

In the first instance, the examination would be of a very general character, covering all the usual points of an external physical evaluation, but with greater emphasis on the functional potential of the individual for physical activity. This would mean that close attention would be given particularly to the examination of the heart, lungs, and musculoskeletal system. Incapacities in locomotion, lack of strength, physical immaturity, shortness of breath, rapid resting pulse rate, and irregularities of the cardiac rhythm would require either rejection from the regular program or at least more careful evaluation by other means. The mental and emotional status could also be of great interest and significance.

As a special examination for the person already identified as not suitable for the regular program, the main focus would be on the nature and extent of the handicapping condition. As detailed a description of this condition and the functional limitations it might impose should be made. The overall fitness of the individual should also be estimated in terms of his ability to respond to the load that might be imposed by the adapted program. It is particularly important to assess the attitude of the individual under consideration toward physical activity, and physical education specifically, in order to ensure his interest and cooperation in the proposed program.

In the examination of the musculoskeletal apparatus, deformity, ranges of active and passive motion, ranges of painfree motion, spasm, contracture, local tenderness, swelling, and strength should be carefully measured or estimated and recorded. These serve not only as guidelines for the prescription of suitable types of exercise but as baselines for evaluation of the effects of the program later on.

C. Laboratory Examinations

If no examinations of this sort have been made before the evaluation for adapted physical education, then, at least, the urine should be examined for sugar, albumin, and its microscopic appearance, and the blood hemoglobin or hematocrit determined and a blood smear stained to identify the differential count of white cells.

What other procedures are done will depend upon the nature of the condition for which the individual is being especially examined. One examination that would not ordinarily be done except as part of a neurological evaluation could be very important in the cases of muscular disorders, that is, the electromyogram. This is helpful in determining the potential of muscles that are currently inactive or greatly reduced in function.

D. X-Ray Examinations

Every candidate for adapted physical education with a musculoskeletal disorder should have X-ray examinations made of the affected parts, if they had not been made very recently and/or were not available for review. In spite of the apparently obvious nature of many of these conditions, X-rays may reveal conditions that are unexpected. This is especially true of conditions involving the lower spine and the knees.

Special studies of joints by the injection of a contrast medium, with or without air, may be necessary to determine exactly the nature of the conditions affecting them. The arthogram of the knee is an example of a procedure that has greatly increased the accuracy of the diagnosis of meniscal injuries.

In the evaluation of heart conditions, especially of a congenital nature, cardiac catheterization may be indicated to complete the evaluation. Coronary angiography may also be done in cases in which coronary occlusion or insufficiency is suspected.

E. Functional Capacity Testing

The primary purposes in testing the functional capacity of the candidate for adapted physical education are to determine strength and endurance. Exact measures of strength are not ordinarily required, but a rough estimation of the dynamic rather than purely static strength is needed in order to determine the individual's ability to carry out certain activities that might be recommended. The determination of endurance is to establish the individual's ability to carry out sustained activity.

Strength can be measured roughly by determining the person's ability to overcome the resistance offered by the examiner's pressure opposing any desired movement. If more exact measurement is required, a hand dynamometer or a strain gauge may be used. A weight and pulley system may also be used for measuring strength in the extremities. The use of an isokinetic device with a recording instrument allows the measurement of strength through a complete range of motion.

Endurance is measured by testing the response of the respiratory and cardiovascular systems to exercise. The best single measure is the oxygen consumption in milliliters per minute per kilogram of body weight during submaximal or maximal exercise. This may be accomplished by using a step-up test (Gallagher *et al.*, 1967), a bicycle ergometer test (Åstrand and Saltin, 1961), or a treadmill test (Balke, 1960) (see also Chapter 19). Close correlations can be obtained among all three methods. The choice of a method will be determined by the time and personnel available to conduct the tests, the availability of the necessary apparatus, and the preference of the tester. The bicycle ergometer is more suitable for candidates who have handicaps in walking.

F. Specialist Consultation

Depending on the expertise and experience of the evaluator, it may be desirable to secure additional opinions or advice from specialists in such fields as neurology, orthopedics, pediatrics, allergy, ophthalmology, and psychiatry before making decisions regarding placement in the adapted program and specific recommendations for activities in that program.

G. Evaluation of Mental and Emotional Status

It is essential for participation in an adapted program that the individual be able to understand in some way what is being asked and expected of him. Even those who are suffering from severe mental retardation may be able to respond to the extent necessary to include them in a special program. If no communication is possible, there is obviously no point in attempting a program. Autistic children are, generally speaking, unsuitable for such a program, as are those persons who are completely out of touch with reality, including severe depressive and catatonic states. The evaluation of the psychologist or psychiatrist is necessary to determine in many instances whether the individual may be able to benefit from the program or not.

H. Evaluation of Attitude toward Physical and Adapted Physical Education

Some individuals who might be entirely suitable from every other standpoint for inclusion in an adapted program have to be excluded because of preconceived and extremely rigid antagonisms toward physical education in general and toward being singled out for special attention in the adapted program in particular. In some cases they have been influenced against all vigorous physical activity of any kind by the well-meaning but misguided warnings of parents and even physicians that exercise will be harmful to them. This appears to be particularly the case with young persons who have severe asthma. They tend, not without some reason, to view every asthmatic attack as a threat to life itself. There is, however, no question that exercise will induce asthmatic attacks in many untrained individuals.

Others are opposed to physical education for the same reasons as they are opposed to any requirements, including education itself, that they feel are imposed on them by society and not freely selected by them. It is not only useless to try to convert these individuals, but, if they are included in the program over their protestations, they will inevitably tend to disrupt it by lack of cooperation and attempts to proselyte others who have already accepted the program to their points of view.

III. RATIONALIZING THE PROGRAM TO THE INDIVIDUAL

A. Potential Contribution of Physical Education to the Individual

The values of physical education to the individual are generally conceived to be those described in Chapter 16. For the handicapped individual the goals of adapted physical education should be:

1. Physiological goal:	To provide an activity program designed to affect the students general physical condition favorably by improving functional capacity
2. Physical education goal:	To help the student explore and widen the potential range of body movements and physical skills
3. Therapeutic goal:	To supplement, on the request of a physician, a strictly therapeutic local treatment with exercise and activity of an enjoyable and conditioning nature
4. Psychological goal:	To provide an opportunity for the student to gain confidence in his own physical proficiency and in the institution which permits him to cope with his handicap complex
5. Educational goal:	To discuss with the student the nature and limitations of the handicap and the possible functional effects of exercise and activity

B. Explanation of the Nature and Purposes of the Program

Very few persons come to an adapted physical education program with a full knowledge of what it includes and what objectives may be as far as they are concerned. Some students actually refer to it as a "baby" program or one for "cripples." Such attitudes imply that compared to a regular program it is not demanding enough to be of interest to them. The use of the latter term suggests that the individual does not see himself as handicapped and would prefer not to be classified with those whose image to him means physical deformation.

The physician may not be familiar with all the techniques that the physical educator may employ to teach the adapted program. Since he is going to make specific recommendations with regard to certain types of activity that should be avoided as well as certain others that should be encouraged, he can indicate to the candidate, in a general way, what might be in store. He might say, for example, to one who might be concerned about having to run that swimming will be used for the development of endurance. If he is concerned about his knee, he could tell him that, although certain games activities will take place, he will not be asked to do anything that might hurt his knee. On the other hand, he will be given some weight resistance work to do to help build up strength in the thigh muscles to help stabilize the knee. Emphasis can be placed on the individual attention of the instructor made possible by working with small groups, and the cooperation of physician and physical educator in planning the program for each person.

The goals of the adaptive program, as outlined in Section III,A, should be discussed with the candidate and related personally by the physician to the candidate's life situation. There may be many doubts and questions that the candidate has regarding the program which can be brought out and discussed at this time. It should be stressed that therapy is not a primary goal of the adapted program, but there may be many gains made as a by-product of the activities involved.

C. Contacts with the Personal Physician

In all those cases where the candidate has indicated that he or she has a personal physician, a summary of the pertinent findings, reasons for selecting an adapted program, and specific recommendations should be sent to this physician. Recommendations for supplementary therapy that can be carried out under the personal physician's direction may also be included. Very often, the acquiescence and cooperation of the personal physician is the key to the acceptance of the program by the candidate.

Many physicians are not familiar with adapted physical education and do not distinguish it from physical or occupational therapy. If the physician has not had any previous knowledge of or experience with the local program, this is a good opportunity to familiarize him with the fact that one does exist and inform him about the program generally.

Follow-up information should go to the physician when the evaluation is made at the conclusion of the program. Recommendations for the type and scope of future physical activities may be made to the physician as well as to the person who has been in the program. Sometimes a recommendation may be made for a continuation of the individual's program for additional periods of time.

If at any time during the program a significant change of an unfavorable nature occurs in the individual's condition, he or she should be referred promptly back to the personal physician, if this is feasible, for his evaluation and treatment.

IV. COORDINATION AND COMMUNICATION
WITH THE PHYSICAL EDUCATOR

A. Examination and Report Form

A copy of the form filled out by the physician at the University of Wisconsin for referral of an undergraduate student to the adapted physical education program is shown in Figs. 1–4. This is the principal source of information that enables the physical educator to set the program for each individual and also tells him those events or reactions for which he should be on the alert. He may supplement this by conversations with both the referring physician and the student as he desires. This form becomes a part of the student's record in the Physical Education Department. It is used in making the final examination of the student for purposes of evaluation.

Identifying the chief reason for which the student is referred seems elementary, but sometimes it is lost sight of due to the interest that develops in other problems the student may have. Sometimes there may be more than one reason. The cause of the condition may not always be apparent, but it is helpful if it is known, since it helps the instructor to relate more directly to the student and to avoid similar activities that might prove harmful to the individual.

The duration of the problem is very significant since it may indicate what can be expected from a prognostic standpoint. It also gives some idea of how much deconditioning has taken place if it has provided a severe handicap. The history of previous or continuing treatment is very important as an index of the extent to which therapy has been or may be useful in restoring the individual to physical activity. The identification of any medications currently being taken is essential both as an aid to encouraging the person to continue his medication regularly, but also in some cases as an index of functional capacity (nitroglycerine, for example, as an indication of angina occurring in response to stress) and a warning to watch for possible side effects (hyperinsulinism in the diabetic).

The physical examination summarizes only the most significant findings that might concern the physical educator in planning his program. The portion relating to the specific problems of the individual is amplified by the physician's description of what significant structural change may have taken place and how the local or general functional capacity has been reduced in very rough terms. If laboratory tests of significance, including X-ray examination have been made, the results are recorded here.

The statement by the individual regarding what physical activities he has engaged in, what sports skills he possesses, and what he feels he cannot do has great significance for the physical educator. The physician may also use this information in shaping his recommendation to the instructor, which appears a little further down on the form. In making these recommendations, the physician cites types of activity he would like to see emphasized but leave the specific selections up to the educator. He may suggest some therapeutic exercise that can be conducted outside of the regular program.

The name and address of the personal physician and any specialist who has been involved in the student's treatment and continued supervision are necessary to facilitate communication with them with regard to the planned program and progress. If they have made any recommendation with regard to what physical education, if any, the student should have, it is also recorded here. Advice against all physical education is frequently given because physicians conceive of such programs as involving only sports and do not understand that an adapted program is available.

Sometimes the advice of a specialist is needed by the referring physician before he makes his final recommendations to the instructor. The information obtained from such consultations is recorded on the last page. The complete evaluation then leads to a classification for physical education which is recorded below this.

B. Personal Contact

A continuing exchange of information regarding the progress of the students between the physician and physical educator is necessary for the success of the program. No one's physical status remains static in such a program. The changes, if favorable, validate the program and help to reinforce future recommendations for persons with similar problems. If things are not going well, some reevaluation of the individual is in order very promptly. Physical and emotional problems that arise from the program or from unrelated sources must be tended to very quickly in order to keep the individual in the program as well as to prevent any of these problems reaching serious proportions.

The physician should visit the adapted class from time to time to observe the progress and to reaffirm that the program agreed upon is being carried out and that there is no immediate need for a change. He may wish also to observe or participate in the functional capacity testing.

C. Individual Case Discussions

Some individuals represent problems that are not easily resolved through the mechanisms outlined above. It is frequently advisable then for the physician and physical educator to hold a formal discussion relating to these problems, sometimes with other specialists in attendance such as an orthopedist or exercise physiologist.

Joint presentations of particular cases may also be made for the benefit of students of physical education or medicine to demonstrate regular or unusual aspects of management for teaching purposes. This may include live or videotaped demonstrations of activity by the students who are involved.

D. Reexamination and Evaluation

At the conclusion of the student's first semester, or comparable period of assignment to the adapted program, his functional capacity should be retested for comparison and a report of progress made by the physical educator to the referring physician. The physician will then probably wish to supplement this himself by a physical examination and perhaps the repeating of selected laboratory tests in order to advise the student regarding his approach to physical activity for the future.

This evaluation may also include some psychological evaluation of the program as seen by the student, in order to allow a continuous reevaluation of the program itself as well as to indicate what approach may best be used to continue the individual's participation in vigorous physical activity.

Some students may wish to or may be advised to select another one or more periods in the program in order to improve their response to a more significant level. At the University of Wisconsin a number of students elect to take a second semester (although only the first is required) and some even a third or fourth.

REFERENCES

Åstrand, P. O., and Saltin, B. (1961). *J. Appl. Physiol.* **16**, 977.
Balke, B. (1960). "The Effect of Physical Exercise on the Metabolic Potential, A Crucial Measure of Physical Fitness, in Exercise and Fitness," pp. 37–81. Athletic Institute, Chicago, Illinois.
Gallagher, J. R., Allman, F. L., Jr., Guild, W. R., Klumpp, T. G., Rose, K. D., Russell, J. C. H., Ryan, A. J., and Hein, F. V. (1967). *J. Amer. Med. Ass.* **201**, 117–118.

Chapter 18

ADAPTED PHYSICAL EDUCATION— THE PROGRAM

SARAH M. ROBINSON

I. INTRODUCTION

Modern philosophies of education and of physical education place heavy emphasis on the value of individually planned instruction.

Adapted physical education can make a direct and practical contribution to an educational program founded on this value premise since the aim of the adapted program is to meet specialized personal needs and to consider individual learning purposes in physical education.

Many special physical education instructional plans exist that have been designed to meet the psychological, physical, or social needs of specific participants. The variation in approach to participation probably reflects differing purposes envisioned by program planners as well as differences among learners. For instance, special instruction is offered for students with low physical fitness, sensorimotor or perceptual deficit, orthopedic or cardiac disability, mental retardation, and neurological and emotional disorders. Adapted activity takes place in many different types of institutions. It seems certain that the major goals of a program must be articulated before activity planning is meaningful.

II. FACTORS INFLUENCING THE STATEMENT OF PURPOSE

Findings in the form of progress reports, activity suggestions, recommendations, and conclusions drawn from special programs are now fairly widely reported in the literature available to physical educators. In order for this information to be most applicable to activity planning, it would be useful to consider the factors that can influence the definition of purpose in the adapted program.

A. Institutional Purpose

A primary influence on the adapted physical education program will be the major philosophical thrust of the institution in which instruction takes place. The content as well as the context of activity will be affected by the careful assessment of institutional purpose. The general categories "educational" and "rehabilitative" can be used to classify, in a gross way, programs that would reflect differing objectives. It is true that most actual program planners aspire to both purposes, but usually one or the other unifying theme must take precedence in establishing priorities for the activity plan.

B. Rehabilitation

The rehabilitative theme in adaptive physical education may be characterized by the statement of objectives that reflect a desire on the part of planners to reduce the immediate handicapping effect of disability. The "limits of disability" are frequently mentioned in a framework of physical or psychological restoration. The intent is improvement of the learner's functioning clearly *with reference to his assessed condition* (Adapted Physical Education, 1969). There is mention of the provision of opportunities for physical, psychological, and social growth, presumably as a result of a regimen of activities therapeutic and recreational in nature. Special care is taken to avoid working at cross purposes with other therapeutic plans. A "rehabilitation team" effort increases the probability of success in amelioration of the handicap. Careful records of status and progress can and should be kept.

An underlying assumption of the possibility and desirability of a prescriptive approach to planning is inherent in the rehabilitative ideal of this form of organization. Cause and effect logic is fundamental to prescriptive practice. The implication is that the specific state of the learner can be assessed. Individual objectives are then derived from the major purposes of the institution. Interventions are proposed and carried out followed by short-term and long-term evaluation. The process results in a reassessment for future individual objectives.

The diagnostic–prescriptive format is basic to the rehabilitative approach and is quite suitable to settings in which rehabilitation, or management, is a stated goal. Physical recreation and physical education programs in hospitals, rehabilitation out-patient centers, and residential care facilities often purport to follow this model. To demonstrate outstanding success, the system depends upon good professional diagnostic support and interpretation of specialized findings and physical education personnel with qualifications in the rehabilitation field.

C. Grouping for Functional Abilities

In settings in which the purpose of the institution is not clearly rehabilitation or management, this approach finds favor as a method whenever task orientation and defined skill acquisition are desired. Examples of educationally based programs that use the method with success are public school programs with the very fearful or naive, perceptual–motor training programs, and routinized plans for the trainably mentally retarded. Group instruction may be more useful under this model if students are grouped according to functional ability. For example, an exercise routine to improve lower extremity range of motion could be executed by all members of a group requiring this practice. A diagnostic label per se may be of very little value in this regard. It seems obvious that not all perceptual–motor problems are tracking problems, for instance. The information of interest is functional *ability* plus *area* of difficulty. Then a prescribed program takes on meaning, for the world of choice is defined for the planner.

D. The Student's Purpose

Within institutions commited to educational, as compared to rehabilitative, purposes, adaptive physical education programs can serve somewhat different ends in the lives of learners. Although not denying the need for specific skills, the newer concepts of learning theory view man as a purposive, exploratory individual (Weber, 1970). This viewpoint emphasizes the importance of environmental transactions and the active processes of human learning. Under this model, the student's own definition of purpose may be accepted as the organizing principle for activity planning. Thus, *choice of experiences is not necessarily directed toward reduction of the handicapping elements of disability,* although in the process of educational change such benefits may accrue.

E. Planning for Motor, Affective, and Cognitive Functions

Delineation of generalized goals for each of the learning domains— motor, affective, and cognitive—may be typical of educationally oriented programs. Many of the adapted physical education objectives will rest with the motor domain. Yet, other worthy objectives for whole groups of learners may be selected from the cognitive and affective schemata. In addition to a focus on generalized human abilities, such as concern for creativity, the educationally oriented setting may postulate goals of broad social or personal relevance.

Adapted physical education plans in such situations take personal limitations into account, but tend to emphasize function and ability. Attempts are made to structure the challenge of situations for active, personal interaction with the environment on the part of the learner at ever higher levels of affective, cognitive, and motor function. In one method that illustrates this transactional logic, several alternative activity problems may be posed by the teacher at a level of presumed competence. However, the choice of act, quality of performance, and type of evaluation and meaning given to the experience may be left to the student's independent judgment. Answers are assumed to be open questions—flexibility of response and openness to new alternatives are desired.

Content is considered appropriate from the whole range of purposive human movement.

F. Preparation of Teaching Specialists

Another factor that influences the stated purposes in various adapted physical education programs available for evaluation relates to the preparation of teaching personnel. Specialized educational experience in work with the atypical is widely varying (Hawkes, 1968). Variation is found in the amount and kind of field experience with differing age and disability groups, theoretical understandings in physical education and rehabilitation, and attitude and behavior toward the atypical. Orientation toward these and other facts of the teacher's professional preparation and work experience will affect his suggestions for desirable practice.

G. Characteristics of the Students

Adapted physical education can serve learners with extremely diverse needs. The characteristics of the students may appear to be too obvious a determinant of program purpose to warrant mention. Yet, to suggest guidelines for the conduct of program without reiteration of this crucial point would be unfortunate. Some disability groups can profit enormously from the special techniques that can be used in physical education to supplement other rehabilitative efforts. The needs of the visually handicapped, for instance, will influence the purposes of the physical education program, and these needs may be very different in basic purpose and in detail of execution from those of the wheelchair bound paraplegic.

H. Age

In consideration of individual needs, the limits of personal disability, and unique aspirations, it is well to consider the student's age also. Many worthwhile activities can be unattractive in the eyes of the learner if he perceives the modification as childish, oversimplified, or an unworthy goal. By the same token, challenges must be planned at a level of realization. The balance is achieved through complete knowledge of the characteristics of the learners for whom the planning is proposed.

III. COMMONALITIES IN ACTIVITY PLANS

Regardless of the major focus of a program, the nature of the specialized preparation of the staff, or the characteristics of the learners, good plans have some similar features.

A. Safeguarding Health and Safety

First, every precaution is taken to safeguard the safety and health of participants. Yet, care is also exercised to avoid the extremes of paternalism that make students unjustifiably anxious about their limitations. The idea is to contribute to the student's maturing judgment by communicating to him a realistic appraisal of the entire situation, of his limits, and of the task demands.

The physical educator must be rigorous in his pursuit of information about questions related to the safety of individuals. Information sources include other professional personnel for task analysis and referring physicians regarding the student's health status. The same is true of the evaluation of the level of complexity of psychosocial demands as well as for the more evident precautions in the motor performance areas.

Administrators' and supervisors' assistance should be sought in the resolution of problems regarding hazards in equipment or facilities.

B. Importance of Preplanning

Second, preplanning is a feature of good programs. Whether the plan is prescriptive or transactional, this step is vital. There will be a difference in the type of data determined relevant, but information will be gathered systematically that will provide variety in an individual's program. In addition, a rational plan for the scope of material, sequence, and progression in the learning experiences or specified tasks will be suggested by this planning stage.

C. Meaningful Evaluation

Third, adequate programs provide for meaningful evaluation. Student progess is assessed periodically, as is teacher behavior and total program effectiveness. Many ways can be found to make record keeping possible. The use of teacher aides might free instructor time. A reasonable method has been found in asking the students to be their own record keepers on suitable objectives and objective measurements. Most students are careful and dependable when they recognize the advantages of accurately gathering information over time. Subjective evaluations are often very helpful, and the suitable use of these should be considered. Tapes and films add another interesting and useful dimension to the evaluation scheme.

D. Individualization of Instruction

Common to the adapted program idea is the central theme of the individualization of instruction. This can be carried out in group settings, but best results occur with favorably low teacher pupil ratios. Exact group size depends upon the nature of instruction, the age of the students, the available facilities, and the type of disability. Sometimes rather large groups are needed for team events. Social recreation goals might call for large and diversified groups to increase appreciation of individual variability and to teach students to function in large group settings. But, by and large, the more intimate and supportive nature of the small group will meet more personal instruction goals.

IV. SPECIFIC TEACHING PROPOSITIONS

Full-length textbooks in this field, such as those by Fait (1972) and Arnheim et al. (1973), emphasize the importance of responsible teaching practice in working with the handicapped. Publications are available from various sources that provide suggestions about the conduct of particular types of activity programs. Articles in the *Journal of the American Association for Health, Physical Education and Recreation* originated through the office of the group's Consultant on Programs for the Handicapped are useful examples. A directory of periodicals is available from this source upon request.

The attempt here will be to propose four principles that apply specifically to education of the disabled. Attention to these propositions could give increased meaning to activity planning for the adapted physical education program.

A. As Much Physical Activity as Possible

First, a basic principle in daily individual program planning is to provide as much physical activity as possible for each participant. In practice this means that students are actively working at a meaningful movement task even when the instructor is occupied with individual questions or demonstrations. The tasks may be exploratory or prescriptive. For too long the handicapped child was assigned the "scorekeeper" role for others' active participation. It is proposed that this is no longer an acceptable use of the disabled person's physical education time.

B. Fostering Independence

Second, an underlying theme of work with the disabled emerges as the principle of fostering independence. In each phase of activity planning, the instructor should consider whether or not the overall scheme contributes to future independence on the part of the student. The goal can be approached slowly and subtly, but the learner can eventually be helped to value the notion that he is capable of making a range of physical education and sports participation choices. He can be led to understand the importance of asking his physician about the advisability of activities that he would like to try as well as the need to heed warnings about areas of participation that he should avoid.

As students grow more independent, they are willing to risk more in competition. Competition can be introduced at all levels of instruction; sensitivity on the part of the instructor will be demonstrated by his handling of the group dynamics of the competitive process. Attention to the ideal of fostering increased independence can be very beneficial to the student in psychosocial development as well as physical improvement. The principle can help organize the instructor's efforts to provide a sound progression of activity.

C. The Importance of Recreation

A third important principle in the teaching of adapted physical education is the realization that recreation plays a vital role in the life of a person. Therapeutic recreation is a recognized ancillary health service profession. The physical education experience should make a contribution to the total functioning of the learner so that he will seek and find satisfaction in physical recreation, sports, and dance *participation* when he is no longer under the guidance of the institution offering the program. Every effort must be made to teach recreational skills, to provide opportunities for fun as well as understanding, and to influence the image of the person in his attitude toward the world of volitional human movement. He should see himself as a competent "mover" and be happy with the vision. In planning a particular program, the instructor needs to use some imagination in projecting the interests and skills of the learner into the future; a recreative, yet instructional, atmosphere in the class contributes to this end.

D. Return to Full Functioning Capacity

The fourth basic idea to be presented here stems from understanding the previous three propositions: activity, independence, and recreative values. This proposition is that rehabilitation and education are not dichotomous in work with the atypical student. There is a need, as was expressed earlier, to discern the main purpose of an institution in order to work effectively within its structure, but in both rehabilitation and education we are interested in assisting a student toward his full functioning capacity. Instructors can and should use the whole range of methodology of the fields of physical education and rehabilitation appropriate to the needs of each student. A range of teaching behaviors may make it possible for more students to gain help from the program. Openness to experience, if expected from the students, should be exemplified by their instructors.

Finally, the coping, positive person with a vision for the possible and a willingness to communicate on all available channels, who is in touch with the realities of his teaching situation, will be able to make significant contributions to real teaching and real learning in this field. He will invest something of himself in the process, and he will also grow.

REFERENCES

Adapted Physical Education. (1969). *J. Health, Phys. Educ. Recreation* **40**, 45–46.
Arnheim, D. D., Auxter, D., and Crowe, W. C. (1973). "Principles and Methods of Adapted Physical Education," 2nd ed. Mosby, St. Louis, Missouri.
Fait, H. F. (1972). "Special Physical Education: Adapted, Corrective, and Developmental," 2nd ed. Saunders, Philadelphia, Pennsylvania.
Hawkes, A. E. (1968). *Amer. Corrective Ther. J.* **22**, 56.
Weber, E. (1970). "Early Childhood Education: Perspectives on Change," p. 34. Jones Publ. Co., Worthington, Ohio.

Chapter 19

FUNCTIONAL CAPACITY TESTING

KARL G. STOEDEFALKE

I. INTRODUCTION

Functional or work capacity may be defined as the physiological response of the cardiovascular and respiratory system to locomotor activity of gradual increasing intensity. The adaptations of the body to the stress of muscular effort is expressed numerically in the amount of oxygen supplied to the tissues and may be determined through indirect methods. These methods include the use of the motor driven treadmill, bicycle ergometer, stepping device, an arm ergometer, and a field test of running. In the laboratory, constant surveillance of the heart rate and arterial blood pressures permit a safe and reliable evaluation of the subject's aerobic capacity. That point at which limitations are observed in the adjustments of the respiratory and circulatory systems to the increased demands of the work is the subject's maximum aerobic power. Maximum aerobic power (V_{o_2} max) is expressed in milliliters of oxygen per kilogram of body weight per minute (ml/kg/min) and provides a meaningful and useful measure for the physician and physical educator.

Need

According to research findings (Stoedefalke *et al.*, 1969), the maximum aerobic power of the disabled school aged poulation is lower than that of the nondisabled student. These differences in performance capabilities have occurred for several reasons. On the one hand, school administrators may consider students with disabilities in physical education classes an unnecessary risk. Accident or injury does occur in physical activity, and a student handicapped by a disabling condition, no matter how minor, could be a more susceptible candidate. Legal reprisal for the administrator, and specifically for the physical educator in the event of negligence, cannot be ignored. On the other hand, the physical educator may not feel comfortable leading students with a variety of disabling conditions. Inadequate professional preparation in understanding the medical aspects of the problem could contribute to the exclusion of the disabled student in physical education classes. The physician often contributes to a student's lowered performance capability by supporting parental or patient requests to excuse the disabled student from any form of organized physical activity and thereby concedes to a cyclic withdrawal from physical education and physical activity (Fig. 1). Or, the physician may judge physical education on the basis of previous experience. If the physician, as a student, had unfavorable experiences in physical education, or has not been informed of the scope and instruction available to the student, he would see little merit to an adapted physical education program in meeting the needs of the disabled. Lastly, repeated unpleasant experiences in physical education as a result of poorly developed motor skills plus a disabling condition contribute to the cycle of inactivity, and lowered performance capability is the result. The needs of students with disabilities can be met if qualified physical educators can enlist the support of the parents, cooperation of the physician, endorsement of the school administrators, and interest of the student. A start toward this goal is to place physical education for students with disabilities on a sound scientific foundation.

The consequences of the inactivity cycle may be averted if physical activity becomes more than a series of ritualistic positions randomly selected. The program must be dynamic, medically approved, and pleasurable to the participant.

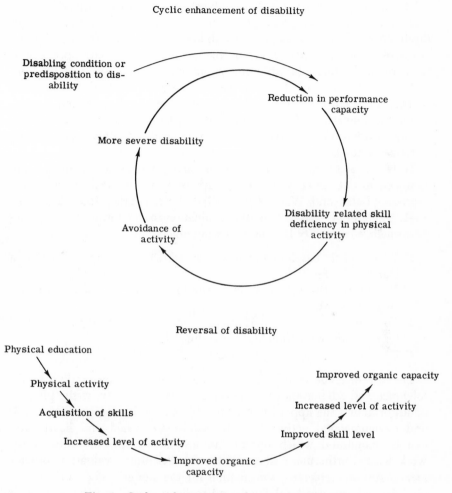

Fig. 1 Cyclic enhancement and reversal of disability

II. FUNCTIONAL CAPACITY

Conducting programs of physical activity for the disabled must be based on more than a trial-and-error method. Neither previous professional experience nor current fashionable exercise techniques are satisfactory. It is important that the physician and physical educator know the performance capabilities of the subject before a physical activity regime is prescribed, or physical exercise of a remedial or developmental nature is recommended.

The consequence of a purely subjective evaluative technique as a basis for an exercise prescription can be deleterious to the subject's disabling condition. Orthopedic disabilities may be aggravated by the stress of improper activity. Or, if the goal of the activity specialist is to increase the muscular strength or endurance capabilities of the subject, intensity or work load as well as duration of the activity must be regulated. Furthermore, a subject may be unduly stressed and thereby suffer the unwarranted effects of discomfort and general fatigue when the justification for the activity is not based on the results of scientifically determined tests.

Tests are available to the physician-physical educator team and are designed to determine a subject's adaptability to physical activity* and exercise (Balke and Ware, 1959; Balke, 1963; Clarke, 1966; Leighton, 1941; Nagle *et al.*, 1965). Scientific evaluation that determines a student's performance capability has the following objectives:

1. To establish baseline measures for activity prescription within a margin of safety
2. To observe the subject's responses to activity, which requires increased energy demands
3. To translate human performance into meaningful physiological terms for the education and counseling of the subject
4. To provide an educational experience for the subject

The key to a successful adapted program is an understanding of the tolerance and adaptation of a subject to physical activity. If the physical educator knows the upper limits of a subject's aerobic power, therapeutic and developmental activity can be safely prescribed and heart rates can be monitored which provide an insight into the intensity of the work load. Furthermore, the results of a scientific evaluation provide meaningful and objective information for the student. The limits of energy expenditure can be defined, and realistic as well as attainable goals may be set.

A. Treadmill Testing

The selection of a treadmill test depends upon the ability of the subject to walk at a speed of from 2 mph to 3.4 mph. In the presence of lower extremity musculoskeletal or neurological problems that impair

---

* For the purpose of this chapter, physical activity embraces all forms of movement with and without objects or the use of equipment. Exercise denotes repetitive movements of a specific nature which are therapeutic or ameliorative.

the timing in walking, other forms of stress testing should be used. These might include the bicycle or arm ergometer.

A number of treadmill tests are available for diagnostic purposes. Each test has common elements. These are a known treadmill belt speed, a series of gradual increases in the treadmill grade, and constant monitoring of the subject's heart rate and arterial blood pressures during the testing session. The Balke Test (Balke and Ware, 1959) is an example of a test that can be safely administered by a physical educator and performed by the majority of people even with mild and moderate physical impairments.

When time permits, it is desirable to have a practice session on the treadmill prior to the testing session. This will allay the anxiety associated with testing, and will inform the subject how the treadmill functions and what will happen during the testing session. Instruction and practice in walking on the treadmill should be done at a variety of treadmill grades and speeds. The anxious reaction of the inexperienced subject will be reflected in elevated arterial blood pressures and heart rates but will usually quickly subside as the subject becomes accustomed to treadmill walking. The sympathetic responses to testing will then disappear.

Balke Test

The Balke Test is a progressive treadmill test in which the treadmill belt speed is held constant and the treadmill grade is elevated by 1% after the completion of each minute of walking. An example of the test recording form is presented in Table I. The grade of the treadmill is set at 1% and the treadmill belt speed at 3.4 mph. After the resting arterial pressures and heart rate are obtained, the subject is asked to walk on the treadmill and informed that the pressures and heart rate will be assessed during the testing session.

a. Blood Pressure Determination. The assessment of accurate arterial blood pressures and heart rates are a critical aspect of the functional capacity testing. The stethoscope should have an extended rubber or polyethylene tube attached to a microphone strapped to the subject's arm. The additional length of tubing is necessary so that the subject may freely swing his arm during the time pressures are not being determined. The placement of the microphone on the subject's arm requires a certain degree of experimentation. The cubital fossa is the site most often used for obtaining the Korotkoff sounds from the brachial artery. In subjects who have a great deal of subcutaneous tissue at this site, it may be necessary to select the medial aspect of the bicipital furrow at a distance of 1 cm from the medial epicondyle. It is a position proximal to the cubital fossa, and for many subjects it is a more favorable place for obtaining a clear sound in auscultation.

Arterial pressures are recorded by inflating the arm cuff of the mercury sphygmomanometer at 30 seconds into each minute of the test. The mercury is raised to a height of approximately 200 mm of mercury, and then pressure is released by turning the thumbscrew permitting a slow steady drop of the mercury until the first phase systolic pressure sounds are heard. This procedure requires 5 to 10 seconds. The pressure is then dropped to approximately 100 mm of mercury while the heart rate is determined. The heart rate count is begun with zero at zero time, proceeds over a 15 second interval, and is reported to a recorder. In the last 5 seconds of the testing minute, the diastolic pressure is obtained, and the assistant is instructed to raise the treadmill belt by 1%. The test proceeds until the criteria for terminating the test are achieved by the subject.

b. RECOVERY. Upon completion of the walking test, the subject remains seated on a chair placed on the treadmill belt, the grade of the treadmill is lowered, and arterial pressure and heart rates are determined and recorded during 3 recovery minutes. The normal testing session requires no more than approximately 30 minutes. Upon completion of the test, the results of the treadmill test are presented to the subject. This baseline measure provides an objective evaluation for leading abled and disabled individuals in a wide variety of physical activities.

c. CRITERIA FOR TERMINATING THE TREADMILL TEST. The purpose of determining maximum aerobic power is to identify the upper limits of a subejct's ability to make satisfactory cardiorespiratory adjustments to gradual increasing work intensities. At the point of optimal work capacity, avoiding exhaustion or overstress of the subject, physiological (objective) and examiner (subjective) criteria terminate the test. These criteria are:

1. Decrease in pulse pressure
    Decrease in systolic blood pressure
    Increase in diastolic blood pressure
2. The achievement of the "critical" heart rate usually of 180 beats per minute (not applicable to the cardiac patient) *
3. Sudden change in color of the ears, lips, and face

* In evaluating the cardiac patient, an ECG is recorded throughout the test, and a physician should be present during the testing session.

4. Labored breathing
5. Observable uncoordinated locomotive efforts
6. Perfuse perspiration
7. A subject reports pain or extreme discomfort

B. Bicycle Ergometer

In subjects who have severe ankle, knee, hip, or back problems, it is often advisable to use the bicycle ergometer as a method of evaluation. The bicycle ergometer provides meaningful results to the adapted physical educator, and many subjects are more comfortable in pedaling the bicycle than they are walking the treadmill. This is particularly true in persons with neurological problems in which the timing involved in walking may not lend itself to maintaining the treadmill belt speed. The mercury sphygmomanometer must be used in bicycle ergometer testing. If an aneroid sphygmomanometer is used, the spring mechanism offers too great variability, and the fluctuations of the needle impair objective reading of the arterial pressures with any degree of accuracy. The protocol for the bicycle ergometer test is found in Table I. Ergometry testing as presented in this table shows the opportunity for a progressive test where the resistance to pedaling is expressed as kilogram meters per minute or watts.

There may be times when the foot must be strapped to the pedal. This can be done either by taping the subject's shoe to the pedal or providing a restraining strap. The subject is instructed to pedal at between 50 and 60 revolutions per minute, as the tester encourages the subject to keep the pace. The bicycle ergometer test proceeds in a similar fashion to the treadmill test. Resting arterial pressures as well as heart rates are obtained, and the subject is instructed to pedal until he can either no longer overcome the resistance or approaches physical discomfort which impairs his cycling rhythm.

It is important that the subject exerts a downward pressure on the pedal with the metatarsal rather than the longitudinal arch. Furthermore, the seat height and arm height should be optimal for the subject's sitting height. If the seat is too low or too high, the mechanics of pedaling are impaired.

To obtain blood pressure readings during the test, the subject is asked to take his left hand off the handle bar and to hold it quietly at his side. With practice, rapid and accurate determinations of blood pressures are possible during the work. After each completed minute of cycling, the resistance is increased by 10 watts or 60 kilogram meters. The test

TABLE I

Functional Capacity Tests

Date_____

Height_____ Weight_____ Age_____

Name_____

Bicycle ergometer		Treadmill grade (%)	Systolic	Diastolic	HR (15 sec)
(kg m/min)	(watts)				
		REST			
300	50				
360	60	1			
480	80	2			
600	100	3			
660	110	4			
720	120	5			
780	130	6			
840	140	7			
900	150	8			
960	160	9			
1020	170	10			
1080	180	11			
1140	190	12			
1200	200	13			
1260	210	14			
1320	220	15			
1380	230	16			
1440	240	17			
1500	250	18			
1560	260	19			
1620	270	20			
1680	280	21			
1740	290	22			
1800	300	23			
	310	24			
	320	25			

Recovery

1			
2			
3			

continues until the subject can no longer overcome the resistance or exhibits other signs which terminate the test. A 3 minute recovery evaluation is also recommended.

C. The Step Test

In the absence of a treadmill or bicycle ergometer, a stepping test may be used. Step tests require a minimal amount of equipment but provide good determinations of aerobic power. A series of steps may be constructed at heights of 10, 20, 30, 40, and 50 cm. The stepping rate is 30 complete 4-cycle trips. To assist the subject in maintaining the proper stepping rate, a metronone can be set at 120. The subject steps for a period of 3 minutes at each level. For subjects with heart disease the test may be started on the level, and the second 3 minute phase of the test is stepping at the 10 cm height. To offset the problem of local muscular fatigue, the subject may vary the lead leg. A procedure of foot tapping to alternate the lead leg can be accomplished with a little practice. The step test also requires that the arterial pressure determination and heart rate be obtained following the procedures suggested for the treadmill and bicycle ergometer tests. Table II relates the stepping to a general estimation of V_{O_2}. The criteria for terminating the test are similar to those presented previously, namely, decrease in pulse pressure, heart rate in excess of 180 beats, or subject discomfort in performing the task. It is also essential that a mercury sphygmomanometer rather than an aneroid type be employed.

D. Field Test

The Balke Field Test (Balke, 1963) is an excellent means of evaluating maximum aerobic power. A stopwatch and a measured running track

TABLE II
Relation of Stepping to a General Estimation of V_{O_2}

Stepping height	Approximate V_{O_2} (ml/kg/min)	Rating
Ground Level	11	Very poor
10 cm	18	Very poor
20 cm	25	Poor
30 cm	32	Below average
40 cm	39	Average
50 cm	46	Above average

or area are the only requirements for testing. The instructions for administration are minimal. As a diagnostic tool, it reveals a great deal about the subject who undertakes 15 minutes of sustained locomotion. As a test, it is applicable to mildly impaired disabled students, especially those who have upper extremity involvement. In subjects with moderate impairments of the hip, knee, and ankle, discretion should be used to avoid aggravating the condition or unwarranted discomfort. Step or bicycle ergometer tests are recommended in these cases.

Instructions to the subject are in the form of a charge. "When I say 'go,' I'd like you to continue to run for 15 minutes; please do not stop. If you have to stop running, continue to walk, and when you feel sufficiently recovered begin running again." Balke reported that as running exceeds a duration of 12 minutes the anaerobic component of the work is 5% of the work accomplished.

As an indirect method of maximum aerobic power, the 15 minute run correlates highly with direct laboratory assessments ($r = .85$). If one considers a measurement error of 5% acceptable, the field test is not only suitable but extremely useful in another way. As a subject runs, the physical educator has the opportunity to observe the subject's mechanics of locomotion, his ability to pace himself, and gains insight into the motivational efforts necessary to accomplish the task. Figure 2 is a synthesis of the Balke report which relates the distance covered in 15 minutes to the mean velocity (in mph), to the time required for 1 mile at a given velocity, and to the oxygen requirements. Table III presents a suggested qualitative rating of the 15 minute test.

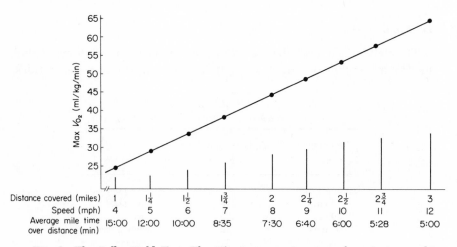

Fig. 2 The Balke Field Test. The 15 minute run is a test of maximum aerobic power.

TABLE III

Balke Rating Scale of Maximum Aerobic Power

Rating	Maximal O_2 intake (ml/kg/min)
Inferior	25
Very poor	25–30
Poor	30–35
Average (Fair)	35–40
Good	40–45
Very good	45–50
Excellent	50–55
Superior	55+

E. Arm Ergometry

Arm ergometry is a means of assessing functional capacity using the technique of cranking. Cranking involves a circular motion of the arms, whereby both arms crank in unison, or alternate in their application of force on the crank handles. As a method of subject evaluation, the arm ergometry testing procedures, as well as the interpretation of the findings, are attractive research challenges. The use of arm ergometry has been confined to the comparison of physiological responses as obtained in standard work tasks of walking and cycling. A promising research area is available to the scientist, particularly those who are involved in evaluating the performance of subjects who have lower extremity disabilities or patients with coronary heart disease (Bobbert, 1960). The efficiency of arm work is less than that for leg work (Bobbert, 1960). The heart rate and minute ventilation are higher for arm work than for leg work of an equivalent oxygen consumption. Maximum oxygen consumption (V_{O_2}) has been determined during arm work at about 70% of maximum V_{O_2} when bicycling. Asmussen and Hemmingsen (1958) report that a linear relationship exists in the heart rate and oxygen uptake in both arm and leg work, but it is not possible to estimate the total aerobic power for leg work from experiments with arm work or vice versa.

A recent report (Clausen *et al.*, 1970) establishes that training performed by arm work on an inverted bicycle ergometer caused a significant reduction of heart rate during arm work but not a reduction of heart rate during leg work. As a developmental or therapeutic exercise technique, arm ergometry may be used. Base line measures could be established using heart rate (telemetered), total number of revolutions, or resistance as the criterion measure. Exercise programs could be prescribed and a retest would provide evidence of the effectiveness of the program and also serve as a motivational technique for the subject. Supplementary to the tests of aerobic power, base line measures and evaluation should be obtained on a subject's muscle strength and flexibility.

III. STRENGTH

Muscle strength is the amount of force a subject can voluntarily apply against a resistance. Man needs muscle strength in his continual battle against gravity as well as for locomotion and daily living. To meet sudden emergencies, he may be required to move rapidly, carry, lift, or push objects or help his fellow man. He climbs up and down stairs and alters his posture hundreds of times during the course of a day. In order to accomplish these tasks a well-developed muscle system is necessary.

With a muscle system deficient in strength, the subject with an orthopedic handicap will lack the ability to maintain the pace of his nondisabled contemporaries, and unnecessary fatigue will result. A low level of muscle strength may also cause an overload and subsequent strain to connective tissue, tendons, and joints. When muscle atrophy occurs, there is inefficient functioning of the peripheral circulation as the milking action necessary to venous return is inhibited. Furthermore, repeated foreshortening of agonists and relaxation of the antagonist muscles may result in functional skeletal changes and unwarranted muscle pain.

Subjects with acquired orthopedic unilateral disabilities may exhibit asymmetry in the girth of a segment as well as a strength deficiency of the involved limb. Therefore, in order to learn more of a subject's performance capabilities, girth and strength measurements should be taken.

The evaluation of strength or muscular work can be obtained by methods that measure dynamic or static muscle force efforts. In dynamic strength measurements, the contracting muscles either shorten (concentric contraction) or lengthen (eccentric contraction). These measurements may be taken by requiring a subject to lift, push, or pull weights through a predetermined range of joint motion. A number of repetitions of the same weight may be required or the weights may be increased in poundage until the subject is unable to move the weight successfully through the "normal" range of motion. It is important that the uninvolved segment be measured so base lines can be established and achievement goals defined for the subject's therapeutic program. Girth measurements should be taken before strength measurements to nullify the possibility of circulatory ischemia in the muscle groups being evaluated. Preselecting an anatomical landmark for girth measurements adds to the objectivity and reliability of the assessment and is necessary to an interpretation of the posttraining test results. Testing for dynamic strength capability provides a challenge to the subject and the investigator. The performance of the subject at heavier work loads is limited by his ability to overcome the inertia of the load as well as his willingness to stress himself maximally. Motivation and pain limit the maximal effort. The above stated limitations to dynamic strength assessment have been of sufficient concern that many physical educators use isometric strength performance as a criterion measure of muscle strength.

In static or isometric muscular work, the muscles exhibit little or a negligible amount of movement. Isometric strength measurements can be obtained through a cable or recording tensiometer (Clarke, 1966) and a variety of segmental angles may be tested. The cable tensiometer (Fig. 3) must be calibrated for reliable measurement. Norms are available but the physical educator should be more concerned with the variance of unilateral measurements and his own objectivity. Body position during measurement is critical. If subsequent measurements of strength of the same muscle groups do not involve the same body or segmental positions, the results of the testing are meaningless. Before and after testing, results become meaningful when the subject is motivated to a maximal effort, the tensiometer is calibrated, and the anatomical positions are held constant.

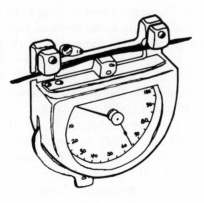

Fig. 3 The tensiometer.

The student with any type of disability must have an average or above average muscle strength capability. This is a realistic goal for the mild to moderately impaired. The general minimum requirements for muscle strength have not been determined for a given population, and a task-oriented investigation would add to man's knowledge of strength. After age 30, man's strength capabilities decrease, and periods of inactivity and illness contribute to this decline. For maintenance and protection, strength evaluation should be a critical part of the assessment of functional capacity.

IV. FLEXIBILITY

Flexibility is defined as the range of motion at a joint. It plays an important part in motor activity and should be of concern to the adapted physical educator as he designs programs of therapeutic exercise for the rehabilitation of orthopedic disabilities. A subject's range of motion is sex dependent and is influenced by muscular, ligamentous and skeletal limitations. Pathological conditions of the bone, ligaments, or cartilage impair the extent of joint mobility.

Man needs flexibility. Perhaps the most important reason for flexibility is to prevent injury to the musculoskeletal systems. As man ages, degenerative changes take place within bone and connective tissue, and sedentary habits lead to muscle atrophy. Muscle or disuse atrophy can be observed in subjects who by the nature of their occupations are required to sit for extended periods of time. This predisposition requires the musculoskeletal system to conform to the stresses to which it is subjected. The result is evident in foreshortened flexor muscles of the hip and leg and a relaxation of the leg extensor muscles. The range of motion at the hip and knee decreases. Unless therapeutic activity is undertaken, functional changes occur leading to further foreshortening of muscles and restricted mobility at the involved joint.

Flexibility also has a qualitative dimension. It contributes to an ease and mechanical efficiency in locomotion which is esthetically attractive. The seemingly effortless fluid and agile movements of the superior performer cannot be compared to the awkward movements of the novice. Flexibility as a factor of motor ability is an asset.

Flexibility may be measured subjectively by an examiner through manipulative efforts (Moore, 1949) or objectively using measurement devices and tests. Manipulation has merit in a clinical setting but lacks the objectivity necessary for the researcher or adaptive physical educator. The goniometer (Fig. 4) and flexometer (Leighton, 1941, 1955) provide reliable results in the hands of the expert.

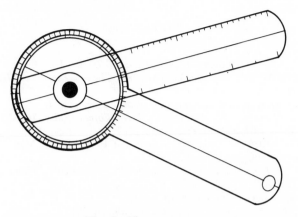

Fig. 4   The goniometer.

The published norms for the normal range of joint motion are variable and give evidence of a lack of agreement among investigators. This variability occurs through the differing measuring devices and objectivity criteria used by different examiners. Reliable results may be obtained if the physical educator accepts the effect of gravity on segmental motion, establishes a protocol for his evaluation, and acknowledges the fluctuations in the axis of motion as the segment moves through its range. If a subject has an acquired unilateral musculoskeletal problem, the physical educator can establish a normal range of motion for that segment by comparing the performance to the corresponding articulation.

In summary, flexibility is important to man's performance capability. It can be measured objectively, and activity of a therapeutic nature can be prescribed.

V. SUMMARY

The success of the team approach to adapted physical education depends upon the mutual respect and cooperation of the medical doctor and the adapted physical educator. Each has an expertise that is complementary to the other. Working as a team, the efforts of both can be effective if the adapted program is based on scientifically determined evaluations. The determination of tolerance and adaptability to activity of a physical nature should be an integral part of the subject's examination. Only then can rehabilitative or developmental activity be safety and objectively prescribed.

REFERENCES

Asmussen, E., and Hemmingsen, I. (1958). *Scand. J. Clin. Lab. Invest.* **10**, 67.

Balke, B. (1960). *In* "Medical Physics" (O. Glasser, ed.), Vol. III, pp. 50–52. Yearbook Publ. Chicago, Illinois.

Balke, B. (1963). *U.S. Civil Aeromed. Res. Inst. Pub. Rep.* 63-6.

Balke, B., and Ware, C. W. (1959). *U.S. Armed. Forces Med. J.* **10**, 675.

Bobbert, A. C. (1960). *J. Appl. Physiol.* **15**, 1007.

Clarke, H. H. (1966). "Muscular Strength and Endurance in Man." Prentice-Hall, Englewood Cliffs, New Jersey.

Clausen, J. P., Trap-Jensen, J., and Lassen, N. H. (1970). *Scand. J. Clin. Lab. Invest.* **26**, 295.

Leighton, J. R. (1941). *Res. Quart.* **13**, 205.

Leighton, J. R. (1955). *Arch. Phys. Med. Rehabil.* **36**, 571.

Moore, M. L. (1949a). *Phys. Ther. Rev.* **29**, 195.

Moore, M. L. (1949b). *Phys. Ther. Rev.* **29**, 256.

Nagle, F. J., Balke, B., and Naughton, J. P. (1965). *J. Appl. Physiol.* **20**, 745.

Stoedefalke, K. G., Balke, B., Ryan, A. J., and Gale, J. B. (1969). *In* "Exercise and Fitness 1969" (B. D. Franks, ed.), pp. 195–200. Athletic Institute, Chicago, Illinois.

Chapter 20

EVALUATION OF THE ADAPTED PROGRAM

ALLAN J. RYAN

I. REEVALUATION OF THE HANDICAPPED INDIVIDUAL

A. Periodic

Due to change in the individual's condition for reasons extrinsic to the program, it may be necessary for the physician to reevaluate him before the conclusion of any stated period, such as a semester. Intercurrent illness or injury or exacerbation of a previously existing condition may require a reexamination. If the matter is of no serious consequence, the individual may resume his program without any change. If it is more serious, then he must be excused from participation either temporarily or for the remainder of the period.

Accidents may also occur in the program itself which bring about a temporary disability. These are of somewhat more serious consequence than those which might occur during a regular program as far as their impact on the handicapped individual is concerned, since his expectation in the adapted program would be that there should be much less chance of an accidental injury occurring. For this reason, he may require considerable reassurance.

Some persons may find, after attempting the program outlined by the instructor, that they are unable to carry it through. This requires a joint reassessment by the instructor and the physician with a view toward modifying the program, or even reaching a decision that the person in question is not really suitable for inclusion in the adapted program, after all. Frank recognition of such a situation by the instructor and admission by both the individual and the physician that the prediction was overoptimistic can lead to the speedy solution of what might otherwise create a very difficult problem.

B. At Conclusion of the Program

Each individual in the adapted program should be reevaluated by the instructor and the physician at its conclusion. This is necessary not only from the standpoint of the individual but as a measure of the success of the program. The evaluation of functional capacity and skills should be made by the instructor, while the physician assesses the effects on the individual's overall mental and physical status, any change in his attitude toward physical education generally and the adapted program specifically, and provides a reclassification for future physical activity.

1. Functional Capacity Testing

The same tests should be employed as were given before starting the adapted program and under conditions as closely similar as possible. Small variations might easily be obscured by making the observations under altered environmental conditions. Some allowance may have to be made for a small degree of improvement resulting purely from a greater familiarity with the test, which the person may have never performed before the initial evaluation.

It should be expected that, if the goals of the adapted program are being met, a significant improvement of the functional capacity should occur. Failure of improvement could be due to interruption of the program by illness or injury. If there was no such occurrence, one would have to suspect that either the program as outlined did not provide sufficient challenge to the individual, that the challenge was too great and the individual could not meet it, or that the individual did not put forth the necessary effort.

2. Skills Estimation

One of the goals of the adapted program is to provide the individual with skills for selected physical activities which will make it possible for him to continue to enjoy these or related activities once he has left the program. If sufficient skill has not been acquired, it may be due to the facts that the skills were too difficult for the handicapped individual to master, that the instruction was inadequate, or that the person did not make sufficient effort to learn the skills.

Ideally skills in all the activities that were taught during the program should be tested. If they were not tested before the activity was started, it may be difficult to evaluate any improvement. For the purpose of determining whether the individual may continue to progress on his own or with the aid of further instruction, rough evaluations by the instructor are probably sufficient.

The results of evaluation of specific skills as well as some estimate by the instructor of the aptitudes of the individual generally to acquire new skills in physical activity can be very helpful to the physician in reclassifying the individual for future activities.

3. Effects on Overall Mental and Physical Status

The physician's evaluation of the effects of the adapted program on the individual's mental status must be to a certain extent subjective and based on his previous interviews with him. Objective evidence can be provided if there has been an initial and final questionnaire to be answered which measures such personality factors as tension, anxiety, depression, etc. Available evidence does not indicate that fundamental changes in mental states can be reliably expected as the result of physical activity programs. For the individual who may have been previously deprived of the experiences of exercise, however, a favorable response would not be entirely unexpected.

The assessment of change in the physical status can be quite objective, based on a comparison with the recorded findings of the initial evaluation. Changes in the status of the handicapping condition as well as changes in such indices of physical fitness as the resting pulse rate, blood pressure, muscle development, and strength may be observed. These observations are of great importance in the planning of future physical activities for the individual as well as determining the success of the program in meeting its objectives.

4. Attitude toward Physical Education and the Adapted Program

As was pointed out in Chapter 19, many candidates for the adapted program have been conditioned by unpleasant experiences, the attitudes of parents and others, unnecessary fear related to some handicapping condition, or an attitude that is opposed to physical education and sports in general. If these attitudes are strongly fixed, the chances of an individual carrying through an adapted program are very slight, and most such persons are excluded. In those who manifest some flexibility, it is possible to include them, but they may enter the program with considerable doubts and reservations.

The majority of individuals who have been persuaded to enter the program in spite of mental reservations about it can be expected to develop a change in attitude that is favorable to physical education if they complete the program. Some actually become so enthusiastic that they elect to continue for one or more additional periods. A few have their doubts and suspicions confirmed, and, although they may complete the program, resume their antipathy to physical education generally.

Attitudes toward the adapted program itself vary considerably even among those who have a favorable feeling about physical education initially. In the beginning, some feel that it may not be demanding enough in spite of their handicap. Others are apprehensive that they may not be able to meet the demands, whatever they may be. If the program is properly planned and conducted, both of these attitudes will be corrected as the result of participation. If they are not, then the physician must acknowledge that there has been a failure of the program as far as the individual is concerned and seek to find out the cause.

5. Reclassification for Future Physical Activity

In the setting of an educational institution, completion of an adapted program to satisfy a physical education requirement should not mean an end to physical activity as far as the student is concerned. There should be intramural, extramural, or even interscholastic or intercollegiate sports and games activities in which the individual can participate safely and effectively consistent with his handicap.

Based upon his reevaluation of the individual's mental and physical status and attitude toward physical education and sports, and on the results of functional capacity testing and skills evaluation by the instructor, the physician should be able to outline a future program for physical activity jointly with the instructor. This is consistent with one of the main goals of the adapted program, which is to encourage the development of a lifelong interest in physical activity on the part of the individual who completes the program. In this regard, it must be pointed out to the student that any improved degree of general physical fitness that has been achieved as the result of the program can only be maintained by regular involvement in physical activity.

The best possibilities for a continuation of physical activity over a long period of time lie in encouraging the individual to participate in walking, swimming, cycling, skiing, and other such individual activities as may be suitable to him. Exclusive reliance on a sports or games program will make him too reliant on circumstances beyond his control.

II. EXTENDED FOLLOW-UP EVALUATION

Some provision should be made, if possible, for a long-term follow-up of individuals who have been involved in the adapted program. Much of the work put into the program will be lost to the handicapped individual who does not accept the challenge to continue regular physical activity. Admittedly, the percentage of those who regularly engage in vigorous exercise after finishing the usual physical education programs is probably relatively small, but the handicapped person may be in much more need of his regular exercise to maintain his state of fitness.

A. Effect on Physical Activity

1. Immediate

What happens to the individual's physical activity during the first year following the conclusion of the adapted program may be critical as far as his future activity is concerned. During this time, if his experience has been favorable, he should be well-motivated toward activity and should have developed some skills that he can use for individual, dual, or group activity.

One would like to know if the activity consists of calisthenic type exercises, weight resistance work, or endurance-type activities such as running, swimming, or cycling. If sports or games are played, are they the ones learned in the program or new ones of a type that has been recommended as suitable? Additionally, it is possible that the person might be participating in sports that were not recommended, and, if so, why?

The regularity of participation is an important consideration in determining the long-term effect. If a diary study showed that there was a trend toward increasing the intervals between participations, some encouragement to be more regular might be appropriate and prove fruitful. Extrinsic factors such as intercurrent injury or illness, might, of course, be responsible, and might dictate an adjustment in the individual's program.

2. Long-Range

Follow-up by interview or questionnaire after five years should provide significant evidence of the lasting effects of exposure of the individual to adapted physical education. By this time, the individual should have established a regular pattern of activity or inactivity. If the former, one would like to find out how it was influenced by the earlier experience; if the latter, what were the factors that caused the individual to withdraw from regular exercise?

B. Change in Physical or Mental Status

1. Related to the Program

Some evaluation of the physical and functional status should be made in the follow-up period to determine if the gains that had been made, if any, were maintained, or if further improvement had taken place. It would be ideal if this could be done after six months, after one year, and after five years.

Changes in mental status could be evaluated by interview or questionnaire or both. It would be most interesting to see if the attitudes toward physical education changed and how these changes, if any, correlated with the continuance or discontinuance of physical activity.

2. Unrelated to the Program

Although many of the handicaps of persons in the adapted program would by their nature be stable, as in the case of an amputation, others might be expected to progress over a period of time, as in hypertension.

Studies over the long-range of the morbidity and mortality of those who had engaged in an adapted program and continued to exercise could be compared with that of those who had been through the program but did not continue and still others who had never been exposed to a regular exercise program.

The effect of intercurrent injury or illness on the ability of the individual to continue the program over a period of time should also be studied. The steady deterioration of a handicapping condition might also seriously impair the ability of the individual to continue.

C. Communication and Recommendations to the Personal Physician

The information given to the personal physician when the individual enters the adapted program should be supplemented by reports of follow-up evaluations. In some cases, where the individual cannot be contacted or return for evaluation, this could actually be done through the personal physician.

The interest and cooperation of the personal physician may be a very important factor in the decision of the individual to continue or discontinue his physical activity. The more this physician knows, therefore, about the program, in general, and his patient's progress, in particular, the better chance there is that this cooperation will be secured.

PART IV

PREVENTIVE MEDICINE

Chapter 21

THE ROLE OF EXERCISE IN DISEASE PREVENTION

FRED L. ALLMAN, JR., and EDWARD W. WATT

I. DECREASED PHYSICAL ACTIVITY AND INCREASED DEGENERATIVE DISEASES

During recent years attention has been drawn to the increase of automation both at work and during leisure. This trend of events has resulted in a drastic reduction of physical energy expenditure which, in general, has not been compensated for by a comparable caloric restriction. As a result, there is an increasing incidence of obesity among many Americans as well as Europeans. Furthermore, the nature of the illnesses that beset us has likewise changed from a situation in which infectious diseases predominated to the present one of increasing degenerative vascular disease, notably, coronary heart disease (CHD) (Wright, 1970).

Numerous studies, as exemplified by those of Morris *et al.* (1953) from England, Kannel (1970), and Keys (1970) from the United States, Vienna Regional Hospital (1956) from Austria, and Karvonen *et al.* (1956) from Finland indicate strong support for the assumption of earlier and greater cardiovascular morbidity among sedentary individuals as compared with those who engage themselves in more physically strenuous occupations. It is not surprising, therefore, that the role of physical exercise has become increasingly meaningful to the middle-aged man in recent years because of the possible association exercise may have in the prevention of CHD. In the United States, investigations pointing to the benefits of exercise training programs were given early impetus by the work of Hellerstein *et al.* (1963). The mechanisms responsible for the improvements observed are as yet not well understood. This is partly due to the paucity of available comparative data on training responses in normal subjects of similar age and experience to the coronary patients. Data on young men and athletes are not directly applicable (Frick, 1963).

II. BENEFITS OF BEING PHYSICALLY CONDITIONED

There is a growing body of evidence that demonstrates the physiological benefits in terms of increased work capacity, slower resting heart rates (bradycardia), lowered systemic blood pressures, decreased premature ventricular contractions, and decreases in fasting serum triglycerides, cholesterol, and blood sugar with accompanying losses in total body fat, all of which are characteristic of the physically conditioned subjects (Holloszy *et al.* 1964). Perhaps the best approach to a definition of a mechanism unique to muscular exercise which might explain the enhanced performance of some "trained" cardiac patients is the hypothesis that physiological stimuli elicited by exercise training operate in the coronary vasculature in a way similar to the development of "optimal" collateral circulation around local arterial obstruction in working skeletal muscle (Naughton *et al.*, 1964). Accordingly, with dogs in which the circumflex coronary arteries were constricted to simulate various stages of CHD, training (possibly through the influence of myocardial isch-emia) resulted in a growth of coronary collateral circulation (Eckstein, 1957). Evidence from coronary arteriograms does not show a consistently similar effect of exercise training in man, although findings of Kattus *et al.* (1965) have shown improved collateral circulation in some patients who participated in an exercise rehabilitation program.

A. Lowered Serum Lipids

In numerous studies, atherosclerosis has been produced experimentally in various animal species by inducing high levels of serum cholesterol (Rowsell *et al.* 1958; Taylor *et al.*, 1959), and an apparent preventive role for exercise training as a means of lowering circulating lipids (pri-marily cholesterol and triglycerides) is strongly suggested (Papadop-oulos *et al.* 1969; Carlson and Froberg, 1969; Gollnick and King, 1969; Gollnick and Taylor, 1969; Simko *et al.*, 1970; Watt *et al.*, 1971). Any po-tentially independent effect of exercise, however, should be viewed with caution in light of findings that demonstrated a negligible change in serum cholesterol with training when body weight and/or diet are held constant (Golding, 1961; Walker *et al.*, 1953). More recent evidence (Nikkila and Konttinen, 1962; Nikkila *et al.*, 1963; Cantone, 1964) has shown the acute effects of exercise on reducing postprandial hyperlipemia (i.e., increased serum triglycerides), a condition that has been implicated in the pathogen-esis of atherosclerosis through its possible effects on accelerating blood clot-ting time, increasing blood viscosity and red cell aggregation (Buzina and Keys, 1956; Williams *et al.*, 1959), and impairing coronary flow and mycardial O_2 extraction (Regan *et al.*, 1961).

B. Decreased Cardiac Oxygen Consumption

Relief or diminution of angina pectoris during daily activities can occur as a result of decreased cardiac oxygen consumption or increased coronary blood supply or from both mechanisms simultaneously (Clausen *et al.*, 1969). Attempts to implicate changes in peripheral cir-culation are not well substantiated by experimental data at this time (Varnauskas *et al.*, 1966). While heart rates at given work loads are generally lower following short periods of training, aortic pressures re-main relatively unaltered. These changes, similar to those training re-sponses in healthy young and middle-aged men, reduce the left ventricu-lar pressure generated per unit time without necessarily reducing the pressure-determined tension effort per stroke. In coronary patients, the left ventricular cavity does not seem to increase in size with conditioning (Clausen *et al.*, 1969), contrary to the training response in young men, but analogous to the response in middle-aged men. Despite the inaccuracy of extrapolating from total heart volume to size of a single chamber, the unresponsiveness of heart size to training suggests that the augmented stroke volume found may not be accomplished through the Frank–Starling mechanism. Both left and right ventricular function have been shown to improve after training in postinfarction patients (Frick and Katila, 1968). Accordingly, stroke volume is presumably augmented due to a more forceful contraction with end-diastolic fiber length unchanged.

In light of animal experiments, this should lead to increased myocardial oxygen consumption. In human coronary artery disease, however, this response is not imperative, since the basis of increased contractility might be, in addition to hypertrophy, increases in cardiac output and coronary perfusion as well as a more synchronous contractile pattern. This would tend to reduce the oxygen demand by decreasing localized systolic bulges and altering favorably the intramyocardial "shunting" of blood from well contracting to poorly contracting areas.

C. Reduced Sympathetic Drive

There is suggestive evidence from experiments with β-receptor blockade in normal men that training reduces the sympathetic drive during exercise (Frick *et al.*, 1967). Judging from reduced heart rates on exertion, the situation is probably similar to coronary patients.

D. Improved Coronary Circulation

Although the issue of improved efficiency is well established, the crucial question remains unanswered, i.e., does a quantitative or qualitative change occur in coronary circulation via collaterals? From the large scale use of coronary angiography, there is now evidence that collaterals do develop as a natural reparative process in coronary artery disease. That hypoxia is the strongest stimulus to collateral development is suggested by the absence of collaterals in patients without angina, and their high prevalence in patients with angina (Forrester *et al.*, 1968). The rationale of increasing the frequency of the hypoxic stimuli by exercise training is logical, but objective evidence for increased collateral development as a direct result of such programs has not been substantiated at this time. Recent studies in dogs with coronary ligations have failed to demonstrate any difference in the X-ray or postmortem pattern of coronary arteries between untrained and trained animals (Kaplinsky *et al.*, 1968).

Although these various investigations have, thus far, afforded only suggestive and often highly speculative evidence, they have nonetheless provided the impetus and rationale for the large scale, interdisciplinary investigations into the effects of exercise as a preventive and/or rehabilitative means of effectively controlling the incidence of CHD.

III. NUTRITION AND ITS RELATIONSHIP TO WORK PERFORMANCE AND HEALTH

So far in our discussion we have talked specifically of the role of physical exercise as a means of increasing cardiovascular efficiency in both health and disease states. Earlier, we made reference to the growing problems of obesity predominant among affluent societies. The constant attention given to diet and physical exercise as a therapeutic means of controlling this "condition" has been well elucidated in the literature. In view of the interrelationships between obesity, hypertension, and coronary heart disease risk, however, and the essential process nutrition performs in maintaining homeostasis, we would now like to consider the role of nutrition and its relationship to work performance and health.

A. Fundamental Principles of Nutrition Related to Exercise

Reviews by Mayer and Bullen (1964) and Van Itallie *et al.*, (1960) have identified some of the few established facts and differentiated them from the large volume of misconceptions that persist regarding diet and exercise. It should be recognized (Davidson and Passmore, 1966) that the nutritional requirements for the athlete in training depend upon the same fundamental principles governing nutrition in general. There are no ordinary foods that man consumes which are either of special value or which are contraindicated in athletic training. Vitamins and minerals that are given over and above those provided by a good mixed diet have no effect on athletic performance. Furthermore, we have found no evidence to support the view that the nutritional value of diets consumed by many athletes should contain excessive quantities of protein. This does not mean that protein requirements are always unaffected by hard physical work (Durnin, 1967), but an intake that allows protein to provide about 11 or 12% of the total calories of the diet seems to be perfectly adequate. Many athletes take larger quantities of protein than this, but it seems to do no particular good. Protein taken into the body in excess of the daily requirements is excreted as urea through the kidneys or converted into fat and stored. For the purpose of this brief review, however, there are two special circumstances in which nutrition has a very direct bearing upon physical well-being and performance. The first is undernutrition, and the second overnutrition leading to obesity. In both of these stages, nutrition may be directly responsible for a condition in which the physical fitness of the individual is less than ideal.

B. Undernutrition

The whole subject of undernutrition in its physiological and psychological aspect is well documented by Keys et al. (1950; Keys, 1955). The loss in fitness of the body may be minimal when the potential energy intake is less than the energy expenditure so long as there is sufficient fat in the body to be mobilized to provide the extra calories required, and provided that there is sufficient protein in the diet to balance the losses of nitrogen. If there is not a balanced intake of protein, and if this amount is less than the requirement, protein is lost from the body and the muscle mass becomes reduced. Muscular power is affected very quickly and the general physical fitness of the body may become quite markedly decreased.

C. Overnutrition

Overnutrition may be described as that condition leading to the development of obesity. It has always been one of the major risks in a society in which affluence reigns and where physical exercise is unnecessary. In the past, such conditions were rare except for the minority of the prosperous. In our present affluent society, obesity is found frequently in childhood and early adolescence. There is considerable evidence to show that obesity is more likely to persist, with minor fluctuations, if it occurs during early childhood (McCance and Widdowson, 1965; Duncan, 1959).

D. Homeostasis

The stability of body weight is one of the ideals of homeostasis for adults (McCance and Widdowson, 1965). This is demonstrated by the fact that many people, year after year, show little or no change in their body weight. The regulation of their calorie intakes apparently meets very satisfactorily their energy expenditures. This is almost independent of the type of food eaten. During the space of a year, a ton of food perhaps has been eaten, whereas the variation in body weight will probably have been little more than a few pounds. The precision of the control cannot be determined by a simple reliance on measurements of body weight, which may show surprising fluctuations in a short period. Groups of young men and women have been weighed each day under standardized conditions, i.e., naked and immediately on rising from bed before any food or drink has been taken but after emptying the urinary bladder (Adam et al., 1961; Robinson and Watson, 1965). Variations in weight of more than 1 kg from day to day are not unusual. These are far too great to be due to a caloric imbalance, and must have been caused by changes in the water content of the body.

Durnin and Passmore (1966) analyzed the records of daily intake and energy expenditure of a large group of individuals, each measured over a period of several days. Many of the subjects displayed marked daily variations in food intake, and only a very small percentage had their food intake controlled to meet requirements on a daily basis. Most of the group, however, balanced intake and expenditure over a period of a week, although in many there was a temporary excess of either intake or expenditure amounting to over 2000 calories before the balance was restored.

When balance is not restored obesity usually results, and fitness may be affected in two ways: physical inactivity brings on obesity and obesity favors physical inactivity.

Obesity often occurs not because of an excessive food intake since many fat people are not excessive eaters. Many are, in fact, abstemious. Most obesity occurs as a result of physical inactivity. While physical exercise should not, therefore, be considered a panacea to ensure maintenance of optimal body weight, it should be regarded as one of the major tools useful in reducing body fat stores once accumulated.

Obese individuals, in general, are less physically well conditioned than they would be if they were not obese. The evidence is indirect (White and Alexander, 1965; Johnson et al., 1956), since it is very difficult to have an entirely satisfactory controlled situation. Indeed, the study of Buskirk and Taylor (1957) might superficially suggest little effect on fitness, although they state that "the obese man is under a substantial handicap in physical performance requiring exhausting work." It seems plain to us that marked obesity is unlikely to be compatible with fitness and is not conducive to maximum efficiency. Ex-

cluding specific athletic events, how often does one see an overfat
athlete?

IV. PSYCHOLOGICAL EFFECTS OF EXERCISE

In the foregoing discussion, we have attempted to underline the
physiological basis of exercise and nutritional patterns associated with
healthful living and CHD prevention. One must also consider possible
psychological changes accompanying regular exercise. These may include
attitudinal, motivational, behavioral, and other psychosocial variables
that are, to say the least, difficult not only to describe precisely but
to measure accurately. Our knowledge is incomplete as to why people
play or participate in exercise, sport, and games, or what the psychosocial
dimensions of physical activity may be.

Personality Characteristics

The literature reveals little research on the attitudes toward involvement in physical activity by adult populations. It has been shown
(McPherson et al., 1967) that normal healthy adult men who exercised
regularly had personality characteristics that differed significantly from
sedentary "cardiacs" (those with asymptomatic acute myocardial infarctions who were referred to the program by their physicians) and sedentary normal adult men. When comparing those who exercised regularly
for four years or longer to those just beginning an exercise program,
the regular participants in exercise experienced a relatively greater increase in energy, patience, aggression, humor, ambition, and optimism.
In addition, they felt sharper, more amiable, graceful, good tempered,
elated, and easy going than those just beginning an exercise program.
Furthermore, it was indicated that subjects induced to exercise for 24
weeks experienced an improved sense of well-being, a gain in self-confidence, a reduction of anxiety and tension, and a better outlook on
life.

It has been suggested (Paivio, 1967) that the psychological effects
of exercise may be dependent upon the individual's interpretation of
the relevance of physical activity to a particular deficiency. Other investigators (Hammett, 1967; Shapiro et al., 1965) have suggested that dis-
crepancies in skill, fitness, and participation levels may be attributed
to differences in life style. The types of physical activities in which
man participates in later life probably become established during youth
(Cratty, 1968).

Buskirk and Counsilman (1960) have suggested that many individuals feel a compulsion to remain inactive when they reach middle age. This may be brought on by fear of the detrimental effects of exercise. Further, since individuals differ with respect to their attitude concerning the importance of exercise, and since daily patterns differ, it would seem unwise in light of the present knowledge to accept the dogmatic dictum that exercise is either good or bad for middle-aged men or women. The psychological and social benefits accrued during middle age through participation in physical activity may be as important as the physiological benefits.

V. TYPES OF EXERCISE PROGRAMS

On numerous occasions we are asked, "What type of exercise program should one follow in order to derive the most benefit?" In general, there is no way of increasing exercise performance[*] (training effect) without inducing physical stress. Furthermore, there is no one conditioning program that will be optimal for all persons, or even for the same person over an extended period of time. Unfortunately, this is an all too often overlooked consideration in exercise training regimens.

The types of exercise programs can and should be varied because of the differences that may exist in a participant's level of fitness, age, health status, and personal interests, as well as the time and facilities available to him. Allowing for these wide variations, consideration of certain principles of work physiology as well as of some practical issues should result in better recommendations of activities for each individual. While the following suggestions pertain primarily to programs for middle-aged men, many of them are applicable to younger age groups, and to women as well.

A. Phases of Exercise Program

An optimal physical activity program should include the following three phases: (1) warm-up (8–10 minutes); (2) main exercise (15–40 minutes); and (3) general warming-down (7–10 minutes).

1. The warm-up should include slow movements, such as walking, jogging, cycling, and some stretching. These activities are aimed at

[*] Refers to physical work capacity only. Neuromuscular changes (skills) are not considered here.

gradually increasing heart rate, respiration, and body temperature so that a transition from rest to work may be achieved less stressfully in preparation for the more strenuous activity associated with the second phase of the program.

2. The main exercise phase involves some type of nonstop rhythmical exercise (e.g., running, cycling, swimming, circuit training, etc.). A gradual build-up in the intensity of the work performed, interspersed with periods of low-intensity exercise, should keep the participant moving, even if slowly, for the total period. It is possible to obtain a conditioning effect from almost any type of exercise (jogging, calisthenics, games, etc.), provided that the intensity and duration of the activity are sufficient to cause an adaptive response. If the intensity is too low, then it is possible that performing the exercise, even for a long time, will not attain much adaptation. On the other hand, if the intensity is too high, then the exercise cannot be continued very long. This may also cause muscle soreness, injuries, or medical probelms in older persons. Therefore, either extreme of the intensity–duration continuum may not be the most practical, desirable, or effective method for conditioning. During the first few months of participation, it is more desirable to exercise longer at a low intensity than vice versa. After the participant has adjusted to the milder forms of exercise, he can then periodically increase the intensity.

3. The general warming-down period should include slow movements, similar to those in the warm-up phase, which allow for a gradual decrease in heart rate, respiration, and body temperature, and recovery from the more strenuous activities of the exercise phase. If an older person stops too quickly after strenuous activity, the need to dissipate body heat may cause pooling of blood in his arms and legs. For one who has a compromised circulatory system, this reduction in central blood volume might result in fainting or circulatory collapse if he abruptly discontinues exercising. Walking and other forms of mild exercise assist the return of blood to the heart and allow the person to recover more gradually.

In oversimplified terms, exercise performed over a long period of time at a low intensity (i.e., low relative to the maximal capacity of the individual) is preferable for programs in which the participant wishes to reduce weight and gain muscular endurance. The high-intensity, short-duration exercises develop speed and/or strength and are used primarily by athletes for those objectives. In a program for middle-aged men, however, development of only moderate speed and strength may be required, while the development of cardiovascular endurance and flexibility is of greater value.

B. Important Factors in Developing Exercise Program

A number of factors should be emphasized in developing an adult exercise program.

1. Proper medical screening of all persons should be done before they participate. People who have medical contraindications should be identified and the necessary precautions taken. Procedures should be established to handle emergencies that may arise. Special cardiovascular and orthopedic problems should be reviewed so that a better, more individualized program can be recommended.

2. After considering the medical problems, the next step to emphasize is that of regular participation in a planned program of activities. A definite schedule should be formulated to individualize the intensity of the exercises, where possible, and to increase gradually the intensity depending on the rate of adaptation. One should attempt a three month program to ensure significant improvement in functional capacity. Also, once one participates regularly, exercise may then become a part of his routine. He will realize that he *can* schedule workouts into his daily routine.

3. By emphasizing those activities that require only the individual (jogging, swimming) or one other person (tennis, handball), programs can be more individualized and easier to schedule. This also allows an individual to exercise when he wants to, and does not force him to depend on the schedules and desires of others. This does not imply that group activities should be neglected, since proper leadership is worthwhile, and even essential, during the early months of the program. Also, the social contacts with other persons of the same age can provide an extra motivation to continue. Group activities (especially such formalized games as volleyball and basketball) should not be relied upon as the main method of conditioning, as the participants may not know what to do when alone. Likewise, a program should not be restricted by special equipment or facilities as they may not always be available. This does not preclude the effective use of equipment as this increases interest and variety.

4. A number of practical considerations have been suggested regarding the conduct of exercise programs for middle-aged persons. In general, working effectively with these people requires an understanding of the special problems, needs, and desires that they may have and how these factors fit into the mosaic of knowledge that is available on work physiology and conditioning. Some of the suggestions made are the result of empirical observations made while working with various

groups of adults with and without special problems. As stated previously, there is no one program or set of programs that will be optimal for all persons or even for the same person over a period of time. Thus, in a particular situation, with its unique combination of personnel, participants, time, and facilities, certain suggestions will be more important or practical while others may be inconsequential.

In conclusion, any topic involving the term physical exercise warrants an entire set of volumes if it is to be covered in depth. Even if one excludes the pseudoscientific beliefs of exercise, the physiological information is both formidable and favorable. Much of our knowledge of exercise performance has been acquired on young individuals and related to athletic performance. This poineer research, however, is being used to benefit those members of society who are aged and more frequently unhealthy than their athletic counterparts.

REFERENCES

Adam, J. M., Best, T. W., and Edholm, O. G. (1961). *J. Physiol. (London)* **156**, 38.

Buskirk, E. R., and Counsilman, J. E. (1960). *In* "Science and Medicine of Exercise and Sports" (W. R. Johnson, ed.), 1st ed. Harper, New York.

Buskirk, E. R., and Taylor, H. L. (1957). *J. Appl. Physiol.* **11**, 72–78.

Buzina, R., and Keys, A. (1956). *Circulation* **14**, 854–858.

Cantone, A. (1964). *J. Sports Med. Phys. Fitness* **4**, 32–35.

Carlson, L. A., and Froberg, S. O. (1969). *Gerontologia* **15**, 14–23.

Clausen, J. P., Larsen, O. A., and Trap-Jensen, J. (1969). *Circulation* **40**, 143.

Cratty, B. J. (1968). "Psychology and Physical Activity." Prentice-Hall, Englewood Cliffs, New Jersey.

Davidson, S., and Passmore, R. (1966). "Human Nutrition and Dietetics," 3rd ed., p. 115. Livingstone, Edinburgh.

Duncan, G. G. (1959). "Disease of Metabolism," 4th ed. Saunders, Philadelphia, Pennsylvania.

Durnin, J. V. G. A. (1967). *Can. Med. Ass. J.* **96**, 715–718.

Durnin, J. V. G. A., and Passmore, R. (1966). "Energy, Work, and Leisure," pp. 115–120. Heinemann, London.

Eckstein, R. (1957). *Circ. Res.* **5**, 230.

Forrester, J. S., Kemp, H. G., and Gorlin, R. (1968). *Clin. Res.* **16**, 229.

Frick, M. H. (1963). *Amer. J. Cardiol.* **22**, 417–419.

Frick, M. H., and Katila, M. (1968). *Circulation* **37**, 192.

Frick, M. H., Elovaini, R. O., and Somer, T. (1967). *Cardiologia* **51**, 46.

Golding, L. (1961). *Res. Quart.* **32**, 499–503.

Gollnick, P. D., and King, D. W. (1969). *Amer. J. Physiol.* **216**, 1502–1505.

Gollnick, P. D., and Taylor, A. W. (1969). *Int. Z. Angew. Physiol. Einschl. Arbeitsphysiol.* **27**, 144–148.

Hammett, V. B. O. (1967). *Can. Med. Ass. J.* **96**, 764–768.

Hellerstein, H. K., Hirch, E. Z., Cumler, W., Allen, L., Polster, S., and Zucker, N. (1963). In "Coronary Heart Disease" (W. Likoff and J. H. Moyer, eds.), Grune & Stratton, New York.

Holloszy, J. O., Skinner, J., Barry, A., and Cureton, T. K. (1964). Amer. J. Cardiol. 14, 761.

Johnson, M. L., Burke, B. S., and Mayer, J. (1956). Amer. J. Clin. Nutr. 4, 37–44.

Kannel, W. B. (1970). N. Engl. J. Med. 282, 1153–1154.

Kaplinsky, E., Hood, W. B., Jr., McCarthy, B., McCombs, H. L., and Lown, B. (1968). Circulation 37, 556.

Karvonen, M. J., Kihlberg, J., Maatta, J., and Virkajarvi, J. (1956). Duodecim 72, 893.

Kattus, A., Hanafee, W. N., Longmire, W. P., Jr., McAlpin, R. N., and Rivin, A. L. (1965). Ann. Intern. Med. 69, 115–136.

Keys, A. (1955). In "Weight Control." (E. S. Eppright, P. Swanson, and C. A. Iverson, eds.), p. 108. Iowa State Univ. Press, Ames.

Keys, A. (1970). "Physical Activity and the Epidemiology of Coronary Heart Disease," Vol. 4, pp. 250–266. Karger, Basel.

Keys, A., Brozek, J., and Henschel, A. (1950). "The Biology of Human Starvation." Univ. of Minnesota Press, Minneapolis.

McCance, R. A., and Widdowson, E. M. (1965). In "The Physiology of Human Survival" (O. G. Edholm and A. L. Bacharach, eds.). Academic Press, New York.

McPherson, B. D., Paivio, A., Yuhasz, M. S., Rechnitzer, P. A., Pickard, H. A., and Lefcoe, N. M. (1967). J. Sports Med. Phys. Fitness 7, 95–102.

Mayer, J., and Bullen, B. (1964). Proc. Int. Congr. Nutr., 6th, 1963 p. 27.

Morris, J. N., Raffle, P. A., Roberts, C. C., and Parks, J. W. (1953). Lancet 2, 1053.

Naughton, J., Balke, B., and Nagle, F. (1964). Amer. J. Cardiol. 14, 837–841.

Nikkila, E., and Konttinen, A. (1962). Lancet 1, 1151–1152.

Nikkila, E. A., Torsti, P., and Penttila, O. (1963). Metab. Clin. Exp. 12, 863–865.

Paivio, A. (1967). Can. Med. Ass. J. 96, 768.

Papadopoulos, N. M., Bloor, C. M., and Standafer, J. C. (1969). J. Appl. Physiol. 26, 760–763.

Regan, I., Binale, K., Gordon, S., DeFazio, V., and Hellems, H. (1961). Circulation 23, 55.

Robinson, M. F., and Watson, P. E. (1965). Brit. J. Nutr. 19, 225.

Rowsell, H. C., Downe, H. G., and Mustard, J. (1958). Can. Med. Ass. J. 79, 647.

Shapiro, S., Weinblatt, E., Frank, C. W., and Sager, R. V. (1965). J. Chronic Dis. 18, 527–558.

Simko et al. (1970). Med. Exp. (Basel) 19, 71–75.

Taylor, C. B., Cox, G., Counts, M., and Yogi, N. (1959). Circulation 20, 975.

Van Itallie, T. B., Sinisterra, L., and Stare, F. J. (1960). "Science and Medicine of Exercise and Sports" (W. R. Johnson, ed.), 1st ed., p. 285. Harper, New York.

Varnauskas, E., Bergman, H., Houk, P., and Bjorntorp, P. (1966). Lancet 2, 8.

Vienna Regional Hospital. (1956). "Wiener Gebietskrankenkasse, Sterbefalle und Sterbegeld, Jahresbericht d. Weiner Gebietskrankenkasse," p. 168. Vienna.

Walker, W. J., Lawry, E. Y., Love, D. E., Mann, G. V., Levine, S. A., and Sture, F. J. (1953). Amer. J. Med. 14, 654–660.

Watt, E. W., Foss, M. L., and Block, W. D. (1971). Circ. Res. 31, 908.

White, R. I., Jr., and Alexander, J. K. (1965). J. Appl. Physiol. 20, 197–201.

Williams, A., Higginbotham, A., and Knisley, M. (1959). Angiology 8, 689.

Wright, I. S. (1970). Circulation 42, 55–A95.

Chapter 22

QUALIFICATION OF THE APPARENTLY WELL PERSON FOR PHYSICAL ACTIVITY

ALLAN J. RYAN

I. INTRODUCTION*

Physicians are frequently asked by patients and even by friends and acquaintances about the advisability of undertaking exercise programs that involve vigorous physical activity. Sometimes physicians are requested to supply a statement of good health for a patient who wishes

* Parts I through VI are adapted from the recommendations of the American Medical Association's Committee on Exercise and Physical Fitness and are reproduced here with their consent and that of the editors of the *Journal of the American Medical Association* in which their statement was published.

to participate in an organized program that has such a requirement. These requests are a reflection of the increased interest of many people today in establishing and maintaining physical fitness.

This presentation is designed to assist the physician in evaluating the apparently healthy person who wishes to undertake vigorous exercise. It attempts to help him to separate those persons whose disease or defect indicates a need for special evaluation before undertaking exercise from those for whom this is unnecessary. It also contains suggestions concerning tests and examinations that may be used in determining whether the patient meets the arbitrary standard of "apparently healthy" and can be so classified. The person, whether young or old, who can be said to be "deconditioned" (out-of-condition) is identified and specific recommendations are made for appropriate reconditioning. Finally, general recommendations are given for those apparently healthy persons who are about to begin an exercise program, including the precautions they should take and the intensity and duration of exercise they should have.

II. MEDICAL HISTORY AND PHYSICAL EXAMINATION

To identify the apparently healthy person of any age, it is necessary to take a medical history and to perform an adequate physical examination. In taking the history, emphasis should be placed on those signs or symptoms indicating the presence of any acute or chronic disease affecting the heart and the circulatory system, the lungs, the liver, and/or the kidneys. It is essential to know whether medications are being taken, especially those that are used to treat disease of the circulatory system. It also is important to know the nature and extent of the individual's current physical activity.

A physical examination, which includes at rest and after exercise evaluations, should be performed on all persons who expect to undertake a vigorous program of physical exercise. This includes those whose medical history does not indicate any reasons for their exclusion from exercise. Defects and diseases that are entirely unknown to the individual may be discovered by this examination. The chief emphasis of the examination should be on the general appearance of the individual, his ability to move about, his weight, his mental and emotional response to the idea of exercise, the blood pressure (seated and supine), heart rate and regularity, heart size, heart sounds, condition of the lungs, enlargement of any abdominal organs, and status of the extremities, especially the lower ones. Diagnostic studies other than a urinalysis and hematocrit need not be performed ordinarily unless suggested by the medical history or physical examination.

III. ELECTROCARDIOGRAM

Arteriosclerotic heart disease is known to have its beginnings in some individuals at a very early age. However, unless the medical history reveals symptoms suggestive of a heart disorder, or some sign of heart or circulatory disease or dysfunction is detected in the physical examination, it is usually not necessary to perform an electrocardiogram on persons who are under 40 years of age. It is advisable, however, to do so on all persons 40 years of age or older because the findings of otherwise undetectable changes in the heart, as reflected in alteration of the electrocardiogram, begin to increase considerably around that age. The electrocardiogram should record the twelve standard leads, should be made at rest, and preferably be repeated immediately following a standard amount of mildly sustained exercise.

IV. THE DECONDITIONED PERSON

Persons under 40 years of age who have not participated in any physical exercise since high school and college days, and who have employment that does not require moderately heavy physical activity on a regular basis have been characterized as being "deconditioned." They should be given a test of functional capacity. A selection of appropriate tests is given in Section VII. These tests are also useful in the evaluation of persons 40 years of age or older who have no history or findings of heart disease, but who give other eivdence of a poor state of physical fitness.

V. REASONS FOR MORE EXTENSIVE EVALUATION

Reasons for considering a further and more extensive evaluation (i.e. more than a medical history, physical examination, and perhaps an electrocardiogram) before recommending an exercise program are as follows:

1. Any acute or chronic infectious disease
2. Diabetes that is not well controlled
3. Marked obesity

4. Psychosis or severe neurosis
5. Central nervous system disease
6. Musculoskeletal disease involving the spine and lower extremities
7. Active liver disease
8. Renal disease with nitrogen retention
9. Severe anemia
10. Significant hypertension (diastolic)
11. Angina pectoris or other signs or symptoms of coronary insufficiency
12. Significant cardiomegaly
13. Arhythmias
    a. Second degree A–V block
    b. Ventricular tachycardia
    c. Atrial fibrillation
14. Significant disease of the heart valves or larger blood vessels
15. Congenital heart disease without cyanosis
16. Phlebothrombosis or thrombophlebitis
17. Current usage of drugs such as
    a. Reserpine
    b. Propanolol
    c. Guanethidine
    d. Quinidine, nitroglycerine, and other vascular dilators
    e. Procaine amide
    f. Digitalis
    g. Catecholamines
    h. Ganglionic blocking agents
    i. Insulin
    j. Psychotropic drugs
18. An apprehensive or extremely negative view regarding exercise and its possible effects

VI. CONTRAINDICATIONS TO EXERCISE PROGRAMS

Reasons for recommending that no exercise program be undertaken include:
1. Active or recent myocarditis
2. Recent pulmonary embolism
3. Congestive heart failure
4. Arhythmias
    a. Third degree A–V block
    b. Fixed-rate pacemakers

5. Aortic aneurysm
6. Ventricular aneurysm
7. Liver decompensation
8. Congenital heart disease with cyanosis

VII. FUNCTIONAL CAPACITY TESTS*

A. General Remarks about Test Procedures

The practical application of tests for the screening of large populations favors simple and short testing procedures. Physiological considerations, however, point to more elaborate and more time-consuming tests. For greatest versatility and utility, therefore, these two conflicting requirements must be optimised.

1. Work Intensity

The test must begin with a work load low enough to be sufficiently submaximal for people in very poor physical condition. The adaptive capacity of the cardiovascular and respiratory systems must be evaluated through continuous work at gradually increasing intensities. Thus, the approach of functional limitations should be detectable with sufficient discriminatory accuracy. Practical considerations suggest the use of the basal—or resting—metabolic rate as the unit by which to gauge the energy demands at the various work loads. The initial work intensity and the following stepwise increments will therefore be defined in "Mets"—multiples of the metabolic rate at complete rest. The physiological units basic to Mets are either the resting oxygen consumptions in ml min^{-1} or their caloric equivalents in kcal min^{-1}.

Since direct control of work intensity by Mets or by their oxygen consumption equivalents during a test would require the display of continuous computation of oxygen consumption by complex instrumentation not readily available at present, the estimation of the oxygen requirements for given types and intensities of work from empirical formulas appears most practical. The predicted values of oxygen requirements for treadmill work from speed and slope, and for step test work from stepping height and rate are in close agreement with values actually

* This section, parts A through D, is adapted from L. A. Larson (1974). "Fitness, Health and Work Capacity: International Standards for Assessment." Reprinted with permission of Macmillan Co., New York.

measured and can serve as the physiological equivalent of the physical effort to which all physiological indices measured during the test are correlated.

2. Test Duration

For adequate test design, the desire for the shortest possible test procedure poses a problem. Tests of too short duration will be lacking in sufficiently discriminatory value while tests of too long duration will activate thermoregulatory mechanisms which will interfere with the assessment of maximum aerobic power. In the standard procedure recommended each work intensity level will be maintained for two minutes. The average time of the actual test might then range from about 10 to 16 minutes.

3. Indications for Stopping Exercise

The test should be terminated whenever:

1. Pulse pressure declines consistently in spite of increasing work intensity.
2. Systolic blood pressure exceeds 240–250 mm Hg.
3. Diastolic pressure rises to more than 125 mm Hg.
4. Symptoms of distress occur such as increasing chest pain, severe dyspnea, intermittent claudication.
5. Clinical signs of anoxia occur such as facial pallor or cyanosis, staggering, confusion, or unresponsiveness to injuries.
6. Following ECG signs occur—paroxysmal superventricular or ventricular dysrhythmia, a succession of ventricular premature complexes occurring before the end of the T-wave, conduction disturbances other than a slight A–V block, and R–ST depressions of horizontal or descending type of greater than .3 mV.

4. Safety Procedures

The subjects should be in a normal state of health as certified by a physician after medical examination. Monitoring the ECG by at least one chest lead is highly desirable in all subjects, but should be compulsory in males beyond the age of 40 years. Regularly repeated blood pressure measurements during the exercise test are a mandatory part of the testing procedure. After termination of the exercise test, the subjects have to be informed about measures preventing dangerous blood pooling in the lower limbs.

5. Contraindications to Exercise Tests

Subjects should be rejected from the test on the following criteria:

1. Lack of a physician's permission to take part in maximal exercise testing
2. Oral temperature in excess of 37.5°C
3. Heart rate above 100 min^{-1} at the end of a sufficient rest period
4. Manifest cardiac failure
5. Myocardial infarction or myocarditis within the past three months, or symptoms and ECG signs showing these conditions, or existing angina pectoris
6. Evidence of an infectious disease including the common cold

Menstruation is not considered a contraindication for exercise testing, but in special cases rescheduling the test may be advisable.

B. The Standard Tests

1. Description of the Basic Procedures for the Standard Tests

Whichever of the three modes of exercise is adopted and notwithstanding whether a submaximal or maximal test is intended the basic procedures for the three standard tests are the same.

The subjects report to the laboratory in light gym clothing and rubber shoes, having abstained from food, coffee, tobacco, etc., for at least two hours.

2. Rest

A preliminary period of at least 15 minutes of rest must precede the exercise test. During this period the subject sits comfortably in a chair while physiological baseline measurements are established.

3. Accommodation Period

The very first test of any individual as well as all subsequent repeats become sufficiently reliable if the actual test is preceded by a short period of exercise at a low work intensity. This accommodation period, (three minutes duration is enough), serves:

1. To familiarize the subject with the equipment and with the type of work required
2. To pre-test the subject's physiological response to a work load of approximately four Mets, or an initial heart rate response of approximately 100 beats per minute
3. To hasten the proper physiological adjustments to the actual test work

4. Rest

The accommodation period is followed by two minutes of comfortable rest in a chair while the necessary technical adjustments are effected.

5. Test

The test begins with the work intensity employed in the accommodation period, (approximately four Mets) and the subject continues to exercise without interruption until the test is completed. At the end of every second minute of work the work load is increased by the equivalent of approximately one Met.

The test stops when:

either 1. the subject is unable to proceed
    or 2. the monitoring of physiological criteria indicates physiological decompensations (see Section VII,A,3)
    or 3. the advanced state of effort permits an extrapolation of maximum aerobic power on the basis of sequential physiological measurements.

6. Scoring

Maximum oxygen intake in ml kg^{-1} min^{-1} is determined directly or is assessed. The methods for its determination vary as do the supplementary techniques used to analyze the individuals physiological capacities. These points are pursued more fully in due course.

7. Recovery

After the cessation of the test exercise, physiological observations are continued for at least three minutes, with the subject again resting in a chair, preferably with legs slightly raised.

Note: The above basic procedure should provide comparable physiological responses to work loads of the same order of magnitude on the treadmill, bicycle, or stepping ergometer. In the following paragraphs the procedure is specifically outlined for each of the testing devices.

C. The Treadmill Test

1. Apparatus

Motor-driven treadmill
Ancillary equipment as required

2. Description

The basic test procedure outlined in Section VII, B, 1 is followed carefully.

The speed of the treadmill, with the subject walking on it, is set to 80 m min^{-1} (4.8 km hr^{-1} or 3 mph). At this speed the energy requirements for walking on the horizontal amount to approximately three Mets, and each increment of 2.5% in slope adds one unit of the resting metabolic rate, i.e., one Met, to the energy expenditure.

TABLE I

Standard Treadmill Test[a]

Test phase	Duration (min)	Energy (Mets)	Requirements V_{O_2} ml/kg/min	% Grade at 80 m/min
Rest	10–20	1	3.5	—
Accommodation period	3	4	14.0	2.5
Recovery	2	1	3.5	—
Actual test	2	4	14.0	2.5
	2	5	17.5	5.0
	2	6	21.0	7.5
	2	7	24.5	10.0
	2	8	28.0	12.5
	2	9	31.5	15.0
	2	10	35.0	17.5
	2	11	38.5	20.0
	2	12	42.0	28.5
	2	13	45.5	25.0
	2	14	49.0	27.5
	2	15	52.5	30.0

[a] From L. A. Larson (1974). "Fitness, Health and Work Capacity: International Standards for Assessment." Reprinted with permission of Macmillan Co., New York.

At the end of the first two minutes the treadmill slope is quickly increased to 5%, after the next two minutes to 7.5%, then to 10%, 12.5%, etc. The entire scheme is presented in Table I.

3. Scoring

The test score is stated as the max V_{O_2} in ml kg^{-1} min^{-1}. It is either measured directly by monitoring the respiratory gas exchanges or estimated by extrapolating the test results. See Table I.

4. General Guide and Regulations

For the accomodation period the treadmill inclination is set at 2.5%. The same grade and speed are maintained during the first two minutes of the actual test—unless the physiological response during the accommodation period is indicative of a superior performance potential. In such case the energy requirements at the speed of 80 m min^{-1} and a 30% grade (assumed limitation for raising the treadmill grade) would not approach the individual's capacity and the test should be modified accordingly (see Table II).

TABLE II

Super-Standard Treadmill Test[a]

Test phase	Duration (min)	Energy (Mets)	Requirement (V_{O_2} ml/ kg/min)	% Grade ($v =$ 100 m/min)
Rest	10	1	3.5	—
Accommodation period	3	6	21.0	4
Recovery	2	1	3.5	—
Actual test	1	6	21.0	4
	1	7	24.5	6
	1	8	28.0	8
	1	9	31.5	10
	1	10	35.0	12
	1	11	38.5	14
	1	12	42.0	16
	1	13	45.5	18
	2	14	49.0	20
	2	15	52.5	22
	2	16	56.0	24
	2	17	59.5	26
	2	18	63.0	28
	2	19	66.5	30

[a] From L. A. Larson (1974). "Fitness, Health and Work Capacity: International Standards for Assessment." Reprinted with permission of Macmillan Co., New York.

b. In case of existing pathological conditions (coronary heart disease, pulmonary deficiency, convalescence after infectious diseases, etc.) a treadmill test modification is recommended.

c. In a test employing walking or running on the motor-driven treadmill, any continuous contact of arms or hands with a fixed object (guard post or rails) is prohibited.

D. The Bicycle Ergometer Test

1. Apparatus

Bicycle ergometer, with calibrated load adjustment facilities.
Ancillary equipment, as required.

2. Description

The basic procedure outlined in Section VII, B,1 is carefully followed. During the test the subject pedals at a predetermined steady rate of 50 or 60 rpm without interruption in time with a metronome.

The intensity of the work load is increased at two-minute intervals as previously indicated. In order to provide on the bicycle ergometer relative work loads comparable to those on the treadmill or stepping ergometer, the body weight should be used for determining both the initial work intensity and the periodic increments of work load, as follows:

a. Set the initial load to 1 watt (6 kg m) per kilogram of body weight
b. Set the increments as ⅓ of the body weight in kg

Example: Subject A = 75 kg; B = 50 kg; C = 25 kg

Subject	Weight	Increments	Initial load	2nd	3rd	4th	. . .
A	75 kg	24 watts	75 watts	100	125	150	. . .
B	50 kg	17 watts	50 watts	67	84	101	. . .
C	25 kg	8 watts	25 watts	33	41	50	. . .

3. Scoring

The oxygen costs for any given intensity of work can be determined by use of the diagram in figure 1 or by the formula:

$$V_{O_2} = (\text{kg m} \times 1.78) + 1.5 \text{ Mets}$$

where: V_{O_2} = oxygen requirement in ml min^{-1}; kg m (or watts $\times$ 6) = work intensity per minute; 1.78 = ml of oxygen required for 1 kg m of work; 1.5 Mets = the approximate oxygen consumption of the individual sitting on the ergometer and pedaling without any load. With increasing resistance more auxiliary muscles are involved, resulting in a rise of this factor to slightly more than two Mets at W = 1800 kg m min^{-1}.

4. General Guide and Regulations

a. Since total oxygen requirements are nearly identical for all individuals working at any given load on the bicycle ergometer, the V_{O_2} in ml kg^{-1} min^{-1} varies considerably in subjects of different weights. In contrast, in work against gravity, treadmill grade walking, and bench stepping, the V_{O_2} requirement per unit of weight are the same but total V_{O_2} varies with total weight.

b. The constancy of the pedaling rate should be monitored by a speed indicator, a revolution counter, or by means of a metronome.

c. The energy costs of riding the stationary bicycle are well established provided that the indicated external load is not markedly offset by undue resistances in the pedal bearings and in the drive chain. Every effort, therefore, should be made to keep these moving parts running freely.

d. The height of the seat should be adjusted individually to allow for an almost completely stretched leg at the lowest pedal position.

e. In case of existing pathological conditions (see Section VIII,A,S) the initial settings should be 25 watts or 150 kg m min^{-1}. The increments after two minutes at each load should be 12.5 watts or 75 kg m min^{-1}.

f. For highly trained athletes the standard procedure is applicable with the only modification that, as in the super-standard treadmill test, the first ten increments of work intensity be done in one-minute intervals to reduce total duration of the test. Beyond a load of 275 watts, or 1650 kg m min^{-1} the switch occurs to 2-minute intervals.

g. Modifications with regard to body position, such as working in a supine instead of the normal sitting position, or cranking instead of bicycling might be feasible in special situations. However, since efficiency for these types of work is different, the "normal" kg m min^{-1} oxygen requirement relationship does not apply and the investigators should state precisely the type of modification utilized.

E. The Ergometer Step Test

1. Apparatus

Adjustable height stepping ergometer in multiples of 4.5 cms
Ancillary equipment as selected

2. Description

The subject, having undertaken the standard rest and warm-up procedure, steps onto and down from the stepping ergometer at the standard rate of 33 mounts per minute. This rate, although slightly faster than comfortable is chosen to keep the stepping heights within tolerable limits at the higher work loads. The initial platform height is 4.5 cm. Each two minutes the height of the ergometer is raised 4.5 cm, without interruption of the stepping rate. This procedure will permit the steady increase of the work load from very mild to most severe, i.e., over an energy expenditure range from two to fifteen Mets.

3. Scoring

The oxygen requirements (V_{O_2}) in ml kg^{-1} min^{-1} for stepping at the frequency of 33 vertical lifts per minute can be predicted or estimated from the following formula:

$$V_{O_2} = (f \times h \times 1.33 \times 1.78) + 10.5$$

where: f = the stepping rate of number of vertical lifts, per minute; h = the height of the step in meters; 1.33 = work involved in the vertical lift + one third for descending; 10.5 = 10.5 ml kg^{-1} min^{-1} extra oxygen requirement for the forward and backward stepping additional to the vertical movement; 1.78 = ml of oxygen required for 1 kg m of work.

4. General Guide and Regulations

a. The energy costs in stepping are made up of the following components: (1) Stepping forward and backward on two counts each. At the proposed metronome setting of 132 total counts ($\frac{132}{4}$ = 33 actual lifts), the energy expenditure for this work is approximately three Mets. (2) lifting the weight of the body to the height of the step level, and (3) descending to the ground. The latter work has been found to be approximately one-third of the work of stepping up.

b. The stepping ergometer procedure is designed so as to be comparable with the treadmill and bicycle ergometer tests.

c. Four counts are taken to complete each up and down stepping cycle: two counts to mount to a completely erect stance on both feet, and two counts to descend to the ground. Frequent changes of the leading leg are encouraged to minimize the development of local muscular fatigue. This can best be accomplished by tapping the descending foot on the floor on the fourth count and immediately lifting it

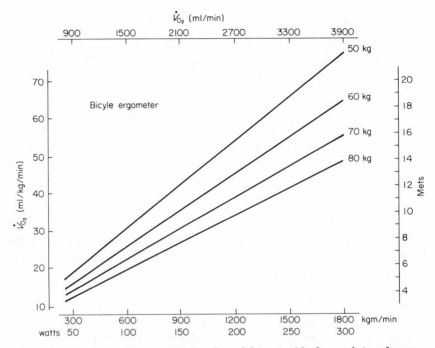

Fig. 1 Oxygen requirements (total and per kilogram of body weight) and energy expenditures in Mets (multiples of the resting metabolic rate) for individuals of different body weight at a wide range of work intensities on the bicycle ergometer. From L. A. Larson (1974). "Fitness, Health and Work Capacity: International Standards for Assessment." Reprinted with permission of Macmillan Co., New York.

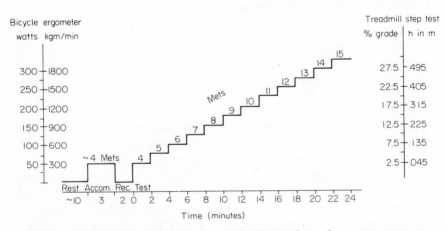

Fig. 2 Standard test procedures for treadmill, bicycle, and stepping ergometer. From L. A. Larson (1974). "Fitness, Health and Work Capacity: International Standards for Assessment." Reprinted with permission of Macmillan Co., New York.

again for the count "one" step-up. With a little practice, especially by establishing a given rhythm, e.g., four mounts leading with the left foot, and then four with the right, the procedure, which does not require any special skill, quickly becomes automatic.

d. As with the treadmill and bicycle ergometer, a great variation of speed (stepping rate) is available. The standard rate of 33 vertical lifts per minute is selected specifically for use with a stepping device like the one described which has an adjustable vertical range from 0 to 50 cm to accommodate approximately 90 percent of any given population. Holding on to any fixed object during the stepping exercise invalidates the test results.

e. When testing individuals in pathological conditions (see Sections VII,C,4,b and D,35) the following modification will provide nearly the same test loads as the sub-standard treadmill test: (1) $f = 22$ vertical lifts per minute; (2) accommodation period and first test load at zero level; (3) all increments at 15 mm as in the standard stepping test. In this case the formula for predicting or estimating V_{O_2} is:

$$V_{O_2} = (22 + 1.33 \times 1.7 \times h) + 7 \text{ (see Section VIII,E,3)}$$

where h = stepping height in meters; $7 = 7$ ml kg^{-1} min^{-1} O_2 required for stepping forward and backward at the rate of $22 \times 4 = 88$ total steps.

F. The Step Test*

One of several tests that measure cardiovascular function is a modification of the Harvard Step Test—the "recovery index"—which is as effective as any and requires little equipment or space.

The patient steps up and down on a bench at a rate of 30 times a minute for four minutes, unless he stops earlier because of fatigue. A suggested height-step scale follows:

Patient's height	Bench height (inches)
Under 5 feet	12
5 feet–5 feet 3 inches	14
5 feet 3 inches–5 feet 9 inches	16
5 feet 9 inches–6 feet	18
Over 6 feet	20

* This section is taken from the statement of the American Medical Association's Committee on Exercise and Physical Fitness, "Is Your Patient Fit?", which was published in *Journal of the American Medical Association* [Vol. 201, 117–118 (1967)], with their permission and that of the editors of the Journal.

Facing the bench or platform, and starting with either foot at the signal "up," the patient places his foot on the bench and steps up so that both feet are on the bench. Then immediately and in rhythm, he steps down again and continues the exercise in a marching count,

TABLE III

Determining the Recovery Index[a]

Total beats	Recovery index	Total beats	Recovery index	Total beats	Recovery index
110	109	142	85	174	69
111	108	143	84	175	69
112	107	144	83	176	68
113	106	145	83	177	68
114	105	146	82	178	67
115	104	147	82	179	67
116	103	148	81	180	67
117	102	149	81	181	66
118	102	150	80	182	66
119	101	151	80	183	66
120	100	152	79	184	65
121	99	153	78	185	65
122	98	154	78	186	65
123	98	155	77	187	64
124	97	156	77	188	64
125	96	157	76	189	64
126	95	158	76	190	63
127	95	159	76	191	63
128	94	160	75	192	63
129	93	161	75	193	62
130	92	162	74	194	62
131	92	163	74	195	61
132	92	164	73	196	61
133	90	165	73	197	61
134	90	166	72	198	61
135	89	167	72	199	60
136	88	168	71	200	60
137	88	169	71	201	60
138	87	170	71	202	59
139	86	171	70	203	59
140	86	172	70	204	59
141	85	173	70	205	58

[a] From "Is Your Patient Fit?" A statement of the American Medical Association's Committee on Exercise and Physical Fitness, published in the *Journal of the American Medical Association* [**201**, 117–118 (1967)]. Reproduced with their permission and that of the editors of the journal. The data in this table are from J. R. Gallagher (1966). "Medical Care of the Adolescent," 2nd ed. Appleton, New York. Reproduced with the author's permission.

TABLE IV

Determining the Response Value[a]

Three 30-second pulse counts total	Recovery index	Response to this test
199 or more	60 or less	Poor
from 171 to 198	between 61 and 70	Fair
from 150 to 170	between 71 and 80	Good
from 133 to 149	between 81 and 90	Very good
132 or less	91 or more	Excellent

[a] From "Is Your Patient Fit?" A statement of the American Medical Association's Committee on Exercise and Physical Fitness, published in the *Journal of the American Medical Association* [**201**, 117–118 (1967)]. Reproduced with their permission and that of the editors of the journal.

"Up-two, three, four." The signal "up" comes every two seconds.

On completing the exercise, he sits quietly. Pulse counts are then taken as scheduled: one minute after exercise for 30 seconds; two minutes after exercise for 30 seconds; and three minutes after exercise for 30 seconds.

The patient's recovery index can then be determined by referring to Table III.

It is recommended that this simple, brief, and practical test be used primarily to measure a person's progress in comparison with the same individual's earlier results; comparison of one person's scores with those of another individual is not as appropriate.

The recovery index (RI) is derived from this formula:

$$RI = \frac{\text{duration of exercise in seconds} \times 100}{\text{sum of 30 second pulse counts in recovery} \times 2}$$

The result is interpreted in Table IV. For example, if a patient exercises the entire four minutes, or 240 seconds, and his recovery pulse counts for 30 seconds are 60 at one-and-a-half minutes, 55 at two-and-a-half minutes, and 45 at three-and-a-half minutes, his formula would read:

$$RI = \frac{240 \times 100}{160 \times 2} = 75$$

This is a good recovery index. However, each individual should be urged to improve his fitness, unless an exercise program is contraindicated.

Chapter 23

PRESCRIBING PHYSICAL ACTIVITY

BRUNO BALKE

I. THE BASIC INGREDIENTS OF TRAINING

The achievement and maintenance of an optimum level of physical competence requires frequent stimulation of the human organ systems through demands that will elicit functional responses in the upper range of their adaptive capacity. The process by which this is accomplished is called "physical training." In general, training includes three slightly different phases of mental and physical activity: (1) a process of learning to acquire an understanding for the sequence of movements and the neuromuscular coordination needed for a specific task or skill; (2)

the frequent practice of this particular task or skill with the aim of achieving a flawless sequence of performance components; and (3) the general conditioning of the entire organism to ensure optimal performance under a variety of environmental factors which may either favor or oppose the perfect task accomplishment.

The planning and prescription of physical activity will, among other things, greatly depend on the priority of any of these three phases. For example, the frequent repetitions necessary for learning the fundamentals of complex human movement may be very tiring and frustrating, therefore requiring a great measure of perfect general physical condition as the basis for adequate energy supply during long practice sessions (e.g., football). In such case a general conditioning training should precede the efforts required for learning specific tasks. In another instance, a certain sport or recreational activity may require a great number of relatively simple movements over a period of time. In such case good physical condition may develop as a by-product of practice in this special activity. It is also possible that the practice of basic movements and the simultaneous achievement of sufficient physical condition is a prerequisite for learning proper techniques essential for optimum performance. In the crew sport of rowing, for example, the learning process involved in developing the correct rhythm, the most effective flow of movements, and the exact timing of power application follows a long practice of a relatively simple basic skill.

Accordingly, appropriate considerations should guide the outline of activity or training programs for people in line with their individual abilities and desires.

II. FORMS OF CONSULTATION, ADVICE, AND PRESCRIPTION

In present days it is not uncommon to hear physical activities and their effects on health widely discussed in social gatherings. Especially among middle-aged men, the word appears to have spread that degenerative organic afflictions, originating in an overly busy but predominantly sedentary life, may be preventable by regular exercise. As the types, advantages, and disadvantages of different exercise programs are discussed, "experts" might be asked for advice in specific cases. However, whatever free advice the expert may have to offer regarding simple and natural exercises as logical choices for a regular exercise program he should not fail to emphasize that the private physician ought to be consulted first. An evaluation of the prevailing health status is essential as a basis for more specific advice whether physical activity will be indicated or not. The physician might, in addition, suggest the type of activity that his client may take up without exceeding safe limits of work tolerance. However, a medical examination performed only at rest will not enable the physician to spell out precisely the patient's tolerance for physical exertion or the intensity of effective training sessions. An adequate activity prescription can only be made up after the client's functional response to energy demands greater than those at rest has been measured and evaluated.

Actually, for the normal healthy individual of any age and sex, a precisely outlined exercise prescription is rarely necessary, and, in many instances, frowned upon. Most people who have the urge and the drive to be physically active will chose for themselves types of activities according to personal likes or dislikes, or because of the social, recreational, or competitive involvement with other people or friends. In such situations, advice or instruction may come from relatives, friends, coaches, or instructors who can teach particular skills properly and who may guide progressing performance with or without elaborate programs.

Who, then, needs special exercise prescription? Actually only two categories of people for whom the achievement of an improved performance level is the major goal of their activity or training program.

The first large group is composed of all the athletes who need the technical advice and detailed training outlines for the development of ultimate performance capacity within their genetic potential. In the past, such training plans have been set up intuitively by coaches on the basis of many years of experience or of active participation in a given sport. Only in recent years has the scientific analysis of the biomechanical and physiological principles involved in sports and athletics contributed to a more rational approach toward training methods and procedures. As before, the performance of the athlete in competition offers the most suitable criterion whether or not a given training plan was successful, and what changes may have to be made to achieve the maximum performance level.

The second group of people, in desperate need of an adequate exercise prescription and of close supervision when exercising, is the one on the opposite side of the fitness scale. To this group belong the persons who, by fate or by neglect, have slipped to such levels of functional degeneration that physical efforts in the range of normal activities might endanger their lives. This is, indeed, a group of people who need precise advice on how to counteract a further degenerative process and how to restore greater functional reserves for a more productive life.

In the following, an attempt will be made to point out the steps required in a program designed to prevent physical and functional disabilities that are basically rooted in overly sedentary living habits.

III. BASIS FOR EXERCISE PRESCRIPTION

As a rule, the general medical status of an individual must have been established by a physician before a program of physical activity can be recommended. Since the normal medical examination is performed at rest only, no assurance is given that the organism will respond to physical stress with adequate functional adjustments. The only "stress test" applied by cardiologists had been for a long time the Master's Step Test (Master and Rosenfeld, 1961; Master and Oppenheimer, 1929). With this test it was possible, at least, to separate people without certain forms of heart disease from those who have. There was no way of using this test for an evaluation of a patient's critical limitations for physical work. However, with the development of more sophisticated exercise tests, using either the motordriven treadmill, the bicycle ergometer, or multistage stepping devices, a concise assessment of physical competence has become possible.

Test methods and test procedures for the determination of "physical fitness" are described in Chapters 22 and 24. In principle, the goal of these tests is the precise measurement of an individual's maximum energy expenditure under overwhelmingly aerobic working conditions. In general, such tests assess the range of cardiac, respiratory, and metabolic adaptability and may point out significant limitations of adaptive mechanisms involved.

The measurement of the individual's maximum oxygen intake (max V_{O_2}) serves as basis for prescribing an exercise program. The wide range of musculoskeletal or organic type handicaps may restrict the use of ordinary testing equipment and testing procedures. Thus, prudent test modifications will become necessary for adequate functional evaluation in special cases, although the use of standardized testing procedures is highly desirable for optimum comparison of results.

IV. FACTORS INFLUENCING EXERCISE PRESCRIPTION

The medical examination preceeding the exercise test is a step necessary for the detection of handicaps that might either rule out certain types of activity or limit performance capacity in others. Age and sex, although generally not advantages or handicaps per se, should neverthe-less be considered as potential modifiers of physical working capacity. The "physiological" age is more meaningful for exercise prescription than the "chronological" age. Sex differences have practically no implica-tions on choice or preference of exercise programs.

Changes of climate can affect work capacity. Prescriptions of exercise may have to be modified according to environmental factors such as heat, humidity, cold, or altitude. Furthermore, considerations should be given to the time of the day most favorably suited for the individual's exercise schedule, and to the type of facility available for the condition-ing program. Not the least, the personal experience gained over past years in sports, games, or various recreational activities should guide the planning of an activity program supposedly to result in highest possible rate of regular attendance and of continued motivation.

V. PHYSIOLOGICAL PRINCIPLES FOR EXERCISE PRESCRIPTION

Attention is directed toward training programs supposedly designed to develop the potentially highest capacity for sustained physical effort. The main factors to be considered in planning such programs are those of intensity, duration, and frequency of training sessions. Since greater than average metabolic stimuli are required to widen the range of physiological adaptability, the intensity of training efforts must be geared to challenge the organ systems to greater responses than they are accus-tomed to producing with ease. An intensity too low may leave the organs unchallenged and, therefore, will not contribute to an improvement of the functional range. A demand too high may exceed the adaptive capa-city, resulting in a failure of making the necessary adjustments. The average level of exercise intensity during any given activity session is to be prescribed as a certain fraction of the maximum aerobic power. The numerical value of this fraction does not seem to be constant, how-ever. For individuals on the low side of the fitness scale, the relative training intensity must be lower than for the more fit persons, and, for those, still considerably lower than for already well-trained athletes. Because of this relation between training intensity and maximum aerobic work tolerance, checks of the latter are required from time to time so that the prescription can be adjusted to the progress made.

The prescription of a certain training intensity may also depend on special training purposes. For instance, for the development of optimum efficiency in energy utilization, we might want to apply a rather low training stimulus for a long period of time, possibly in excess of one hour. Or we might want to elicit quick maximal adjustments of blood flow and pulmonary ventilation, and may approach this by means of relatively short bursts of maximal efforts, followed by periods of recovery just sufficient for paying back the greater portion of an oxygen deficit incurred. Thus, in addition to intensity of energy expenditure, its duration is an important factor in spelling out an exercise prescription.

A very convenient and most effective way of combining the advantages of the low but sustained stimulus with those of the high intensity but short duration stimulus is available in the much favored use of the *interval exercise principle* that employs low and high demands alternatingly. Although each intermittent phase is relatively short, the total workout may last up to one hour or more. The special purpose of the training will not only determine the intensity and duration of the intervals but also the number of repetitions. Finally, the frequency, i.e., the number of physical activity sessions per week has to be taken into consideration, not only from the standpoint of desirable physiological results but also from the standpoint of time and opportunity available to the advice seeking client.

One basic experience must be emphasized, though: there is no shortcut to attaining and maintaining such desirable physical attributes as slimness, strength, relaxation, quickness, and flexibility, and to having, in addition, fatigue-defying staying power. The individual endowment for developing these characteristics to optimum level varies greatly among people. One should, therefore, not judge achievement by absolute athletic standards. The middle-aged man, for example, who has such odds as high blood pressure, considerable overweight, high blood cholesterol values, electrocardiographic abnormalities, and a life full of psychosomatic disturbances working against his health may not be able to achieve athletic standards by any means, however long he trains. But the return and continuous dedication to a more active life might at least restore an average level of physiological reserves for stressful life situations, might prevent him from the fate of a crippling heart attack, and might give him a feeling of confidence and well-being. These are the individuals who most of all need exercise prescriptions fitted to their handicaps, risks of health, and functional limitations. The basic principles in designing training plans for either this type of person or for a champion athlete are, however, much the same.

Adequate exercise prescription follows a certain sequence of consideration. These pertain to (1) the type of exercise to be recommended, (2) the before-mentioned intensity, duration, and frequency of exercise sessions, (3) motivation for regular attendance, and (4) periodic reevaluation.

VI. TYPES OF EXERCISE

A regular exercise program may have the following threefold purpose: (1) to improve the ability of the organ systems to adjust more efficiently and with a greater endurance to increased energy demands; (2) to keep the body machinery in such condition that it is able to maintain an adequate equilibrium between energy intake and output, i.e., to keep a reasonable weight balance; and (3) to provide sufficient physical distraction and recreation from the psychophysiological stresses of daily life, thereby counteracting or removing the impact of tension buildup, anxieties, and frustrations. These purposes seem to be fulfilled in activities that engage the major muscle mass in movements of the entire body. The simple use of the legs for walking, jogging, running, skipping, and jumping provides the most efficient basic form of exercise. These activities may become more interesting and challenging when utilized in the form of games and relays. Additional use of arms and of other body parts will contribute to an augmentation of total work load. Other types of desirable activities for general conditioning are bicycling, skating, skiing (especially cross-country skiing), mountain hiking, rowing (using the racing-type shells), rope jumping, and dancing. Swimming provides sufficient metabolic challenge only to the proficient swimmer. The unskilled swimmer can usually not perform at the effort required for sufficient conditioning of the cardiovascular system.

There are a number of individual games that fulfill the purpose of general conditioning very closely. Such games are handball, squash, paddle ball, badminton, and tennis. However, considerable skills must be acquired in most of these games before they can be performed in a more continuous flow and pace of body movement. Bowling and golf are definitely not activities that could result in an acceptable training stimulus for the heart and body of a recreational player.

Activities of highly competitive character and those of the quick go-and-stop type should be avoided by individuals who undertake exercise with the intent to compensate for the accumulation of nervous tensions or to relieve anxieties and frustrations. The tennis player who becomes upset because of a long string of bad strokes should not neglect to follow up his game of tennis with a two-mile run to rid himself from the overdose of accumulated epinephrine.

To be sucessful in a given sport, one must be in the best possible physical condition in order to perform this sport efficiently and untiringly. Otherwise, the fun may be missed, and the sport may become "work" of an unpleasant nature.

VII. INTENSITY OF EXERCISE

The work intensity is the most important factor in the establishment of a conditioning program. As mentioned earlier, energy demands at certain fractions of the measured aerobic power will be selected. But what is the physiological dose of exercise that will provide an adequate stimulus for the heart and respiratory system to "learn" to adjust more efficiently, or more vigorously, to greater than usual demands?

A clue for selecting the proper training dosage might be derived from the relationship of an individual's total daily energy expenditure to the energy expended during several hours of actual work on the job or in recreational activities. As an example, Table I presents average values of caloric costs for rest and work periods over a 24-hour span for two persons with different job requirements.

To simplify the comparison of the energy demands between these two individuals, the assumption was made that both would have the same duration of resting and sleeping periods, and that 10 more hours would be filled with relatively undemanding activities. In both cases, more severe energy demands were assumed for a duration of 4 hours. During that period of time these amount to 25% of the 24-hour energy expenditure for Subject A, and to about 30% for Subject B.

TABLE I

Estimated Energy Requirements for the Job of an Office Worker (Subject A) and a Laborer Involved in Moderately Heavy Physical Work (Subject B)[a]

Activity	Subject A			Subject B		
	Mets	Hours	Total kcal	Mets	Hours	Total kcal
Sleep and rest	1	10	750	1	10	750
Sedentary activities	1.4	10	1050	1.4	6	630
Physical work, light	2	4	600	2	4	600
Physical work, heavy	—	—	—	3.5	4	1050
		24	2400		24	3030

[a] Both subjects are assumed to have the same body weight of 75 kg and the same height. The resting metabolic rate, one Met, was estimated at 1.25 kcal per minute.

When tested for maximum aerobic power, Subject A attained a maximum aerobic work tolerance of 8 Mets, Subject B one of 11.5 Mets. Since the average intensity of energy expenditure during the 4 hours of greatest work output was 2 Mets for Subject A and 3.5 Mets for Subject B, the former worked during that period of time at 25% and the latter at 33% of their maximum aerobic power, respectively. One could hypothesize, therefore, that the maximum intensity of aerobic work (max Mets) depends greatly on the highest average level of work that an individual maintains for a period of approximately 4 hours. Thus, one may draw the conclusion that any exercise performed at levels of 25 to 33% of max Mets will not result in a functional improvement of any kind. It seems that the minimum demands in training must be at least 40% of max Mets.

Having established the minimum training intensity, the next concern should be the assessment of the maximum level of work that will utilize the maximum rate of oxygen transport functions. The maximum energy expenditure that can be maintained for a period of 12–20 minutes is usually between 80 to 90% of maximum aerobic power established in a standard test procedure of 4–6 minutes duration. Thus it appears reasonable to limit the maximum training intensity to about 85% of max Mets. The relatively short duration (12–30 minutes) of work performance at that intensity points to the fact that this work has still a high anaerobic component, leading to an accumulation of oxygen debt and acid metabolic by-products. In order to keep cardiorespiratory adjustments for a longer period of time at the level that ensures maximal oxygen transport, a brief period of low intensity work is in order to eliminate a major part of the oxygen debt. After an intermittent period at minimum training requirement, the high-intensity work is taken up again until major discomfort ensues. Thus, work at low and high intensities alternates in periodic intervals, and this type of training procedure ensures maximal cardiorespiratory responses without the occurrence of insurmountable fatigue. In such type of interval training, the periods of low intensity work may be accomplished at 40% of max Mets, and the periods of high intensity work at about 85% of max Mets. The resulting average work intensity, therefore, should usually amount to about 66% of max Mets. Approximately the same level of energy demands would be utilized in a type of training that prefers continuous work at a steady state over a long period of time.

Slight modifications of the average training intensity are desirable, however, because of the dependency of the optimum level of submaximal work intensity on the maximum aerobic work tolerance. On the basis of the author's own training experiences and observations of successful middle- and long-distance runners in training, the following sliding scale is suggested for prescribing an acceptable training intensity:

$$\text{Training Intensity} = \frac{60 + \text{max Mets}}{100} \times \text{max Mets}$$

For example, if maximum aerobic power had been determined as 6 Mets, the training intensity would be prescribed as $(60 + 6)/100 \times 6 = 4$ Mets. In case of a max Mets of 10, training intensity would be $.7 \times 10 = 7$; in case of max Mets being 15, the average training effort should be 11.5 Mets.

One major problem remains, however, namely, the quick determination of the energy demands of a given physical activity. For the simple activities of walking, jogging, and running, a close estimate of energy costs can be made when time and distance are measured. For these activities, a close and nearly linear relationship exists between the average speed attained and energy demands. For quick orientation this relationship has been expressed in numerical values in Table II.

In these basic human movements of walking and running, the efficiency of work varies only relatively little in comparison with almost all other activities. Even in walking and running, the slightest incline or softness of the ground will give rise to increased metabolic demands.

TABLE II

The Energy Costs of Walking, Jogging, and Running

Energy cost of walking (Mets)	Speed		Energy cost of jogging/ running (Mets)
	(mph)	(meter/min)	
2	1	27	—
3	2.5	65	—
4	3.3	90	6
5	4.2	113	7.5
—	5.2	140	9
—	6	160	10
—	6.75	180	11
—	7.5	200	12
—	8.25	220	13
—	9	240	14
—	10.25	260	15

In other activities, the variability of external and internal factors such as friction, wind or water resistance, ground slope changes, or particular equipment characteristics make the task of prescribing work intensities with a sufficient degree of accuracy very difficult if not almost impossible. This problem, however, has a chance of being solved by using the heart rate count as a measure of energy demands.

Heart Rate as an Indication of Work Intensity

When metabolic demands increase, an adequate oxygen delivery to the active tissue is accomplished by greater extraction of oxygen from the arterial capillary blood and/or by augmentation of blood flow by means of increased heart rate and increased stroke volume of the heart. The variability in the extent to which any of these functional factors becomes involved in making the proper adjustments seems to prevent the potential use of only one of these factors for the prediction of estimation of metabolic loads. Generally, however, these three factors contribute simultaneously in relative proportion of their adaptive capacity to increased oxygen delivery. This explains the fact that in experimental investigations involving a great number of people a linear relationship has been found between heart rates and levels of energy expenditure. Since the individual response of heart rate to progressive work demands has been assessed by the test for physical competence mentioned previously, a strictly individualized prescription of given heart rates for desired work intensity levels becomes feasible. For finding the heart rates for the minimum (40% max Mets) and maximum (85% max Mets) training intensity, one adds to the resting heart rate 40% or 85%, respectively, of the difference between the heart rates at max Mets and at rest. Similarly, the heart rate for the average training intensity is calculated by using the appropriate factor $(60 + \text{max Mets})/100$. The three examples in Table III illustrate this suggested procedure.

With some practice, heart rates can readily be counted by palpation of the pulse over the radial, carotid, or temporal artery. Instructions of how to count properly can be obtained from the private physician or from the activity instructor. The count should be taken for a 15-second period and multiplied by four. Since it is impossible to count the pulse during running or during many other more violent exercises, it is suggested to assume temporarily a comfortable exercise intensity and begin counting as quickly as possible. Usually the heart rate will remain quite constant for about 30 seconds. To make sure that one really measures the heart rate that existed during the period of greater effort, one can

TABLE III

Estimation of Heart Rate (HR) for Various Training Intensities

		Training intensities		
		Minimum (40%)	Maximum (85%)	Average (60 + max Mets) %
Subject C.P. (max Mets: 5)				
HR at max Mets	130			
HR at rest	84	84	84	84
HR difference	46	15	39	31
Training HR		99	123	115
Subject L.S. (max Mets: 8)				
HR at max Mets	156			
HR at rest	76	76	76	76
HR difference	80	32	68	54
Training HR		108	144	130
Subject W.T. (max Mets: 14)				
HR at max Mets	184			
HR at rest	56	56	56	56
HR difference	128	51	109	95
Training HR		107	165	151

break down the 15-second count into three 5-second counts to become aware of a possibly existing quick recovery.

The procedure to adjust the training intensity to the heart rate level prescribed is simple enough but may require a considerable period of time. If the heart rate has not yet attained the value prescribed, the physical effort must be increased, usually by increasing the speed of movement in walking, running, cycling, swimming, rowing, etc. If the heart rate is found to exceed the set limit, the duration of the minimum training intensity must be extended and that of the higher intensity work shortened.

VIII. DURATION OF EXERCISE

After the training intensity has been established, consideration must be given to the duration of exercise in the alternating periods of interval training as well as for the total duration of an exercise session. Immediately coming to one's mind is the question whether or not there is a physiological criterion by which the extent and the duration of an adequate training period could be assessed.

Although proof is still lacking, it appears that the energy expenditure in training sessions should at least amount to approximately 10% of the normal daily caloric output. For example, if the latter was 2400 kcal (see Subject A in Table I), the metabolic demand in training should amount to 240 kcal. According to the value of 8 Mets at maximum aerobic work tolerance, an average training intensity of 5.5 Mets was prescribed (68% of 8 Mets). The caloric equivalent for 5.5 Mets in this particular case is 5.5×1.25 kcal/minute, i.e. 6.9 kcal/minute. This means that the prescribed energy expenditure of 240 kcal, accomplished at a rate of 6.9 kcal/minute, requires a total time of 35 minutes.

It is understood by now that people with high daily caloric outputs will range high in fitness level. Accordingly, their metabolic demands in training must also be higher. Thus, the duration of a training session will remain about the same. Assuming a man with a 4000 kcal daily energy output spends 400 kcal in training at a prescribed rate of 10 Mets or 12.5 kcal/minute, he will need 32 minutes for accomplishing this task. Thus, adding a few minutes for "warm up" and for "cooling down," a normal period of physical conditioning will usually require 45 minutes. This theoretical assessment of the time factor very closely agrees with the experiences and observations in training practices.

The duration of alternating work intensities during interval training can not be standardized but must be adapted to the fitness level of the individual. A very practical schedule for interval work provides 30-second periods of exercise alternating between high and low effort. The intensity of effort is geared to the heart rate response. To attain or to maintain the prescribed exercise heart rate, it might be necessary to make many adjustments in speed or in duration of work intervals.

Repetition of Exercise Intervals

In the type of conditioning training advocated here, the number of repetitions at low and high work intensity is, for all practical purposes, automatically decided by the duration of each single work interval and by the total duration of the exercise session.

As a rule of thumb, one could say that the high intensity work interval should stop when fatigue becomes unnecessarily painful and begins to affect negatively the coordinated flow of movements. The heart rate count at that point will serve as the objective criterion as to whether or not the discontinuation of work at the high rate had been justified from a physiological point of view.

IX. FREQUENCY OF EXERCISE SESSIONS

If it is theoretically acceptable that the energy spent in physical conditioning should amount to approximately 10% of the normal daily caloric output, then six days per week should be dedicated to exercise. Such a schedule would have several advantages: (1) the time needed each day would be relatively short, possibly 30 minutes only; (2) a habit pattern is more easily established and maintained; (3) the activity program can be made more versatile and enjoyable—various types of sports may be included in an alternating sequence; (4) the intensity and duration of each exercise session can vary freely according to time, facilities, and companionship available; and (5) the tension-relieving effects of daily physical activity may be highly desirable.

Any shortening in the number of weekly training days requires a lengthening of each session, as the total metabolic load must be increased to conform to a given exercise prescription. Reducing the daily exercise schedule, for instance, to a three times per week program practically doubles the time requirement to approximately one hour per session. In practice, such a schedule might turn out to be most economical and sufficiently effective. In many cases, it may be supplemented by more active living habits during the rest of the week.

A twice-weekly activity program, although better than none, cannot be expected to become enjoyable when trying to cramp into these two exercise sessions the total weekly training load. Nearly two hours of continuous exercise at the prescribed intensity level would be required, and that is too much for many reasons. The resulting fatigue would quickly kill the best intentions for regular adherence.

Generally, a frequency of three to four exercise sessions per week is preferred. In athletic training for maximum sport performance, however, the latest trend is not only one but two periods of *daily* training, especially for events that require a combination of great power and endurance. One of these daily sessions is usually dedicated to power training, the other to endurance training. One should not forget, however, that energy sources are limited. After a long grinding morning work-out, the exhausted energy stores may not have been sufficiently replenished and the second afternoon training period may, in fact, bring more harm than benefit in the long run.

Certain physical or physiological handicaps may require special consideration. If, for example, regular exercise is prescribed in a weight-reducing program, the intensity and frequency of exercise sessions should be kept low at the outset to allow for a slow adjustment of joints and rarely used muscles to the unusual strains. In time, the work load is slowly increased until, eventually, a regular daily program might be established.

X. ACTUAL ENERGY EXPENDITURE OF PRESCRIBED EXERCISE

The "Mets" concept introduced in the terminology of stress physiology simplifies work evaluation and exercise prescription. It assumes that the energy requirements of the human body at rest are nearly constant for a given unit of body mass. On the average, the oxygen requirement for one kilogram (1 kg = 2.2 pounds) of body weight is 3.5 ml/minute during rest, i.e., at 1 Met. Depending on the source of fuel utilized (fat and/or carbohydrates), the caloric equivalent for one liter (or 1000 ml) of oxygen amounts to 4700–5000 gramcalories (cal). Thus the caloric equivalent of 1 Met is, on the average, 17 cal/minute per kg of body weight. The hourly caloric equivalent of 1 Met is then 1000 cal or 1 kcal (kilocalorie) per kg. Assuming that an exercise prescription calls for an average training intensity of 10 Mets, the hourly energy requirement becomes 10 kcal per kg, or a total of 750 kcal for a person with a weight of 75 kg. Since this particular person is expected to spend only 350 to 400 kcal per training session, a 30-minute work-out at the prescribed intensity would fulfill this requirement. Thus, the prescribed Met value, for all practical purpose, is identical with the one-hour value of energy requirement, in kilocalories per kilogram body weight and allows for a quick estimation of actual caloric energy expenditure over time.

One example may be in order to illustrate the factors leading to an appropriate exercise prescription (Table IV).

XI. SUPERVISED OR UNSUPERVISED PHYSICAL ACTIVITY

People may decide to take up "vigorous" physical activity for many reasons. If they do, some will seek out well-reputed ongoing programs, but some will try it on their own. If the latter know what they are doing and adhere to adequate exercise prescription, they will be as well off as those who let themselves be guided professionally. In danger are only those who had physically "fallen apart" over many years and one day decide to get back "into shape" quickly. Unfortunately, this happens rather frequently and the resulting accidents are tragic. Imagine

TABLE IV

A Sample Prescription for Exercise

Subject: middle-aged male, sedentary, no indication of health risks.

Height: 182 cm   Weight: 100 kg   Relative Weight: 122%

Average daily energy expenditure: 2750 kcal/day

Maximum aerobic work tolerance: 8 Mets

Training intensity: 5.5 Mets

Energy requirement of activity program: 275 kcal/day

                                        or: 1650 kcal/week

Heart rate: 70 at rest   170 at max Mets   138 during training

Prescribed type of training work:
    Alternating walking (at 3 mph) and jogging (at 4.6 mph) for periods of 30 seconds each, i.e., 30 seconds at 3 Mets followed by 30 seconds at 8 Mets, averaging 5.5 Mets.

Training effort to be guided by an average heart rate of 138/min

Frequency and duration of training sessions:
    Either 6 days/week for 30 minutes at 275 kcal/session
       or 5 days/week for 36 minutes at 330 kcal/session
       or 4 days/week for 45 minutes at 412 kcal/session
       or 3 days/week for 60 minutes at 550 kcal/session

---

a 33-year old man with family, in the prime of life but too busy to spend even a little time for health maintenance. Considerable overweight and some chest discomfort under exertion make him decide one day to go back to the gymnasium and to try for a physical comeback. For reasons unknown, he does not consult his physician and does not utilize the cardiac stress test facility available to him. His own chosen exercise program is about the worst for his condition: violent pull-ups, push-ups, sit-ups, frequent short sprints, or other bursts of overload exercises. Several days after he had taken up these self-inflicted ordeals, he collapsed under the chinning bar, and, before others in the gymnasium realized that something must have gone wrong, it was too late for successful resuscitation attempts. Although there was postmortem evidence of progressive atherosclerotic disease of the coronary arteries of the heart, this incident in an apparently healthy young man was certainly premature, and might have been prevented. In all probability, with the right type of functional evaluation, the degree of cardiac limitations would have been defined, and, with the right type of a preventive activity program, the progress of disease might have been stopped or even reverted.

The advantages of a supervised activity program are manyfold. First of all, it will be more diversified and more fun because the professional instructor has many variations of exercises and games at his fingertips. He knows the ranges of energy expenditure for many activities and has learned to assess the work effort of his charges from many signs. He will either encourage the "loafer" to do better, or will insist on sufficient recovery periods when he recognizes approaching limitations. Of course, he is guided by the prescription of training intensity and heart rate and teaches his participants to make frequent checks of pulse counts.

In a supervised training program, several people usually work together in a group. Many of them may have similar problems and may influence each other to maintain a regular exercise schedule, to work at the required intensity level, to avoid habits that are opposed to the purpose of training, and to enjoy a relaxing atmosphere.

Many people, however, never develop a liking for regular exercise in groups and prefer to be "loners" in their chosen training programs. This applies as well to patients who exercise on doctor's orders as to people of all ages who maintain a certain exercise ritual as basic conditioner for their special sport programs, and, last but not least, to the athlete with great ambition for top performance. Nothing is wrong with this temporary isolation as long as the training effort, in intensity and duration, is physiologically geared to gradual achievement of the nearest goal set. The goals, however, should be set by those who have the background and knowledge to prescribe the right type and amount of exercise on the basis of adequate functional evaluation, can detect positive or negative changes in performance levels, and, thus, can make necessary changes in the training plan.

XII. EXERCISE PRESCRIPTION AND MOTIVATIONAL FACTORS

People differ greatly in their likes and dislikes for active expressions of human life. To the physically, mentally, and morally healthy individual a life filled with activities is a natural phenomenon. A tendency to detest any sort of hard physical work may indicate a step toward degeneration. In a free society with a "live and let live" philosophy, problems may arise only if the consequences of insufficient use of the body organs over a long period of time lead to health hazards on a population-wide level. But even then, the individual must be assured of his freedom to decide his own road, either to a possible premature decay or to a more desirable maintenance of sufficient organic reserves for long years of enjoyable life. In recent years, the public awareness of health benefits ascribed to more active living habits has considerably increased. "Run for Your Life" has become a slogan outlasting temporary "fads." The belief of millions of people that it is wiser and healthier to save energy wherever and whenever possible has been especially shattered by those who have experienced the first symptoms of crippling atherosclerotic heart disease or have survived a heart attack. When these people learned that the heart can be retrained to operate faithfully for many years without a repeat of the fearful experience, they became the most faithful adherents to regular exercise programs. More and more the observation is made that motivation for physical exercise can be created and maintained much more easily in individuals who have lived through the anxious moments of a faltering heart than in others who already have the early signs and symptoms of myocardial degeneration but still believe that a heart attack could never happen to them.

Once it comes to the point of exercise prescription, the problem is not anymore how to motivate people to take the first step toward a more active life but to keep motivation alive. This requires a training program that will keep the new participant in a spirit of expectation as well as accomplishments. The most potent motivational factors for continuing exercise on a regular schedule are possibly the following:

1. Exercise programs that result in a subjective improvement of physical well being

2. Exercise programs that offer great variations in physical activity, and are presented in an enjoyable form

3. Establishment of social ties among participants

4. Individual attention by exercise leaders and other staff members conducting the program

5. Periodic evaluation of progress, demonstrating improvement or lack of it, both of which need to be known in order to plot the new course of action

6. The realization that regular exercise helps in reducing the tensions accumulating from a score of stressful impacts in daily life with the disappearance of previous symptoms of early fatigue during routine work

XIII. A FINAL CHALLENGE

This chapter was written as the result of many years of experience and observations in designing and conducting training programs for people of normal and abnormal health of almost all age ranges. Some parts of the presentation are very much of a hypothetical nature rather than based on hard facts. Much research will still be needed to establish the physiological training programs which are most meaningful and the most effective exercise prescriptions. The author is convinced that he is far from the optimal solution, but hopes that some of the suggestions made will help in establishing an acceptable basis for further work on physiological training programming.

REFERENCES

Master, A. M., and Oppenheimer, E. T. (1929). *Amer. J. Med. Sci.* **177**, 223.
Master, A. M., and Rosenfield, I. (1961). *N.Y. State J. Med.* **61**, 1850.

Chapter 24

EVALUATING THE EFFECTS OF PHYSICAL ACTIVITY

FRANCIS J. NAGLE AND NEIL B. OLDRIDGE

It is fair to say that the evidence for regular physical training as a preventative in disease and/or premature aging is inconclusive. This is due primarily to the many uncontrolled factors in the numerous studies that have focused on the problem. A need continues to exist for well-controlled, longitudinal studies of meaningful human physiological responses under precisely defined evaluative testing and physical training conditions. It will be our purpose to discuss the issues of exercise testing and meaningful physiological responses in evaluating the effects of physical activity, referring the reader to Chapter 23 for details on the physical training prescription.

I. EVALUATIVE TESTING

While we will focus on exercise test procedures, it should be said at the outset that the total test record should include a living habit and medical history, a psychological profile, and data on body size and composition as well as physiological responses to an exercise stress.

A wide variety of test procedures are available (Costill and Fox, 1969; Hermansen and Saltin, 1969; Taylor *et al.*, 1955) for evaluations of exercise tolerance, most designed to measure or estimate the maximal aerobic capacity (MAC). While such a determination is valuable, as we shall see shortly, there are other critical assessments that should be made during exercise test procedures. This requires a test design that lends itself to routine monitoring of a wide range of physiological parameters which may include blood pressure, electrocardiogram (ECG), lung diffusing capacity, cardiac output, and blood chemistry. Of importance, too, would be the advantage of being able to relate these various exercise responses to the intensity of the metabolic stress being tolerated.

Balke and Ware (1959) introduced a progressive treadmill test procedure for measuring the MAC of "normal" individuals allowed to adapt to increasing work loads up to maximum. This procedure was further refined by Balke (1970) and by Naughton *et al.* (1966) with the setting of continuously increased work loads calculated to demand single increments of the rest metabolic rate (taken to be 3.5 ml/kg/minute). The procedure has been extended for use on a bicycle ergometer and step device by Nagle *et al.* (1971). This test design appears particularly appropriate for use in longitudinal studies for numerous reasons:

1. A metabolic standard (multiple of rest metabolic rate) of reference is established for interpretation of physiological functions over a range of submaximal to maximal work stresses.
2. The condition for continuous monitoring of physiological functions (blood pressure, pulse, ECG) employing small work increments allows for greater safety in test procedures.
3. Assessment of maximal aerobic capacity is possible, if necessary.
4. The test procedure accommodates subjects displaying a range of physical conditions from the pathological to the superior, endurance athlete.

The test loadings for the treadmill, bicycle and step device beginning at energy requirements of 3 times the rest metabolic rate (3×3.5 ml/kg/minute) are presented in Table I.

Bruce *et al.* (1963) have reported on the merits of a Multistage Exercise Capacity Test (Table II). The rationale for the treadmill test is similar to that reported above, insofar as allowance is made for observations of submaximal work adaptations before maximal loads are imposed.

TABLE I

Treadmill, Bicycle, and Step Test Loads[a]

	Treadmill (3 mph)	Bicycle (50–60 revs/min)	Step device (30 steps/min)
Initial work	0% grade	35 watts	2.5 cm step height
Increment every 2 minutes	2.5% grade	25 watts	4.5 cm step height

[a] Work loads established to demand unit increments of the rest metabolic rate (3.5 ml O_2/kg/min).

TABLE II

Work Loads and Energy Requirements of Bruce Multistage Exercise Test[a]

Stage	Speed (mph)	Grade (%)	Duration (minutes)	O_2 intake (liters/min)
1	1.7	10	3	1.1
2	3.4	14	3	2.2
3	5.0	18	3	3.0
4	6.0	22	to exhaustion	3.5

[a] From R. A. Bruce, J. R. Blackman, J. W. Jones, and G. Strait (1963). Exercising testing in Adult normal subjects and cardiac patients. *Pediatrics* **32**, Suppl., 742–756. Copyright 1963. Used with permission of C. C Thomas Publishing Co., Springfield, Illinois.

Work increments, however, are relatively large from stage to stage, thereby limiting the number of observations that can be made, especially on the more functionally impaired individual.

II. MEANINGFUL PHYSIOLOGICAL FACTORS

The most revealing factor relating to an individual's fitness, or state of training, is his maximal O_2 capacity corrected for body weight. Buskirk and Taylor (1957) state that the ratio of oxygen uptake per kilogram of body weight provides a measure of the immediately available oxidative energy that can be supplied to move a kilogram of body weight from one place to another.

The maximum O_2 capacity (amount of O_2 delivered to active tissue per unit time) may be increased with training from 7% to 33%. Data

TABLE III
Maximal Oxygen Uptake Data from Training Studies[a]

Authors	Number of subjects	Control	Maximal O₂ uptake (liters/min)	
			After bed rest	After training
Robinson and Harmon, 1941;				
Dill *et al.*, 1966	9	3.36		3.90 + 16%
Knehr *et al.*, 1942	14	3.45		3.69 + 7%
Taylor *et al.*, 1949	2	3.85	3.18 − 17%	
Rowell, 1962	7	3.47		3.93 + 13%
Ekblom *et al.*, 1968	8	3.15		3.68 + 16%
Saltin *et al.*, 1968	3	2.52	1.74 − 31%	3.41 + 33%
Saltin *et al.*, 1969	42[b]	2.90		3.43 + 18%
Saltin *et al.*, 1969	8[c]	2.25		2.67 + 19%

[a] From P. O. Åstrand, and K. Rodahl, (1970). "Textbook of Work Physiology." McGraw-Hill, New York. Copyright 1970 by McGraw-Hill, Inc. Used with permission of McGraw-Hill Book Company, New York.
[b] Aged 34 to 50 years.
[c] Aged 50 to 63 years.

from representative training studies compiled by Åstrand and Rodahl (1970) are shown in Table III. The wide range of changes is apparently due to differences in the initial training states. Those highly trained at the outset experience little improvement, and, conversely, initially sedentary subjects experience changes of considerable magnitude.

Figure 1 shows that there is a decrease in maximal aerobic capacity with age, and that at any age level the aerobic power of the female is less than that of the male, even when a correction is made for differences in body weight. The figure also shows that the loss of aerobic power with age is reduced by physical training. Hollmann (1964) showed that over a 15-year period from 1949 to 1964 seventeen active sportsmen experienced reductions in their maximum aerobic capacities from 45 to 38 ml/kg/minute, while thirty-nine nonsports subjects declined from 42 to 26 ml/kg/minute in aerobic power. Costill and Winrow (1970) reported on two distance runners aged 45 and 49 with measured maximal aerobic capacities of 63.7 and 65.1 ml/kg/minute, respectively. This far exceeds the normal measured values of 44–53 ml/kg/minute found in many young adults 20–29 years of age (Cummings, 1967).

Because the MAC is, in turn, dependent on certain dimensional factors and functional capacities of the respiratory and circulatory systems, it

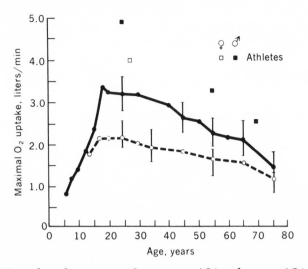

FIG. 1 Maximal aerobic power in German men (●) and women (○) in relation to age. The figure also includes data for male and female athletes (long distance runners). From W. Hollmann, (1963). "Hockst- und Deuerleistungsfähigkeit des Sportslers." Barth, Munich.

is singularly indicative of the functional status of the systems which we will now discuss.

A. Respiratory System

The oxygen transporting capacity of the human organism depends on a number of respiratory factors. Two important ones are (1) the minute ventilation of the lungs (V_E, the amount of air moved out of the lungs per unit time) and (2) the level of diffusion of oxygen at the alveolar–lung capillary surface. Figure 2 shows the effect of training and age on the minute pulmonary ventilation in exercise. In general, the higher the state of training, the lower the V_E at a given submaximal O_2 uptake. At maximal O_2 uptake, the V_E is higher in the trained than in the untrained. Figure 2 also shows that older people may exhibit somewhat higher ventilations at the same O_2 uptake than younger individuals. However, the maximum V_E decreases with age (Grimby and Saltin, 1966). The direction of V_E changes with training, and age tends to make interpretation of ventilatory observations somewhat complex.

Lung diffusion capacity (D_L) is measured by determination of the movement of oxygen or carbon monoxide across the lung–blood interface and is expressed in milliliters of gas diffused per millimeter of gas pres-

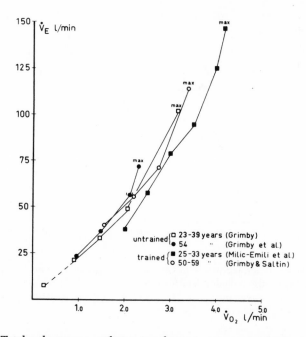

FIG. 2   Total pulmonary ventilation in relation to oxygen uptake in young sedentary and well-trained subjects, in 53 men from a population study in the city of
Gotesburg, Sweden and in a group of still active, very well-trained middle-aged
athletes. From G. Grimby. (1969). Respiration in exercise, *Med. Sci. Sports* 1, 9–14.

sure. The D_L is influenced by such factors as (1) the size of the alveolar
capillary surface area, (2) the thickness of the membranes through which
the gases diffuse, (3) the alveolar to capillary gas pressure gradient, (4)
the pulmonary blood flow and, (5) the pulmonary capillary blood volume
at a given time. Turino *et al.* (1963) have shown that higher D_L values
are measured at rest and in exercise when O_2 is used rather than CO.
However, with use of either gas, D_L increases linearly with the oxygen
requirement of exercise (Reuschlein *et al.*, 1968). Hanson (1969),
Shephard and Anderson (1968), Reuschlein *et al.* (1968), and Reddan
et al. (1969) have shown that D_L is not affected by training. It has been
demonstrated that some trained athletes have higher D_L values than
untrained subjects, but this is apparently due to differences in such
factors as body size, lung dimensional factors, total hemoglobin, and
blood volume (Hanson, 1969).

Donevan *et al.* (1959) have reported that diffusion capacity decreased
with age at rest and at various levels of work. This is believed to be
due to a lower pulmonary blood flow at rest and work in the older

age groups. One could assume that, with aging, training would decrease the rate with which the loss in diffusion capacity occurs as is true for the maximal oxygen capacity. However, the authors have found no reports to confirm this assumption.

B. Cardiovascular System

The dimensional factors of heart volume (HV), blood volume (BV), and blood hemoglobin (Hb) content contribute to the O_2 transport capacity of the cardiovascular system. Representative mean values for Scandanavian men and women physical education students and soldiers aged 21–30 are shown in Table IV. Similar values for HV and BV and slightly higher values (1.0 gram %) for Hb were reported by Holmgren and Åstrand (1966) for 10 college men and 10 college women. Heart volume increases with training. Calculating heart volume from biplane roentgenograms, Ekblom and Hermansen (1968) reported values as high as 1150 ml in competitive, endurance athletes. Aging (Åstrand, 1968) and various cardiovascular diseases, e.g., mitral, aortic stenosis, and hypertension, increase heart size. These conditions must be marked by qualitative differences in the enlargement occurring with training. In the last century, Morpurgo (1897) postulated that the differences were marked by greater homogeneity of muscle fiber sizes and more desirable fiber-to-capillary ratios in enlargement resulting from physical training.

The blood volume constitutes approximately 8% of the body weight. Saltin *et al.* (1968) have reported that blood volume increases with physical training and it is also known to increase with age (Åstrand, 1968). Apparently training does not appreciably influence relative blood hemoglobin levels (Hb per 100 ml blood) but total hemoglobin is elevated (Åstrand, 1956). Ekblom and Hermansen (1968) reported mean values of 14 grams % for competitive distance athletes, a figure similar to that reported for normal males in Table IV. Aging is accompanied

TABLE IV

Mean Values for Heart Volume, Blood Volume, and Blood Hemoglobin

Author	Sex	Number	Heart volume (ml)	Blood volume (liters)	Hb (grams %)
Åstrand and	♀	11	637 ± 50	4.5 + 0.5	12.2 + 0.6
Rodahl, 1970			(585 − 755)	(3.7 − 5.4)	(11.2 − 13.5)
Ahlborg, 1967	♂	39	849 + 86	5.6 + 0.7	13.9 + 1.0
			(680 − 1070)	(4.2 − 7.1)	(12.4 − 15.7)

a Estimated from measured plasma volumes.

by an increase in blood hemoglobin levels up to at least the fifth decade
(Åstrand, 1968).

In addition to the dimensional factors, the transport of O_2 in the
cardiovascular system depends on a functional capacity identified as
the cardiac output (Q). Its contribution to the O_2 uptake capacity is
clearly described by the Fick equation in which $V_{O_2} = Q \times$ artery to
vein O_2 difference. Since Q is the product of the heart rate (HR) and
the stroke volume (SV), the equation may be expressed as

$$V_{O_2} = \text{HR} \times \text{SV} \times (\text{a} - \text{v } O_2 \text{ difference})$$

which then identifies all the cardiovascular factors contributing to oxygen
uptake. For the intact human the a — v O_2 difference is the venous O_2
content (measured in the right ventricle or pulmonary artery) subtracted from the arterial O_2 content (measured in any systemic artery).
The functional relationship of all these factors in acute exercise of increasing intensity is illustrated in Fig. 3. Physical training increases the

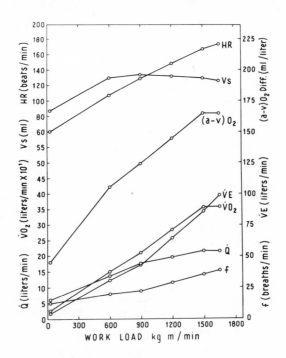

FIG. 3 Respiratory and cardiovascular response to increasing work loads on
a bicycle ergometer. Each work load up to 1500 kgm/minute was performed for 10
minutes. Work duration of 1650 kgm/minute to voluntary fatigue ranged from 5
minutes to 10 minutes. From J. A. Faulkner. (1970). *In* "The Physiology and Biochemistry of Muscle as a Food" (E. J. Briskey, R. J. Cassens, and B. B. Marsh,
eds.), Vol. 2. Univ. of Wisconsin Press, Madison. Copyright 1970 by the University
of Wisconsin. Used with permission.

maximal cardiac output. Mean values as high as 36.0 liters/minute have been reported by Ekblom and Hermansen (1968) for highly trained, endurance athletes. Since maximum heart rates were in a normal range (190 beats/minute, mean for nine subjects) the high Q values are attributed to very high stroke volumes (189 ml, mean for nine subjects). Various controlled training studies (Saltin et al., 1968) show that, while maximum cardiac outputs were increased from 4 to 16%, maximum heart rates decreased from 0.5 to 3.6%, stroke volumes increased from 8.5 to 16.7%, and a — v O_2 differences increased from 3.6 to 16.4%. Aging is marked by a decrease in maximum Q, heart rate, and stroke volume, but the rate of decline is probably diminished by physical training. This observation would appear to follow from the slower loss of total aerobic power with aging in those who continue to exercise.

At any submaximal work level at which the older individual exhibits a heart rate response similar to that of the younger individual, the work must be marked by a higher a — v O_2 difference in the older individuals (Granath et al., 1970). It is instructive to point out that not all investigators are agreed on the direction of change in Q and SV with age. Becklake et al. (1965) reported increases in Q and SV at given work loads with increasing age in males and females.

1. Blood Pressure

Saltin et al. (1968) showed that a period of bed rest followed by extended physical training for five normal subjects resulted in no significant change in mean arterial blood pressure at rest or during exercise. It has been shown (Åstrand, 1968) that older men had consistently higher systolic and diastolic pressure than younger men at rest and during exercise. Granath et al. (1970) attribute this to the reduced elasticity of the aorta in older men despite the fact that the increased aortic volume (also an age effect) would tend to offset the effect of the lost elasticity.

Johnson and Grover (1967) reported that regular physical training failed to change the rest blood pressure responses in four hypertensive subjects. Other investigators have reported a reduction in systolic and diastolic blood pressures following training (Boyer and Kasch, 1970). The influence of psychological factors and the lability of blood pressure in some subjects may contribute to the disparity in results.

The magnitude of the blood pressure response is related to the type of work performed. Work performed with the arms results in a higher blood pressure response than does work of the same intensity performed with the legs; this also holds for the heart rate response. Donald et *al.* (1967) have shown that relatively moderate and localized isometric work can cause a far higher pressure component than that observed in dynamic work. Such observations have serious implications for the selection of desirable forms of physical activity for normal and especially for physiologically impaired adult groups.

2. Electrocardiogram

In the clinical situation, exercise is used to impose a metabolic stress on cardiac muscle. In turn, a blood flow deficit (ischemia) in the heart muscle may be indicated by changes in the electrical impulse transmission pattern as recorded by the ECG tracing. Physical training has little if any influence on the normal ECG. It has been reported that well trained competitive athletes may exhibit high amplitude R and T waves as a result of left ventricular hypertrophy, and minor intraventricular conduction defects are also common (Åstrand and Rodahl, 1970).

It is widely held that regular physical training tends to change the ECG tracings of subjects who suffer from documented ischemic heart disease (Hellerstein *et al.*, 1967; Radke *et al.*, 1970) probably through increasing the collateral circulation of the myocardial tissue. Radke *et al.* (1970) state that improvement in physical fitness in patients with arteriosclerotic heart disease is associated with a decrease in ST-J segment displacements of the ECG. Such observations are suggestive of beneficial, qualitative change in heart muscle function, but do not provide conclusive evidence of such. Here again, only long duration regulated studies of ECG patterns and survival rates on matched groups with and without heart disease will provide definitive answers to this problem.

3. Systolic Time Intervals

These determinations provide another tool in assessment of the functional state of the heart muscle. In the technique, which is noninvasive, the carotid pulse wave, ECG, and heart sounds are related to reveal preventricular and ventricular ejection time intervals (Blumberger and Meiners, 1959; Diamant and Killip, 1970; Weissler *et al.*, 1961; Wiggers, 1922). Left ventricular ejection time (LVET) varies inversely with heart rate and directly with stroke volume in normal individuals. In patients with cardiovascular disease, particularly aortic valvular disease, the LVET is prolonged in relation to the severity of the disease (Weissler *et al.*, 1961).

Heart rate change is the most important determinant of LVET with aging; there is a slight but significant prolongation of LVET that amounts to approximately 2 milliseconds/decade (Willems *et al.*, 1970). This is attributed to left ventricular dysfunction (Weissler *et al.*, 1968), specifically a decline in sympathetic nervous tone (Rabb, 1966; Urschell *et al.*, 1968), and myocardial contractility (Strandell, 1964; Urschell *et al.*, 1968), as well as aortic impedance (Willems *et al.*, 1970). With aging there is no significant change in LVET when corrected for heart rate (Harrison *et al.*, 1964; Weissler *et al.*, 1968), the ratio LVET/HR being identified as the ejection time index (ETI) (Weissler *et al.*, 1968).

At rest it appears that LVET and ETI do not differentiate between normal individuals and those with ischemic heart disease, provided they are not hemodynamically disabled (Pouget *et al.*, 1971; Whitsett and Naughton, 1971; Willems *et al.*, 1970). It is suggested that the measurement of systolic time intervals can be made more sensitive and precise by determination of the intervals with a standard exercise test.

When normals and those with ischemic heart disease are compared, there is a greater difference in LVET and ETI following exercise than at rest (Pouget *et al.*, 1971; Whitsett and Naughton, 1971). This is true for both sedentary and active groups. Active individuals, normals, and those with ischemic heart disease, respond to exercise with a significant shortening of ETI, while sedentary normals show minimal shortening, and sedentary diseased individuals show a significant prolongation of LVET and ETI (Frank and Kinlaw, 1962; Hanson *et al.*, 1968; Pouget *et al.*, 1971; Whitsett and Naughton, 1971).

Both aging and cardiovascular disease, including ischemic heart disease, cause prolongation of ETI following exercise. Shortening of ETI following exercise is most pronounced in normal and diseased individuals who are active. This shortening is ascribed to an improved left ventricular function.

4. Blood Chemistry

Physical training has been reported to influence various lipid compounds, e.g., blood serum free fatty acids (FFA), triglycerides (TG), and cholesterol (C) which have also been implicated in the genesis of athroschlerotic heart disease. Saltin *et al.* (1968) showed that after 21 days of bed rest followed by 53 days of physical training, control FFA, TG, and C serum concentrations were not influenced. Numerous other studies of the influence of training on serum cholesterol specifically have revealed rather equivocal results (Fox and Haskell, 1967; Grimby *et al.*, 1971; Skinner, 1968). A large population study (Rosenmans, 1970) showed that TG levels were significantly lower and C levels slightly lower in male adults who adhered to an exercise regimen. Grimby *et al.* (1971) showed also that TG levels were significantly reduced with physical activity and increased aerobic power while cholesterol showed no difference with training. It has been shown that weight change also affects serum lipid levels of TG and C (Albrink *et al.*, 1962) with increasing weight associated with elevated levels of blood lipid. Skinner (1968) states that, if weight can be stabilized over a period of years with increased activity, this may in turn have a beneficial effect on lipid concentrations.

5. Body Composition

Studies of young adults who habitually exercise and those who were sedentary showed that activity was associated with a greater lean body mass and less fat (Buskirk *et al.*, 1955). It was found that body fat was inversely related to the extent of participation in physical activity. Keys and Brozek (1953) found that a physically active adult group showed a lower estimated body fat content than a sedentary group. Christian *et al.* (1964) have reported that the change with training in adults is due only to loss of fat. However, this is difficult to reconcile with numerous other studies, of which that of Leedy *et al.* (1965) is representative, where physical exercise alone did not result in a significant loss in weight. It has been shown that weight determination is not a good guide to fat loss because fat loss may be compensated by an increase in muscle density due to exercise (Kireilis and Cureton, 1947).

Sprynarova and Parizkova (1965) demonstrated that training and dieting in preadolescent boys decreased the absolute maximum oxygen capacity, but not the maximum O_2 capacity corrected for body weight. The change in O_2 uptake capacity was thereby attributed to body composition changes, a factor of some significance in interpreting O_2 uptake changes resulting from physical training.

Excess body weight has been implicated in the etiology of various diseases and this is discussed in detail in Chapter 27. Suffice it to say here that it is well documented that regular physical activity helps regulate body weight (Mayer, 1968) and in this way may well provide a safeguard against excess fat deposition and disease through the adult years.

REFERENCES

Ahlborg, B. (1967). *Försvarsmedicin* 3, Suppl. I.
Albrink, M., Meigs, J., and Granoff, M. (1962). *N. Engl. J. Med.* 266, 484.
Åstrand, P. O. (1956). *Physiol. Rev.* 36, 307.
Åstrand, P. O. (1968). *J. Amer. Med. Ass.* 205, 729.
Åstrand, P. O., and Rodahl, K. (1970). "Textbook of Work Physiology." McGraw-Hill, New York.

Balke, B. (1970). "Advanced Exercise Procedures for Evaluation of the Cardiovascular System," Monograph. Educ. Dept., Burdick Corp., Milton, Wisconsin.

Balke, B., and Ware, R. W. (1959). *U.S. Armed Forces Med. J.* 10, 675.

Becklake, M. R., Frank, H., Dagenais, G. R., Ostigery, G. L., and Guyman, C. A. (1965). *J. Appl. Physiol.* 20, 938.

Bergman, H., and Varnauskas, E. (1970). In "Physical Activity and Aging" (D. Brunner, ed.), p. 138. Univ. Park Press, Baltimore, Maryland.

Blumberger, K. J., and Meiners, S. (1959). In "Cardiology: An Encyclopedia of the Cardiovascular System" (A. Luisada, ed.), p. 4. McGraw-Hill, New York.

Boyer, J. L., and Kasch, F. W. (1970). *J. Amer. Med. Ass.* 211, 1668.

Bruce, R. A., Blackmon, J. R., Jones, J. W., and Strait, G. (1963). *Pediatrics* 32, Suppl. 743.

Buskirk, E., and Taylor, H. L. (1957). *J. Appl. Physiol.* 11, 72.

Buskirk, E., Taylor, H. L., and Simonson, E. (1955). *Int. Z. Angew. Physiol. Einschl. Arbeitsphysiol.* 16, 83.

Christian, J. E., Combs, L. W., and Kessler, W. V. (1964). *Clin. Nutr.* 36, 156.

Costill, D. L., and Fox, E. L. (1969). *Med. Sci. Sports* 1, 81.

Costill, D. L., and Winrow, E. (1970). *Res. Quart.* 41, 135.

Cummings, G. R. (1967). *Can. Med. Ass. J.* 96, 868.

Diamant, B., and Killip, T. (1970). *Circulation* 42, 579.

Dill, D. B., Phillips, E. E., Jr., and MacGregor, D. (1966). *Ann. N.Y. Acad. Sci.* 134, 760.

Donald, K. W., Lind, A. R., McNicol, G. W., Humphreys, P. W., Taylor, S. H., and Staunton, H. P. (1967). *Circ. Res.* Suppl. 1, p. 1.

Donevan, R. E., Palmer, W. H., Varvis, C. J., and Bates, D. V. (1959). *J. Appl. Physiol.* 14, 483.

Ekblom, B., and Hermansen, L. (1968). *J. Appl. Physiol.* 25, 619.

Faulkner, J. (1970). In "Physiology and Biochemistry of Muscle as a Food" (J. Briskey, R. Cassens, and B. Marsh, eds.), Chapter 27, pp. 555–575. Univ. of Wisconsin Press, Madison.

Fox, S. M., and Haskell, W. L. (1967). *Can. Med. Ass. J.* 96, 806.

Frank, M. N., and Kinlaw, W. B. (1962). *Amer. J. Cardiol.* 10, 800.

Granath, A., Jonsson, B., and Strandell, T. (1970). In "Physical Activity and Aging" (D. Brunner, ed.,), Chapter II, pp. 48–79. Univ. Park Press, Baltimore, Maryland.

Grimby, G., and Saltin, B. (1966). *Acta Med. Scand.* 179, 513.

Grimby, G., Wilhelmsen, L., Bjornthorp, P., Saltin, B., and Tibblin, G. (1971). In "Muscle Metabolism During Exercise" (B. Pernow and B. Saltin, eds.), pp. 469–81. Plenum, New York.

Hanson, J. S. (1969). *Dis. Chest.* 56, 488.

Hanson, J. S., Tabakin, B. S., Levy, A. M., and Nedde, W. (1968). *Circulation* 38, 783.

Harrison, R. T., Dixon, K., Russel, R. O., Birdwar, P. S., and Coleman, H. N. (1964). *Amer. Heart J.* 67, 189.

Hellerstein, H. K., Hornsten, T. R., Goldbarg, A. N., Burlando, A. G., Friedman, E. H., Hirsch, E. Z., and Marik, S. (1967). *Can. Med. J.* 96, 901.

Hermansen, L., and Saltin, B. (1969). *J. Appl. Physiol.* 26, 31.

Hollmann, W. (1964). *Proc. Int. Congr. Sports Sci.*, p. 91, Tokyo, 1966.

Holmgren, A., and Åstrand, P. O. (1966). *J. Appl. Physiol.* 21, 1463.

Johnson, W. P., and Grover, J. A. (1967). *Can. Med. Ass. J.* 96, 868.

Keys, A., and Brozek, J. (1953). *Physiol. Rev.* 33, 245.

Kireilis, R. W., and Cureton, T. K. (1947). *Res. Quart.* **18**, 123.
Knehr, C. A., Dill, D. B., and Neufeld, W. (1942). *Amer. J. Physiol.* **136**, 148.
Leedy, H. E., Ismail, A. H., Kessler, W. V., and Christian, J. E. (1965). *Res. Quart.* **36**, 158.
Mayer, J. (1968). "Overweight." Prentice-Hall, Englewood Cliffs, New Jersey.
Morpurgo, B. (1897). *Arch. Pathol. Anat. Physiol. Klin. Med.* **150**, 522.
Nagle, F. J., Baptista, G., Allieya, J., Howley, E., and Balke, B. (1971). "Compatibility of Progressive Treadmill, Bicycle, and Step Tests Based On Oxygen Uptake Responses." *Med. Sci. Sports* **3**, 149.
Naughton, J., Shanbour, K., Armstrong, R., McCoy, J., and Lategola, M. (1966). *Arch. Intern. Med.* **117**, 541.
Pouget, J. M., Harris, W. S., Mayron, B. R., Naughton, J. P., and Urschell, C. W. (1971). *Circulation* **43**, 289.
Raab, W. (1966). *Sports Med. J.* **6**, 38.
Radke, J. D., Hellerstein, H. K., Salzman, S. H., Maistelman, H. M., and Ricklin, R. (1970). *In* "Physical Activity and Aging" (D. Brunner, ed.), pp. 168–194. Univ. Park Press, Baltimore, Maryland.
Reddan, W., Forster, H., Thoden, J., and Balke, B. (1969). *Fed. Proc., Fed. Amer. Soc. Exp. Biol.* **28**, 593.
Reuschlein, P. S., Reddan, W. G., Burpee, J., Gee, J. B. L., and Rankin, J. (1968). *J. Appl. Physiol.* **24**, 152.
Robinson, S., and Harmon, P. M. (1941a). *Amer. J. Physiol.* **132**, 757.
Robinson, S., and Harmon, P. M. (1941b). *Amer. J. Physiol.* **133**, 161.
Rosenmans, R. H. (1970). *In* "Physical Activity and Aging" (D. Brunner, ed.), pp. 267–273. Univ. Park Press, Baltimore, Maryland.
Rowell, L. B. (1962). Thesis, Univ. of Minnesota, Minneapolis.
Saltin, B., Blomquist, G., Mitchell, J. H., Johnson, R. L., Wildenthal, K., and Chapman, C. B. (1968). *Amer. Heart Ass. Monogr.* **23**.
Saltin, B., Hartley, L. H., Kilbom, Å., and Åstrand, I. (1969). *J. Scand. Clin. Lab. Invest.*
Shephard, R. J., and Anderson, T. W. (1968). *Fed. Proc., Fed. Amer. Soc. Exp. Biol.* **27**, 379.
Skinner, J. (1968). *In* "Exercise Physiology" (H. B. Falls, ed.), Chapter VIII, p. 219. Academic Press, New York.
Sprynarova, S., and Parizkova, J. (1965). *J. Appl. Physiol.* **20**, 934.
Strandell, T. (1964). *Acta Physiol. Scand.* **61**, 279.
Taylor, H. L., Buskirk, E., and Henschel, A. (1955). *J. Appl. Physiol.* **8**, 73.
Taylor, H. L., Henschel, A., Brozek, J., and Keys, A. (1949). *J. Appl. Physiol.* **2**, 233.
Turino, G. M., Bargofsky, E. H., Goldring, R. M., and Fishman, A. P. (1963). *J. Appl. Physiol.* **18**, 447.
Urschell, C. W., Covell, I. W., Sonnenblick, E. H., Ross, J., Jr., and Braunwald, E. (1968). *Amer. J. Physiol.* **214**, 298.
Weissler, A. M., Peller, R. G., and Roehill, W. H. (1961). *Amer. Heart J.* **62**, 367.
Weissler, A. M., Harris, L. C., and White, G. D. (1963). *J. Appl. Physiol.* **18**, 919.
Weissler, A. M., Harris, W. S., and Schoenfeld, C. D. (1968). *Circulation* **37**, 149.
Whitsett, T. L., and Naughton, J. (1971). *Amer. J. Cardiol.* **27**, 352.
Wiggers, C. J. (1922). *Amer. J. Physiol.* **56**, 439.
Willems, J. L., Roelandt, J., DeGeese, H., Kesteloot, H., and Joossens, J. V. (1970). *Circulation* **42**, 37.

PART V

THERAPEUTIC EXERCISE

Chapter 25

EXERCISE AS A THERAPEUTIC MODALITY

VOJIN N. SMODLAKA

Physical exercise is the most important
therapeutic modality of physical medicine.

I. HISTORY

Very early in the prehistoric era, man realized, through experience, that exercising improves the physical ability of a hunter, warrior, worker, and, later, competitor. He also discovered that exercising helps the in-

541

jured regain his physical condition and working capacity. This was the first therapeutic exercise.

Three thousand years ago in ancient China, a physical exercise system was in use called *Cong Fou*. It was a ritual in which men took positions and followed motions prescribed by priests for the relief of pain and other symptoms of diseases (Licht, 1958).

A similar use of exercise as therapy is indicated in ancient manuscripts from India—the Athava-Veda and Ayur-Veda.

Early Grecian medical writing contains many recommendations for the use of exercise to promote health and cure diseases. Hippocrates in his book, "On Regimen," describes the use of exercise in medicine. For centuries his writings were most influential in medical education. From Greece, medical knowledge was disseminated to Ancient Rome and throughout the Middle East. Through the translations of the Arabic physicians, Greek and Roman medicine were transmitted to the Europe of the Renaissance.

The great Greco-Roman physician, Galen, wrote in his book, "On Hygiene," about treatment with exercises. Roman physicians used to combine therapeutic exercises with hydrotherapy, giving massage in natural spas.

In the Middle Ages, there was a gradual decline in the use of exercise due to Christian views of that time, but, during the Renaissance, physical exercise once again gained importance. Educators, philosophers, and physicians have advocated the use of physical exercise ever since.

The Swedish teacher, Per Henrik Ling, had a great influence on the modern use of exercise. His Royal Gymnastic Central Institute in Stockholm, organized in 1813, was the center from where his students dispersed to publicize his system throughout the world. The Ling Gymnastic System, known later as the Swedish System, was introduced and used in the United States.

As a result of the World Wars, particularly World War II, medical and paramedical personnel delved deeper into the problems of rehabilitating the injured veterans, thus developing today's rehabilitation medicine. After World War I, a new specialty in medicine, physical medicine, appeared and became established in different countries. Under the title, physical medicine and rehabilitation, it was granted specialty status in the United States in 1947.

II. MODERN CONCEPTS OF REHABILITATION MEDICINE

In a Report of the Joint Committee of the Public Health Service, the Vocational Rehabilitation Administration, United States Department of Health, Education and Welfare (1963), the following definitions of Rehabilitation Medicine are given:

> Rehabilitation is a dynamic process of re-establishment of the disabled person's capacity to sense and participate in his environment and communicate with others; to adapt to the physical world, which includes ability to tolerate physical energy expenditure while resuming activities of daily living; and to utilize fully his intellectual, social and vocational potentialities.
>
> Rehabilitation is the process of restoring the disabled to optimal physical, mental, social, vocational and economic usefulness.
>
> Rehabilitation Medicine has frequently been termed the "third phase of medicine," following "preventive medicine" and "curative medicine and surgery." It is the period when the "fever is down and the stitches are out" (Rusk, 1964). The goal is to eliminate, reduce or alleviate the disability, to train and teach the person "to live and to work within the limits of the disability but to the height of his capabilities." Rehabilitation is "the restoration through personal health, services of handicapped individuals to the fullest physical, mental, social and economic usefulness of which they are capable, including ordinary treatment and treatment in special rehabilitation centers" (Krusen et al., 1966).

III. THERAPEUTIC EXERCISE

Therapeutic exercise is an important modality in the process of physical and medical rehabilitation. It helps to develop and maintain the general physical condition and muscle function, especially in strength and endurance; it prevents disuse atrophy; it helps restore proper posture and body alignment; and it improves cardiopulmonary function.

In combination with sports and recreational activities, formal exercises help the subject to develop coordination of movements and the skill to perform complex tasks.

The positive effect of therapeutic exercise is based on the biological principle that "function develops the organ." Use develops and disuse atrophies an organ. Immobilization of the entire body or any of its parts has negative effects, causing atrophy and deterioration of the physical condition and qualities. Such negative effects manifest themselves in a decrease of muscle mass, muscle strength, heart volume, heart diameter, and oxygen intake, and an increase in heart rate and secretion of nitrogen, calcium, potassium, sodium, or phosphate through the urine, feces, etc. (Deitrick et al., 1948; Taylor et al., 1949).

Physical exercise affects the organ in two ways, morphologically and functionally. Usually, the morphological values increase and the functional values decrease. The muscles, lungs, heart, bones, etc., increase

TABLE I

Classification of Muscle Strength by Manual Evaluation Recommended by the
National Foundation for Birth Defects and Poliomyelitis[a]

0. 0	Zero, 0%	No evidence of contraction
1. T	Trace, 10%	Evidence of contraction but not of joint motion
2. P	Poor, 25%	Full range of motion; gravity eliminated
3. F	Fair, 50%	Full range against gravity
4. G	Good, 75%	Movement against gravity and moderate resistance at least 10 times without fatigue
5. N	Normal, 100%	Full range against gravity and full resistance

[a] Adapted from T. F. Hines. (1958). Manual muscle examination. *In* "Therapeutic Exercise" (S. Licht, ed.), Vol. III, Chart III, p. 170. Elizabeth Licht, New Haven, Connecticut.

in size. The circulation time, heart rate, cardiac output, blood pressure, respiration rate, etc., decrease in their resting values in both healthy individuals and patients.

IV. EVALUATION OF EXERCISE EFFECTS

The medical control of healthy persons and patients is based on periodic examinations in which the physician evaluates the morphological and functional qualities and compares them to study the effect of regular training. For example, the heart rate, which decreases at rest as a result of exercise during a reconditioning program, is the parameter most commonly used to evaluate the physical condition of the subject.

The Manual Muscle Test is recommended by the National Foundation for Infantile Paralysis to evaluate muscle strength (Table I).

In order to evaluate the range of motion of a joint, we use a goniometer.

V. CLASSIFICATIONS OF FUNCTIONAL CAPACITIES

There are different clinical classifications for emphysema pateints, cardiacs, and amputees. Classifications help us to evaluate the patient and to follow the progress of the patient's malady or rehabilitation (Tables II, III, and IV).

TABLE II

Classification of Emphysema Patients according to Their Work Capacities[a]

Grade I:	Can keep pace walking with person of same age and body build on the level without breathlessness but not on hills or stairs
Grade II:	Can walk a mile at his own pace without dyspnea, but cannot keep pace on the level with normal persons
Grade III:	Becomes breathless after walking about 100 yards or for a few minutes on the level
Grade IV:	Becomes breathless by dressing or talking

[a] H. W. Harris, G. R. Meneely, A. D. Renzetti, Jr., J. D. Steele, and J. D. Wyatt. (1962). A statement by the chairman of the Committee for Non-Tuberculous Respiratory Diseases. *Amer. Rev. Resp. Dis.* **85,** 762–768.

TABLE III

Classification of Cardiac Patients according to Their Functional Capacities and by the Amount of Physical Activity Recommended[a]

Functional Capacity Classification

Class I:	No limitation of physical activity
Class II:	Slight limitation of physical activity
Class III:	Marked limitation of physical activity
Class IV:	Unable to carry on any physical activity without discomfort

Therapeutic Classification

Class A:	No restriction to physical activity
Class B:	Moderate restriction of severe efforts
Class C:	Restriction of ordinary physical activity; strenuous efforts should be discontinued
Class D:	Ordinary physical activity should be markedly restricted
Class E:	Patient confined to bed or chair—complete bed rest

[a] Adapted from Criteria Committee of the New York Heart Association (1964). "Diseases of the Heart and Blood Vessels—Nomenclature and Criteria for Diagnosis," pp. 112–114. Little, Brown, Boston, Massachusetts.

TABLE IV

Classification of Amputees with Prostheses according to Their Functional Capacities in the Use of the Prostheses[a]

Class I:	Full restoration; patient is disabled but not unable
Class II:	Partial restoration
Class III:	Self-care; can walk but works in the wheelchair
Class IV:	Self-care but needs help
Class V:	Cosmetics

[a] Adapted from A. Russek. (1961). Management of lower extremity amputees. *Arch. Phys. Med.* **42,** 687–703.

VI. THERAPEUTIC EXERCISES

A. Passive Exercises

Passive exercises are performed without the active participation of the patient. The physical therapist moves a part of the paralyzed body through its full range of motion to preserve motion of the particular joint.

B. Active Assistive Exercises

Active assistive exercises are performed with the help of a therapist when the patient has some voluntary motion.

C. Active Exercises

Active exercises are performed by the patient alone, going through a full range of motion, if possible. They are performed as needed to increase the range of motion, muscle power, and endurance of the particular part of the body.

D. Progressive Resistive Exercises

Progressive resistive exercises are performed by the patient with resistance supplied by the therapist, or with the resistance of weights, pulleys, dynamometers, ergometers, or other such gym equipment and apparatus.

E. Sports and Games

Coaches, in the process of conditioning their athletes, face the problem daily of how much exercise to prescribe and when. Some use very intensive training, others more moderate training, but all with seemingly similar results!

VII. GUIDELINES FOR PRESCRIBING EXERCISES

The exact dosage of exercise, indications, and contraindications, or, to be more precise, the pharmacology and pharmacopeia of exercise, is yet unknown. Future research will give us a thorough pharmacology of exercise. There are some guidelines, however, based on clinical experience, to follow in prescribing therapeutic exercise.

It is accepted that a daily physical educational lesson for general reconditioning should last 45 minutes. If work is to be done on a small group of muscles, the session may be shorter. Each session may be performed daily, or it may be repeated two or three times a week.

The best results while reconditioning patients with low cardiopulmonary reserve (i.e., cardiacs, the very old, or emphysema patients) appear to come with three sessions a week. These patients need one day of rest between exercise sessions.

Fatigue is the enemy of training. Exercise should stop when fatigue occurs.

As a general rule, the duration and intensity of the exercise should be increased gradually. To increase the endurance, the length of the session should be increased.

A reconditioning program for a young, robust patient should last at least six weeks. For an older patient with low potentials, the program must last longer—perhaps 12, 18, or 24 weeks.

The process of adaptation takes time. For example, it takes at least six weeks for an alpinist to adapt to the high altitude of the Himalaya Mountains!

VIII. THERAPEUTIC EXERCISES IN SKELETAL AND JOINT DISEASES

Fractures, amputations, bone diseases, osteoporosis, dislocations, and subluxations are customarily treated in acute, subacute, and some in chronic stages with immobilization, bed rest, splinting, casting, traction, and nonweight-bearing. For these reasons, the immobilized structures atrophy, losing morphological and functional qualities.

To prevent atrophy through disuse, physicians shorten the time of immobilization as much as possible. As soon as it is indicated, the physician prescribes passive, active assistive, active, and finally, progressive resistive exercises to preserve or regain full joint range of motion, strength, endurance, and skill to the affected structures. A gradual increase of the range of motion and resistance to muscle contraction is the general routine.

IX. THERAPEUTIC EXERCISES IN CARDIOPULMONARY DISEASES

Patients with cardiopulmonary diseases such as congenital anomalies, arteriosclerotic heart disease, coronary heart disease, angina pectoris, myocardial infarction, hypertension, peripheral vascular disease, asthma, pulmonary fibrosis, emphysema, postpneumonia, and postpleurisy states and patients who have undergone surgery for these conditions require a well-organized rehabilitation program to recondition them to their former capacities.

This gradual program consists of general calisthenic exercises for the musculature, breathing exercises for the chest muscles, and walking, jogging, and cycling for the cardiovascular system. Training may be performed using either the continuous or interval training method.

The interval training method is recommended for patients with low cardiopulmonary reserve, using short intervals of work (30 seconds) and short intervals of rest (60 seconds), intermittently 30 times in a daily exercise session of 45 minutes (Smodlaka, 1966).

Patients with low cardiopulmonary reserve and poor physical condition should perform their daily activities in short intervals of work and rest. They may walk one short block and stop to recover, or they may stop to recover after taking several steps in walking to the upper floors to their apartments. After a period of well-balanced work and rest sessions, the patients reach the upper floors without difficulty.

Working in intervals is a natural method for these patients. Under laboratory conditions, the bicycle ergometer is used, permitting resistance to be applied gradually to measure the exact work load of the reconditioning training program. Later the exercise may be replaced by walking, jogging, cycling, or swimming. These activities may be prescribed quite accurately.

X. THE PRINCIPLE OF SUBSTITUTION

In the process of rehabilitating a disabled patient, emphasis is placed on keeping the normal organs functioning well rather than on improving the disabled organs. The normal organs have to be trained to take on the added load and to continue to work. Hypertrophy will be achieved through therapeutic exercises.

REFERENCES

Deitrick, J. E. *et al.* (1948). *Amer. J. Med.* 4, 3–36.
Krusen, F., Kottke, F. J., and Ellwood, P. M. (1966). *In* "Handbook of Physical Medicine and Rehabilitation," p. 1 Saunders, Philadelphia, Pennsylvania.

Licht, S., ed. (1958). "Therapeutic Exercise," Vol. III, Chapter 16, pp. 380–422. Elizabeth Licht, New Haven, Connecticut.

Report of the Joint Committee of the Public Health Service and the Vocational Rehabilitation Administration. (1963). "Areawide Planning of Facilities for Rehabilitation Services," p. 1. U.S. Department of Health, Education, and Welfare, Public Health Service, Washington, D.C.

Rusk, H. (1964). In "Rehabilitation Medicine," 2nd ed., p. 11. Mosby, St. Louis, Missouri.

Smodlaka, V. N. (1966). In "Prevention of Ischemic Heart Disease: Principles and Practice." (W. Raab, ed.), Chapter 44, pp. 351–358. Thomas, Springfield, Illinois.

Taylor, L. H. et al. (1949). J. Appl. Physiol. 2, 233–239.

Chapter 26

TEAMWORK IN EXERCISE THERAPY

VOJIN N. SMODLAKA

I. THE PHYSICIAN

The complete rehabilitation of a patient takes the combined effort of many professionals from the medical, paramedical, and social fields. This entails teamwork under the leadership of a physician, generally, a physician specialized in rehabilitation medicine. A physiatrist spends three years as a resident in an approved department of rehabilitation medicine. In addition, he is required to pass the two parts of the Specialty Board examination, the second part taken after practicing two years in the field.

Others who may lead the team work are orthopedic surgeons, general

551

practitioners, or such specialists as consultants in internal medicine, neurology, pediatrics, surgery, psychiatry, etc.

In most instances, the family physician takes care of the patient. He may refer the patient to a specialist for consultation. If the patient needs a particular rehabilitation program, he may be referred to a rehabilitation department, unit, institution, or a physiatrist who will establish the program and work with his own rehabilitation team.

II. PARAMEDICAL WORKERS

Such a team consists of physical therapists, nurses, occupational therapists, specialists in communicative disorders, recreational therapists, clinical psychologists, social workers, prosthetists, physical educators, and vocational counselors. Of these, only the physical, occupational, and recreational therapists, physical educator, prothetist, and clinical psychologist are ordinarily directly involved in exercise therapy.

A. The Physical Therapist

The physical therapist is the professional who applies physical therapy and therapeutic exercises, prescribed by the physician, to the patient. He may use all the therapeutic modalities, which include heat, cold, light, hydrotherapy, electrotherapy, and therapeutic exercises. His educational requirements consist of a Bachelor's degree or a certificate in physical therapy. Many physical therapists have taken postgraduate courses and hold a Master of Science degree. In order to practice physical therapy, the therapist must be licensed and have passed the State Board examination. Some physical therapists have been trained in physical education.

B. The Occupational Therapist

The occupational therapist uses work as therapeutic activity. He will stimulate the affected part of the patient's body to work, move, exercise, and produce. The patient is psychologically involved in the productive process. In order to provide all the facilities necessary for a diversified program, the occupational therapist should have a workshop with all the necessary equipment. These therapists require a Bachelor of Science degree in addition to passing the National Board examination to obtain a license to practice.

C. The Recreational Therapist

The recreational therapist organizes recreational activities for patients in the hospital. He serves those patients who are in a chronic stage and those whose hospital stay is lengthy. These activities may be performed at bedside or in rooms assigned for recreational activities, thus helping the patient enjoy his hospital stay. A Bachelor's degree is the requirement for a recreational therapist. The organization and supervision of games activities involving considerable physical activity may be the responsibility of the recreational therapist.

D. The Clinical Psychologist

The clinical psychologist works with patients, evaluating their mental and emotional status. He performs psychotherapy, either individually or in groups. These workers are psychologists with special postgraduate training in clinical psychology with either a Master's degree or a doctorate. He fills an important role in orienting the patient to the need for physical activity as a key part of his rehabilitation.

E. The Prosthetist

Prosthetists are professionals who make prostheses, braces, splints, and other necessary supports for disabled persons. They are craftsmen who work along with other members of the rehabilitation team to fit the patient with the best designed supports. This equipment must be designed in such a way as to facilitate exercise activity.

F. The Physical Educator

The physical educator may be a member of the rehabilitation team in situations in which sports and games are used in the rehabilitation process. The modern approach to patients with myocardial infarctions, cardiac conditions, and other high-risk factors is to have physical educators teach the patients sports and games. He works closely with the physical and recreational therapists.

G. The Patient

Finally, the most important member of the rehabilitation team is the patient. The patient's rehabilitation depends very much on his motivation, his mental disposition, and physical level of ability.

A very important factor involved is motivation. How to motivate a patient or even a normal person is the problem in rehabilitation as it is in education. Members of the team try to motivate the patient by establishing a good personal relationship, collaborating with him, and helping him become active and participate in the program. It is an art to motivate people to physical activity.

III. FACILITIES

In order to perform a well-organized program of rehabilitation, a rehabilitation team should have at its disposal a gymnasium, appropriate space for hydrotherapy, electrotherapy, speech therapy, psychotherapy, workshops for occupational therapy, and a spacious, well-lit recreation area.

The better centers around the world have indoor and outdoor facilities, with playgrounds and swimming pools within parks surrounded by grass and trees. In such centers, the program is comprehensive, diversified, dynamic, and complete.

This is one of the reasons why many old spas have been transformed into rehabilitation and recreational centers. There, balneological and climatological factors and modalities are combined with modern concepts and modalities of physical medicine and rehabilitation.

The Gymnasium

The most important facility is the gymnasium. This is a room in which a small number of individuals may exercise under the supervision of physical therapists. It may be very large, depending on the number of therapists working there. The equipment includes the usual items used in physical education, but, in addition, other appropriate equipment for use by the disabled is included.

Gymnasium Equipment

a. Parallel Bars. In order to teach a patient how to stand, walk, and transfer independently, parallel bars are most useful.

b. Mats. For exercising in the lying or sitting positions and for general reconditioning of body muscles, mats are used for almost all patients.

c. Pulleys. In order to perform progressive resistive exercises, different weights are used, beginning with a collection of dumbbells, bags, and pulleys. Using an appropriate position, a muscle or a synergist muscle group may be exercised and trained. The therapist knows the functional anatomy and is able to train each affected muscle.

d. Balls. Finally, balls of various sizes are used for appropriate exercises of the body parts or the entire organism. The therapist has to adapt the games to a patient's disability and specific needs by organizing the appropriate games.

IV. GROUP THERAPY

Each patient requires much personal attention, supervision, and assistance. Handling one patient at a time is very common. There are a large number of apparatus and machines that are used in the process of reconditioning. These machines save time and allow the therapist to treat more patients at one time.

Where there are a large number of patients involved with the same or similar pathology, group therapy may be organized. They would form "shoulder," "elbow and hand," and "knee or ankle" groups. Usually, eight to twelve patients are selected and they exercise together. The therapist saves time and the patients are psychologically stimulated while exercising in groups. Here, the competitive factor becomes involved.

V. CONTINUITY OF REHABILITATION

After a disease or injury, the patient may recover completely without any disability, defect, invalidism, or functional deficit. Others are affected for life. Young persons have to face their disability and learn to live with it. The rehabilitation program, therefore, must be designed to fit the patient's situation, age, and status.

A young, disabled person may have to have a long rehabilitation program and be under constant supervision until he is an adult. Once he reaches the plateau of his capabilities, the disabled person has to have a "maintenance program" to preserve the achievement.

The aging process affects the disabled patient more than a normal person. For this reason, the aging disabled subject has to work harder at his conditioning program.

VI. SPORTS FOR THE DISABLED

In countries with high standards of physical culture, disabled persons, invalids, veterans, cripples, etc., are organized to exercise and participate in all sports activities and compete in local, national, and international championships.

Today we have the parolympics movement of competition by paraplegics in many sports, skiing by amputees and the blind, and swimming by many others.

In the history of sports, many disabled persons have competed with success and were national and international victors.

People must be made aware that disabled persons can be rehabilitated and educated to live with their disabilities and compete with other "normals" in their daily, professional, and recreational life. This is the final goal of rehabilitation.

Chapter 27

EXERCISE AND OBESITY

J. A. DEMPSEY

I. INTRODUCTION

Is muscular exercise an important determinant in the etiology, prevention, and treatment of obesity? This hypothesis is (1) readily confirmed by the exercise evangelist who would lump coronary artery and chronic lung disease under the same "exercise-is-good-for-you" umbrella; (2) explicitly denied in print, or most important in practice, by most clinicians or (3) given a highly qualified and usually skeptical "nonanswer" from the biochemist, endocrinologist, physiologist, or morphologist. Unfortunately, solutions to both the stated hypothesis and condition in question remain unresolved. However, in the last decade laboratory findings of significance, some even classical, based on current fact rather than tradition, and, indeed, the very controversy and skepticism alluded to above have stimulated a vigorous, multidisciplinary attack on the problem of obesity. This chapter provides a brief review of recent findings and concepts concerning the recognition, causes, consequences, treatment, and prognosis in obesity. Then, application of these findings to the question of exercise and obesity is attempted, with specific emphasis on exercise pathophysiology and implications for treatment.

II. OBESITY—A PERSPECTIVE OF RECENT FINDINGS*

A. Recognition

It is probably correct to define obesity as a chronic disturbance in homeostatic function—in this case, "excessive fatness." The controversy in this area stems from an apparent need for further delineation of what characterizes excessive fatness. To devotees of the study of statistics and body composition, the popular usage of body weight standards or percent overweight for height and age represents a gross oversimplification of the obese state. These "average" body weight standards (drawn from data on life insurance policy holders) have received a variety of criticisms including inaccurate measurement and sampling procedures, failure to differentiate among variations in body type or somatotype, and, most importantly, the fact that total body weight is simply too gross an index for purposes of assessing body composition, e.g., excessive fatness versus excessive muscularity. Several alternate methods of body composition assessment are currently available. Most readily applicable to clinical situations are relatively simple caliper measures of skin fold fat. Population studies in Britain (Tanner and Whitehouse, 1962) and the U.S. (Corbin, 1969) have yielded quantitative data on age trends in skin fold fat from early childhood to middle age. In addition, Pryor (1959) has established "normative" weight standards across various ages which consider interindividual somatotype variation based on simple measurements of body diameter and stature.

To the physician faced with the 5 foot 7 inch, 460 pound, 25-year-old patient, or to the housewife experiencing "creeping overweight" in middle age, recognition of "excessive fatness" hardly requires sophisticated assessment techniques or, in fact, any objective measurements at all.

*The brevity of this review permits only highly selective reference to recent findings. The interested reader is referred to recent reviews of specific topics by Gordon (1969, 1970), Wilson (1969), Penick and Stunkard (1970), and Bray (1971). Jean Mayer has also recently provided a comprehensive review of his work (1968).

While in most cases of obesity in adults, then, the argument over precise definition of excessive fatness is probably superfluous, there are a number of situations in both clinical practice and research where credence should be paid to reported findings concerning anatomical characterization of the obese state.

1. Evaluation of Findings

Considerable confusion in the iterature has been perpetuated through failure to recognize the complexity of the obese state. For example, widely different concepts concerning the psychogenic nature of obesity have been ardently advocated by groups who were actually investigating grossly dissimilar populations of "obese" children, i.e., outpatients seeking psychiatric care versus those persons who were "selected" because they exceeded the average weight norm by two standard deviations (Bruch et al., 1958). Furthermore, it has been difficult to evaluate the relative effects of various treatment regimens because the reporting of total body weight changes fails to reveal the highly complex fat and/or "fat-free" and/or fluid composition of the weight loss or gain.

2. Ideal Body Weight

Attempts to define anatomically or to predict an individual's so-called "ideal" or desirable body weight have developed because of the obvious inadequacy of average height–weight tables for this purpose. Essentially, this approach individualizes the definition of obesity by stipulating a chosen range of fatness that is permissible in relation to frame size and muscular development (Behnke, 1969). This concept of individualized ideal body weight is certainly worth consideration, particularly in defining realistic goals for the patient. At the same time, such concepts are inherently dangerous if oversimplified by the practitioner. For example, purely literal translation of this morphological definition of "ideal" body weight (1) ignores a multiple etiology for the obese state and, hence, a disregard for such desirable and realistic therapeutic goals as a return toward normal cardiopulmonary function, physical performance capability, psychiatric "normalcy," etc., or (2) overlooks the critical observation that simple "stoutness" or moderate obesity is (in the adult or particularly in the young adolescent) not necessarily undesirable or less than ideal in functional terms. Surely, the decision to impose the "risks" of such common measures as dietary restriction and/or drug therapy and to what extent should be based on broadly based criteria that recognize morphological–functional relationships.

3. Obesity and Maturation

It is the area of obesity in childhood to which valid principles of obesity recognition should be most carefully applied. Those observations alone which show (1) that 50% or more of obese adults were obese children and (2) that 75–80% of those with juvenile obesity became obese adults clearly point to a need for early diagnosis. Some findings concerning the question, "How are children fat?" may be helpful: (1) two age peaks for the onset of juvenile obesity have been identified, 0–4 years and 7–11 years; (2) maturation rates are usually slightly abnormal, the obese showing earlier menarche by about one year, greater height, and advanced bone age; (3) the excess body weight and fat in the obese child may or may not be accompanied by an increased fat-free body mass depending on the age of onset of excessive fatness. There is, however, unanimous agreement with the concept that endomorphy is a basic trait in the body type of the obese child; (4) the obese child who becomes an obese adult shows a relatively progressive increase in body fat throughout childhood and adolescence above the normal growth curve, with little or no differentiation between sexes. In normal weight children, however, a "physiological fat spurt" is often observed at pubescence, and during adolescence a sex differentiation occurs with females continuing to develop adiposity at an increasing rate, and males decreasing or plateauing in body fat content.

An awareness, then, that the growth process is a highly complex, dynamic process points to the necessity for longitudinal assessment of abnormal deviations in body weight and fat content throughout all phases of childhood. Such an approach together with an appropriate regard for family history should play a dual role in both recognizing early onset obesity and preventing the all too common error of mistaking a physiological fat spurt for the pathological onset of chronic obesity.

B. Etiology

Conventional clinical thinking easily assigns the cause of obesity to the intake of more calories than are expended during the time of their consumption. Aside from being a confession of faith in the first law of thermodynamics, this concept tends to confuse a result with a cause. As has been pointed out on a number of occasions one could as well say that the *cause* of edema is a gain of salt and water to the body, or that the *cause* of alcoholism is excessive consumption of spirits. A multitude of regulatory, metabolic, endocrine, and nutritional disorders has been hypothesized. Accumulation of research findings does, however, permit some separation of cause from effect, leaving few possibilities that may be considered as primary or initiating causes.

As is now common clinical practice in determining the risk "factors" in coronary artery disease or diabetes, the possibility of a genetic basis for obesity has gained some recognition primarily from the results of animal studies (Bray, 1971). The numerous studies in humans completed on this topic all suffer from an inability to distinguish conclusively between genotype and phenotype (Mayer, 1965). Nonetheless, accumulated evidence does permit at least the tentative conclusion that genetic factors dictate a predisposition toward overweight. The major question, then, is really one of labeling or defining the genetic trait or predisposing factor that stimulates the genesis of obesity. Although several classifications of causative mechanisms in obesity have been postulated, they may be conveniently broken down into endocrine and metabolic and regulatory. Much of what has been recently uncovered in these areas fits poorly with traditionally accepted concepts concerning the pathogenesis of obesity.

1. Regulatory

When the food intakes of obese and normal weight individuals are accurately studied and compared, the average obese person is shown to be euphagic (Penick and Stunkard, 1970). Furthermore, psychiatric study of unselected groups of obese individuals shows a wide spectrum of emotional adjustment from stability to incapacitating mental illness. More recent findings reveal that hyperphagia in the obese is manifested only in an environment which presents completely unrestricted food supply (Schacter, 1968). These analyses hardly fit the oversimplification that all obese persons present a picture of voracious overeating which drives the patient in a way that a desire for narcotics drives the addict.

2. Endocrine and Metabolic

Although one occasionally encounters the BMR test as part of the routine diagnostic workup in clinical obesity, it is now widely recognized that hypothyroidism is rarely, if ever, a cause of obesity. Similarly, *in vitro* studies of human adipose tissue have dispelled earlier theories that the obese possesses a decreased ability for fatty acid mobilization or excessive enzymatic activity associated with lipogenesis (Hood and Bjornthorp, 1966; Shrago *et al.* 1967; Mosinger *et al.*, 1965).

3. Other Possible Causes

What then is available as a basic mechanism that may serve as a true precursor of obesity? Two possibilities have arisen from recent findings that, while speculative at present, serve to illustrate the sophistication with which these problems are being attacked.

a. The prevalence of childhood obesity has been clearly linked with excessive weight gain in the first six months of life (Eid, 1970). Furthermore, a series of studies in man and animals has established that, the earlier (in life) obesity onset occurs, the greater the development of adipose tissue cell number. Thus, excessive adiposity comprises an approximately threefold greater than normal adipose tissue cell number when the age of onset is less than 10 years, but only a cellular hypertrophy or augmented lipid content per cell with adult onset obesity. Further findings revealed that the cellular hyperplasia, once established, was irreversible, and that total fat reduction was achieved only through reduction of cell content and size (Salans et al., 1971; Hirsch and Knittle, 1970). What stimuli are available to initiate cellular hyperplasia in adipose tissue? In adipose tissue, as in other organ systems, it is now clear that early under- or overnutrition in animals is a critical factor in regulating permanent changes in cell number (Knittle and Hirsch, 1968; Pace and Rathburn, 1945; McCance, 1962). Cheek et al. (1970) attributed the effects of early overnutrition on cell size and number (in human fat and muscle tissue) to hormonal factors. Furthermore, in vitro analyses have described an augmented synthesis of DNA (in resonse to human serum) in the adipose tissue of obese persons.

b. Another possibility for a primary defect in obesity concerns recent findings on the long-held concept of an interindividual variability in metabolic or thermodynamic efficiency. The glycerophosphate pathway in liver and adipose tissue serves as a critical regulator of the efficiency with which oxidation and phosphorylation are coupled, as α-glycerophosphate is an essential precursor in adipose tissue for triglyceride synthesis from glucose. Recent work has shown that the adipose tissue of obese persons is characterized by an excessive lipogenesis from glucose and an increased supply of α-glycerophosphate secondary to a deficiency of intramitochondrial glycerophosphate dehydrogenase (Bjornthorp, 1966; Galton and Bray, 1967; Bray, 1969). That this deficiency in mitochondrial oxidation of α-glycerophosphate might be a true primary cause of obesity is supported by its presence in obesity of early onset and its absence in obese patients with regulatory obesity secondary to intracranial lesions. On the other hand, the activity of the glycerophosphate pathway is also affected by diet—both by amount and type and by thyroid hormone (Bray, 1969).

These recent findings at the cellular and subcellular level present exciting hypotheses to the beleaguered search for an objective metabolic etiology for obesity. The practical application for such postulates and the firm establishment of their validity as true precursors to human obesity awaits future work into the stimulus role of endocrine, behavioral, genetic, and nutritional factors, or their combination.

C. Consequences

1. Psychosociology

The older psychiatric literature has served to confuse the field, in the main primarily because of its attempt to define a "basic" set of sociopsychological traits or "familial constellation" of factors in the obese through the study of highly selective yet diverse patient populations (Bruch, 1963; Mendelson, 1964). The evidence has, however, clearly pointed out that "some" of these persons do indeed suffer in reaction from the everpresent pressure of society's derogatory attitude toward excessive fatness. Accordingly, the marked onset of weight gain in some patients has been traced to a traumatic social event. Peer status is significantly lacking in the obese child, claims of widespread discriminatory social practices with the obese adolescent are akin to minority group discrimination, and, recently, socioeconomic status and obesity have been shown to bear a close, inverse relationship to each other (Morello and Mayer, 1963; Borjeson, 1962; Silverstone et al., 1969; Goldblatt et al., 1965). A recent series of studies by Stunkard and Burt (1967) and Glucksman and Hirsch (1969) were concerned with the question of disturbances in body image—one of the few psychopathological characteristics specific to obesity. These studies showed basic disturbances in body image (in about 50% of the randomly selected group of obese persons) to occur in three areas: in an almost revolting view of their own body; in an intense self-consciousness and even misconception of how others viewed them; and in a self-consciousness in relation to the opposite sex, promoting a behavior that ranged anywhere from avoidance to hateful devaluation. These disturbances in body image were largely confined to persons who were obese during their impressionable adolescent years. In addition, studies during weight reduction in obese adults suggest that the internalized image of the body size of these patients was relatively fixed. It could not be altered nearly as easily as the actual change in body configuration.

2. Pathophysiology

Primarily as a result of epidemiological evidence and patient case studies, obesity has been associated with a wide variety of health hazards, although definitive knowledge of cause–effect relationships is lacking. The high mortality rate of overweight individuals is well documented, and is most often attributed to cardiac dysfunction. Epidemiological investigation permits three generalizations concerning obesity and systemic hypertension (Kagan, 1963; Bjerkedahl, 1957): hypertension is more prevalent in the obese; the obese person experiences a greater risk of coronary artery disease when either or both hypertension or hypercholesteremia are also present; and mortality rates for obese persons who are hypertensive are higher than for obesity or hypertension alone. Alexander's definitive studies show a high incidence of systemic and pulmonary hypertension in the obese, but an even more consistent cardiac enlargement secondary to left ventricular hypertrophy which often lead to congestive heart failure (Alexander *et al.*, 1962; Alexander and Pettigrove, 1967; Alexander and Petersen, 1968; Amad and Alexander, 1965). The increased volume work load on the heart is probably due to the high cardiac output and blood volume in the obese which serve higher flow and metabolic requirements of an excessive adipose tissue mass. The degree to which hemodynamic deterioration is manifested and intensified in the obese adult is greatly diminished in the absence of progressive fat accumulation (Alexander and Lufschanowski, 1969).

Pulmonary dysfunction in the obese has been greatly misunderstood. It is probably correct to conclude that excessive fatness (and, hence, increased intra-abdominal pressure) usually causes a decreased expiratory reserve volume and lung compliance, high mechanical work rates, and an increased metabolic cost of respiration (Sharp, 1964; Naimark and Cherniack, 1960). With less confidence, it may be expected that gross obesity will often be accompanied by nonuniform ventilation to perfusion distribution, and, hence, by varying degrees of arterial hypoxemia (Holley, 1967). The source of confusion in this area resides in the prevalence of the so-called "Pickwickian syndrome" in obesity, which involves alveolar hypoventilation, somnolence, periodic respiration, cyanosis, polycythemia, pulmonary hypertension, right ventricular hypertrophy, and failure. From the time of the first case description in 1955, it has become the popular notion that all obese patients who were somnolent were "Pickwickians." However, studies of the unselected obese population clearly show that alveolar hypoventilation develops in only about 10% of extremely obese adults, that the degree of hypercapnia is severe in less than 5% and is uncorrelated with "excess" body weight, and that a portion of this latter group has coincident pulmonary (airway) disease (Bedell *et al.*, 1958; Alexander *et al.*, 1962). Furthermore, isolated right ventricular hypertrophy and failure probably occurs rarely, if at all, in obese persons and has never been documented at necropsy (Amad and Alexander, 1965).

Finally, obesity most likely exerts an important compounding influence on established diseases. This synergistic effect is most obvious in such states as the physical immobilization accompanying arthritis and other varieties of bone and joint disease, with the ventilatory limitations of chronic obstructive lung disease, and with the insulin insensitivity of adult-onset diabetes. It is instructive to remember with respect to the majority of abnormalities outlined above that their incidence and severity bears no linear relationship to the degree of excessive fatness over a wide continuum. Nor is there sufficient knowledge concerning the natural history of the various diseases coincident with obesity, such as their time of onset, their progression, or, in fact, in most cases, their true causal relationship to excessive fatness.

3. Self-Perpetuation of Obesity

Without question, the evidence is overwhelming that the most severe consequence of obesity is its self-perpetuation. This statement is generally supported from longitudinal clinical studies which have shown the remarkable stability of the obese state once initiated. The odds against an obese child becoming a normal weight adult are 4 to 1. For an obese adolescent, they are 28 to 1, and, with this progressive attainment of adult obesity, there is, approximately, less than a 90% probability that one will (with frequent but only transient relief) spend the remainder of his years in this state. While many factors (including a variety of "self-protective" psychogenic manifestations) have been proposed in an attempt to explain this treadmill of corpulence, recent findings point to two specific physiological mechanisms.

a. CELLULAR HYPERPLASIA. Alluded to earlier as a "primary" precursor in the pathogenesis of obesity is the concept that there is a critical period during the growth cycle (in childhood or in infancy) during which obesity develops via irreversible adipose tissue cell hyperplasia. It has been shown further that the person with adult-onset obesity reduces his excessive fatness "simply" by emptying his adipose tissue cells of their excessive load of fat. One suffering from juvenile-onset obesity, however, might be able to achieve a similar degree of weight loss only by decreasing the fat content of the excessive number of adipose tissue cells to abnormally low concentrations. Clinical experience accords well with these predictions, i.e., juvenile-onset obesity is much more resistant to treatment than obesity beginning in adult life.

b. INSULIN INSENSITIVITY. Disordered glucose metabolism is commonly observed in obesity, and kinetic studies of utilization in obese patients have demonstrated a reduction in the disappearance rate and uptake of glucose from the blood (Grodsky, 1969; Franckson, 1966). That this disorder is attributable to the presence of insulin resistance of both fat and muscle tissue is well documented by the common observation of hyperinsulinemia in the obese nondiabetic (Bagade *et al.*, 1967; Salans *et al.*, 1970) and by *in vivo* and *in vitro* studies of peripheral tissue insulin resistance in both spontaneous and experimentally induced obesity (Horton *et al.*, 1970). The nature of the insulin resistance is determined at least in part by the expansion of adipose tissue cells, although the state of nutrition and growth period might also be contributing factors (Bray, 1969; Salans and Dougherty, 1971). The precipitation of disordered glucose metabolism by obesity is clear, that is, weight loss and/or reduction of fat cell size returns circulating insulin levels and pancreatic insulin production, glucose tolerance, and peripheral insulin resistance all to within normal levels (Grodsky, 1969).

D. Treatment and Prognosis

Extensive reviews of the results of treatment for obesity over the past three decades have revealed discouraging yet consistent conclusions. Most obese adults will not enter formal treatment; of those who do, almost all will lose weight as hospitalized inpatients, but few on an outpatient basis; and, of those who lose weight during the formalized treatment, less than 15% will maintain the loss, approximately 5% will reduce further, and 1–2% will approach their "ideal" body weight (Stunkard and McLaren-Hume, 1959; Glennon, 1966). Less extensive long-term study of the obese child reveal similar findings (as pointed out earlier), with the result that the adult with juvenile-onset obesity has undergone a long series of treatments and failures—a typical life style appropriately coined "the rhythm method of girth control" (Mullins, 1959; Abraham and Nordsieck, 1960).

Why is obesity, by statistical criteria, incurable, when it is obviously controllable in the short-term through manipulation of one's environment? Certainly there are metabolic and psychological bases, as outlined in the previous section, for expecting difficulty with either sustaining fat reduction in established obesity or preventing fat accumulation in adolescent obesity. Recent reviews, however, have been unanimous in their condemnation of popular and traditional therapeutic practices:

> Recent evaluations by the FDA show ". . . an almost unbelievable amount of quackery occurring regularly in the field of weight control"; which is, perhaps, ". . . a natural occurrence in a country that can boast of the highest incidence of obesity in the world" (Gordon, 1970).

> Therapeutic maneuvers aimed at the result of a disturbed physiology, while often satisfying to the physician, are never as effective as those that succeed in adjusting the underlying mechanisms (Wallace, 1964).

> The [traditional medical] model defines an authoritarian role for the physician, who prescribes a diet and appetite depressing medication. The patient loses weight to please the doctor and to meet his expectations. When the relationship is terminated or attenuated, the patient discontinues the diet and regains weight (Penick and Stunkard, 1970).

Recent research findings in the area of obesity treatment have not as yet had sufficient time nor clinical trial to be judged worthy of practical application. However, they do provide a basis for some speculation in terms of the direction future therapeutic programs should pursue.

1. Prevention

The arguments in favor of prevention are overwhelming. Summarizing earlier discussion in this review concerning the "treadmill of corpulence," it is now clear that there is a firm metabolic and psychogenic basis for either avoiding the onset of obesity or controlling its progress at the time of onset. However, the call for preventive medicine is hardly unique to obesity, and attempts to educate physicians, public health personnel, and patients toward preventive action in such areas as cardiovascular and pulmonary disease have met with limited success. The goal does, then, present a formidable task, which has recognition of impending obesity as its basis. Accordingly, the risk factors for juvenile-onset obesity are clearly reflected in the child's family history of obesity and/or diabetes and in his body type classification; and impending obesity is readily recognized through a close attention to longitudinal growth data. Similarly the risk for adult-onset obesity has been shown to be enhanced during periods when one's mode of life undergoes change, such as at school graduation, marriage, occupational advancement, or with development of such debilitating diseases as arthritis or emphysema. Hence, although the means for recognition of the impending problem are at least adequate, unfortunately, implementation of appropriate preventive measures requires a complete overhaul of current philosophies guiding clinical medicine.

2. Behavior Modification

A reordering of priorities toward the underlying causes rather than the manifestations of hyperphagia has been attempted through systematic application of the principles of the new field of behavior modification to the treatment of established obesity (Krasner and Ullmann, 1965; Stuart, 1967). As recently outlined by Stuart, initial efforts in this individualized treatment regimen are directed toward helping the patient gain control over the time and circumstances of his eating habits. A variety of devices are used such as detailed records of the time, nature, and quantity of food intake, carefully scheduled interruption of each meal for varying periods of time, and making eating a "pure experience" paired with no other "conditioning" behavior. Only after a variety of such techniques of self-control had been mastered did weight loss become a major focus of treatment. Another departure from tradition in obesity treatment emphasizes group over individualized therapy and supplants the authoritarian role of the physician with the self-help of the patient. Recent, widespread organization of self-help groups combines these approaches with a potentially effective aim of teaching behavioral control of eating. Initial reports claim results that rank with the best reported in the medical literature (Penick and Stunkard, 1970).

3. Caloric Restriction and Drug Therapy

Some progress has been made in the traditional mode of treatment of the obese inpatient. Gordon has recently reveiwed this topic in detail (1969, 1970). Of particular interest is what appears to be a more rational approach to the use of drugs in obesity treatment.

a. The problems of fluid retention in the obese and the effects of over- and underfeeding are now adequately described, and appropriate individualized diuretic therapy may now be prescribed acutely and chronically as an important supplement to weight-reducing programs.

b. The futility and even danger of widespread indiscriminant use of appetite depressants (primarily of the amphetamine family) is now established. However, their use as a supplement to dietary therapy taken sparingly and at times coincident with the patient's peaks in appetite may be useful.

c. Except in highly exceptional and carefully diagnosed cases, elimination of thyroid substances from the therapeutic armamentarium in obesity has been strongly recommended (Gordon, 1970).

d. Most intriguing is the as yet theoretical postulate that (unspecified) pharmacological agents be developed for the inducement of thermogenesis, that is, producing wasted energy as heat through "speeding up" the lipolysis–fatty acid esterification cycle, accelerating the glycerophosphate shuttle, uncoupling oxidative phosphorylation, or increasing the urinary loss of partially metabolized food stuffs (Gordon, 1970; Stirling and Stock, 1968).

4. Controversial Procedures

Frustration with traditional dietary methods has lead to the recommendation and practice of two somewhat drastic and controversial techniques, prolonged fasting and small bowel bypass, in "intractable obesity in an otherwise normal healthy individual not responding to conservative or conventional methods" (Questions and Answers: Total Fast Program, 1965; Scott and Law, 1969).

In practice, the therapeutic use of "zero calorie diets" usually consists of a prolonged fast of 3–4 days to 2–3 weeks with unlimited use of noncaloric fluids, followed by a sustained low carbohydrate, low calorie diet, interspersed with an occasional day of fasting. A variety of findings contraindicate widespread use of prolonged fasting:

a. A delayed hyperinsulinemia has been observed and "starvation diabetes" claimed as a result of the fast (Unger et al., 1963; Tzagournis and Skillman, 1970).

b. Weight reduction with fasting occurs at the expense of ("nonsurplus") lean body tissue, particularly when the fasting program is prolonged (Ball et al., 1967; Benoit et al., 1965; Gilder et al., 1967).

c. Refeeding after the fast may precipitate marked and prolonged retention of sodium and water or "refeeding edema" (Billich, 1968).

d. An inability to maintain weight loss following the fast indicates that total fasting provides no opportunity for reeducation of the obese person's eating habits (Parsons, 1966).

On the other hand, the prolonged fast has gained in popularity as a therapeutic tool and various case studies report substantial although sporadic short and long-term success (Drenick et al., 1970). Of particular interest is the finding from biopsy studies of a progressive dimunition of fatty infiltration of the liver in obese patients accompanying weight loss during short periods of fasting or carbohydrate deprivation (Rosenthal, 1967; Westwater and Fainer, 1958; Drenick *et al.*, 1970; Cahill, 1970). Cahill (1970) has recently explained this finding by a remarkable metabolic adaptation during fasting whereby the body derives over 95% of its energy needs from fat, including the brain, which "learns" to utilize ketone bodies derived from fatty acid oxidation. Hence, body protein stores are spared (i.e., muscle catabolism drops from 75 to 20 gms/day), gluconeogenesis in the liver almost ceases, essential amino acids are conserved, and fat does not accumulate in the liver. While the pros and cons of fasting are still debatable and the possibilities for its clinical application deserve further study, recent findings provide no justification for the surgical procedure of small bowel bypass in the treatment of obesity. Several authors report severe hepatic liver degeneration or liver enlargement with this procedure (Bondar and Pisesky, 1967; Maxwell *et al.*, 1968; Drenick *et al.*, 1970), possibly attributable to absorption from the colon of toxic amounts of a secondary bile acid (lithocholic acid) (Carey, 1966).

II. THE RELATIONSHIP BETWEEN EXERCISE AND OBESITY

The foregoing review of recent findings reveals the complexity of the obese state—its etiology, consequences and treatment; the slow, but certain, refutation of entrenched yet malconceived traditional concepts concerning obesity treatment and etiology; and the considerable degree of depth, breadth, and objectivity with which investigators in a variety of disciplines are attacking the problem. Keeping these broad observations in mind, this section will attempt a brief critical examination of findings pertaining to physical exercise and its contribution to the emerging new concepts of obesity.

A. Exercise Pathophysiology

The varied consequences of a pathophysiological nature attributed to the obese state become most evident when a mass of some 200 kg, of which some 40–50% may be comprised of fat, is "made to move." Certainly, any attempt at even the most superficial or transient interjection of physical activity into any chronic treatment regimen requires some knowledge of the response characteristic of the patient to acute application of exercise.

1. Physical Work Capability

In measurement terms the "max V_{O_2}" has gained popular, routine usage in clinical and exercise physiology laboratories throughout the world as *the* criterion for physical fitness. Properly defined, it is that relatively steady-state O_2 consumption achieved when the V_{O_2}–work rate relationship plateaus, or departs from linearity. More usually, in practice, the max V_{O_2} is assumed to equal that V_{O_2} obtained at the highest work load achieved through "maximum" volitional effort (on a stationary bicycle or treadmill). Not unexpectedly, the physical work capacity of obese individuals (in common terms of maximum oxidative energy available to move a kilogram of body weight) has been shown repeatedly to occupy a position at the lower extremes of the fitness continuum (15–30 ml/kg compared to the normal range in nonathletic young men of 38–50 ml/kg) (Moody *et al.*, 1969b; Dempsey *et al.*, 1966; Buskirk and Taylor, 1957). By these criteria the young adult, sedentary, obese male shares a position on the fitness continuum with those suffering from such debilitating diseases as mitral stenosis or chronic obstructive lung disease. Furthermore, increasing obesity, above 30% of total weight as fat, bears a fairly close inverse relationship with working capacity (Dempsey *et al.*, 1966; Dempsey, 1964b). Subnormal work capacity in the obese child and adolescent is also prevalent (Borjeson, 1962; Mocellin and Rutenfranz, 1971; Parizkova and Rutenfranz, 1971).

The multiple consequences of a pathophysiological nature in obesity render almost impossible any attempt at the popular practice of defining "limiting factors" to performance capability. It is, however, obvious that excess body fat presents a substantial handicap to work capability in its role as a relatively metabolic inert, noncontributory load. Any independent effect of excessive adiposity on gas transport system adaptability to severe exercise appears to be evident only in the grossly obese adult or child ($>$ 100 kg weight, $>$ 30% of weight as fat). That is, when max V_{O_2} is expressed per kilogram of fat-free body mass, such indexes are similar among normal and moderately obese individuals but are depressed in the grossly obese adult and child.[*] Among a variety of possible resistances operative along the entire gas transport chain, such

---

[*] According to Buskirk and Taylor, who found a near-perfect correlation between max V_{O_2} and fat-free body weight among normal sedentary young men, max V_{O_2}/kg fat-free weight expresses the capacity of the cardiorespiratory systems to fulfill maximal metabolic demands of active tissue. Thus, by discounting body fat as noncontributory to the work performed, and by holding constant the influence of the working muscle mass on (absolute) max V_{O_2}, maximal functional capacities may be quantitatively compared among individuals (Buskirk and Taylor, 1957).

known factors as increased left ventricular volume load, pulmonary hypertension, blood flow redistribution and heat discipation, high elastic resistances to the lung-thorax system, and exertional dyspnea probably play *some* "limiting" role in *some* obese people.

2. Energy Costs

In both acute and chronic states, the intensity of function in organ systems concerned with gas transport bears a close association with (if not dependency on) total body metabolic rate. Hence, a consideration of the energy cost or requirement of exercise in obesity must introduce, and in this case dominate, a discussion of the "cost" of cardiopulmonary, vascular, or metabolic factors in their role as dependent adaptations. An evaluation of "mechanical efficiency" provides a useful concept for analyzing the basis for individual differences in the energy cost of exercise, i.e.,

$$\text{Mechanical efficiency} = \frac{\text{useful energy delivered}}{\text{total energy supplied}}$$

$$= \frac{\text{external work completed (kcal)}}{\text{total energy cost} - \text{resting metabolism (kcal)}}$$

An interpretation of the total energy cost (usually measured simply as the exercise V_{O_2}) hinges upon an awareness that the measured entity is but the sum total of a series of energy-consuming reactions, including each of those functions concerned with maintenance and adaptation of body processes and homeostatic systems, in addition to the great amounts of energy consumed by muscles engaged directly in "productive" work.

Concern over the disposition of dietary calories has prompted considerable interest in the mechanical efficiency of the obese. Findings from these and related studies are summarized here.

a. More than $\frac{2}{3}$ of the total basal metabolic rate (BMR) is contributed by organ MR which comprise less than 10% of the body weight (liver, brain, heart, and kidney). Although adipose tissue is indeed metabolically active, its contribution to the total MR is barely measureable ($< 10\%$). Hence, the increase in BMR with increasing fatness is not in proportion to increasing body weight, but is more closely related to a heavier fat-free body mass (Margen, 1969; Dempsey, 1964c).

b. Limited findings, which eliminated any energy contribution serving a weight supportive or body stabilization function, indicate that the efficiency of skeletal muscle engaged directly in productive, external work is normal in obese persons (McKee and Bolinger, 1960). Less well controlled findings of a reduced efficiency of respiratory musculature in the obese suggest that this conclusion may not apply to all muscle groups (Cherniack and Guenter, 1961).

c. It is generally true that the external work produced in locomotive non-weight-supported activities is critically dependent upon the weight of the mass displaced (external work = magnitude of mass displacement $\times$ force acting in direction of displacement). It follows, then, that in simple tasks which are performed with little interindividual variation in mechanical deficiency (walking, marching, and climbing at moderate speed of 2–3.5 mph), energy costs will, with some qualification (Workman and Armstrong, 1963), bear a direct linear relationship with body mass (Dempsey, 1971; Malhotra, 1962). Furthermore, during simple task performance the increased V_{O_2} observed in obese persons (up to 164 kg), or in normal weight persons with up to 20 kg added to their upper backs, is a direct linear extrapolation of the established V_{O_2}–body weight correlation in normal subjects (Buskirk, 1963; Dempsey, 1971; Goldman and Iampietro, 1962). Hence, the mechanical efficiency with which the grossly obese lifts and transports his mass to accomplish a simple everyday task is indeed normal. Nonetheless, the crucial comparisons of obese and lean in "real life" terms reveals that the lean man (70 kg) accomplishes an evening stroll at approximately 60% of the energy cost required for the obese (150 kg), and that the lean individual completes a 7 minute mile run incurring an energy expenditure identical to that which the obese person requires for a moderate walk up a slight incline.

d. In work tasks of increasing complexity, body mass continues as an important determinant of energy costs, but its predictive ability is diminished by the overriding involvement of factors that contribute "extra work" of a static or dynamic nature to the completion of the task. Under these situations, interindividual variations in the ratio of total to productive work and, hence, in mechanical efficiency, are great. The obese individual is at a distinct disadvantage. For example:

i. Energy requirements in weight-supported exercise, such as stationary bicycle ergometry, are proportional strictly to the preset pedaling resistance, until body weight exceeds 100 kg, at whch point energy costs in the obese exceed normal by 30–90% (Dempsey, 1966). During actual cycling, where body mass must be transported and energy cost bears a relatively steep linear relation to body weight in the nonobese (Malhotra, 1962), it might be expected that the obese will exhibit even a greater subnormal mechanical efficiency than with stationary ergometry.

ii. Load carriage studies show that the speed with which simple loco-motion is accomplished (>3.0 mph) interacts with body mass (>100 kg total weight) in producing a steep rise in the body weight–V_{O_2} relation, and, hence, a reduced mechanical efficiency.

iii. The distribution of a carried load (and conceivably of adipose tissue) has a marked effect on mechanical efficiency if even a small portion of the extra weight is located on the limbs.

iv. Limited findings suggest that the high energy cost of hard work (>50% max V_{O_2}) in obesity may be even higher than estimated from exercise V_{O_2} measurements, secondary to an abnormally large and pro-longed O_2 debt or "repayment" period following the exercise (Dempsey and Gordon, 1965).

In summary, the obese individual requires an abnormally high energy expenditure for all work tasks, attributable solely to the increased body mass transported in simple locomotive tasks, to the additional factor of "extra" (supportive) work and, thus, a decreased mechanical efficiency in more complex tasks, to a greater recovery V_{O_2} in strenuous work, and to a minor contribution from an elevated resting metabolic rate un-derlying all activities. A marked individual variation in energy expenditure has been observed when lean, skilled persons of comparable weight engage in sport activities such as tennis, handball, swimming, paddleball, etc. Although similar data are not available for the obese, it seems reason-able to expect that their need for supportive, nonproductive work, their subnormal mechanical efficiency, and their energy requirement must attain its highest peaks during athletic endeavors.

3. Exercise Intermediary Metabolism

The relative roles of glucose and fatty acids as substrates for working skeletal muscle and the neurohumoral-morphological factors that deter-mine their mobilization and utilization have been intensely investigated in recent years (Pernow and Saltin, 1971). However, all the parts of this highly complex metabolic puzzle remain at least partially unac-counted for in the normal individual at work and are almost completely unknown in the obese. The wide spread incidence of tissue insulin "resis-tance" in obesity provides a rational basis for testing the normalcy of fatty acid (FFA) mobilization and glucose uptake during exercise. In insulin-dependent diabetics, "prediabetics," and in the nondiabetic obese, FFA mobilization is abnormally high during and, particularly, following exercise of moderate or heavy intensity (Dempsey and Gordon, 1965; Schwarz, 1969; Ostmann, 1971). These changes were not associated with abnormal release of such FFA mobilization factors as circulating insulin or growth hormone, and were tentatively attributed to changes in adipose tissue "sensitivity." Skeletal muscle probably represents an important site of insulin insensitivity and resistance to glucose uptake in the obese. Plasma glucose levels are, however usually stable during exercise in the obese, unless obesity is accompanied by prediabetic characteristics (of insulin resistance), in which case exercise results in a steady rise in both plasma glucose and insulin levels (Schwarz, 1969). The whole question of obesity and exercise metabolism remains highly speculative. The need is obvious for well-controlled studies of substrate turnover rates during exercise of varying intensity and duration, and for a delineation of the effects of "pure" obesity from diabetes.

4. Gas Transport System Adaptation to Exercise

Detailed, well-controlled studies concerned with cardiopulmonary adaptation to exercise in obesity are in short supply. From the available evidence it is clear that the physiological costs of work are indeed high in obese persons. Yet, the multifaceted nature of the disease also prevents any attempt at categorizing obese persons in terms of a homogeneous adaptation of any single aspect of cardiovascular–pulmonary function to increased energy demands. For present purposes, three general areas of cause are proposed in an attempt to "explain" the high physiological cost of exercise in obesity.

a. HIGH ENERGY COST PER TASK. As pointed out earlier, the total energy requirement dictates with considerable precision the degree of organ system adaptation in the healthy, uncompromised gas transport system during exercise. Predictably, then, the high V_{O_2} per work task inevitably incurred by the obese usually elicits abnormally high levels of pulmonary ventilation, cardiac output, and heat production. Such adaptations (on a per task basis) have been observed in obesity regardless of sex or age. These consequences are manifested generally in a greater subjective effort on the part of the obese worker, contributed to in part through exertional dyspnea, high levels of cardiac work and systemic blood pressures, and an elevated core body temperature. Dyspnea on exertion has been labeled as a prime contributor to the avoidance of physical activity in the obese child. Furthermore, it is anticipated that the high cardiac demands of exercise would contribute substantially to a chronic high volume and pressure work load on the heart in obesity, a factor that has been implicated as a major precipitant of myocardial hypertrophy and, eventually, congestive heart failure.

b. Precipitating Factors Peculiar to the Pathophysiology of Obesity. Specific pathophysiologic consequences of longstanding obesity may contribute to an abnormal response to exercise which is somewhat independent of the high energy requirement. It is important to clarify that these adaptations are highly heterogeneous within the limited samples of obese persons studied to date.

i. Cardiovascular. During relatively mild exercise with near-normal cardiac output per liter V_{O_2} and normal arterial blood gases, pulmonary hypertension and increased left ventricular diastolic pressures occurred in over 50% of a grossly obese adult population. Their occurrence was usually accompanied by left ventricular hypertrophy, and bore some relationship to the degree of excess adiposity. In many cases, pressures were within the normal range under resting conditions. It is to be expected that any attending alveolar hypoventilation (i.e., respiratory acidosis and hypoxemia) would precipitate an even greater pulmonary hypertension through local vasoreactive mechanisms. Rest or exercise ECG findings were not indicative of the hypertensive response to work (Alexander and Petersen, 1968). Indirect evidence exists to suggest that the redistribution of systemic flow during exercise may be compromised in obesity. The high cardiac output and circulating blood volume has a low-normal distribution to vital organs at rest, with the large adipose tissue mass receiving slightly more than its rightful share. During exercise, even a normal increase in skin flow for heat dissipation purposes might be sufficient in an already over-burdened circulation to deprive working muscles (heart and skeletal) of much needed flow and O_2 transport.

ii. Pulmonary. The increased intraabdominal pressure, limited diaphragmatic excursion, high mechanical work rates, and the low lung volumes at which the obese person breathes may precipitate an abnormal pulmonary response to exercise. Limited evidence suggests three areas of potential problems. First, young obese but asymptomatic adults display a widened alveolar to arterial pO_2 difference and a low alevolar–capillary diffusion during light through heavy exercise, although pulmonary gas exchange is often within normal limits at rest. This abnormal response probably reflects an inability (at low lung volumes) to redistribute ventilation to perfusion relationships more uniformly during exercise [an adaptation that is typical and essential in a normal individual in order that arterial blood gas homeostasis may be preserved in the face of a precipitous fall in mixed venous oxygen saturation and red cell transit time through the pulmonary capillaries (Dempsey and

Rankin, 1967)]. A good predictor of this abnormal ventilation to per-fusion distribution in the obese may be obtained through the simple measurement of expiratory reserve volume at rest. Secondly, when lean and obese persons are compared at equal V_{O_2}, the obese were found to hyperventilate (to low arterial pCO_2) with abnormally high breathing rates, low tidal volumes, and mild to severe sensations of dyspnea. Their unconscious choice of this respiratory pattern probably represents an attempt to avoid the high elastic forces of inspiratory work. Their hyper-ventilatory response, which is specific to exercise conditions, must arise from some as yet unknown source of respiratory center stimulation. An increased autonomic activity via lung receptor sites is known to accom-pany both a hypertensive pulmonary vasculature and an inelastic pul-monary parenchyma. Thirdly, the grossly obese individual may experi-ence alveolar hypoventilation with CO_2 retention and arterial hypoxemia during exercise of mild to heavy intensity (Dempsey et al., 1966; Demp-sey and Rankin, 1967). This uncommon occurrence exemplifies an anom-aly which results from a combination of "stress" factors in obesity. The critical factors are an increased CO_2 production (per work task) and a high mechanical work of (or resistance to) breathing, which, when super-imposed on a respiratory control system with an inherently low "sensitiv-ity," results in alveolar hypoventilation. Longitudinal case study data sug-gest that alveolar hypoventilation on exertion may represent the early manifestation of an impending CO_2 retention at rest, i.e., Pickwickian syndrome. When yet an additional "stress" on the respiratory control sys-tem is added, such as bronchial asthma in the obese, CO_2 retention and hypoxemia during exercise are severe. Removing just one of these stress factors through fat reduction results in a normal exercise hyperpnea and arterial blood gas homeostasis.

iii. Temperature regulation. During intermittent exercise of short dura-tion in a neutral environment, temperature regulation is usually relatively precise in the normal individual. Failure of homeostatic mechanisms for heat dissipation during exercise results in a severe limitation to per-formance capability through both an increased physiological cost of exercise (hyperventilation, tachycardia, and hypertension) and a com-promised blood flow to working muscles for purposes of peripheral heat removal. Theoretically, the obese should adapt poorly to the metabolic heat load of exercise, especially in a hot, humid environment (Buskirk et al., 1969). Excessive adipose tissue alters the body contour, decreases the ratio of body surface area to mass, and reduces the exposed surface for evaporative heat loss. The low water fraction of adipose tissue ren-ders it a poor heat conductor. The density of heat activated sweat glands is decreased in obesity. Heat production per work task is higher in the obese. During exercise the obese show a steeper rise in core body temperature and sweat rate, particularly during mild environmental heat stress, and especially when obese and lean individuals are compared under the more realistic "equal task" (rather than equal heat production) conditions. The differences in temperature regulation between obese and lean persons are smaller than predicted theoretically, a finding that the authors attribute in part to the reduced body surface area to mass ratio in the obese, which would prevent excessive heat gain from the environment when ambient temperature greatly exceeds skin temperature. Nonetheless, if a lesson may be taken from evidence showing a clear aggravation of mild states of congestive heart failure through heat exposure (Burch, 1956; Burch and Hyman, 1957), then the important interpretation here is that the obese can ill afford any extra burden on his already compromised, "fully-loaded," cardiovascular system. Summarizing a number of considerations, it seems reasonable and instructive to speculate that the greatest requirement for heat dissipation and the most pronounced net gain of an internal heat load would occur when the obese person participates in skilled locomotor activity on a hot humid day; and that the conditions that precipitate heat stroke fatalities, in supposedly well conditioned yet "endomorphic" football linemen (Fox, 1966; Buskirk et al., 1969), are not that far removed from the potential hazards presented to the grossly obese, sedentary, competitive businessman who is about to initiate his "reconditioning" program with a midsummer tennis game.

If there is an advantage to excessive amounts of adipose tissue, it is its insurance of an efficient physiological response to a cold environment. The rotundness of successful channel swimmers has long been cited as testimony to the importance of adiposity for survival under such extreme competitive conditions. Under laboratory conditions, Buskirk and co-workers (1969) demonstrated that upon prolonged exposure to cold air or water a certain degree of obesity (approximately 20% of weight as fat) prevents an adaptive rise in total body metabolic rate or a loss of body heat. It is probably also true that exercise in the cold would generate an improved mechanical efficiency in the obese. Apparently, the greater thermal insulation in the obese reduces his rate of body heat loss to such an extent that only a small amount of heat production can maintain core body temperature.

c. NARROW PHYSIOLOGICAL "COST-CAPACITY MARGIN." It has been emphasized throughout this discussion that specific physiological responses to exercise are highly heterogeneous among the obese population, and, indeed, many cardiopulmonary parameters are well within the normal measured range. A somewhat unique characteristic of all obese persons during the performance of a routine task is their high "relative" cost of work. That is, the obese person performs with a physiological cost that is markedly greater than normal, and yet has a capacity for energy expenditure that is less than normal. Many recent findings point to a close association between relative work intensity and the intensity of physiological stress adaptation (i.e., body temperatures, heart rate, pulmonary ventilation, plasma lactate concentration, etc.). Hence, yet another factor is available, somewhat independent of a high absolute energy cost per task or specific pathophysiological characteristics to explain the tremendous burden undertaken when an obese mass is "made to move." At high relative work rates, it is known that precise homeostatic regulation of organ system function, optimal blood flow distribution, heat dissipation, etc., is difficult to maintain even in the physically trained individual. Accordingly, the obese person is probably unable to sustain hemeostasis or "steady-state" conditions during prolonged work at even what might appear to be a routine work intensity as in industry. In these practical terms, the true "functional performance capacity" of the obese person is even more severely limited than suggested by laboratory testing techniques.

B. Obesity Etiology and Voluntary Energy Expenditure

The classical expression of energy balance dictates a theoretically important role for voluntary energy expenditure.

Energy intake = energy expenditure $\pm$ stored energy $-$ excreted energy

1. Evidence to support a truly quantitative contribution of inactivity to the etiology of obesity has emerged from a variety of studies and observations.

   a. Empirically, a causative role for exercise is assumed from observations that many obese persons have apparently normal caloric intakes and those who participate in regular physical activity have less body fatness. Such retrospective data obviously greatly oversimplify the problem of obesity etiology, and, although popularly quoted, contribute little to an objective understanding of obesity–exercise relationships.

   b. A critical question of long-standing concerns the manner in which appetite or satiety mechanisms are coupled with energy turnover. Popular notions would ascribe a negative, self-defeating role for exercise, i.e., the more the exercise the higher the caloric intake. Available evidence does not support this assumption.

i. Animal studies demonstrate that moderate through heavy rates of exercise provide precise regulation of energy intake in maintaining "optimal" body weight. Chronic activity below a minimum rate was, however, imprecise, and optimal intake levels were not maintained.

ii. This regulatory concept is supported by the relatively high caloric intakes and body weights observed in sedentary occupations as opposed to those requiring greater energy expenditures (Mayer *et al.*, 1956). Although no supportive data are available, an exception to this precise regulation via occupation may be found during the retirement stage in the once highly trained, mesomorphoic professional athlete.

iii. Longitudinal well-controlled studies of exercise training in animals reveal a concomitant reduction in caloric intake which contributes significantly to the observed loss of total body fat (Oscai and Holloszy, 1969). Such studies, although difficult, must be conducted at several levels of energy expenditure in man before a definitive argument may be made in support of a role for chronic activity in the autoregulation of energy intake and balance.

c. The major evidence usually cited in support of a role for habitual physical activity in the etiology of obesity is based on the numerous comparisons of voluntary energy expenditure between lean and obese children and adults. Most findings suggest that the obese person walks fewer miles daily, and routinely engages in less strenuous forms of physical exertion (Buskirk, 1969, summary of findings). Many of these studies were, however, conducted in settings (summer camp, gymnasia) that were somewhat unnatural for the participants. When data were obtained during more routine daily living in housewives, a marked variability was observed in energy expenditure among obese persons, and no systematic differences were obtained between obese and lean in terms of the fraction of their time spent in "light" or "moderate" activities (McCarthy, 1966; Margen, 1969). Despite these contradictions, it seems logical to speculate, solely from the standpoint of physiological cost or subjective effort, that the obese individual must spontaneously participate rarely, if at all, in skilled motor activities. Furthermore, the "creeping overweight" experienced with increasing age in the adult population must have some contribution from a change in life style in general and spontaneous activity patterns specifically.

The major objection to all such data is its purely retrospective nature; that is, there is probably as much or more rationale to suspect that the observed sedentary existence is a consequence rather than a cause of the obese state. More correctly, the lack of voluntary energy expenditure in the obese probably represents yet another vehicle through which established obesity is self-perpetuated and intensified.

2. Two sets of recent findings contribute substantially to an objective understanding of obesity etiology–physical activity relationships.

a. Development of adolescent adiposity was the subject of Parizkova's recent study (1968). A sample of 96 healthy nonobese, initially prepubescent boys who were highly homogeneous in terms of body mass, skeletal dimensions and composition, socioeconomic conditions, and family history were followed longitudinally over five years. A clear relationship (or in this case an "effect") was established between the time spent in sports activities and the development of body fat, lean body mass (LBM), and working capacity. The greater the participation, the more was the progressive loss of body fat and gain in LBM. The "inactive group," who still experienced some degree of sports participation, maintained relatively steady levels of percent body fat. None achieved (by age 15 at least) what might be classified morphologically as obese proportions. Apparently, the relatively gross obesity developed in the caged, maturing rat (Mayer, 1953) is not paralleled in human society by assuming a relatively sedentary existence as one grows into adolescence. This study demonstrates clearly, then, the positive effect of chronic sports participation in normal adolescents on body composition. It does not suggest that a relatively low level of daily physical activity in an unselected healthy population leads to chronic obesity.

b. The study of Rose and Mayer (1968) was concerned with the question of inactivity as a true "precursor" to obesity development during infancy. The relationships between caloric intake, spontaneous daily activity (i.e., mechanical monitoring of arm and leg activity in two planes), and body weight and skin-fold fat were determined in 31 healthy infants during four to six months of age. Although the correlation coefficients were not particularly impressive, it was generally true that fat and weight gain were greatest in the least active, and unassociated with a wide range of caloric intakes and that inactivity was linked to characteristics of "placidity" in the mother. The obvious hypotheses emanating from these findings deserve the close, critical attention of pediatricians and investigators alike. Is inactivity in infancy sufficient, independently, to produce significant changes in adipose tissue morphology that will be manifested in childhood-onset obesity? Is a predisposition toward habitual inactivity, and, hence, toward obesity or at least "creeping overweight" dictated in the first few months of life? What contribution do genetic factors make toward an early sedentary existence, and how might such inactivity interact with metabolic and regulatory factors as potential precursors to obesity development?

C. Exercise in the Treatment of Obesity

1. Exercise and "Weight Control" in the Nonobese

The once-held notion that the relatively low caloric expenditure required for exercise rendered it ineffective as a determinant of caloric balance has been adequately dispelled (Mayer, 1968). This important contribution of regular daily exercise and/or athletics has been demonstrated most clearly within the "normal" (or nonobese) population. The absence of excessive fatness in habitually active middle-aged men is well documented, and the consistent effects of well-planned physical training programs in this age range confirm a true "effect" of exercise on optimal weight control, at least within the time limits imposed by the various studies (Keys, (1955; Moody et al., 1969a; Kilbom et al., 1969; Parizkova and Rutenfranz, 1971; Thompson, 1959). Despite a dearth of substantative, longitudinal data, it seems reasonable to postulate a vital role for regular physical exercise in the control of "creeping overweight" (Mayer, 1968). Furthermore, the recently mentioned longitudinal data of Parizkova (1968) together with a number of short-term "training" studies serve as convincing evidence that exercise and participant oriented athletics contribute substantially to the "normal" regulation of body composition during critical periods of maturation. Recent animal studies revealed that almost one-third of a substantial weight reduction achieved via daily exercise was attributable to a voluntary suppression of caloric intake (Crews et al., 1969; Oscai and Holloszy, 1969). Although comparable data from long-term studies in man are not available, appetite suppression through habitual, vigorous exercise may explain much of the remarkable success and even some of the wide individual variation in weight reduction observed as a result of various physical training studies.

Finally, the evidence is fairly consistent in support of a protein-sparing effect during the production of a negative caloric balance and weight loss through chronic exercise (Oscai and Holloszy, 1969; Keys, 1955). Hence, body fat is reduced and (densitometrically determined) lean body mass maintained, increased, or only slightly decreased as a result of physical training in children, adolescents, and young or middle-aged adults (Parizkova and Rutenfranz, 1971; Buskirk, 1969; Dempsey, 1964a,b,c). This preservation of lean tissue is most evident when comparisons are made between exercise and caloric restriction regimens that produce comparable degrees of weight loss. Loss of "nonfat tissue" via caloric restriction in normal or obese adults was shown to comprise more than one-third of the total observed weight reduction (Oscai and Halloszy, 1969; Keys, 1955; Young and Digiacomo, 1965). Indirect evidence suggests (Oscai and Halloszy, 1969) that the protein-sparing effects of physical training may be attributable to an exercise-induced lipolysis (Rodahl et al., 1964) operative both during and following exercise bouts, in combination with amino acid conservation and protein synthesis via a direct effect of exercise on skeletal muscle (Hamash et al., 1967). Concerning the popular and highly publicized concept of a "site-selective" action of muscular work on lipolysis, i.e., "spot reduction," recent data comparing dominant (and hypertrophied) and less-active upper arms in tennis players have confirmed previous findings that fail to support this concept (Gwinup, 1971).

2. Exercise in Established Obesity

Buskirk (1969) has recently provided an excellent summary of the limited findings available concerning the effects of exercise in established adult obesity. Generally speaking, daily exercise was capable of effecting statistically significant effects on body composition: exercise and sports training programs with unrestricted caloric intake decreased body weight and fat content with little or no change in fat-free weight; when, under carefully controlled experimental conditions, exercise, and dietary restrictions were combined in varying amounts, exercise was consistent in enhancing weight loss almost independently of the level of reduced caloric intake; in a clinical setting, Strong et al. (1958) similarly demonstrated the positive effects on weight loss of diet and exercise combinations.

Apparently, then, physical training may offer a critical contribution to the therapy of established obesity, as postulated above for the control of "creeping overweight" in the "normal" population. However, a more critical review of findings does not permit this conclusion since the weight or fat loss attributable to exercise even in highly intense programs was usually quite small when viewed in relation to the eventual goal in grossly obese adults; exercise effects were highly variable among subjects (and in many cases negligible) and the variation in fat reduction was not apparently related to the initial degree of obesity or to the intensity or duration of training; a compensation to the treatment regimen occurred in some cases, in that energy expenditure was decreased (below normal) at times of the day when training sessions were not scheduled, or spontaneous caloric intake was increased following training sessions, with the result that energy balances were more stable and weight loss curtailed; most discouraging is the impression that, like the traditional formal in-patient therapeutic programs, exercise therapy (for as long as five months) was of little permanent value in effecting permanent change in activity habits or body composition. Realistically, it is probably illogical to expect one to adopt a way of life that he has so carefully avoided, with certainly adequate personal justification, most of his life. Perhaps, there is some rationale for programs to be developed that combine such promising techniques as psychiatric counseling and behavior modification, individually planned activity and diet menus, drug therapy, etc., although variations on this theme have met with little success in the long term (Gordon, 1970). One is forced, then, to conclude that at present established obesity in adults is, by statistical criteria, incurable.

3. Exercise in Developing Obesity—"Prevention"

If exercise and sports participation are to offer a significant contribution to the control of obesity, the most logical target group must be children. It is during maturation that daily, vigorous physical activity is society's norm, that peer group status is dependent more on motor performance than on body configuration (Borjeson, 1962), that self-degrading concepts of one's body image have not yet been ingrained (Penick and Stunkard, 1970), and that the physiological cost of exercise and their "effort" manifestations have not yet reached intolerable proportions. The avenues are then, at least, open, and theoretically the motivation high for the acceptance of physical activity and slimness as a way of life. An additional important factor to be considered, particularly in the growing child, is the protein-sparing action of chronic exercise. Caloric restriction of even moderate proportions during maturation may cause significant loss of lean body mass and even growth retardation (Vamberova, 1958; Mayer, 1968).

Although published data are extremely limited in this very difficult area of research, some tentative hypotheses may be formed from available findings concerning treatment effects in children with obvious obesity, and preventive effects in the infant and "overweight" child.

a. Parizkova and associates are, once again, responsible for the definitive work done in the treatment of the grossly obese, preadolescents, and adolescents (Parizkova and Rutenfranz, 1971; Sprynarova and Parizkova, 1965; Parizkova and Vamberova, 1967). The therapeutic regimen employed by these investigators is multifaceted, emphasizing "complete" occupation of the child's time in a summer camp setting with exercise and sport, moderate caloric restriction (1500–1700 kcal/day), and education. Short-term studies confirm the predicted effects of exercise on fat reduction with results that were usually quantitatively more substantial than reported for adults. Lean body mass was usually preserved or declined insignificantly with weight loss. Furthermore, greater fat loss with preservation of lean tissue was more consistently achieved in the prepubescent child than in the adolescent. A recent longitudinal study followed a small group of severely obese children from pre- to post-pubescence who were treated intensely in the summer camps along with intermittent therapy on an out-patient basis during the school year. The success of short-term intense treatment was short-lived. Body weight returned almost to its (high) projected growth curve during the school year, resulting in consistent annual fluctuations which exceeded 10–15% of total weight. There was a tendency for the proportion of total body fat to decrease over the entire four-year experimental period, but all subjects clearly maintained their status among the grossly obese—now, however, as adolescents. These limited findings permit the tentative interpretation that exercise therapy is capable of modifying the otherwise inevitable tide of increasing corpulence in the obese child. On the other hand, the negative findings prevent any claim of "curative powers" and point to the discouraging possibility that the obese child might be only slightly better motivated than his adult counterpart toward a self-discipline of habitual exercise.

b. A group of Swedish investigators have devoted much of the last decade to the study of exercise therapy in "preobesity," i.e., the pre-adolescent or early adolescent child with a body mass for age that is in the heaviest 2–3% of the unselected, "nonpatient" population (Borjeson, 1962; Sterky, 1971; Blomquist *et al.*, 1965). Clinically, their therapeutic program emphasized activity and sports, with an initial intense summer camp session of short duration followed by twice-weekly training sessions. Their aim was a regulatory rather than a curative one, i.e., to prevent the onset of gross obesity and thus avoid the self-perpetuating attainment of obesity's metabolic consequences. Their initial attempts with once-weekly training sessions over a short term were (as presently interpreted) clearly negative. Weight development was not different from a nontraining matched control group, and absences from scheduled therapy sessions were high. However, more recent findings from a slightly more structured program showed some substantial effects of training on an "out-patient" basis. Over a two-year period, 90% of the projected change in body weight (from control group data) was prevented, all subjects significantly decreased both the degree of overweight and the (absolute) amount of skin-fold fat, and, up to one year after the formal program terminated, the lesser degree of overweight was maintained. Additional studies strongly indicated that regular exercise also resulted in an increased "insulin sensitivity" and lower fasting plasma insulin levels. These series of findings, if expanded and confirmed by further work of a longitudinal nature, definitely suggest a highly realistic application of exercise in obesity regulation.

c. Finally, some brief speculation may be made concerning the possible role of energy expenditure in a truly preventative sense. Is "exercise" capable of preventing adipose tissue cellular hyperplasia in infancy? Animal studies show a definite effect of "undernutrition." Similarly, Mayer's early studies (1953) in rats revealed that even genetically determined (Goldthioglucose) obesity in mice was preventable in infancy through vigorous, "perpetual" exercise (which was also genetically stipulated by inbreeding the "waltzing" gene into the same mice). Hence, such measures show the obvious capability for prevention, but can hardly be accepted as realistic evidence applicable to the human infant. The studies of Rose and Mayer (1968) outlined earlier represent an initial attempt at such application. The need for further work at both the clinical and experimental levels during this critical period bears reemphasis.

4. Exercise and the Pathophysiology of Obesity

A solution to the morphological dimension of obesity through weight reduction is generally assumed as the key to alleviation of attending consequences of a pathophysiological nature. Clinical case-study reports generally confirm the reversibility in the obese adult (at least on a short-term basis) through caloric restriction and weight loss of hyperinsulinemia, systolic systemic hypertension, hypervolemia and edema, and of low lung compliance, ventilatory work, and respiratory acidosis. On the other hand, several exceptions to these "effects" of weight loss have been noted, particularly with reference to the irreversibility of pulmonary hypertension, pulmonary ventilation to perfusion nonuniformity, and of irregularities in ventilation regulation (Bedell *et al.,* 1958; Alexander and Lufschanowski, 1969; Sharp, 1964; Vogel, 1967; Dempsey and Rankin, 1967).

In discussing the resistance of functional cardiac derangements to weight reduction in the obese patient with established myocardial hypertrophy, Alexander and associates (Alexander and Petersen, 1968; Alexander and Lufschanowski, 1969) emphasize the importance of applying treatment, on both an acute and chronic basis, which is specific to the cardiovascular consequences in the obese patient, rather than merely relying on the assumption that fat reduction offers a universal panacea to all of his maladies. Somewhat analogous to this concept are attempts to modify "underlying causes" before launching direct attacks on weight reduction itself. Hence, the psychiatrist and psychologist attempt to modify the eating behavior of the hyperphagic obese adult (Penick and Stunkard, 1970; Stuart, 1967), and the pediatrician and physical educator work together to upgrade the motor skills of the obese or "preobese" child before initiating him into the more formalized training program (Sterky, 1971; Blomquist et al., 1965).

Considerable evidence has accumulated which indicates that physical training may contribute to alleviation of the pathophysiological consequences of obesity through effects that are somewhat independent of those attributable to fat reduction alone.

a. Physical training programs from five weeks to four years in duration and of wide variation in content and intensity consistently demonstrate a marked increase in max V_{O_2} (milliters per kilogram body weight and milliliters per killigram fat-free weight). This effect on performance capacity occurs regardless of the age, sex, or initial degree of obesity, and (while usually not as marked an effect) is evident even in those who experience little or no change in body weight or fat (Buskirk, 1969; Parizkova and Rutenfranz, 1971; Blomquist et al., 1965; Parizkova, 1968; Bjornthorp et al., 1970). The effects of weight reduction on the physiological cost per work task are also well documented, at least in terms of a concomitant lowering of pulmonary ventilation, cardiac output, systemic hypertension, heart rate, and plasma lactate concentration. Quantitatively, the major contribution to these changes in physiological adaptation to submaximal work rates are mediated primarily through weight reduction and a lower energy cost per task. However, training most certainly produces a relative bradycardia and less anaerobic glycolysis even at comparable (pretraining) energy expenditures. The overall result is that the "trained" obese individual completes a given task at a lower relative work intensity, at a wider exercise "cost-capacity" margin, and with an increased "functional" work capacity. These findings are consistent with the breakdown of the linear relationship between physical performance capability and body fat content in trained subjects (Buskirk and Taylor, 1957; Dempsey, 1964b), and fit well with the high levels of competence displayed by some obese athletes in endurance sports such as free-style wrestling.

b. Limited evidence exists to support a positive role for chronic exercise in effecting a disordered metabolism and substrate supply to metabolizing tissue in established obesity. From as yet highly indirect findings, claims have been made that exercise training both enhances lipolysis from adipose tissue and suppresses liposynthesis (Parizkova and Rutenfranz, 1971; Sonka, 1961; Schwarz, 1969). Most convincing are reports of a highly independent effect of physical training on insulin insensitivity, a factor that contributes substantially to perpetuation of the obese state via depressed tissue glucose utilization. Sterky (1971) observed increased glucose tolerance and reduced fasting plasma insulin levels following training in overweight boys. In grossly obese adults who maintained their fat, fat-free, and total body weight throughout eight weeks of heavy exercise training, tissue insulin resistance was markedly reduced, i.e., "the transport of glucose from blood stream to tissues occurred with a much smaller amount of produced insulin" (Bjornthorp *et al.*, 1970). The investigators attributed this training effect to both an acute and a chronic effect of exercise on skeletal muscle: (1) acutely, glucose transport into muscle would be enhanced through a decrease in muscle stores of glycogen and lipid, and/or through a direct "insulin-like" effect of exercise which increases sugar transport over muscle cell membranes and (2) chronically, exercise may increase the enzymatic activity important for glucose uptake in muscle via an increase in the total oxidative capacity of muscle cells (Mole and Holloszy, 1970; Gollnick *et al.*, 1971; Holloszy *et al.*, 1971). These findings offer important implications for the application of exercise training to "diabetic-like" diseases.

c. The protein-sparing effects of exercise training were emphasized earlier, with particular reference to a comparison with the loss of lean body tissue during caloric restriction and the implications for treatment of obesity during maturation. Oscai and Holloszy (1970) recently extended this comparison to the heart. Marked weight loss in obese male adult rats produced a reduction in heart weights of food-restricted animals regardless of the protein content of the diet. Exercise training with identical weight loss prevented a significant decline in heart weight or myocardial content below normal levels. The authors hypothesized, from the results obtained in obese humans by Alexander *et al.* (1962), that the decrease in the mechanical work rate of the heart (and hence in myocardial protein synthesis) associated with body weight reduction was "compensated for by an increase in myocardial work brought about by the swimming program."

The overriding implication of these last sections has been that exercise training offers some independent, possibly even unique, relief to the pathophysiological consequences of obesity. This conclusion certainly appears valid with reference to the known effects on work capacity, and, upon further confirmation through future work at the cellular level, may even apply to those hypotheses pertaining to training-mediated effects on insulin sensitivity and glucose utilization. Do these findings also suggest clear-cut endorsement for the widespread use of physical training in the treatment of obesity? Certainly the literature contains ample precedence for such a decision as may be found in the popular application of physical training programs on both an in- and out-patient basis to the rehabilitation of patients with coronary heart disease and chronic obstructive pulmonary disease. The major finding in these applications (and the principal evidence which has served to perpetuate them) has been that chronic exercise training increases the capacity to exercise.

There are, however, pertinent questions of some complexity which have yet to be answered. Do the training sessions impose a cumulative "volume load" on the heart which is hastening progress toward permanent myocardial hypertrophy, pulmonary hypertension, and perhaps even overt interstitial pulmonary edema and/or congestive heart failure? Are there safe, noninvasive diagnostic tests, more sensitive than the various indexes of work capacity, which are capable of some prognostic value through their adequate assessment of the patient's exercise pathophysiology? Can individualized training programs be devised, with appropriate monitoring, which are sufficient to promote only the beneficial effects of stress adaptation and avoid chronic maladaptation? While answers are not presently available, limited findings concerning acute exercise effects in the grossly obese would dictate a cautious approach. Moreover, the high attrition rate with any therapeutic program in established obesity prompts the conclusion that the potential for (transient, if any) benefit through physical training is outweighed by the risk. On the other hand, in preobesity or overweight in the child or adult, or in "developing obesity" in the preadolescent or adolescent, most evidence suggests that the potential for exercise therapy appears promising, and the risk with appropriate pretreatment assessment techniques, low. Finally, it cannot be stressed enough that childhood obesity is perpetuated best through repeated failure, and that traditionally much of the responsibility for failure in this area must be assigned to the therapist with tunnel vision. The obese child does not need yet another evangelist!

ACKNOWLEDGMENTS

I am indepted to Mrs. Patricia Renzelman for her invaluable assistance in the preparation of this manuscript.

For much of the original work reported here, much appreciation is expressed to Dr. John Rankin who provided the facilities for this research; to Drs. Rankin, William G. Reddan, G. A. doPico, and H. V. Forster for their many hours of discussion, always thoughtful advice, and technical assistance; and to the National Institutes of Health, the Wisconsin Heart Association, and the University of Wisconsin Medical and Graduate Schools for financial assistance.

REFERENCES

Abraham, S., and Nordsieck, M. (1960). Pub. Health Rep. 75, 263.
Alexander, J. K., Amad, K. H., and Cole, V. W. (1962). Amer. J. Med. 32, 512.
Alexander, J. K., and Lufschanowski, R. (1969). Circulation 39/40, Suppl. III, 98.
Alexander, J. K., and Petersen, K. H. (1968). Postgrad. Med. 44, 1967.
Alexander, J. K., and Pettigrove, J. R. (1967). Geriatrics 22, No. 2, 101.
Amad, K. H., and Alexander, J. K. (1965). Circulation 32, 740.
Bagade, J., Bierman, E. L., and Porter, D. (1967). J. Clin. Invest. 46, 1544.
Ball, M. F., Canary, J. J., and Kyle, L. H. (1967). Ann. Intern. Med. 67, 60.
Bedell, G., Wilson, W., and Soebohm, P. M. (1958). J. Clin. Invest. 37, 1049.
Behnke, A. R. (1969). In "Obesity" (N. J. Wilson, ed.), pp. 25–54. Davis, Philadelphia, Pennsylvania.
Benoit, F. L., Marton, R. L., and Watten, R. H. (1965). Ann. Intern. Med. 63, 604.
Billich, C. O. (1968). Clin. Res. 16, 279.
Bjerkedahl, T. (1957). Acta Med. Scand. 159, 13.
Bjornthorp, P. (1966). Acta Med. Scand. 179, 229.
Bjornthorp, P., DeJounge, K., Sjostrom, L., and Sullivan, L. (1970). Metab. Clin. Exp. 19, 631.
Blomquist, B., Borjeson, M., Larsson, Y., Persson, B., and Sterky, G. (1965). Acta. Paediat. Scand. 54, 566.
Bondar, C. F., and Pisesky, W. (1967). Arch. Surg. (Chicago) 94, 707.
Borjeson, M. (1962). Acta Paediat. Scand. 51, Suppl. 132.
Bray, G. (1969). J. Clin. Invest. 48, 1413.
Bray, G. (1971). Physiol. Rev. 51, 597.
Bruch, H. (1963). Nutr. News 26, 13.
Bruch, H., Nielson, N. O., Quaade, F., Ostergaard, L., Iversant, T., and Tolstrop, K. (1958). Acta Psychiat. Neurol. Scand. 33, Suppl.
Burch, G. E. (1956). J. Chronic Dis. 4, 350.
Burch, G. E., and Hyman, A. (1957). Amer. Heart J. 53, 665.
Buskirk, E. R. (1963). Ann. N.Y. Acad. Sci. 110, 918.
Buskirk, E. R. (1969). In "Obesity" (N. J. Wilson, ed.), pp. 165–175. Davis, Philadelphia, Pennsylvania.
Buskirk, E. R., and Taylor, H. L. (1957). J. Appl. Physiol. 11, 72.
Buskirk, E. R., Bar-Or, O., and Kollias, J. (1969). In "Obesity" (N. J. Wilson, ed.), pp. 119–140. Davis, Philadelphia, Pennsylvania.
Cahill, E. F. (1970). N. Eng. J. Med. 282, 668.
Carey, J. B. (1966). Medicine (Baltimore) 45, 461.
Cheek, D. B., Schultz, R. B., Paira, A., and Reba, R. C. (1970). Pediat. Res. 4, 268.
Cherniack, R. M., and Guenter, C. A. (1961). Can. J. Biochem. Physiol. 39, 1215.
Corbin, C. B. (1969). Amer. J. Clin. Nutr. 22, 7.
Crews, E. L., Fuge, K. W., Oscai, L. B., Holloszy, J. O., and Shank, R. E. (1969). Amer. J. Physiol. 216, 359.
Dempsey, J. A. (1964a). Res. Quart. 35, 275.
Dempsey, J. A. (1964b). Res. Quart. 35, 288.
Dempsey, J. A. (1964c). Rev. Can. Biol. 23, 1.
Dempsey, J. A. (1967). Can. Med. Ass. J. 96, 784.

Dempsey, J. A. (1971). *In* "Encyclopedia of Sports Medicine" (L. A. Larson, ed.), pp. 196–202. Macmillian, New York.

Dempsey, J. A., and Gordon, S. G. (1965). *Res. Quart.* 36, 96.

Dempsey, J. A., and Rankin, J. (1967). *Amer. J. Phys. Med.* 46, 582.

Dempsey, J. A., Reddan, W., Balke, B., and Rankin, J. (1966). *J. Appl. Physiol.* 21, 1815.

Drenick, E. J., Simmons, F., and Murphy, J. F. (1970). *N. Engl. J. Med.* 282, 829.

Eid, E. E. (1970). *Brit. Med. J.* 2, 74.

Evans, J., Ellison, L., and Capen, E. (1958). *J. Phys. Ment. Rehabil.* 12, 56.

Fox, E. L. (1966). *Res. Quart.* 37, 332.

Franckson, J. (1966). *Diabetologia* 2, 96.

Galton, D. J., and Bray, G. (1967). *J. Clin. Endocrinol. Metab.* 27, 1573.

Gilder, H. *et al.* (1967). *J. Appl. Physiol.* 23, 304.

Glennon, J. (1966). *Arch. Intern. Med.* 118, 1.

Glucksman, M. L., and Hirsch, J. L. (1969). *Psychosom. Med.* 31, 1.

Goldblatt, P. B., Moore, M. E., and Stunkard, A. J. (1965). *J. Amer. Med. Ass.* 192, 1039.

Goldman, R. E., and Iampietro, P. F. (1962). *J. Appl. Physiol.* 17, 675.

Goldstein, M. S., Mullick, V., Huddlestum, B., and Levine, R. (1953). *Amer. J. Physiol.* 173, 212.

Gollnick, P. D., Ianuzzo, C. D., and King, D. W. (1971). *In* "Muscle Metabolism during Exercise" (B. Pernow, and B. Saltin, eds.), pp. 69–86. Plenum, New York.

Gordon, E. S. (1969). *Med. Times* (Port Wash. N.Y.) 97, 142.

Gordon, E. S. (1970). *Advan. Metab. Disorders,* 4, 229–296.

Grodsky, G. M. (1969). *In* "Obesity" (N. J. Wilson, ed.), p. 67. Davis, Philadelphia, Pennsylvania.

Gwinup, G. (1971). *Ann. Intern. Med.* 74, 408.

Hamash, M. M., Lesch, M., Baron, J., and Kaufman, S. (1967). *Science* 157, 935.

Hirsch, J., and Knittle, J. (1970). *Fed. Proc., Fed. Amer. Soc. Exp. Biol.* 29, 1516.

Holley, H. S. (1967). *J. Clin. Invest.* 46, 475.

Holloszy, J. O., Oscai, L. B., Mole, P. A., and Don, I. J. (1971). *In* "Muscle Metabolism during Exercise" (B. Pernow and B. Saltin, eds.), p. 56. Plenum, New York.

Hood, B., and Bjornthorp, P. (1966). *Acta Med. Scand.* 179, 349.

Horton, E. S., Runge, C. F., and Sims, E. A. (1970). *J. Clin. Invest.* 49, 45a.

Kagan, A. (1963). *Ann. N.Y. Acad. Sci.* 97, 883.

Keys, A. (1955). *In* "Weight Control" (E. S. Eppright, P. Swanson, and C. A. Iverson, eds.), pp. 18–28. Iowa State Univ. Press, Ames.

Kilbom, Å., Hartley, L. H., Saltin, B., Bjure, J., Grimby, G., and Åstrand, I. (1969). *J. Clin. Lab. Invest.* 24, 315.

Knittle, J., and Hirsch, J. (1968). *J. Clin. Invest.* 47, 2091.

Krasner, L., and Ullmann, L. P., eds. (1965). "Research in Behavior Modification." Holt, New York.

McCance, R. (1962). *Lancet* 2, 621.

McCarthy, M. C. (1966). *J. Amer. Diet Ass.* 48, 33.

McKee, W. P., and Bolinger , R. E. (1960). *J. Appl. Physiol.* 15, 197.

Malhotra, K. (1962). *J. Appl. Physiol.* 17, 433.

Margen, S. (1969). In "Obesity" (N. J. Wilson, ed.), pp. 79–90. Davis, Philadelphia, Pennsylvania.

Maxwell, J. E., Richards, R. C., and Albo, D. (1968). Amer. J. Surg. 116, 648.

Mayer, J. (1953). Physiol. Rev. 33, 472.

Mayer, J. (1965). Ann. N.Y. Acad. Sci. 131, 412.

Mayer, J. (1968). "Overweight—Causes, Cost and Control." Prentice-Hall, Englewood Cliffs, New Jersey.

Mayer, J., Roy, R., and Mitrank, P. (1956). Amer. J. Clin. Nutr. 4, 169.

Mendelson, M. (1964). Fed. Proc., Fed. Amer. Soc. Exp. Biol. 23, 69.

Mocellin, R., and Rutenfranz, R. J. (1971). Acta Paediat. Scand., Suppl. 271, 77.

Mole, P. A., and Holloszy, J. O. (1970). Proc. Soc. Exp. Biol. Med. 134, 789.

Moody, D. L., Kollias, J., and Buskirk, E. R. (1969a). Med. Sci. Sports 1, 75.

Moody, D. L., Kollias, J., and Buskirk, E. R. (1969b). J. Sports Med. Phys. Fitness 9, 1.

Morello, L. F., and Mayer, J. (1963). Amer. J. Clin. Nutr. 13, 35.

Mosinger, B., Kulne, I., and Kujalova, V. (1963). J. Lab. Clin. Med. 66, 380.

Mullins, A. G. (1959). Nutr. Rev. 17, 99.

Naimark, A., and Cherniack, R. (1960). J. Appl. Physiol. 15, 377.

Oscai, L. B., and Holloszy, J. O. (1969). J. Clin. Invest. 48, 2124.

Oscai, L. B., and Holloszy, J. O. (1970). Amer. J. Physiol. 219, 327.

Ostmann, J. (1971). In "Muscle Metabolism During Exercise" (B. Pernow and B. Saltin, eds.), pp. 529–536. Plenum, New York.

Pace, N., and Rathburn, E. (1945). J. Biol. Chem. 158, 685.

Parizkova, J. (1968). Hum. Biol. 40, 212.

Parizkova, J., and Rutenfranz, J. (1971). Acta Paediat. Scand., Suppl. 271, 80.

Parizkova, J., and Vamberova, M. (1967). Develop. Med. Child Neurol. 19, 202.

Parsons, W. B. (1966). Circulation 33, Suppl. III, 24.

Penick, S. B., and Stunkard, A. J. (1970). Med. Clin. N. Amer. 54, No. 3, 745.

Pernow, B., and Saltin, B., eds. (1971). "Muscle Metabolism During Exercise." Plenum, New York.

Pitts, G. C. (1963). Ann. N.Y. Acad. Sci. 110, 11.

Pryor, H. B. (1959). In "The Child in Health and Disease" (C. C. Grulee, ed.), p. 101. Williams & Wilkins, Baltimore, Maryland.

Questions and Answers: Total Fast Program. (1965). J. Amer. Med. Ass. 192, 71.

Rodahl, K., Miller, H. I., and Issekutz, B. (1964). J. Appl. Physiol. 19, 489.

Rose, H. E., and Mayer, J. (1968). Pediatrics. 41, 18.

Rosenthal, P. (1967). Amer. J. Dis. 12, 198.

Salans, L. B., and Dougherty, J. W. (1971). J. Clin. Invest. 50, 1399.

Salans, L. B., Horton, E., and Sims, E. (1970). Clin. Res. 18, 463.

Salans, L. B., Horton, E., and Sims, E. (1971). J. Clin. Invest. 50, 1005.

Schacter, B. (1968). Science 159, 1254.

Schwarz, D. J. (1969). Metab., Clin. Exp. 18, 1013.

Scott, H. W., and Law, D. H. (1969). Amer. J. Surg. 117, 246.

Sharp, J. T. (1964). J. Clin. Invest. 43, 728.

Shrago, E., Glennon, J. A., and Gordon, E. S. (1967). J. Clin. Endocrinol. Metab. 27, 679.

Sills, F. D. (1960). In "Science and Medicine of Exercise and Sports" (W. R. Johnson, ed.), 1st ed., p. 44. Harper, New York.

Silverstone, J. T., Gordon, R. P., and Stunkard, A. J. (1969). Practitioner 202, 682.

Sonka, J. (1961). *Acta Univ. Carol., Med.* 3, 353.
Sprynarova, S., and Parizkova, J. (1965). *J. Appl. Physiol.* 20, 934.
Sterky, G. (1971). *In* "Muscle Metabolism during Exercise" (B. Pernow and B. Saltin, eds.), pp. 521–528. Plenum, New York.
Stirling, J. L., and Stock, M. J. (1968). *Nature (London)* 220, 801.
Strong, J. A., Passmore, R., and Ritchie, F. J. (1958). *Brit. J. Nutr.* 12, 105.
Stuart, R. B. (1967). *Behav. Res. Ther.* 5, 357.
Stunkard, A. J., and Burt, V. (1967). *J. Amer. Med. Ass.* 192, 1039.
Stunkard, A., and McLaren-Hume, M. (1959). *Arch. Intern. Med.* 103, 79.
Tanner, J. M., and Whitehouse, R. H. (1962). *Brit. Med. J.* 155, 446.
Terjung, R., and Tipton, C. M. (1971). *Amer. J. Physiol.* 220, 1840.
Thompson, C. W. (1959). *Res. Quart.* 30, 87.
Tzagournis, M., and Skillman, T. G. (1970). *Metab. Clin. Exp.* 19, 170.
Unger, R. H., Eisentraut, A. M., and Madison, L. L. (1963). *J. Clin. Invest.* 42, 1031.
Vamberova, M. (1958). *Rev. Czech, Med.* 4, 135.
Vogel, J. H. (1967). *Circulation* 36, Suppl. II, 258.
Wallace, W. M. (1964). *Pediatrics.* 34, 303.
Westwater, J. O., and Fainer, D. (1958). *Gastroenterology* 34, 686.
Wilson, N. J., ed. (1969). "Obesity." Davis, Philadelphia, Pennsylvania.
Workman, J. M., and Armstrong, B. W. (1963). *J. Appl. Physiol.* 18, 798.
Young, C. M., and Di Giacomo, M. (1965). *Metab. Clin. Exp.* 14, 1084.

Chapter 28

EXERCISE AND CARDIOVASCULAR DISEASE

JOHN L. BOYER AND FRED W. KASCH

I. INTRODUCTION TO THE CARDIOVASCULAR DISEASE PROBLEM

A. The Occurrence of Arteriosclerotic Heart Disease

Cardiovascular disease, principally atherosclerotic coronary heart disease, has been described by the World Health Organization as potentially the greatest epidemic the world has ever faced. There are 1,200,000 cases of myocardial infarction in the United States each year; 600,000 of those affected die. Of the 600,000 who survive, 100,000 to 300,000 do not rehabilitate adequately. By this is meant they do not return to their usual and former occupation, or remain incapacitated because of exertional angina or an impaired myocardium. The survivors of a myocardial infarction have a 13 times higher eventual coronary heart disease death rate than those who have not had an infarction (Most and Peterson, 1969; Statistical Abstract of the United States, 1970). In addition to these 1,200,000 cases of myocardial infarction, there are each year 1,000,000 persons with angina pectoris who have arteriosclerotic heart disease but have not shown evidence of a myocardial infarction. These persons have a death rate from coronary heart disease five times greater than normal.

In addition to the victims of arteriosclerotic coronary heart disease, over 500,000 persons are found to be hypertensive each year. These individuals are predisposed to strokes and heart attacks in that order, since most of them also demonstrate some degree of arteriosclerosis (Report of the Inter-Society Commission for Heart Disease Resources, 1970).

One out of four men between 40 and 59 years of age will develop a myocardial infarction by 60 years of age if the trend in this country today continues (Stamler, 1966).

B. The Cost of Cardiovascular Disease

The direct expense, meaning the direct cost of medical care, for these cardiovascular disease victims is $4 billion per year. This is $11 million a day. The indirect cost, meaning labor loss and absence from job, is $4.5 billion per year or $12 million a day (Report of the President's

Commission on Heart Disease, Cancer and Stroke, 1964). Thus, the economic costs alone are staggering. The economic costs, however, do not take into account the personal and human elements when the wage earner and head of the family is a heart attack victim in the prime of life. The personal tragedy of the victim and the immense impact on the family can never be expressed in economic terms. People move from productive roles to semidependency and restricted capacity. From the time the individual has his heart attack, the life pattern of the family unit changes and rarely returns to its former style.

C. The Atherosclerotic Process

The common denominator of cardiovascular disease is the atherosclerotic plaque. The striking thing about atherosclerotic disease is that it is a relatively new disease. The pathological and clinical features were reported for the first time by Herrick (1912). We know from the medical literature that the disease existed before this time, but it was not recognized often enough for the physicians to have identified it frequently. Even in the middle 1930's, coronary heart disease was so rarely recognized that Paul Dudley White (1964) could publish a series of individual cases with heart attacks as a contribution to the medical literature. By the time of the Korean conflict, atherosclerotic coronary disease had become widespread in our population. Autopsy studies of battle casualties with an average age of 22 showed that 70% had gross anatomic evidence of fatty deposits in the coronary arteries and 3% of these young men had complete occlusion of one of their coronary vessels (Harrison, 1970). Since then, large numbers of cases of young people with this disease have been recorded, and we recognize that it occurs at an early age and extends throughout a lifetime. We realize that its origin is in early childhood. Actually it is a pediatric disease, for, by the time it is clinically recognized in the adult, it is the end process of a metabolic disorder that has been present for at least two decades.

The deposition of fatty plaques in the arteries is the pathological expression of the disease process itself. Myocardial infarction, angina pectoris, aortic aneurysm, and occlusive peripheral disease are clinical manifestations of the underlying disorder. The present concept of the etiology of the deposition of fatty plaques in the arteries is that it is an expression of our total living pattern, our modern life style. Similar patterns of this disesase are seen in all industrialized nations of the world. In Great Britain, for example, the incidence of coronary heart disease is approximately the same as in the United States.

D. Coronary Risk Factors

Certain conditions have been thought to predispose to the development of coronary heart disease (CHD). Whether these conditions really are predisposing, which would mean a causal association, or are only characteristics associated with the later development of heart disease is still open to debate. Until more solid data regarding the cause and effect of these conditions are available they should be called "risk factors." In all probability, atherosclerosis is a multifactorial process. Even though all of these factors are unknown, there are individuals with certain characteristics who are heart attack prone. These factors that increase the risk of CHD are an elevation of the blood lipids, a diet high in saturated fat, cholesterol calories, hypertension, cigarette smoking, sedentary living, obesity, a family history of premature atherosclerotic disease, certain personality traits and psychosocial tensions, and certain metabolic disorders such as diabetes and hypothyroidism (Report of the Inter-Society Commission for Heart Disease Resources, 1970). Of these risk factors, five are of particular importance and are considered cardinal factors for CHD risk-taking behavior patterns. These five cardinal factors are hyperlipidemia, hypertension, cigarette smoking, obesity (increased percent of body fat), and physical inactivity.

Prevention of CHD is dependent upon a change in risk-taking behavior patterns. Dietary habits must be changed to a restricted intake of saturated fats, carbohydrate, and calories to control hyperlipidemia and obesity. Reforms in the dairy and food industries are needed to replace the high saturated fat commercial food products now available with nonfat or polyunsaturated items. Continued antismoking campaigns and clinics are mandatory. Early detection of hypertension by regular medical checkups is important for this is the one risk factor that can be controlled by medication. The role of physical inactivity in the development of CHD has received increasing interest. Though dating back only to 1951, the specific literature on the subject has become voluminous. Despite the lack of unequivocal proof, there is almost universal acceptance in the medical literature of the harmful cardiovascular effects of sedentary living.

No direct, proven evidence exists that control of the risk factors has a causal relationship to the prevention of atherosclerotic vascular disease. Nevertheless, the experiential and epidemiological evidence seem to be significant, and physicians have been treating patients empirically since the beginning of medical therapy. Doctors have stopped smoking in large numbers simply on the basis of epidemiological evidence. They have concerned themselves with weight reduction, lowered dietary saturated fat intake, and the reduction of elevated blood pressure. There is growing indication that we should act as forcefully with respect to exercise and fitness as we do with hyperlipidemia, obesity, and cigarette smoking. This seems of greatest importance in the area of primary prevention beginning in childhood and continuing throughout the lifetime of the individual.

II. THE EFFECT OF EXERCISE ON THE ATHEROSCLEROTIC PROCESS

Since the primary process of heart disease is atherosclerosis, a most interesting hypothesis would be that exercise would significantly reduce the atherosclerotic process that had already started, or at least delay it significantly, so that the consequences and complications of that process would not occur in later life. This, however, does not appear to be the case. Studies indicate that once the atherosclerotic plaque has formed on the inner wall of the artery, exercise does not alter the process in any way. It appears, however, that physical activity does have a significant influence on the amount of damage to the heart muscle which may be due to atherosclerosis. Available data show that the physically active and physically fit individual has fewer complications of the underlying disorder. He suffers less vascular occlusions, less exertional angina, and less peripheral disease. Of even greater significance is the apparent finding of less serious results if coronary artery occlusion occurs (Lamb, 1970). There is a higher initial survival rate following myocardial infarction in the fit individual than in the unfit. In addition, there are fewer complications such as cardiogenic shock or the development of arrhythmias. There also appears to be less myocardial damage at the time of the occlusion, and the infarcts are not as extensive as in the untrained individual. The previously fit individual has a more rapid recovery following a myocardial infarction than the unfit, and is more likely to return to his previous occupation and usual activities. In general, the physically fit individual seems to have a better adaptation to the underlying disease process itself, diminishing the possibility of severe disability or fatality.

III. THE EFFECT OF EXERCISE ON CARDIAC FUNCTION

There are three main mechanisms by which the heart is improved by physical exercise. The first is an improved relationship between myocardial oxygen supply and demand. The second is an improved power function of the heart. The third is an improved efficiency of the oxygen transport system.

A. Improved Balance between Myocardial Oxygen Supply and Demand

In the past, the adequacy of myocardial oxygenation has been evaluated exclusively in terms of blood supply to the heart itself. This failed to take into account the fact that the adequacy of the blood supply of any organ is dependent as well on its requirements. The oxygen requirement of the heart depends on the amount of work performed by the heart. The oxygen economy of the myocardium, therefore, is best defined by the ratio oxygen supply over oxygen demand, or vascular oxygen supply over myocardial oxygen consumption. What are the factors that influence this oxygen economy of the heart? The first is the heart rate. The relation between myocardial oxygen consumption and heart rate under a constant workload is that it increases with the increases of heart rate. The efficiency of the heart continues to increase with the increase in rate until a maximum rate is achieved. This maximum rate of efficiency is highest in young adults and decreases with age (Braunwald *et al.*, 1968). When the rate of maximum efficiency is exceeded, performance decreases.

Second, the type of mechanical strain imposed on the heart exerts an influence on oxygen consumption. There is a sharp increase of oxygen consumption connected with work of the heart against increasing arterial pressure. Thus, the economy of cardiac work can be substantially improved by lowering the mean arterial pressure. Third, an augmentation of myocardial oxygen consumption is caused by adrenergic neurohormonal influences (Raab, 1956; Valori *et al.*, 1967). Since heart rate and work of the heart muscle against pressure are governed by the chronotropic and inotropic influences, respectively, of the autonomic system, it follows that myocardial oxygen requirements are reduced by mechanisms inhibiting the sympathetic tone and augmenting cardiac vagal tone. Another important factor in increasing oxygen demand is the disturbance of the peripheral circulatory economy. Poor vascularization of the muscles, inadequate coordination of muscular action and blood distribution during exercise, and a reduced effectiveness of muscular effort cause an augmented total oxygen requirement of the body as a whole to impose an additional strain on the heart, to which it responds primarily with acceleration of the heart rate.

The prophylaxis and therapy of coronary heart disease depend almost entirely on modifications of myocardial function and metabolism rather than on change in coronary vascular structure. This is comparable to the symptomatic effectiveness of drugs in angina pectoris. The nitrites do not produce their beneficial effects primarily by coronary dilatation but rather by decreasing ventricular volume which lowers myocardial wall tension. This reduces cardiac work and improves the relationship between myocardial oxygen demand and myocardial oxygen consumption.

It is known that systematic physical training of the persistent and vigorous aerobic activity type reduces the resting cardiac sympathetic tone and excitability and raises vagal tone. This is manifested by a slow heart rate, a change in cardiac output, and a lower systolic blood pressure; consequently, the oxygen consumption of the heart at rest is diminished (Raab, 1956).

In addition, regular exercise improves the distribution of blood supply in the body according to the demands of physical activity. The training effect is to decrease the arteriolar resistance of the coronary bed, the exercising muscles, and the skin. However, the resistance of the renal, hepatic, and splanchnic areas is increased. If it were not for this peripheral shunting of blood, a much greater cardiac output and work of the heart would be required for any given level of exercise. One of the major benefits of training is an enhanced efficiency of this altered distribution. The net effect of the regional alterations in flow is to decrease the total resistance to ejection.

In summary, the availability of oxygen to myocardial tissue is defined by the ratio of vascular oxygen supply over myocardial oxygen consumption. Any form of this quotient below one signifies myocardial ischemia. This occurs where diminished oxygen supply is available as in coronary artery stenosis, arterial hypotension, or low oxygen saturation of the blood. It will also occur in augmented myocardial oxygen consumption under an exaggerated influence of sympathetic catecholamines. It is often the result of a combination of both factors. The trained individual is more capable of improving the relationship between supply and demand than the untrained.

B. Increase in Size and Capacity of the Heart

The second benefit of exercise is to increase the volume capacity and volume size of the heart. Since the heart is a volume organ, the size and capacity of the heart itself are important factors in pump efficiency. The hemodynamic changes that occur during exercise are well known.

The exercise hyperventilation, the pumping action of large skeletal muscle groups, and the increase in tone of the capacity vessels all augment ventricular filling. At the same time increased sympathetic nerve impulses to the heart, an increased concentration of circulating catecholamines, and the exercise tachycardia all increase the contractility of the myocardium. Vasodilation of the resistance vessels in the exercising muscles reduces the peripheral vascular resistance and the aortic impedance. All of these interactions result in a greatly increased cardiac output during exercise primarily as a result of increased stroke volume.

In the trained individual, these factors increase the capacity of the heart as a pump and the myocardial reserve and power function of the heart itself. The heart is thus able to respond to a sudden demand placed upon it in a way not possible in the untrained heart. Under physical strain, the trained heart works at a lower rate and ejects a larger stroke volume than the untrained heart. It requires, for a given work load, a lesser amount of oxygen than that of a sedentary individual. This improved power function of the myocardium (a stronger pump with more horsepower) is one of the most important aspects of training.

C. Improved Oxygen Transport System

The third major benefit of exercise is its effect on the oxygen transport system. The total oxygen transport system can be effectively measured by the maximal oxygen uptake. Improvement in the maximal oxygen uptake is the third adaptive mechanism by which physical training improves the heart. The oxygen uptake is the amount of oxygen metabolized by the body to meet the demands of a given work load. The maximal oxygen uptake (V_{O_2} max) is the measurement that characterizes the upper limit of aerobic work capacity in man. Many studies have shown improved V_{O_2} max in individuals on an endurance type training program such as walking, jogging, swimming, or cycling. The improvement in oxygen consumption indicates an improved capacity of the circulatory system to transport oxygen. A large oxygen transport capacity requires optimal function of the components of the cardiovascular system to maintain a high cardiac output and to distribute it adequately throughout the body (Holmgren, 1967).

D. Other Beneficial Effects of Training

There are some additional benefits of physical training. One is an increase in myocardial vascularization. This may be the result of an

TABLE I
The Effects of Exercise on Cardiac Function

Decreases	Increases	Improves
Resting heart rate	Vagal tone	Oxygen transport system
Arterial pressure	Peripheral shunting of blood	Myocardial vascularization
Sympathetic tone	Power function of the myocardium	Other risk factors

increase of collateral vessels in the coronary artery tree or an increase in capillary/myocardial fiber ratio from capillary proliferation. Another is the beneficial effect of exercise on the other CHD risk factors. Exercise has a positive effect on lowering the blood lipids, particularly triglycerides, decreasing the percent of body fat in obesity, lowering the resting blood pressure, and in helping to abstain from cigarette smoking.

These combined metabolic and dynamic effects of training protect the heart against myocardial ischemia even in the presence of some degree of coronary atherosclerosis. The greatest benefit of these protective mechanisms, however, is in primary prevention. For this reason regular, aerobic endurance exercise should start in childhood and continue throughout life. Table I summarizes the effect of exercise on cardiac function.

IV. SELECTION OF CANDIDATES FOR EXERCISE THERAPY

A. Potential Candidates for Therapeutic Exercise

The indications for prescribing a supervised exercise therapy program are shown in Table II. Of these candidates, the healthy subjects who are coronary prone show the best response to a regular exercise program. Along with physical activity, they should receive help in modifying their other risk factors. They should have a weight reduction program with skin fold measurements to estimate percent of body fat. They should have diet counseling, especially if hyperlipidemia is present, and their blood lipid pattern classified and periodically evaluated. An intensive antismoking program should be started. Blood pressure records before and after exercise sessions should be kept in those with hypertension. They should be encouraged to have regular medical follow-up examinations by their physicians. A change in risk-taking behavior patterns may change these persons from a high CHD risk status to a lower

TABLE II
Potential Candidates for a Therapeutic
Exercise Program

Apparently healthy persons
  High in coronary risk factors
  Manifesting low levels of physical fitness
  Suffering from neurocirculatory asthenia
Persons with cardiovascular disease
  Ischemic heart disease
  Selected individuals with hypertension
  Peripheral vascular disease
    Intermittent claudication
  Selected pre- and postoperative patients

one. This change is one of the primary objectives of a conditioning program. Persons with clinically recognized ischemic heart disease and selected individuals with mild essential hypertension are also excellent candidates for exercise therapy.

B. Contraindications to Exercise Therapy

The contraindications to an exercise program are listed in Tables III and IV. Certain medical problems are absolute contraindications to phy-

TABLE III
Absolute Contraindications to an Exercise Program—
No Exercise Program Recommended

Recent or impending myocardial infarction
Changing patterns of angina pectoris
Recent pulmonary embolus
Severe valvular heart disease
Gross cardiomegaly
Certain arrhythmias:
  paroxysmal ventricular tachycardia
  untreated atrial fibrillation
  frequent ventricular premature beats with exercise
  second and third degree heart block and fixed rate pacemakers
Cor pulmonale and severe chronic obstructive lung disease
Congestive heart failure
Uncontrolled metabolic disease (diabetes, thyrotoxicosis, myxedema)
Severe anemia-hemoglobin below 10 grams
Uncontrolled hypertension
Acute infectious disease
Myocarditis or cardiomyopathy within a year

TABLE IV

Relative Contraindications to an Exercise Program—Exercise under
Medically Supervised Rehabilitation Program Only

Myocardial infarction after 3 to 6 months
Angina pectoris
Moderate to severe hypertension (BP greater than 160/100)
Massive obesity
Deforming arthritis or musculoskeletal problems
Severe varicose veins
Any recent bleeding problem
Certain drugs that may interfere with the normal cardiovascular response to exercise, e.g.,
   Propranolol
   Reserpine
   Guanethidine
   Quinidine
   Procaine amide

---

sical conditioning while others are only relative. These latter cases, however, require careful medical supervision and frequent monitoring during and after the exercise session. There are a number of reported cases of cardiovascular collapse in the shower after the exercise session was completed (Doan *et al.*, 1965). A test–retest protocol is necessary to follow the progress of these selected persons with relative contraindications to exercise. If progress is not shown on regular testing, the exercise program is discontinued and the medical problem reevaluated. The improvement from physical reconditioning of these individuals is often rewarding. The exercise program may also enhance any other therapy they are receiving.

V. THE PREEXERCISE PHYSICAL EXAMINATION

The primary objective of the preexercise physical examination is to determine the presence of medical problems that make subsequent exercise stress testing or the exercise program inappropriate. Special emphasis is on the evaluation of the cardiovascular system. This increases in importance with age. If disease is present, physical activity is prohibited or modified.

The health history is as important as the physical examination. Background medical information will disclose the established physical activity pattern as well as past medical problems and any familial disorders. Motivation for fitness and an indication of possible adherence to the program can be determined.

Ideally, all persons should have an annual physical examination. Those of school age, or up to 30 years without apparent disease, can probably exercise without restraint. After age 30 the following requirements are recommended prior to embarking on an exercise program:

Age 30–40:   a complete history and physical examination with both resting and exercise ECG within the preceding three months

Age 41–59:   a complete history and physical examination with both resting and exercise ECG within the preceding two months

Age 60 and over: a complete history and physical examination with both resting and exercise ECG immediately prior to starting a fitness program

It must be emphasized that a resting ECG is of limited value in discerning coronary heart disease (Bruce *et al.*, 1963; Kattus, 1968). Exercise tests yield more significant data. Occult disease can often be found only after an exercise stress test.

VI. EXERCISE STRESS TESTING

A. The Selection of Stress Tests

A variety of tests has been designed for stressing the human subject as a means of evaluating the circulatory system. These tests range from very mild to maximal effort. The three most common methods have been the step bench, bicycle ergometer, and the treadmill. One of the most common tests for evaluating the ischemic response of the myocardium is the Master's two step ECG test (Master, 1950). The ECG is recorded with the subject supine after a standard exercise load. An ST–T segment depression of 0.05 mm is considered a positive test. Due to the mildness of the Master's test, and, thus, its low yield of positive results, many investigators have designed their own more vigorous tests. Any valid test must be sufficient intensity and duration to call upon the cardiac reserve. Exercise at low heart rates (HR) often fails to produce an ischemic response. The best means of accomplishing the necessary stress is by a multistage test of three to six minutes per stage, and usually three to five stages. Each stage must be of sufficient duration (3 minutes) to permit the physiological adjustment to occur.

In addition to discerning ischemia, stress tests also act as a reference to indicate functional capacity, and can be used as a basis for aerobic exercise prescription, either by using the percent of capacity, or by expressing it in multiples of the resting metabolic rate (Mets). Submaximal tests may be erroneous and misleading. They often underestimate or overestimate an individual's work capacity, so he is either understressed or overstressed during training. It is during training that exercising subjects get into difficulty and *not during carefully monitored maximal laboratory tests*. Investigators who are not familiar with the signs of circulatory insufficiency *should not do stress testing*. It is suggested that they learn the techniques from other investigators thoroughly before attempting to use them.

B. Standardization of Test Conditions

Standardization of conditions is essential to secure valid results in any type of stress test. The subject must avoid smoking, coffee, tea, drugs, and food for 3–4 hours prior to being stressed. The laboratory environment (temperature, humidity) and time of day must be constant. The subject must be free of infection or other stimulating factors. The basal state is preferred.

C. Precautions in Stress Testing

The ECG should be monitored continuously in all stress tests, particularly if any circulatory abnormality is suspected.

Stress tests carry a minimum of hazard, yet certain precautions are necessary. A physician should be present. The laboratory must be equipped with an oxygen supply, a defibrillator, and resuscitative drugs. The test should be terminated if the subject appears to be in any danger.

D. Types of Stress Tests

1. Submaximal Tests

In addition to the Master's two-step test, other sub-maximal tests have been designed by Åstrand (Åstrand and Rodahl, 1970), Rhyming (Åstrand and Rhyming, 1954), Gallagher *et al.* (1967), Kattus (1968), Kasch (1961), Sheffield and Reeves (1965), and Sjöstrand (Wahlund, 1948).

a. Åstrand's Test. The well known bicycle ergometer stress test by Åstrand requires the subject to reach a HR range of 120–170 under a load of 300–1500 kilopond-meters (KPM). The max V_{O_2} is predicted for men and women from tables intersecting HR and KPM. As HR is not linear to max V_{O_2} in heterogeneous subjects, according to Åstrand, predictions must be guarded.

b. The Sjöstrand Ergometer Test. This test consists of three stages of six minutes each at 300, 600, and 900 KPM for women, and 600, 900, and 1200 KPM for men. An attempt is made to reach 170 HR during the last stage. Sjöstrand recommends maximal stress unless it is not feasible. If the pulse is below 170 per minute, then the line intersecting the HR at each of the three stages is extended to the 170 level and the max V_{O_2} predicted from the graph (Fig. 1).

c. Gallagher's Test. The American Medical Association Committee on Physical Fitness modified the Harvard Step Test, fitting the bench height to the stature of the subjects (Table V). The step rate is 30 per minute and the duration up to four minutes. Each step has four counts or movements, i.e., up, 2, 3, 4, etc. After completing the exercise, the subject sits down and his pulse is recorded at $1\frac{1}{2}$ minutes, $2\frac{1}{2}$ minutes, and $3\frac{1}{2}$ minutes. The score or Recovery Index is derived by formula

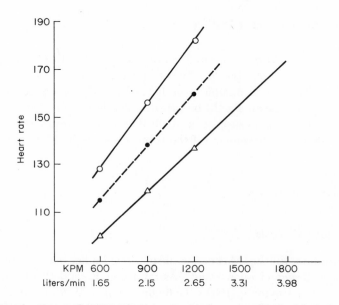

Fig. 1 The Sjöstrand PWC 170 Test. ◯, Cardiac cases; ●, healthy subjects; △, athletes.

TABLE V
Subject and Bench Heights for Modified
Harvard Step Test

Subject's height (inches)	Bench height (inches)
Under 60	12
60–63	14
63–69	16
69–72	18
Over 72	20

TABLE VI
Calculation of Recovery Index for
Modified Harvard Step Test

$$RI = \frac{\text{duration of exercise in seconds} \times 100}{\text{sum of three pulse counts} \times 2}$$

Sum of 3 counts	RI	Value
199+	60 or less	Poor
171–198	61–70	Fair
150–170	71–80	Good (75 = M)
133–149	81–90	Very good
132 or less	91 or more	Excellent

TABLE VII
Classification of Results for Kasch
Pulse-Recovery Step Test

0–1 Minute recovery HR	Classification
71–78	Excellent
79–83	Very good
84–99	Average
100–107	Below average
108–118	Poor

(Table VI). Although the ECG is not usually used with the Harvard Step Test, it would be more valuable if this were done.

d. THE KASCH PULSE-RECOVERY STEP TEST. This test uses a 12-inch bench, and lasts three minutes at a 24 step per minute rate. A one minute recovery HR is counted in the lying position (Table VII). The

ECG during exercise can be added to this test, thus making it more definitive.

2. Maximal Tests

Numerous maximal stress tests have been reported (Åstrand, 1952; Balke, 1968; Kasch *et al.*, 1966; Mitchell *et al.*, 1958; Taylor *et al.*, 1955) using the open system or Douglas Bag Method, with max V_{O_2} being the criterion of maximal exertion.

a. BALKE's TEST. The treadmill is set at 3.4 MPH, and 0% grade (Balke and Clark, 1961). It is then elevated 1% after each minute of testing until exhaustion. The HR, ECG, and blood pressure (BP) are monitored at one minute intervals and expired air to determine max V_{O_2} is collected near the end of the test.

b. BRUCE's MULTISTAGE TREADMILL TEST (BRUCE, 1956; BRUCE *et al.*, 1963) (TABLE VIII.).

c. MODIFIED ÅSTRAND–SJÖSTRAND MULTISTAGE BICYCLE ERGOMETER TEST (KASCH AND BOYER, 1969). This test has been used for normal and cardiac subjects. A Monark ergometer is used with counter and metronome. Revolutions per minute (RPM) are held at 50 until the final stage, at which time they are increased to about 80–100. The duration is usually 27 minutes. The V_{O_2} collection by the Douglas Bag can be made at one of the five stages, or only during the maximum portion of the test. The test is long, giving ample time for warm-up, which appears to be a safe approach for both cardiac and normal subjects. The general protocol is seen in Fig. 2.

TABLE VIII
Protocol for Bruce's Multistage Treadmill Test

Stage	Speed (mph)	Grade (%)	Duration[a] (min)	V_{O_2}[b] (liters/minute)
1	1.7	10	3	1.1
2	3.4	14	3	2.2
3	5.0	18	3	3.0
4	6.0	22	To exhaustion	3.5

[a] Now changed to 4 minutes.

[b] V_{O_2} collection is made at the end of each stage. ECG, HR, and BP are monitored throughout the test.

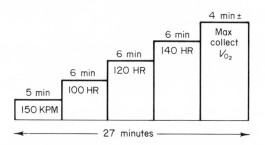

Fig. 2 The Kasch-Boyer Modified Stress Test.

ECG, HR, and BP (by auscultation) are monitored throughout the test. Tension Time Index (TTI) can be estimated from HR and BP and related to the KPM of work (TTI)/(KPM). Also, max V_{O_2} can be predicted, using Åstrand's and/or Sjöstrand's methods.

E. Problems of Stress Testing

Data collection is easier on the bike than by other method. The instrument is portable, inexpensive, easy to use, almost noiseless, and the subject is at ease. Work loads are easy to calculate and reproduce. One drawback has been postexercise hypotension. Placing the subject supine after exercise appears to minimize this problem.

Obtaining acceptable ECG tracings during exercise has been a problem for years. This is virtually eliminated by sanding the skin and using small cupped electrodes with minimal amounts of jelly. The electrodes are placed as follows: C lead in V5, right arm on right thorax, and right leg on the manubrium. The ECG is used in the V or Lead I position usually at one-half standard. Any ECG may be used to obtain excellent tracings for monitoring purposes during maximal exercise in the laboratory. Telemetering is not needed, but is very helpful in the field. It is not without error and technical problems.

1. Indications for Termination of Stress Tests

Any test whether maximal or submaximal may need to be terminated. Conditions for termination include hypotension, pallor, syncope, bradycardia, tachyarrhythmias, ventricular premature beats, weakness, and incoordination. ST segment depression in itself is not usually a reason for termination.

2. ST–T Changes on the Electrocardiogram

The simplest method of observing myocardial ischemia is with the ECG during stress testing. A tracing with horizontal or downsloping ST segment depression of one mm or more and of 0.08 to 0.12 milliseconds duration is considered significant (Mattingly, 1962). Persons showing these phenomena have positive electrocardiographic evidence of myocardial ischemia.

F. Field Tests

The Harvard Step Test or its modification (Gallagher *et al.*, 1967) is a helpful field test. We have found the Balke 15 minute run test (Balke, 1960a) more meaningful and easier to administer to large groups. It is unwise to use these with untrained coronary-prone middle-aged subjects. We prefer the 2 or $2\frac{1}{4}$ mile run to the 15 minute run because of its ease of scoring. Shorter runs of $1\frac{1}{2}$ miles are more anaerobic (15%) and, thus, more likely to cause myocardial problems, whereas 15 minute to 20 minute runs are less anaerobic, being 9% and 7%, respectively. Scoring for either the 2 or $2\frac{1}{4}$ mile runs is shown in Table IX. It must be noted that subjects of low aerobic or circulatory capacity cannot score on this test as 134 meters per minute is the minimum level.

VII. THERAPEUTIC EXERCISE PROGRAMS

A. Determination of Training Level

A main purpose of exercise or physical training is to improve myocardial function and the oxygen transport system by increasing the max

TABLE IX

Scoring for Two and One-Quarter Mile Run

2 Mile run (minutes)	$2\frac{1}{4}$ Mile run (minutes)	Meters/minute	V_{O_2} (ml/min/kg)	Mets
24:00	27:00	134	34	10
21:27	24:08	150	37	11
16:05	18:06	200	45	13
12:52	14:29	250	53	15
10:23	12:02	300	61	17

V_{O_2}. This is usually accomplished by stressing the heart and circulation above 60% of the aerobic capacity as determined by a stress test. (Karvonen *et al.*, 1957; Bouchard *et al.*, 1966) have shown that about 60–70% is the stress level that is needed to bring about changes in aerobic power.

With CHD or other cardiac problems, it is not essential to stress the subject to more than 40–60% of his capacity. As hypoxia is the primary stimulus, valuable therapeutic changes may occur at reasonably low training levels. The use of the HR level at which an ischemic ST segment depression first occurs is a simple approach. The subject is given an HR, which he is *not* to exceed during training. He continually monitors his pulse using a 10-second count multiplied by six for a minute value. If, for example, 108 is the man's ischemic HR, or point on the ECG at which one mm ST segment depression first appears, the subject is told to run or walk, stop, count a 10 second HR and multiply it by 6 for a minimum value ($18 \times 6 = 108$). If the HR goes to 19, he has been overstressed and his exercise is curtailed to reduce the HR to 18 or 108.

Balke (1960a) uses caloric cost or Mets for exercise prescription. Each activity is categorized in relation to one Met or resting V_{O_2} (3.5 ml/min/kg). The subjects V_{O_2} max is known and a load below this level is selected within the person's capacity.

Periodic reassessment of max V_{O_2} is essential as an indication for changing the prescription, to follow progress, and for motivation.

B. General Principles of Cardiovascular Training

Warm-up, musculoskeletal and cardiovascular, is essential to most exercise programs. Minor musculoskeletal injuries are one of the problems in physical training. The reconditioning of muscles and joints is needed if one is to stress his O_2 transport system, particularly by running. The use of movement and stretching (Ingelmark, 1957) is helpful in the preparation of musculoskeletal tissue for increased work. A warm-up of 10–15 minutes is needed for preparation of the cardiorespiratory system if it is to be stressed from 60 to 90% of its capacity.

When embarking on a training program, it is necessary to use interval training to allow the cardiorespiratory system to adjust. The HR should be counted for 10 seconds and multiplied by six to give a minute value, and it should be within the 60–70% level. After any cardiovascular exercise bout, the HR should return to 120 within two minutes, or, if the age is over 50 years, then to 18×6 or 108 per minute. A cool-down period of interval work should cover 5–10 minutes, including stretching exercises. Hot showers and steam or sauna baths are to be strictly avoided immediately after exercise due to the demand of the body to rid itself of excess heat.

Persons beginning a physical training program, particularly those with heart disease, need supervision to control the amount. Most adults do not know how to exercise. They desire supervision and motivation (Hellerstein *et al.*, 1967). Subjects with CHD should be started at about 40% capacity and progressed where applicable to a maximum of 80%, while "normals" start at 60% and increase to 90% of their capacity. Higher levels during continuous work cause chronic fatigue and retrogression.

Supervisory personnel should be instructed in resuscitation techniques, i.e., mouth-to-mouth respiration, external cardiac massage, and defibrillation. Emergency drugs should be available in case of cardiac arrest.

C. Types of Training Programs

A wide variety of training means are available for developing fitness in a large population. Sports are not the answer to fitness. Sports should be encouraged for the fit individual, but must remain secondary to fitness because of their often spasmodic-anaerobic nature, the need for equipment and facilities, and the lack of monitoring of the subject.

Optimal training frequency is 3–4 times per week for all means.

Swimming has been shown to be as effective as jogging (Kasch, 1970b) in producing aerobic changes in middle-aged men during a six-month period (V_{O_2} 30 to 37 ml/min/kg). The average swimmer spends the same training time as a runner, but covers only about one-fifth the distance.

Run–walk or jogging programs are the simplest and easiest to administer. They have the advantage of being easy to prescribe and monitor in exact dosages. The leader has excellent control and can minimize overdoing. Interval training appears best for the first 3–6 months. Thereafter, continuous running of 15–20 minutes may be instituted within 80–90% of capacity (10–20 Mets), using HR as a guide. Pollock *et al.*, (1971) have found walking up to 3.25 miles per session at 4.74 mph to be as effective as running. His subjects worked between 65–75% of their capacity, or about 7–9 Mets. Again, monitoring is relatively simple. Facilities are easily obtainable for either walking or running programs.

Treadmill running is equivalent to horizontal running and may be substituted for it.

Cycling varies between 4–9 Mets and should be continuous for approximately 20–25 minutes. Stationary cycling at 900 KPM is about 8 Mets,

1200 KPM = 11 Mets, and 1500 KPM = 14 Mets. The duration should be 15–25 minutes.

Rowing at 3.5 mph equals 8 Mets, while at 11 mph it is equivalent to 13 Mets. Again, the duration should be about 15–25 minutes.

Ski machines elevate the metabolism to about 7–8 Mets. A crawling device, EXER-COR,* varies from 4–9 Mets. Three months training in sedentary middle-aged females showed a 22% increase in max V_{O_2} (Balke, 1960a).

All types of training means must work the subject above 65% of his capacity to produce training effects. In CHD cases, however, we believe that a range of 40–80% of maximum capacity is of greatest value and less likely to cause chronic fatigue.

Most types of physical training programs benefit from careful monitoring and data tabulation. This permits control of the exercise prescription, safety, and motivation. The distance, rate, or Mets should be recorded at each exercise session as well as the maximum HR and two-minute recovery HR. Any notable changes or signs should also be recorded.

D. Exercise Symptoms Requiring Medical Review

The following signs or symptoms should be subject to medical review when they appear in any person on a therapeutic exercise program (Hellerstein and Hornsten, 1971):

1. Any chest pain or pain referred to teeth, arm, jaw, ear, or back
2. Syncope, vertigo, light headedness
3. Irregular pulse
4. Persistent fatigue lasting more than one hour after exercise
5. Unusual weight loss
6. Nausea and/or vomiting
7. Failure of pulse to recover in three minutes to 120 or less
8. Change in medication dosage (hypotensive drugs, insulin, digitalis)
9. Musculoskeletal problems.
10. Chronic fatigue when cardiac work levels remain within the 49–80% range and normals within 60–90% of maximum.

E. Follow-Up and Reevaluation

A monthly review of the training data and body weight should be made with the exercise leader and the subject. Revision of the prescrip-

* Available from Flick-Ready Corp., Chicago, Illinois.

tion or a variation in the exercise program may be of help in motivation. Subjects with CHD need reevaluation of their capacity or status at least each three months, while normals can go six months ·between laboratory stress evaluations. Any and all findings and training data need continual review because of changing needs and disease patterns.

F. Lack of Training Response (Exercise Failures)

In a certain number of subjects, particularly those with CHD, there is a lack of training response. This lack of response is readily observed during training by laboratory evaluation; i.e., by changes in max V_{O_2}, O_2 pulse, BP, TTI, ECG, HR, and KPM. In such cases, it may be advisable to conduct further studies such as apex cardiograms, coronary arteriography, or hemodynamic evaluation. Should these prove to be positive, further help may be needed such as a saphenous vein bypass for a blocked coronary artery.

G. Rehabilitation following Surgery

Rehabilitation after surgical intervention should include daily walking in the hospital up to the point of fatigue. After discharge, the patient may increase his walking at the fourth week from one-quarter to one-half mile per day. By the fifth week, he can walk one mile per day, and thereafter increase the distance one-half mile per week up to four miles per day. HR should be monitored and maintained within 40–60% of maximum capacity. Walking at 2 mph is about 2.3 Mets with a caloric cost of 85 calories per mile.

REFERENCES

Åstrand, P. O. (1952). "Experimental Studies of Physical Working Capacity in Relation to Sex and Age." Munksgaard, Copenhagen.

Åstrand, P. O., and Rhyming, I. (1954). *J. Appl. Physiol.* 7, 218.

Åstrand, P. O., and Rodahl, K. (1970). "Textbook of Work Physiology." McGraw-Hill, New York.

Balke, B. (1960a). "Exercise and Fitness," pp. 73–81. Athletic Institute, Chicago, Illinois.

Balke, B. (1960b). *In* "Medical Physics" (O. Glasser, ed.), Vol. I, pp. 50–52. Yearbook Publ. Chicago, Illinois.

Balke, B., and Clark, R. T. (1961). "Health and Fitness in the Modern World," pp. 82–89. Athletic Institue, Chicago, Illinois.

Bouchard, C., Hollmann, W., Venrath, H., Herkenrath, G., and Schussell, H. (1966). *World Congr. Sports Med. 16th, 1966* p. 202.

Braunwald, E., Ross, J., Jr., and Sonnenblick, E. H. (1968). "Contraction of the Normal and Failing Heart." Little, Brown, Boston, Massachusetts.

Bruce, R. A. (1956). *Mod. Conc. Cardiovasc. Dis.* **25**, 321–326.

Bruce, R. A., Blackmon, J. R., Jones, J. W., and Strait, G. (1963). *Pediatrics* **32**, Suppl., 742–756.

Doan, A., E., Peterson, R. D., Blackmon, J. R., and Bruce, R. A. (1965). *Amer. Heart J.* **69**, 11–21.

Gallagher, J. R., Allman, F. L., Jr., Guild, W. R., Klumpp, T. G., Rose, K. D., Russell, J. C. H., Ryan, A. J., and Hein, F. V. (1967). *J. Amer. Med. Ass.* **201**, 117–118.

Harrison, R. T. (1970). "Principles of Internal Medicine," 6th ed. pp. 1143 and 1208. McGraw-Hill, New York.

Haskell, W. (1970). "Current Knowledge Effects of Conditioning on Humans," Adult Physical Fitness Symp. San Diego State College, San Diego, California.

Hellerstein, H. K., and Hornsten, T. R. (1971). *In* "The Encyclopedia of Sports, Sciences and Medicine" (L. Larson, ed.), pp. 1428–1431 Macmillan, New York.

Hellerstein, H. K., Hornsten, T. R., Goldbarg, A., Burlando, A. G., Friedman, E. H., Hirsch, E. Z., and Marik, S. (1967). *Can. Med. Ass. J.* **96**, No. 12, 758–759.

Herrick, J. B. (1912). *J. Amer. Med. Ass.* **59**, 2015.

Holmgren, A. (1967). *Can. Med. Ass. J.* **96**, No. 12, 697–702.

Ingelmark, B. E. (1957). *F.I.E.P. Bull.* **27**, 37.

Karvonen, M., Kentala, E., and Mustala, O. (1957). *Ann. Med. Exp. Biol. Fenn.* **35**, 307–315.

Kasch, F. W. (1961). *J. Ass. Phys. Ment. Rehabil.* **15**, 35–40.

Kasch, F. W. (1970a). *17th Ann. Meet. Amer. Coll. Sports Med.*

Kasch, F. W. (1970b). "Exercise Physiology Laboratory Manual." San Diego State College, San Diego, California.

Kasch, F. W., and Boyer, J. L. (1968). "Adult Fitness." All-American Publications, San Diego State College, San Diego, California.

Kasch, F. W., and Boyer, J. L. (1969). *Med. Sci. Sports* **1**, 156–159.

Kasch, F. W., and Carter, J. E. L. (1970). *J. Sports Med. Phys. Fitness* 225–234.

Kasch, F. W., Phillips, W. H., Ross, W. D., Carter, J. E. L., and Boyer, J. L. (1966). *J. Appl. Phys.* **21**, 1387–1388.

Kattus, A. A. (1968). "Coronary Arteriography." Exercise and Heart Disease, Amer. Coll. Cardiol. Pacific Medical Center, San Francisco, California.

Kemp, G., and Ellestad, M. (1967). *Calif. Med.* **107**, 409.

Lamb, L. (1970). "Physical Fitness for Today's Adult," Phys. Fitness Symp. San Diego State College, San Diego, California.

Master, A. M. (1950). *Ann. Intern. Med.* **32**, 842.

Mattingly, T. W. (1962). *Amer. J. Cardiol.* **9**, 395–409.

Mitchell, J. H., Sproule, B. J., and Chapman, C. B. (1958). *J. Clin. Invest.* **37**, 538.

Most, A. S., and Peterson, D. R. (1969). *J. Amer. Med. Ass.* **208**, No. 13, 306.

Pollock, M. L., Miller, H. S., Janeway, R., Linnerud, A. C., Robertson, R., and Valentino, R. (1971). *J. Appl. Physiol.* **30**, 126–130.

Raab, W. (1956). "The Adrenergic-Cholinergic Control of Cardiac Metabolism and Function." *Advances in Cardiology* Karger, Basel.

Primary Prevention of atherosclerotic diseases. Report of the Inter-Society Commission for Heart Disease Resources. (1970). *Circulation* 42, A55-A95.

Report of the President's Commission on Heart Disease, Cancer and Stroke, (1964). U.S. Gov. Printing Office, Washington, D.C.

Sheffield, L. T., and Reeves, J. T. (1965). *Mod. Conc. Cardiovas. Dis.* 34, 1.

Sonnenblick, E. H., and Skelton, C. L., (1971). *Mod. Conc. Cardiovasc. Dis.* 40, 9-16.

Stamler, J. (1966). *Med. Clin. N. Amer.* 50, 229.

Statistical Abstract of the United States. (1970). Table 73, p. 58.

Taylor, H. L., Buskirk, E. R., and Henschel, A. (1955). *J. Appl. Physiol.* 8, 73.

Valori, C., Thomas, M., and Shillingford, V. (1967). *Amer. J. Cardiol.* 20, No. 5, 605-617.

Wahlund, H. (1948). *Acta. Med. Scand. Suppl.* 215, 1-77.

White, P. D. (1964). *In* "Fitness for the Whole Family." Doubleday, Garden City, New York.

Chapter 29

EXERCISE AND RESPIRATORY DISEASE

HARRY BASS

I. INTRODUCTION

The primary function of the lung is to bring *oxygen* to the organism for metabolism and eliminate *carbon dioxide,* the waste product of metabolism. Its structural parts are so designed that air and blood are brought into close proximity of one another but remain in compartments separated by tissue layers.

The nose and mouth meet in a common cavity, the posterior pharanx, and continue into two systems, the respiratory system and gastrointestinal system. Airways in humans have a dichotomous branching pattern, each branch beginning with the trachea divides into two branches (bronchi), the length and diameter of which are not always equal but are always smaller in diameter than the bronchus from which they originated. Total cross-sectional area and volume of airways increases progressively over twenty-three branching generations. In the last four to six generations, side chambers (*alveoli*) increase the airway volume and the lung's surface area. The alveoli spaces in which the air is exposed to blood, comprise about 50% of the entire lung volume.

The lungs sit within a body cavity, the *thorax*, which also contains the heart. The thorax is enclosed by soft structures, the diaphragm, and by bony structures (ribs, sternum, clavicle, scapulae, and spine). A membrane, the pleura, lines the inner side of the chest wall and the outer surface of the lungs. The space between the two lining layers containing a small quantity of fluid is called the pleural space. The diaphragm separates the thoracic from the abdominal cavity (Figs. 1 and 2).

The lung has two *blood supplies,* one from the *pulmonary artery* (an artery is a blood vessel which conducts blood from the heart) and the second from the *bronchial circulation.* The pulmonary artery origi-

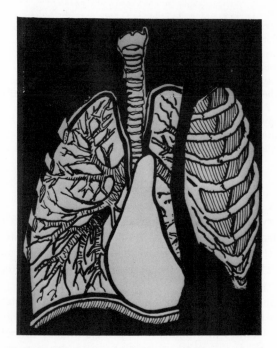

Fig. 1 On the left, the trachea and the bronchial tree. On the right, the ribs and costal cartilages showing the intercostal muscles.

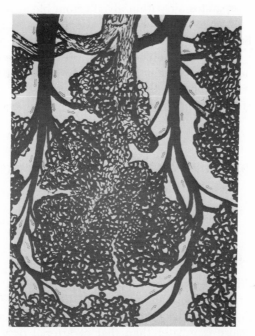

Fig. 2   A gas exchange unit including the terminal nonrespiratory bronchiole and alveolus, and capillaries receiving blood from the right heart via the pulmonary artery and delivering blood to the left heart via the pulmonary vein.

nates at the point of exit of blood from the right side of the heart. The bronchial arteries originate from the aorta, the blood vessel which directs flow away from the left side of the heart bringing oxygenated blood to the lungs for their nutrition. Pulmonary arteries branch in parallel with the bronchial tree and have similar dimensions. At the smallest branches of the tracheobronchial tree where alveoli and atria meet, small arteries give off numerous branches which lead directly into a dense network of small blood vessels, capillaries. In alveoli, air is trapped like "bubbles" and, in capillaries, blood is spread into a thin film insuring contact between blood and air. *Pulmonary veins* (a vein is a blood vessel conducting blood *to* the heart) collect blood from the dense capillary network and conduct it to the left heart.

Airways are lined by an uninterrupted layer of cells called *epithelium* and blood vessels by a layer of cells called *endothelium*. At the periphery, the two systems are separated by these cells and other tissue called interstitial tissue. This forms a tension skeleton composed of strands of connective tissue. Alveolar cells and capillaries sit upon a basement membrane that separates air within alveoli from blood within capillaries. Ascending the airways, the thickness of walls increases and more tissue is present (fibrous connective tissue, smooth muscle, and cartilage). Ascending the circulatory system, either arterial or venous vessels increase in diameter and contain progressively more muscle and fibrous connective tissue. Ascending the airways from alveoli, or vessles from capillaries, the total tissue barrier separating air and blood increases.

II. BLOOD FLOW, VENTILATION, AND GAS EXCHANGE AT REST AND DURING EXERCISE

A. Rest

1. Blood Flow through the Lungs

There are differences in blood flow between the bottom and top of the lung in normal erect man; in fact, at least three lung zones can be defined (Fig. 3). In the upper one-third of the lung, the influence of alveolar pressure is greater than that of arterial or venous pressure, and capillaries narrow or close forming high resistance pathways for blood flow. Descending the middle portion of the lung, arterial pressure exerts a progressively greater influence and alveolar pressure a progressively smaller influence on blood flow. Arterial and alveolar pressure exceed venous pressure in the middle portion of the lung, and blood flow is determined by the magnitude of pressure difference between arterial and alveolar pressure. In the lowest third of the lung, arterial pressure exceeds both venous and alveolar pressures, and the pressure difference between arterial and venous pressure becomes the major determinant of blood flow. Isotope studies in humans have shown these regional differences in blood flow with the greatest blood flow in the lower lung zone and the least in the upper zone (Anthonisen and Milic-Emili, 1966).

2. Ventilation of the Lungs

The volume of air per alveolus is greater at the top compared to the bottom of an upright lung at most lung volumes, due to a more negative pleural pressure at the top compared to the bottom of the lung (Fig. 4). Conversely, ventilation per unit volume of lung during normal breathing is greater at the bottom compared to the top of the

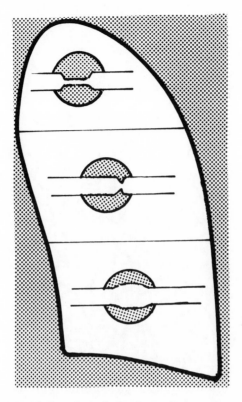

Fig. 3 Regional blood flow through the lung of erect man. In the upper third of the lung, alveolar pressure exceeds arterial pressure, and alveolar and arterial pressure exceed venous pressure, resulting in narrowing or closure of capillaries in this zone and poor blood flow. Descending the middle third of the lung, arterial pressure increases and alveolar pressure decreases. Both arterial and alveolar pressure exceed venous pressure and blood flow is determined by the arterial alveolar pressure difference. Arterial and venous pressure exceed alveolar pressure in the lower lung zone, and blood flow is determined by the arterial venous pressure difference.

lung; during normal breathing, air is delivered preferentially to the lowest lung zone (Milic-Emili *et al.*, 1966).

3. Gas Exchange in the Lung

Gas transfer is most efficient when ventilation and blood flow are evenly matched. Ventilation in excess of blood flow or blood flow in excess of ventilation is inefficient. In normal man, resting in the erect position, the decrease in blood flow from bottom to top of lung is greater than the decrease in ventilation from the bottom to the top of the lung,

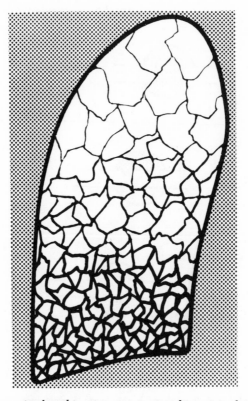

Fig. 4 During quiet breathing in erect man, volume per alveolus is greater at the top compared to the bottom of the lung due to a more negative transthoracic pressure at the top compared to the bottom of the lung. Ventilation is greater at the bottom than the top of the erect lung, and during quiet breathing, inspired air is preferentially delivered to the bottom of the lung. Capillaries surrounding alveoli are thinner and contain less blood at the top than at the bottom of the lung.

and, as a result, gas exchange is maximal and most efficient in the lowest lung zone.

B. Exercise

During exercise, arterial pressure increases, eventually exceeding alveolar pressure. The distribution of blood flow becomes uniform throughout the lung, and blood flow is determined by arterial venous pressure difference. Hyperpnea occurs during exercise; the system controlling this response is imperfectly understood, but it has been attributed

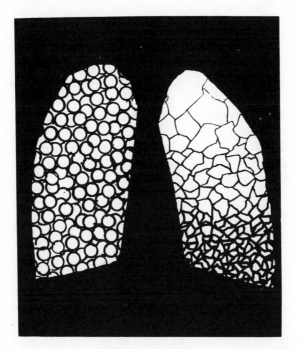

Fig. 5   The drawing on the left shows the lung of an erect man during exercise, with uniform blood flow and ventilation from the top to the bottom of the lung. On the right, is seen the lung of an erect man at rest, with maximal blood flow at the bottom of the lung.

to impulses originating in the cerebral cortex or in exercising muscles and then transmitted humorally or neurally to the respiratory centers. Nevertheless, with hyperpnea, ventilation becomes more uniform throughout the lung. Uniform distribution of ventilation and blood flow throughout both lungs leads to an increase in the number of gas exchange units (alveoli and capillaries) and increased transfer of oxygen and elimination of carbon dioxide (Bryan *et al.*, 1964) (Fig. 5).

III. RESPIRATORY DISEASES ALTERING THE RESPONSE TO EXERCISE

A. Introduction

Chronic lung disease cripples over a million people in the United States. First visits to physicians, disability payments, and reported deaths due to obstructive pulmonary disease have been increasing at a faster rate than most other health problems (Department of Health, Education, and Welfare, Public Health Service, 1966; U.S. Department of Health, Education, and Welfare, 1968).

Although much attention and study has been directed toward management of patients with acute respiratory problems, little attention has been given to management of patients with chronically disabling pulmonary disease. Investigations to elucidate the pathophysiology of chronic lung disease are in their infancy, and little is available in the armamentarium of drugs to treat afflicted patients. Appropriate treatment of disease depends upon knowledge of causation of the specific disease or diseases in each patient.

B. Diseases Interfering with Ventilation

1. Pulmonary Emphysema

Emphysema is an anatomic alteration of the lung characterized by abnormal enlargement of air spaces distal to the terminal nonrespiratory bronchiole which may be accompanied by destructive changes of alveolar walls (American Thoracic Society, 1962). Increased size of air spaces arises from hypoplasia, atrophy, overinflation, and destruction. The description of emphysema depends upon the location of the disease. In *panlobular* emphysema, all clusters of alveoli in a region of lung are equally involved to a greater or lesser extent (the disease is generalized for that particular segment, lobule, lobe, or lung) (Fig. 6). In *centrilobular* emphysema, those alveoli directly contiguous to a respiratory bronchiole are affected (Fig. 7). A *respiratory bronchiole* is the first order of bronchiole into which alveoli open; it is the earliest division of the airways in which gas exchange may take place.

When panlobular emphysema results in selective parenchymal and vascular destruction of the lower lobes, patients have shortness of breath at an early age. Man is most dependent on his lower lung zones for gas exchange in the erect position. Selective parenchymal and vascular destruction of both upper lobes does not often evoke dyspnea until the disease is advanced and lower lobe involvement with emphysema or other disease develops (Fig. 8).

Loss of elasticity is the underlying defect in emphysema. Total elastin and collagen in the lungs of patients with emphysema is normal; it is the loss of normal architecture and the resultant loss of airway support that leads to air trapping, ventilation/perfusion abnormalities, and shortness of breath. Although a few large air spaces may exist, the gross

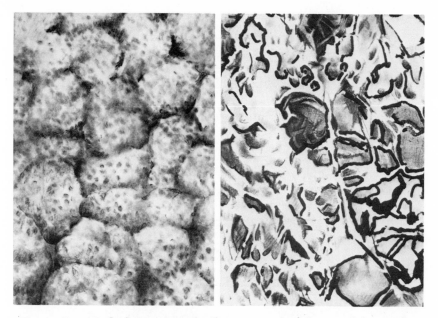

Fig. 6 Retouched photomicrographs showing, on the left, normal lung and, on the right, the picture of panlobular emphysema.

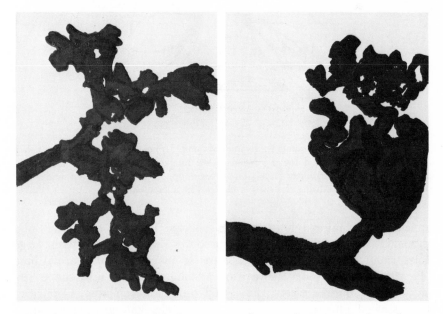

Fig. 7 Drawing on the left shows a normal terminal airway. On the right, one involved with centilobular emphysema.

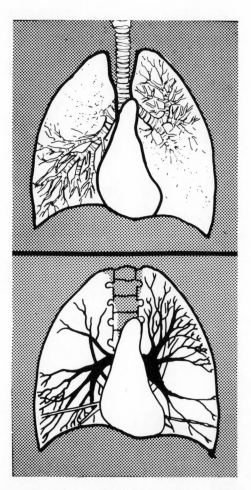

Fig. 8 Emphysema limited to regions of lung. Upper panel, emphysema upper portion of right lung and lower portion of left lung causing destructive changes in parenchyma of lung. Lower panel, emphysema upper portion of right and lower portion of left lung causing destructive changes in microcirculation.

appearance of normal lung is homogeneous. The appearance of lung with widespread emphysema demonstrates heterogeneity with large holes, small holes, and intermixed areas of compacted and normal lung (Fig. 6). In emphysema, airways are no longer held open by the tethering effect of normal elastic tissue and thus easily collapse. Capillaries are "pinched off" if not destroyed completely, and gross inequalities in the matching of ventilation to blood flow occur.

2. Chronic Bronchitis

Chronic bronchitis is a disease defined arbitrarily as chronic 'or recurrent productive cough which must be present clinically on most days for a minimum of three months in the year and for not less than two successive years (American Thoracic Society, 1962). The criteria used to diagnose chronic bronchitis clinically are arbitrary, and pathological abnormalities found in chronic bronchitis can be found in patients without cough or sputum. These abnormalities include hypertrophy of mucous glands, hypersecretion of mucous, and ulceration and damage of structures within the bronchial and bronchiolar walls as well as scarring of these walls. At times, total obliteration and destruction of small air passages occurs. Damage to the surface epithelium of the larger bronchi is more common than damage to the deeper part of the bronchial wall. Damaged surface epithelium is replaced by metaplastic squamous epithelium, and, at times, bronchial polyps are found.

Recurrent infection is common in patients with chronic bronchitis, resulting from bacterial proliferation in mucous. Bacteria growing in intraluminal mucous attract white blood cells which migrate between bronchial epithelial cells and produce pus. With infection, clear mucous is transformed into yellow or green mucopus.

Clear mucous within the bronchial lumen does not imply infection invading the bronchial wall, and it may not be accompanied by a host response manifested by a rise in antibody. However, mucopurulent inflammation may be invasive and cause ulceration and destruction of bronchiolar walls. Repair later results in formation of granulation and fibrous tissue in the wall and replacement of the normal ciliated epithelium with flattened stratified epithelium.

The structural abnormalities resulting from bronchitis may be local or scattered. Scarring develops in small bronchi and narrowing occurs, leading to airway obstruction. In addition to scar formation, bronchioles are weakened and dilate, and some are totally destroyed. Severe damage in the bronchioles accompanied by peribronchiolar extension of infection may lead to damage of the microcirculation of the bronchial and pulmonary arterial systems and eventually to the development of pulmonary emphysema.

3. Bronchial Asthma

Bronchial asthma is a disease characterized by increased responsiveness of the trachea and bronchi to various stimuli, manifested by a widespread narrowing of the airways that changes in severity either spontaneously or as a result of therapy (American Thoracic Society, 1962). Clinically, patients have episodes of shortness of breath and wheezing and symptom free intervals. Many factors influence the development of asthma including genetic factors, infection, stress, and exercise. These stimuli produce bronchospasm and increased mucous production. Sensitivity of the airways to these factors varies day to day. Drugs resulting in relaxation of bronchial smooth muscle and decreased mucous production help alleviate shortness of breath in patients with asthma. Increased mucous production in patients with asthma often results in recurrent and frequent episodes of bronchitis.

Within the lungs of patients dying of bronchial asthma are found mucous plugs, denudation of bronchial epithelium, increased size of mucous-producing cells, hypertrophy of smooth muscle, and thickening of basement membrane underlying epithelial cells.

C. Diseases Interfering with Blood Flow through the Lungs

1. Pulmonary Embolism

A decrease in blood flow through a region of the lung often occurs secondary to obstruction by blood clot (embolism). When obstruction causes a regional decrease in blood flow, ventilation remains normal in the poorly perfused lung zone (Bass, 1970b). When there is death of tissue (pulmonary infarction) in addition to pulmonary embolism, regional hypoventilation still is less than regional hypoperfusion and there is excessive ventilation in reaction to perfusion in the zone of infarcted lung.

2. Heart Failure

In patients with left heart failure and preexisting normal lungs, hydrostatic forces produce a relatively higher venous pressure in the lower compared to the upper lobes. Transudation of fluid occurs selectively at the lung bases producing increased interstitial pressure and narrowing or closure of lower lobe vessels. High resistance pathways to blood flow develop in the lower lobe and blood flow is redistributed (West et al., 1965).

When left heart failure occurs in a patient who has emphysema localized in unusual regions, physical findings are bizarre, the interstitial pattern seen on chest roentgenograms unusual and abnormalities noted on lung function tests variable. In these patients interstitial fluid forms in areas of normal perfusion, leading to regional differences in compliance and an increase in interstitial pressure which causes narrowing of extra-alveolar vessels and ultimately redistribution of perfusion away from originally well-perfused regions (Bass, 1970a).

D. Other Diseases Causing Abnormal Relationship of Ventilation to Blood Flow in the Lung

Breathing involves coordinated function of the brain, peripheral nerves, bony thorax, muscles, and lungs. Disease affecting any of these organs can alter the optimal relation of ventilation and perfusion.

IV. THERAPY FOR PATIENTS WITH CHRONIC RESPIRATORY DISEASE

Rational therapy is based upon understanding of pathophysiological processes that produce disease. Pharmacologic or physical agents that halt or alter adverse processes can then be administered. Better understanding of the pathophysiological processes resulting in pulmonary disease is needed. What is known can be applied to the care of afflicted patients.

Bronchial asthma, a disease in which there is spasm of bronchial smooth muscle and increased mucous production, is characterized clinically by intermittent episodes of shortness of breath with wheezing and symptom-free intervals which can occur spontaneously or as the result of therapy. Elimination of the agent triggering acute asthma, if this can be identified, is of prime importance. Pulmonary infection, particularly bronchitis, is frequently the agent triggering muscle spasm and increased mucous production. Mucous in lower airways is a good culture media for bacterial growth resulting in a vicious cycle of increased mucous, infection, and asthma. Therapy for patients with bronchial asthma must include effective clearance of mucous. Cough most effectively removes mucous from small airways and productive cough requires a strong chest wall and liquid mucous. Water and other fluids help expectoration by keeping the tracheobronchial tree liquid. If one drinks little fluid and mouth-breathes during sleep in a poorly humidified and overheated room, secretions dry out and obstruct airways. A cold vaporizer humidifies the environment and prevents drying of airways.

Drugs that decrease spasm of bronchial smooth muscle, bronchodilators, are useful in the treatment of asthma and used frequently for this purpose are ephedrine or xanthene derivatives. Drugs are best administerd in pill, suppository, or intravenous form in asthmatic patients. Although aerosols effectively deliver drugs to the lungs, they can irritate the bronchial mucosa and trigger increased asthma.

Patients with chronic bronchitis have inflammation of bronchial mucosa and increased mucous production. Cigarette smoking is the most common offending agent causing chronic bronchitis. Discontinuation of smoking is a prerequisite for other therapy to be effective. As in patients with bronchial asthma, mucous within airways serves as a culture media for bacterial growth. Organisms most frequently found in sputum cultures of patients with chronic bronchitis include *D. pneumonia* and *H. influenza*. Viral and mycobacterial infections often cause an acute exacerbation in patients with chronic bronchitis and these infections are soon complicated by bacterial superinfection (Fisher *et al.*, 1969). Tetracycline and amphicillin are effective antibiotics for treatment of exacerbations of chronic bronchitis. Both are effective against *D. pneumococcus* and *H. influenza* (Chodosh, 1967). Clearing the tracheobronchial tree of mucous in patients with chronic bronchitis follows the same principles as discussed for patients with bronchial asthma, i.e., adequate hydration, a strong chest wall, and expectorants if needed.

Patients with emphysema often have coexisting bronchial asthma or chronic bronchitis and these coexisting diseases must be treated in order to prevent further destruction of lung parenchyma. Therapy for patients with emphysema relies upon treatment of coexisting pulmonary or nonpulmonary disease and on graded exercise training.

Heart failure or pulmonary embolism may be responsible for a sudden increase in shortness of breath in patients with preexisting respiratory disease. Therapy for heart failure includes use of drugs that improve cardiac function or that eliminate fluid (diuretics) which is retained in patients with heart failure. When pulmonary embolism occurs, anticoagulants can be used and ligation or the vena cava (the vein through which blood clots most frequently reach the lungs) might be advocated. Therapy of pulmonary embolism is directed toward the elimination of factors predisposing to embolism and toward aiding resolution of clot.

V. EXERCISE THERAPY FOR PATIENTS WITH RESPIRATORY DISEASE

Shortness of breath limits the activity of patients with chronic obstructive pulmonary disease, and the resultant lack of activity leads to an unfit state and increased dyspnea, a vicious cycle. Therapy for patients with pulmonary emphysema is limited. Preventive measures such as discontinuation of smoking and the use of antibiotics to prevent or treat respiratory tract infection can help preserve existing function; mucolytic and expectorant agents help patients who cough effectively, and, when bronchospasm is present, bronchodilators can be used. Specific therapy to improve myocardial function or eliminate increased fluid can relieve shortness of breath in patients with heart failure. Anticoagulation, ligation, or clipping of the vena cava and measures directed at eliminating causative factors can help patients with pulmonary embolism.

In all of the conditions discussed, the structural abnormality results in a ventilation to blood flow imbalance, increased work of breathing, and shortness of breath.

Exercise causes ventilation and blood flow to be more uniform throughout the lungs leading to more efficient gas exchange in normal subjects and most patients with respiratory disease. When exercise causes gas exchange to deteriorate, serious disease is often present in a patient who has lost his reserve of blood vessels and/or airways needed for increased gas exchange during exercise.

Early studies employing exercise in patients with chronic obstructive pulmonary disease were concerned with the question, "Can oxygen breathing enable a breathless patient to do more?" (Barach, 1959; Committee on Public Health, 1962). Results of oxygen supported exercise programs revealed that patients had subjective improvement, but yielded little, if any, objective evidence that improvement occurred. It was impossible to ascertain whether subjective improvement was related to breathing air enriched with oxygen, exercise, or whether it was entirely a psychological effect. Later work evaluating the pulmonary, cardiac, and peripheral effects of graded exercise training in patients with chronic obstructive pulmonary disease revealed that subjective and objective improvement could be achieved using graded exercise alone. The form of exercise chosen for patients studied was riding a stationary bicycle, a task that can be performed daily, regardless of weather. Before admission into a graded exercise program as therapy for chronic obstructive pulmonary disease, complete medical evaluation should be performed and treatable pulmonary or nonpulmonary abnormalities corrected. Motivation to lead a more active life is a necessary prerequisite for successful exercise training (Bass, et al., 1970).

Bicycles used for training should be equipped with odometer and variable wheel tension. At the start of the exercise program, patients should be instructed to pedal for the length of time that they consider work, but not to exhaust themselves. The suggestion that a tension permitting five to seven minutes of exercise at the first session is helpful. Thereafter, exercise should be performed at the same tension two or three times a day, increasing the time of daily sessions each morning until twenty minute sessions are achieved, after which tension should be increased to a higher level and the entire process repeated. Patients should keep a diary and record time pedaled, tension setting on bicycle, and miles achieved at each exercise session. Comments about activities of daily living should be recorded.

Patients performing graded exercise training experience subjective and objective improvement within three to six weeks. Objective improvement after training includes ability to perform at an increased work load, a decrease in heart rate at rest and during exercise, increase in the amount of air that can be breathed in from the end of a normal breath, and an increase in maximal voluntary ventilation. The ventilatory equivalent for oxygen (V_EO_2) (liters breathed to consume 100 ml oxygen) decreases after training in some, but not all patients. V_EO_2 is not a good index to gauge training in patients with ventilation to blood flow imbalance. It is dependent upon the determinants of oxygen consumption and minute ventilation. When patients have bronchospasm during an exercise study, minute ventilation increases more than oxygen consumption in the trained state and V_EO_2 increases. Ventilation perfusion abnormalities secondary to pulmonary disease are often aggravated by left heart failure. Heart failure can cause deterioration in ventilation to blood flow relationships with an increase in oxygen consumption greater than the increase in minute ventilation and a resultant decrease in V_EO_2. Irregardless of their effect on V_EO_2, bronchospasm and left heart failure do not limit successful exercise training in patients with respiratory disease (Bass *et al.*, 1970).

The diary is useful to physicians and patients. Patients claim that they are encouraged by their progress and that the diary serves as an incentive to perform increased amounts of exercise. Physicians can use the diary to quantify home performance. Also, a decrease in daily activities, as reflected in the diary, is often an early sign of infection (Fig. 9).

Subjective improvement reported by patients was that they "could do more" with "less shortness of breath." Their claim of increased activities of daily living was validated by analysis of their diaries. Heart rate at rest or during exercise is a sensitive gauge of fitness, a lower heart rate being associated with better health (Fig. 10). Heart rate can be used to follow the fitness of patients in a graded exercise program. After achieving the trained state, an increase in the resting heart rate

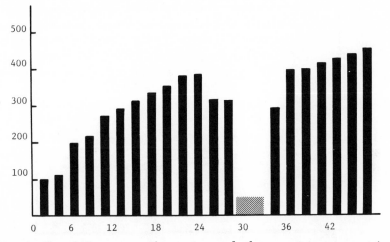

Fig. 9 Plot of diary score. The *y*-axis records the percent improvement in activities of daily living; the *x*-axis, the months of exercise training. Zero represents the score on week prior to training. The stippled zone represents no activity due to illness caused by acute bronchitis.

can be the harbinger of acute respiratory infection or other illness. Other changes noted in physiological indices confirmed clinical observations that patients were stronger and could do more. Significant increases in inspiratory capacity and maximal voluntary ventilation after training reflected increased muscle strength. Improvement in chest wall strength resulted in improved ventilation distribution and the ability to cough more effectively.

More efficient distribution of ventilation after training, together with more efficient cardiac performance, leads to improved gas exchange and decreased work of breathing. Decrease in the work of breathing reduces oxygen requirement. In the trained state, patients with respiratory disease are better able to handle nonrespiratory illness or surgery without respiratory complications.

To achieve continued improvement, graded exercise must be performed indefinitely. Patients exercising at a constant work load will improve initially and then achieve no further improvement. Patients who stop exercise lose their fitness.

Graded exercise training for patients with chronic obstructive pulmonary disease improves ventilation, cardiac efficiency, and gas exchange, and decreases the work of breathing and lowers oxygen requirement. It is a valuable tool in the treatment of patients with respiratory disease.

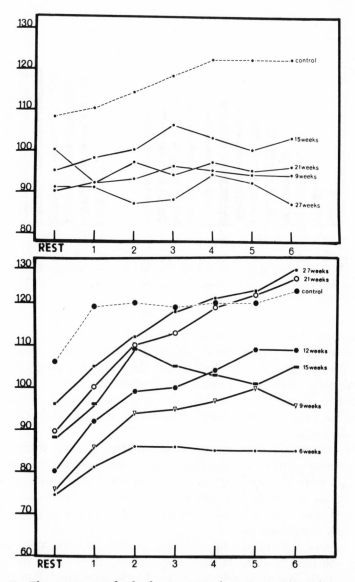

Fig. 10 The *y*-axis records the heart rate in beats per minute; the *x*-axis, the resting value and value at each of six minutes of exercise. In the upper panel, the heart rate is shown at rest and during six minutes of exercise at baseline work load (50 kg/m/min) at time of the control study, and at 9, 15, 21, and 27 weeks after initiating exercise training. In the lower panel, similar values of heart rate for control week exercise at 50/kg/m/min are shown, and for values measured at higher work loads on subsequent studies at 6 weeks (200 kg/m/min), 9 weeks (250 kg/m/min), 12 weeks (300 kg/m/min), 15 weeks (350 kg/m/min), 21 weeks (400 kg/m/min), and 27 weeks (450 kg/m/min) after initiating exercise training.

REFERENCES

American Thoracic Society. (1962). *Amer. Rev. Resp. Dis.* **85**, 762.

Anthonisen, N. R., and Milic-Emili, J. (1966). *J. Appl. Physiol.* **21**, 760.

Barach, A. L. (1959). *Dis. Chest* **35**, 229.

Bass, H. (1970a). *Amer. J. Med.* **48**, 413.

Bass, H. (1970b). *Bull. Physio-Pathol. Resp.* **6**, 123.

Bass, H., Forman, R., and Whitcomb, J. (1970). *Chest* **57**, 116.

Bryan, A. C., Bentivoglio, L. G., Beerel, F., Macleich, H., and Zidulka, A. (1964). *J. Appl. Physiol.* **19**, 395.

Chodosh, S. (1967). *Med. Clin. N. Amer.* **51**, 1169.

Committee on Public Health. (1962). *Bull. N.Y. Acad. Med.* [2] **38**, 135.

Department of Health, Education, and Welfare, Public Health Service. (1966). "Vital Statistics of the U.S., Mortality," Vol. II, Part A. Department of Health, Education, and Welfare, Washington, D.C.

Fisher, M., Akhtar, A. J., Calder, M. A., Moffat, M. A. J., Stewart, S. M., Zealley, H., and Crofton, J. W. (1969). *Brit. Med. J.* **4**, 187.

Milic-Emili, J., Henderson, J. A. M., Dolowitch, M. B., Trop, D., and Kaneko, K. (1966). *J. Appl. Physiol.* **21**, 749.

U.S. Department of Health, Education, and Welfare. (1968). "Monthly Vital Statistics ,Report, Provisional Statistics, Annual Summary for the U.S. (Births, Deaths, Marriages, and Divorces)," Vol. 16, p. 3. U.S. Dept. of Health, Education, and Welfare, Washington, D.C.

West, J. B., Dollery, C. T., and Heard, B. E. (1965). *Circ. Res.* **17**, 191.

Chapter 30

EXERCISE AND MUSCULOSKELETAL DISEASE

VEIDA BARCLAY

I. INTRODUCTION

Rehabilitation has as its objective the restoration to health of an injured person so that he may resume his normal life by becoming physically, mentally, technically, and socially as strong and capable as he was before his injury. Rehabilitation is essentially the work of a team of specialists each of whom is an expert in his own field, and whose efforts reinforce and supplement those of the other members of the team. Thus, throughout the various stages of treatment, from the earliest to the posthospital, the closest possible cooperation and consultation between the physician or surgeon and the technical experts is imperative.

The most important member of the team is the patient himself. If the combined efforts of the medical and technical experts are to be completely successful, it is essential that the wholehearted cooperation of the patient be obtained. Full and frank discussions with the patient at all levels throughout the course of treatment will help to develop mutual trust and confidence, banish fear, and foster the patient's determination to do well.

Rehabilitation is largely based upon a "do-it-yourself" concept in so far as the patient is concerned, while for the therapist it is a case of taking the horse to water and persuading it to drink. The point to stress is that the patient should do the work. He must cooperate with all concerned; otherwise, recovery is delayed or may never occur.

Exercise as a therapy in the treatment of musculoskeletal disorders has been used by the medical profession for many years, and should be commenced as soon as possible after the injury has been sustained. It does not end until the patient is fit enough to return to gainful occupation.

Figure 1 shows the relative position of the various aspects of the rehabilitation curriculum. The best results are obtained when the various treatments are combined in the correct proportions, although in different phases of the patient's recovery one may be used more than the others. The type of exercise used will depend on the results desired. All activity aims at the normal patterns of movement of everyday actions. Thus, the patient is encouraged to develop those motor skills that form the basis of his everyday living, be he a miner, industrial worker, or housewife.

One of the major elements of the rehabilitation program is exercise therapy, which can be subdivided into specific exercises and recreational activities. A great deal has been written about specific exercises and their employment in the rehabilitation of the injured. Little attention, however, has been given to the use of recreational activities such as

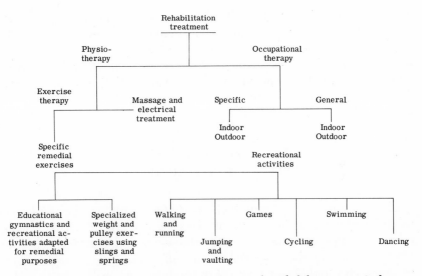

Fig. 1 The position of recreational activities in the rehabilitation curriculum.

games, cycling, swimming, and dancing; it is the intention of this chapter to concentrate upon their use within the rehabilitation program.

Recreational activities adapted for remedial purposes play an important part in the scheme of rehabilitation. While not taking the place of specific remedial exercises, they have an important role in supplementing them. It has been found that patients become interested in what seems to them to be a novel and enjoyable form of treatment. From being merely interested, they become enthusiastic, using their limbs spontaneously and expediting their recovery. In this way, the wholehearted cooperation of the patient is assured.

Recreational activities provide a challenge most patients find difficult to resist. No less important is the fact that psychological stimuli can take the body beyond its physiological limits. Accordingly, the basis of this form of treatment lies in the implementation of these two facts. The aims of treatment are, therefore, physical and psychological in character.

II. THE PSYCHOLOGICAL VALUE OF
RECREATIONAL ACTIVITIES

The psychological value of recreational activities lies in the fact that by producing excitement and enjoyment they help the patient to forget his injury and enable him to regain his lost confidence. Thus, the mental outlook is improved together with the physical condition. Equally, seeing other patients with similar injuries performing at a more advanced stage of recovery, the patient is stimulated to reach a similar stage. Furthermore, patients may be taught recreational activities they have always wished to play but for which they have previously lacked the opportunity. The desire to learn something new increases the effort to become physically stronger.

III. THE PHYSICAL VALUE OF RECREATIONAL ACTIVITIES

Their physical values lies in their ability to provide specific and general remedial exercises in the guise of everyday activities, such as walking, running, jumping, lifting, carrying, throwing, and catching. They are most effective in the mobilization of stiff joints, the strengthening of weak muscles, and the toning up of the body as a whole.

Recreational activities may be divided into two groups: those producing specific movements and those producing general movements of the body.

A. Specific Movements

The specific remedial value of recreational activities lies in producing the movement desired through the careful teaching of the technique of the recreational activity in which the patient is taking part. Thus, if abduction and outward rotation of the hip joint are required, and the activity is swimming, then the leg kick of the breast stroke would be taught; or, if the quadriceps muscle lacked strength, the low drive in soccer.

B. General Movements

The general value of recreational activities lies in the performance of the activity after the technique has been mastered and is embraced within the whole activity, e.g., the breast stroke leg kick and swimming the breast stroke, or kicking a soccer ball and playing the game of soccer. Recreational activities provide the therapist with an extensive repertoire of games and sports from which to choose suitable activities for each stage of the recovery process.

IV. THE CHIEF POINTS TO BE NOTED IN THE ORGANIZATION OF ANY FORM OF RECREATIONAL ACTIVITY

For any form of recreational activity to be a success, every precaution must be taken to ensure the safety of the participants. All the possible dangers must be anticipated and steps taken to prevent their occurence. Each activity has its own specific dangers that must be noted, but there are a few rules that apply to most, if not all, activities. Roughness in any form must be prevented. The teacher must have complete control of the class at all times. Each patient must have complete confidence in his own ability to perform whatever is required of him. Patients must be graded into classes according to specific criteria that will depend upon the number of patients attending the department, the number of trained staff, the space and facilities available and the length of time for each patient's treatment.

V. GRADING CRITERIA

A. The Location of the Injury

Back, arm, and leg injuries provide three groups that may require different types of activities. Within these regions, further subdivision may be required, e.g., the leg class could be further subdivided into foot and knee classes, and the arm class into shoulder, arm, forearm, and hand classes.

B. The Sex of the Patient

There are many arguments in favor of separating the sexes for many activities. Men generally are stronger than women. Many women do not wish to appear in mixed company in shorts or other sporting dress (this is particularly true of the nonathletic persons). Certain activities appear to be better suited to men than women and vice versa.

C. The General Fitness of the Patient

During the initial stages of recovery the patient should be involved in a progressively planned set of specific exercises aimed at increasing his general level of fitness. Only when an optimum level has been reached, should he be asked to take part in sports and games.

D. The Recreational Background of the Patient

The patient's experience in physical recreation must be a determinant in the choice of activities employed in his treatment.

E. Stages of Recovery

Each rehabilitation department has its own method of grading patients according to their stage of recovery. The following has been found to be both easy and practical. All classes are divided into three grades: early, intermediate, and advanced.

1. The early grade consists of those patients who may be in or out of plaster. They may be non-weight-bearing or partial weight bearing. Patients who have had menisectomies might be included up to the fourteenth postoperative day.

2. The intermediate grade includes those patients who can walk and perform a heel-and-toe run. All patients should reach this stage of performing recreational activities.

3. The advanced grade is for those in the final stage of recovery, when the duration and severity of the activity will approximate very closely that experienced under normal conditions. In other words, few if any restrictions would be imposed either on the activity or upon the patient.

V. GENERAL PRINCIPLES OF APPLICATION OF EXERCISE THERAPY

The general principles regarding exercise therapy apply to all areas of the body, especially the back, arms, and legs, but, for the sake of brevity and to avoid repetition, the examples given will refer to activities for lower limb injuries.

A. Walking and Running

Walking and running are the basic forms of human movement. Their correct execution is fundamental to all other forms of recreation performed on foot. It is essential, therefore, that from the moment the patient is ambulatory he is taught to walk and, later, to run. The characteristic limp of the leg injury must not be allowed to manifest itself.

From the beginning of the patient's treatment, it will be found useful to enlist his cooperation by teaching him the simple mechanics of walking and running so that he understands what he is trying to do. The position of the pelvis is all important. It must be kept level and not allowed to dip as weight is taken on the injured limb.

If the limb is encased in plaster, it is essential that the cast is strong, light, and comfortable, and, except in cases of fracture of the foot, that the cast should only extend to the metatarsal heads, thus promoting good forefoot joint movement. A below-knee plaster should allow for good knee movement of at least 90°. In a full-length plaster, from toes to groin, the knee should be held straight with very few exceptions. A semiflexed knee produces a semiflexed hip in order to bring the center of gravity of the body over the base.

The specific remedial value of walking and running lies in the careful teaching of the following:

1. Walking

The reeducation of walking may be divided into three parts: the stage of no weight bearing; weight bearing with some support; and full weight bearing.

a. NON-WEIGHT-BEARING OR PARTIAL WEIGHT BEARING. From the beginning, the injured limb is on the ground although little weight may be taken by the limb. The patient then produces the normal walking action and never loses the proprioceptive sensation of touch. To assist the patient, crutches are used. The patient is taught the three-point rule, forming a wide triangular base (Fig. 2).

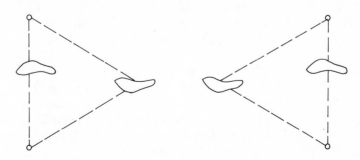

Fig. 2 The uninjured leg forms the apex of the triangle at each step.

Short even steps should be insisted upon. If the patient is on partial weight bearing, the weight is taken by the injured limb and the crutches at the same time. Walking in a long leg plaster (toes to groin) involves a special technique, that of drawing up the hip to allow the foot to swing clear of the floor during the recovery stage. When this has been taught, the patient walks employing the three-point rule but, instead of flexing the knee during the recovery stage, he raises the hip.

b. WEIGHT BEARING WITH PARTIAL SUPPORT. The support is two crutches; one crutch is *never* used. At this stage the patient has gained confidence and often tries to progress faster than he is able to by taking long strides with the injured limb and short ones with the sound leg. Short steps of even length must be insisted upon. The position of the feet must be watched to ensure they are not turned out.

c. FULL WEIGHT BEARING. Full weight bearing cannot be allowed until the patient can walk without a limp. He should then discard both crutches and be encouraged to take short, even steps, stressing the push off with the toes. Walks should be taken daily, the distance depending upon the stage of recovery. All walks should be supervised.

d. FAULTS TO BE NOTED. Absence of heel and toe gait, irregular rhythm, uneven spacing of the feet, walking with the toes turned out, walking with a stiff knee or ankle from force of habit, and dipping of the pelvis when weight is taken on the injured limb should all be corrected by the therapist as soon as they are detected.

2. Running

The patient begins to run when he reaches the intermediate stage of recovery. Running may be divided into three stages: (1) heel and toe running; (2) toe and heel running used for short distances; and (3) toe running or sprinting used for quickness.

a. HEEL AND TOE RUNNING. The patient is able to manage a heel and toe run long before he is able to run on his toes. This type of running is used to enable the patient, when he is unable to run on his toes without a limp, to move at a faster pace than walking. Normal walking is taught first. Then the pace is increased, still keeping an even rhythm. Walking and heel and toe running should be combined at first. For example, twenty walking steps are taken followed by an equal number of heel and toe running steps. The speed and distance should be developed progressively.

b. Toe and Heel Running. This is taught when the patient is able to walk evenly on the toes but before he is able to sprint. The toe of the pushing-off foot is placed on the ground under the body's center of gravity. As the push is made, the knee extends and the heel just brushes the ground. There is a shorter recovery period than in heel and toe running, and the recovery period is higher in preparation for the push. It is taught to enable patients to move quickly, to mobilize the ankle joints, and to strengthen the calf and quadriceps muscles.

c. Toe Runinng. Toe running, or sprinting, is only taught to patients in the advanced stage of recovery. This type of running is used over short distances and should be combined with heel and toe running.

The ability to walk and run enables the patient to take part in a variety of activities and to enjoy many forms of outdoor exercise.

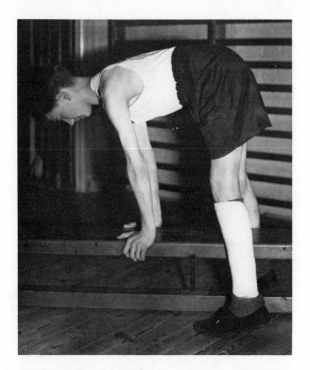

Fig. 3 Stage 1 in jumping exercise; most of the weight is taken on the arms. The patient has had 8 weeks previously an unstable oblique fracture of the middle third of the left tibia and fibula fixed internally with two screws in the tibia and the leg encased in plaster.

B. Jumping

The ability to jump and land from a height is an essential movement. The patient learns these two movements as soon as he has reached the intermediate stage of recovery, when he is able to take his weight evenly on either foot and can walk without the aid of crutches. The basic progression is from the first stage until the patient is able to jump from a height of several feet.

1. Stage 1

Most of the weight is taken by the arms and the patient learns rhythm and relaxation (Fig. 3). Initially the patient learns heel raising and lowering in a bouncing movement. Gradually, as confidence is gained, the feet leave the floor (Fig. 4), and, when the feet touch the floor from the landing, the knees bend. With a little more effort, the feet

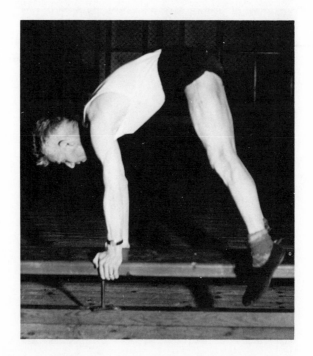

Fig. 4 Stage 1 in jumping exercise; now the feet leave the floor, and when they touch on landing, the knees bend. The patient has had 6 weeks previously an intertrochanteric fracture of the left femur fixed internally with a plate and a Smith–Peterson nail.

can be jumped onto the form and back onto the floor in a rhythmical movement (Fig. 5). In order to sustain the interest, the feet may be moved from side of the bench, or the hips may be raised as high as possible (Fig. 6). This is an important stage for the patient, since he learns to absorb his body weight when landing.

2. Stage 2

The body weight is taken chiefly by the feet and the support is gradually removed. The patient stands facing a firm support (Fig. 7), and the exercises of stage one are repeated, until the patient has confidence to let his feet leave the floor and he can perform a simple jump without support (Fig. 8). As soon as this stage is reached, more complicated jumps may be attempted.

3. Stage 3

This stage is jumping from a small height. Before attempting to jump from a height, the patient should practice stepping from a bench using alternate feet. The initial jump should be with support (Figs. 9 and 10), which may be the physiotherapist or another patient. The jumping

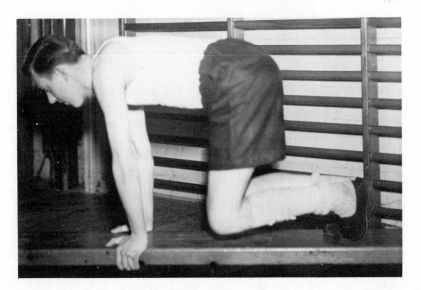

Fig. 5 Stage 1 in jumping exercise; the feet are jumped onto the bench and back onto the floor in a rhythmical movement. The patient has had a closed reduction of fractures of the midshaft of the left tibia and fibula 12 weeks previously.

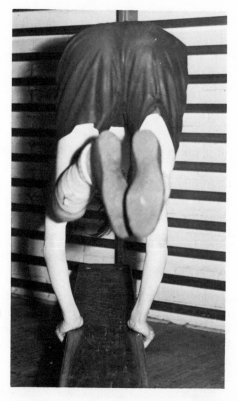

Fig. 6 Stage 1 in jumping exercise; the hips are now raised as high as possible in jumping from the floor above the bench. The same patient as in Fig. 5.

movement is repeated until the patient has enough confidence to jump without support (Fig. 11). When the support is removed, it is essential that the patient is told to bend his knees fully on landing, and to touch the floor with the hands, thus ensuring that he lands on his toes with his body weight forward (Fig. 12). The next stage is to face the form, and, placing one foot on the form, to push off and jump over to land on the other side. The jump should be practiced with alternate feet, and, as confidence increases, walking, and later running, toward the form should be introduced. Patients should be encouraged to get a good upward jump off the form. This stage is the important one in the progression because, when the patient can jump and land correctly from a height of 12 inches or so, he will do equally well from increasing heights. From this stage the height can be gradually raised, until the patient can land from a Swedish vaulting box (Fig. 13). This type of box may be used in a variety of ways, with the weight either on

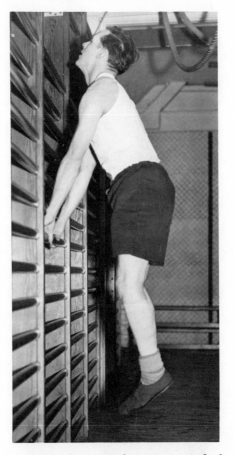

Fig. 7 Stage 2 in jumping exercise; the patient stands facing a firm support and the Exercises of Stage 1 are repeated. Patient has had a spiral fracture of the left tibia with a comminuted fracture of the fibula treated by two-screw fixation of the tibia 9 weeks previously.

the hands or the feet (Fig. 14). Here, the patient learns to land from awkward angles, which is very necessary if his job entails working at a height and he should fall.

C. Cycling

Cycling is an activity that may be enjoyed by patients of all ages and stages of recovery. The distance cycled depends upon the stage of recovery, the age of the patient, and the time available. The rides should be carefully planned to include places of interest. The patient

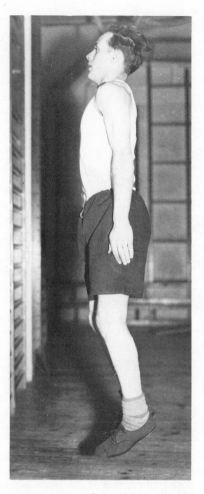

Fig. 8 Stage 2 in jumping exercise; the patient now makes simple jumps without support. Same patient as in Fig. 7.

should know where he is going and what is expected of him. He should be supervised at all times.

Before being allowed to use a normal bicycle, each patient should be tested on a stationary bicycle. This gives the teacher the opportunity to explain the basic fundamentals of cycling, and the patient the time to develop the necessary confidence.

The specific values of cycling are (1) to increase the power of the calf and quadriceps muscles and (2) to increase the mobility of the ankle, knee, and hip joints.

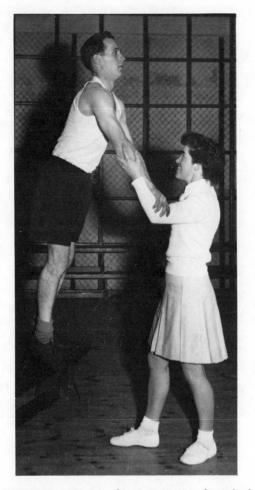

Fig. 9 Stage 3 in jumping exercise; the patient jumps from the bench with some support offered by the therapist. Same patient as in Fig. 8, 1 week later.

Increased power of the calf and quadriceps muscles is produced by the correct method of using the feet in cycling. Great care must be taken to see that the patient does not cycle with the instep on the pedal, in which case there is no movement of the ankle joint, all the work is done by the quadriceps muscle, and the patient quickly tires.

Correct cycling technique improves the mobility of the ankle joint. Equally, when the mobility of the knee joint is increased, the range of the hip joint is also automatically improved. In order to cycle on a regular bicycle, it is necessary to have a 100° or more of knee flexion

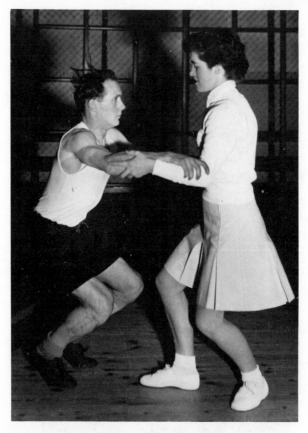

Fig. 10 Stage 3 in jumping exercise; the patient bends his knees in landing and is partially supported by the therapist. Same patient as in Fig. 9.

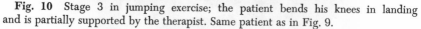

when the saddle is at the normal height. Acceptance of this range of movement automatically excludes a large number of patients who would derive benefit from cycling. Accordingly, two adjustable cranks have been devised, one with a swinging pedal, and one with a fixed pedal.

1. An Adjustable Crank with a Swinging Pedal

The crank with the swinging pedal may be attached at any distance from 2 to 7 inches from the bottom bracket axle. In the vertical position, the pedal of the adjustable crank is at its lowest point and is vertically opposed to the other pedal (Figs. 15 and 16). As the crank moves off the vertical, the swinging pedal remains parallel but is offset (Fig. 17), and as the crank of the swinging pedal moves into its highest point the

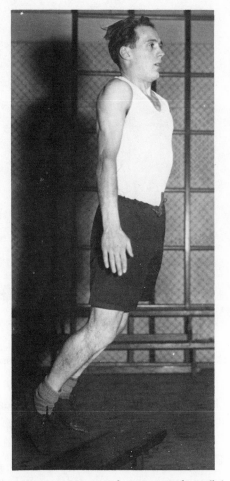

Fig. 11 Stage 3 in jumping exercise; the patient takes off from the bench with no support. Same patient as in Fig. 10, a few days later.

pedal is only ½ inch above the bottom bracket axle. As seen in Fig. 18, the center of the circle through which the pedal passes is 1¼ inches below the bottom bracket due to the fact that the pedal passes only ½ inch above the bottom bracket axle. This type of pedal is only useful for cycling on the flat; otherwise, there is too great a strain on the good leg.

The adjustable crank with a swinging pedal enables patients with approximately 70° of knee flexion to cycle. No muscle work is required from the injured limb. Knee flexion appears to improve quickly, probably because the patient knows that, as soon as he is able, he will be allowed

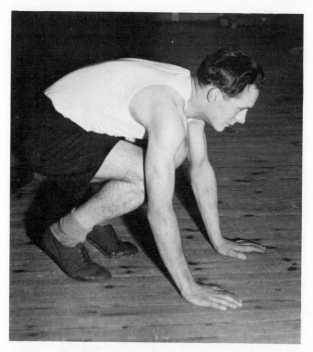

Fig. 12 Stage 3 in jumping exercise; in landing the patient bends his knees fully and touches his hands so as to keep his body weight forward. Same patient as in Fig. 11.

to cycle using a bicycle equipped with a single pedal. He will then be able to cycle farther afield and negotiate hills.

2. An Adjustable Crank with a Fixed Pedal

The adjustable crank with the fixed pedal may be attached 1 to 7 inches from the bottom bracket axle. When the pedal is at its lowest point, it is vertically opposed to the normal pedal (Fig. 19). As the crank moves off the vertical, since the crank is fixed, it continues to remain vertically opposed (Fig. 20). When the crank is at its highest point, the pedal is the same distance above the crank as it was below (Fig. 21). Thus, the end of the crank moves through a circle of 7 inches radius while the pedal moves through a circle of 1 inch radius (Fig. 22). It has been found, however, that, when the crank is fixed 1 inch from the bottom bracket axle, the foot slips on the pedal. Since toe straps are not recommended for patients, it is better to attach the fixed pedal 2 inches from the bottom bracket axle. Both cranks are easily adjusted by unscrewing one nut.

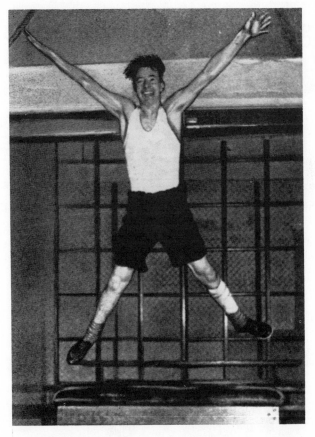

Fig. 13 Stage 3 in jumping exercise; the patient makes a star jump and lands from a Swedish vaulting box. The patient has had an oblique fracture of the midshaft of the left tibia treated by internal fixation 9 weeks previously and is wearing a plaster cast.

This crank offers a progression from the previous one. There is strong muscle work for the injured limb and patients require approximately 75° or more of knee flexion to use it. When the fixed attachment can be fitted to the end of the crank, the patient is ready to use a bicycle with a normal crank.

By using the adjustable crank with either the fixed or swinging pedal, patients are able to enjoy cycling long before they would normally do so. Patients on crutches have a very limited range of travel, but on a bicycle they can cover distances of many miles comfortably. Patients regain their confidence by renewing their ability to cycle, and, later, to encounter traffic.

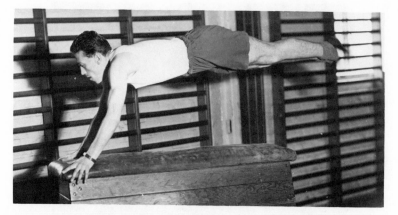

Fig. 14 Stage 3 in jumping exercise; the patient jumps from a springboard to a hand rest on the vaulting box and lands on his feet to one side of the box. This patient has had a closed reduction of a fracture of the left tibial plateau with displacement 10 weeks previously.

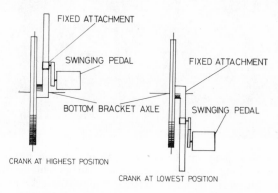

Fig. 15 An adjustable bicycle crank with a swinging pedal attached 2 inches from the bottom bracket axle. Frontal view.

D. Games

Games are of value in the rehabilitation of the injured because they produce free, spontaneous movement. Patients who think they cannot move quickly forget their fears in the excitement of the game. By means of suitably chosen games, patients who are not sports minded gradually gain in confidence and proficiency, and are more able to enjoy their classes.

The patient must first learn to handle the implement with which he will be playing. This is usually a ball. From a sitting or standing position,

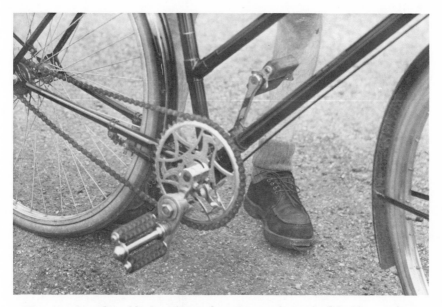

Fig. 16 An adjustable bicycle crank with a swinging pedal. The crank is at its lowest point and the pedal is 2 inches from the bottom bracket axle.

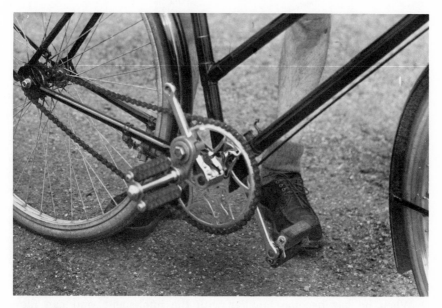

Fig. 17 An adjustable bicycle crank with a swinging pedal. The crank has just moved off the vertical axis. The pedal is parallel but offset and is also $\frac{1}{2}$ inch from the bottom bracket axle.

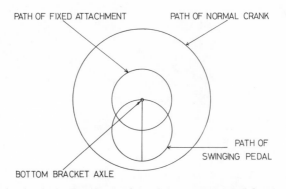

Fig. 18 An adjustable bicycle crank with a swinging pedal. The center of the circle through which the pedal passes is 1½ inches below the bottom bracket axle since the pedal passes ½ inch above it.

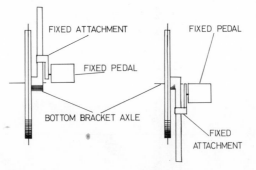

Fig. 19 An adjustable bicycle crank with a fixed pedal. At its lowest point the pedal is vertically opposed to the normal pedal and parallel. Frontal view.

depending on his stage of recovery, he finds out what he can do with the ball by throwing and catching, using both hands to catch, and then one to throw and one to catch. By using the space around him, he finds out the limits to which he can move in order to catch the ball. When he uses the space behind him he has to twist his body. Many find this difficult. From a stationary position, he then learns to move in the space around him, to stop and start, to change his speed of movement, sometimes very quickly, to disguise his movement, and to twist and turn.

When he has become familiar with the implement, and can move safely in the space around himself, he is ready to play with a partner. He throws the ball where his partner can catch or trap the ball with

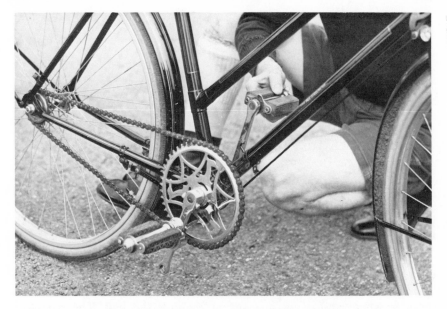

Fig. 20 An adjustable bicycle crank with a fixed pedal. As the crank moves off the vertical the pedal remains parallel and opposed.

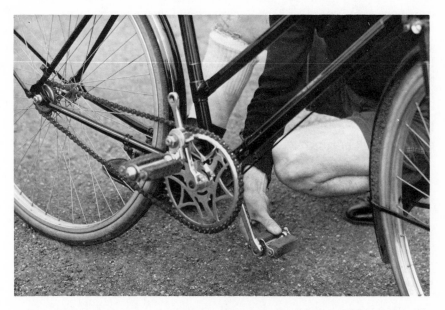

Fig. 21 An adjustable bicycle crank with a fixed pedal. At its highest point the pedal is still the same distance above the bottom bracket axle as it was below.

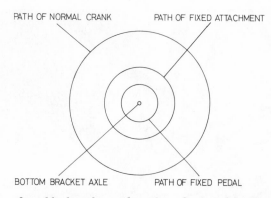

Fig. 22   An adjustable bicycle crank with a fixed pedal. The diagram shows that the end of the crank moves through a circle of 7 inches radius while the pedal moves through one of 1 inch radius.

his feet, hands, or body. His partner makes this easy by indicating where he requires the ball. The players then move. The thrower now has to consider where and when his partner requires the ball. The strength of the throw will depend upon the distance between the two players. The catcher decides where he will move in space, in a straight line or on a curved pathway, and the speed at which he will travel. He may move at top speed, or he may hesitate and then move.

The partners are now ready to play against an opponent. Games such as "Two against One," "Pig in the Middle," etc., where two players have the ball and the third player tries to intercept the ball, are very suitable at this stage, and may be adapted for use with the ball on the ground as in soccer, or in the air as in basketball.

Games have much in common, and the techniques and tactics learned in one game can be adapted for use in another. For inclusion in the rehabilitation programme, they may be divided into three groups:

1. Individual Games

In bowls, golf, darts, croquet, and similar games, the player has only to think about beating himself or outwitting an opponent. There is no body contact, and he therefore feels completely safe.

2. Noncontact Games

In these games the player is either protected by a net, but plays in a team, as in deck quoits or volleyball, or one player plays against the rest of the opposing team, as in rounders, softball, nonstop cricket, or cricket. Here again, the player is protected against being pushed over.

3. Contact Games

Body contact may occur in basketball, ringing the quoit, sitting-down handball, and soccer, but within reason.

4. Selection of Games

Individual, noncontact, and contact games may be played by patients at varying stages of their recovery, but they must be carefully chosen to suit the class. Sitting-down handball, where the player stays in the sitting position, may be played by patients who are non-weight-bearing, but strict rules must be adhered to—specifically, no body contact is allowed. Soccer, on the other hand, is only to be played by those in the advanced stage of recovery and whose technical skill is adequate.

5. A Typical Games Lesson

A typical games lesson should include (1) an activity wherein the patient will learn to use his implement and the various ways of moving; (2) the development of the required movement through careful teaching before it is incorporated into a game; and (3) the final or major game that involves the whole class. An activity specific to the injury should be demonstrated and learned. For example, if a good inversion and eversion of the foot is required, then dribbling a soccer ball or other small ball using the inside and outside of the foot is appropriate. First, the correct position of inversion and eversion with the good foot is taught; then, with the injured limb using a stationary ball. The exercise is first taken at walking pace, the ball being propelled along by the eversion and inversion of the foot, or by alternate movements. Further motivation and interest may be secured by employing the movement in a relay race around suitably placed objects.

An activity relevant to the final game is then added. The activity in this section should consist of the practice of one of the techniques or skills of the final game. For example, if the final game is heading tennis, the skill to be taught would be heading the ball.

6. Progression between Lessons

The progressive development of the patients' skill and the experience of a variety of games is desirable, and all efforts should be made to achieve this whenever possible. Progression will depend upon whether the teacher has the same patients for successive classes. This is difficult whether dealing with in- or out-patients because of schedule conflicts and the changing list of patients.

7. Points to Be Noted in the Organization of a Games Lesson

  a. The number of patients involved
  b. The type of injuries of those taking part, and therefore the aim of each game
  c. The ages and experiences of the patients: a patient of sixty years who has been athletic in his youth can be allowed to take part in quite an advanced game, while a nonathletic person of forty years would be a liability in the same class
  d. The available apparatus
  e. The playing area, including its shape, size, and the type of surface, whether wood, grass, asphalt, concrete, or whatever
  f. Players should be suitably clothed. If soccer or hockey is being played, shin pads and correct footwear should be worn. If the games are played out of doors and the weather is cold, a warm sweater is required (a cold muscle is more prone to injury than a warm one).

8. Additional Information

Space does not permit here the further elaboration of the principles underlying the use of games in the rehabilitation of the injured. Readers requiring additional information are advised to consult "The Adaptation of Recreational Activities for Men" (Barclay, 1956).

E. Swimming

Swimming as a remedial exercise has few rivals, since water, by eliminating gravity, enables patients at all stages of recovery to take part in this activity. Many excellent books are available on the teaching of swimming, but, if it is to be successfully employed in the rehabilitation program, certain aspects need to be emphasized.

No stylized strokes should be taught until the patient has come to terms with the water. Only in exceptional circumstances should artificial aids be used, because of their tendency to upset the balance of the body. This is especially true of the patient who has a paralyzed limb. Many patients dislike immersing their faces in the water. Simple activities such as blowing bubbles in the water or placing the face in the water and counting the tiles on the bottom of the pool should be employed. Confidence activities of all types should be a prominent feature of this initial introduction to the water.

1. Balance and Flotation

Initially, the patient must be taught how to regain his feet from a supine and prone position. Having mastered this, with or without the assistance of another patient, he must now begin to learn what he can do in the water. He should learn not to fight the water, but to allow it to support his weight in various positions, vertical, supine, and prone. He should appreciate that it is easier to balance if the body shape is a wide one and should learn to make small adjustments to his body position in order to maintain a floating position. If the legs have a tendency to sink in the supine stretched floating position, this can be rectified by raising the hands out of the water by flexing the wrists. Since the weight of the body is heavier out of the water, added weight on one end may lift the feet at the other end.

2. Propulsion—The Body Moving in Water

The patient discovers he can propel his body through the water by using various parts of his anatomy, for example, his arms or legs, moving together or alternately. The pelvis also can initiate movement. He soon discovers that he can move by either pushing or pulling the water. He finds that he can move on the surface or on the bottom of the pool, feet first or head first, so that he has a variety of ways of traveling between the two surfaces. Swimming strokes are a narrowing down of the patient's experience in water and should only be taught after he has experienced the balance, flotation, and propulsive phases.

3. Breathing

It is essential to teach the patient to breath in the first lesson. Both trickle and explosive breathing should be taught and the patient can then choose which suits him best.

4. Entry and Exit

Entering and leaving the water while protecting the anterior surfaces of the body by streamlining the body, and curling the body forward or gently lowering it into the water are techniques that should be mastered in early lessons.

5. Diving

Diving head first is not allowed until the patient can enter the water feet first and feel the tension necessary to hold the body in a straight line. A patient in the early stage of recovery should not dive from one leg.

F. Track and Field Sports

The three throwing events—discus, javelin, and shot—are very useful in the production of strength, but they are very one-sided exercises. Their greatest use is probably with the wheelchair patient.

G. Dancing

Dancing is a very popular activity that gives a great variety of movement. It is especially useful during the winter months when inclement weather prevents outdoor activities such as games, cycling, and walking. The specific value of dancing lies in the teaching of the basic steps of the dance to produce the movement required, as, for example, the pas de bas in Scottish dancing for outward rotation of the hip joint. Dancing has a strengthening effect on all the muscles of the lower limb, particularly the calf muscle. The patient learns poise, rhythm, relaxation, coordination, and control. Dancing is regarded as an entertainment and not as an exercise to be mastered. The patient, therefore, loses any fear that he might not be able to take part in an activity he may have enjoyed before his injury.

VII. SUGGESTED PROGRAMS OF TREATMENT

There can be no hard and fast rules as to when exercise therapy may be started. No two patients ever react in exactly the same way to any injury or recover at exactly the same rate, although they may be undergoing the same treatment. Progression in all forms of recreational activity should be gradual, so that the class passes from the simple to the more difficult and demanding activities with comparative ease. The following two examples illustrate the average times that recreational activities should be started following routine menisectomy in the knee and surgical repair of a fractured shaft of the tibia with internal fixation.

A. Following Routine Menisectomy in the Knee

Taking 130 cartilage operations treated at one hospital over a period of two years, it has been found that the average time from operation to return to work was 35 days. These 130 cases included:

- 78 cases which had no effusion when they arrived at the hospital
- 23 cases with effusion of the knee joint on arrival at the hospital
- 3   cases with removal of both the internal and the external semi-lunar cartilage on the same knee
- 27 cases with complications as follows:
  - 7 by cystic cartilage
  - 8 by rupture of the anterior cruciate ligament
  - 1 by rupture of the posterior cruciate ligament
  - 2 by a large hematoma under the scar
  - 8 by osteochondritis dessicans
  - 1 by developing an abscess in the popliteal fossa

The average times when recreational activities may be started following routine menisectomy are given in Table I. Swimming should be a daily activity.

B. Following Internal Fixation of a Fracture of the Shaft of the Tibia

A considerable proportion of fractures of the tibia are treated by internal fixation either by a plate or screws. This method of treatment is adopted in the case of unstable fractures or where perfect apposition cannot be obtained. Taking 34 cases at one hospital over a period of 2 years, the average length of time from operation to return to work was 4 months. Twenty-six of the thirty-four cases were simple fractures; the other eight were compound comminuted. The average times when recreational activities may be started are given in Table II.

VIII. CONCLUSION

Recreational activities contain a wide range of movements many of which can be employed in the treatment of musculoskeletal injuries.

TABLE I

Recommended Recreational Activities following a Routine Menisectomy

Duration of treatment after operation (days)	Ambulant stage	Class stage	Recreational activities recommended
1–10	Treated in hospital		Physiotherapy; ward classes
12–21	Full weight bearing	Early leg	Early games (20–45 minutes daily). Walking up to one mile. The progession of walking may be taught in the specific remedial class. Swimming. N.B. Cycling is not recommended at this stage of recovery as it has been found that cycling is a possible cause of effusion in the early stage.
21–28	Full weight bearing	Intermediate	Intermediate games, including the early technique practice of football—the trap with the sole of the foot, and the low drive. Progression of jumping up to Stage 4, jumping from a springboard. Cycling progressed from 10 minutes to one hour. Walking up to two miles. Running. Swimming. Ballroom dancing.
28–35	Full weight bearing	Advanced	Advanced games (40–60 minutes). Full vaulting. Cycling up $1\frac{1}{2}$ hours. Walking and running up to 3 miles. Swimming. Ballroom and Scottish dancing.

The response of patients to these activities has been found to be so cooperative and purposeful that many of the more stereotyped remedial exercises formerly used have been discarded. The use of sports and games, however, must be governed by discretion and an appreciation of certain fundamental principles. The patient must be taught the correct movement. The daily program must be adapted to the needs of the patient. Interest must be maintained by the use of a varied program. Finally, the patient must have complete confidence in his teacher and in his own ability to do whatever is asked of him.

REFERENCE

Barclay, V. (1956). "The Adaptation of Recreational Activities for Men, in the Rehabilitation of Lower Limb Injuries," Bell, London.

TABLE II

Recommended Recreational Activities for a Fractured
Upper Shaft of Tibia with Internal Fixation

Duration of treatment after operation (days)	Ambulant stage	Class stage	Recreational activities recommended
1–10	Tibia plated, treated as an in-patient in hospital		
11–21	Admitted to rehabilitation. Plaster of Paris toes to groin. Non-weight-bearing or on crutches	Early	Early games and the progression of walking on crutches.
21–28	Plaster of Paris replaced by a back slab, malleoli to groin, very slight weight bearing on crutches	Early	Early games. Walking. Swimming, the back slab being removed and replaced on the edge of the bath.
28–42	Full weight bearing on crutches. Back slab only used for sleeping in and when playing games	Early	Early games. Swimming. Walking.
42–56	Walking with two sticks	Early	Early games. Walking. Swimming. Cycling slowly progressed.
56–63	Walking with two sticks, gradually discarding these. (The two sticks are discarded together.)	Early	Early games. Cycling (distance increased). Swimming. Walking.
63–84	Full weight bearing	Early intermediate	Early intermediate games. Cycling (distance increased). Swimming. Walking progress to heel and toe running. Progression of jumping, Stages 1a, 1b. Ballroom dancing.
84–98	Full weight bearing	Advanced intermediate	Advanced intermediate games. Swimming. Walking and heel and toe running. Vaulting, Stages 1, 2, 3, 4. Ballroom dancing.
98–112 onwards	Full weight bearing	Advanced	Advanced games. Progression of jumping, Stage 5. Simple vaults according to the ability of the patient. Swimming. Running long distances. Ballroom and folk dancing.

Chapter 31

EXERCISE AND MENTAL DISORDERS

WILLIAM P. MORGAN

I. OVERVIEW

The value of physical activity and sport in maintaining mental health, as well as its therapeutic efficacy, is emphasized throughout the rehabilitation and physical fitness literature. Such views are holistic in nature and emphasize the totality of mind and body. This position is consonant with expectations derived from organismic theory, and, teleologically at least, such somatopsychic explanations have historically been quite popular.

Unfortunately, such views have not been supported by a wealth of objective psychometric data. Indeed, support for such beliefs has been largely intuitive or anecdotal in nature. For example, the catharsis theory of physical activity, which holds that exercise will reduce anxiety, aggression, and hostility, not only lacks objective support, but there is some evidence that suggests that physical activity evokes increments in such states. The purpose of the present chapter will be to examine the objective evidence pertaining to the psychological effects of sport and physical activity, as well as to examine the role of physical activity in the major mental disorders.

II. PSYCHOLOGICAL EFFECTS

A number of investigators have directed their attention toward an understanding of the psychological effects of acute and chronic physical activity and/or sport. These reports will be reviewed in the present section.

A. Acute Physical Activity and Sport

In one of the first investigations dealing with this topic, Johnson and Hutton (1955) administered a protective test (H-T-P) to college wrestlers before the season, five hours prior to an important match, and the day following this same match. A decrease in functioning intelligence, increase in anxiety, and prominence of neurotic signs characterized the wrestlers in the prematch setting. From a mental health standpoint, these observations suggest that anticipation of approaching competition evokes undesirable psychological states. On the other hand, whether such changes are undesirable from a performance standpoint is another matter. More importantly, however, the wrestlers returned to their preseason "baselines" by the following morning.

Morgan (1970a) evaluated the state anxiety of college wrestlers during the preseason and one hour prior to an easy and difficult match. He observed a significant *reduction* in anxiety for both prematch settings. More recently, however, Morgan and Hammer (1974) assessed state anxiety in college wrestlers during early season, four hours before, one hour prior to, and fifteen to thirty minutes following a state tournament. The wrestlers were characterized by a significant *increase* in anxiety one hour prior to the tournament, and a significant *decrease* in the postmatch period. As a matter of fact, the postmatch level was actually lower than the base-line measure obtained in early season. Morgan and Hammer (1974) also reported that these college wrestlers scored appreciably lower than published norms under the base-line conditions. Therefore, the observed reduction following competition is even more remarkable.

The influence of exercise on various treadmill exercise bouts on anxiety and depression levels of male and female college students and male professors has been evaluated by Morgan et al. (1971). They have reported that neither acute aerobic or anerobic physical activity influenced anxiety or depression levels. At the same time, the majority of the subjects in their experiments reported a sensation of "feeling better" after the exercise.

These investigations have been concerned with individuals who have been presumably normal.* The findings indicate that competitive sport of an acute nature is associated with significant fluctuations in psychic states. Physical activity in noncompetitive settings has been associated with the commonly reported "feeling better" sensation, but not with shifts in behavioral manifestations such as anxiety or depression. There is considerable evidence that suggests that this may not be the case for anxiety neurotics.† Individuals suffering from anxiety neurosis exhibit abnormally high blood lactate responses to light work, and muscular exertion of even a mild nature is frequently associated with anxiety attacks in such persons. Also, Pitts and McClure (1967) have demonstrated that lactate infusion provokes anxiety attacks in such patients. In short, their work not only suggests that physical activity does not reduce anxiety, but it is apparently contraindicated in persons suffering from anxiety neurosis! While this position may not be of appeal to physical culturists, it is quite clear that no single form of somatotherapy qualifies as a panacea for mental illness. However, it has more recently been demonstrated that vigorous physical activity can consistently provoke decrements in state anxiety in normals, as well as anxiety neurotics (Morgan, 1973).

B. Chronic Physical Activity and Sport

There have been very few studies directed toward an understanding of the psychological effect of chronic physical activity and sport. However, the several longitudinal and cross-sectional investigations that are available seem to be in agreement on several points, and these studies will be reviewed in the present section. The longitudinal investigations to be reviewed have ranged from six weeks to four years in duration.

* Approximately 10% of the "normals" in our investigations have had anxiety and depression levels regarded as clinically significant.

† The diagnosis of anxiety neurosis has been used interchangeably with Da Costa's syndrome, effort syndrome, neurocirculatory asthenia, vasoregulatory asthenia, nervous tachycardia, neurasthenia, vasomotor neurosis, nervous exhaustion, irritable heart, and soldier's heart.

In a cross-sectional study, Schendel (1965) administered the California Psychological Inventory (CPI) to ninth grade, twelfth grade, and college athletes. These CPI scores were compared to those of nonathletes at each educational level. Differences between the athletes and nonathletes were observed at each level. This finding tends to support the view that athletes and nonathletes differ early in life. The alternative explanation, of course, would be that sport modifies the personality of participants. However, since these athletes and nonathletes were found to differ at each level, a gravitational explanation seems more reasonable.

Werner and Gottheil (1966) compared freshmen cadets at West Point who had participated in high school athletics and those who had not. The groups were found to differ on seven of the sixteen variables at the time of entrance to the Academy. These same cadets were tested four years later at which time those freshmen who had been classified as nonathletes had since participated in four years of athletics. They reported that four years of athletic participation did not change the personality of either group.

The Junior Eysenck Personality Inventory (JEPI) was administered to junior high school males who had never participated in organized athletics by Lukehardt and Morgan (1969). Those students who subsequently elected to participate in interscholastic football were found to be significantly more extraverted than those who did not. Also, when these students were tested following the season, the athletes and nonathletes still differed, and the season of sport participation had no influence on personality. This observation is similar to the finding of Morgan and Hammer (1974) who reported that three months of athletic participation had no influence on anxiety levels in college wrestlers.

Naughton *et al.* (1968) administered the MMPI to postinfarct patients before and after a six month physical activity program. These patients did not experience psychological changes as measured by any of the MMPI scales.

The Self Rating Depression Scale (SDS) was administered to a group of adult males by Morgan *et al.* (1970b) before and after a physical activity program lasting six weeks. Each of the eleven subjects who was depressed at the outset experienced a reduction in depression. However, significant alterations in depression were not observed for the nondepressed subjects.

It is commonly felt that chronic physical activity improves the mental health of hospitalized patients. However, research offered in support of this view has been characterized by statistical and design inelegancies. Investigations concerning this topic have been reviewed by Layman (1955). Also, the inferred role of chronic physical activity in the development and maintenance of mental health will be examined in Section IV.

III. MENTAL HEALTH AND THE ATHLETE

Numerous investigators have reported that athletes tend to be quite stable as measured by various tests of neuroticism–stability (Morgan, 1968b, 1972). Indeed, stability seems to be a prerequisite for high-level competition. Also, it would appear that participation in sport does not produce such stable profiles, but rather, those athletes who tend toward neuroticism drop out of sport as the level of competition increases; that is, selective mortality appears to occur. Such an explanation is based upon Eysenckian theory and the work of Yanada and Hirata (1970) who reported that students who dropped out of sport clubs were more neurotic, depressive, and manic than those who continued.

Despite the fact that investigators have consistently observed that athletes are characterized by stability, there are frequent reports in daily newspapers and lay journals regarding aberrant behavior manifested by professional athletes. Also, books by Beisser (1967) and Ogilvie and Tutko (1966) contain numerous case studies of athletes they have treated for psychological problems.

Carmen et al. (1968) reported that athletes used the Harvard Psychiatric Service less frequently than nonathletes. However, those athletes who requested treatment tended to have more problems than did the nonathletes. A later report by Pierce (1969) corroborated this observation. Pierce (1969) suggested that differences between athletes and nonathletes were related to the ability to assume the role of patient rather than actual degree of pathology. In a recent paper entitled "The Athlete's Neurosis—A Deprivation Crisis," Little (1969) reports a similar finding. He compared neurotics with athletic and nonathletic backgrounds and found a number of interesting differences. First, there was an absence of neurotic markers in the life histories of those patients scoring high on athleticism, whereas the converse was true for the nonathletes. Secondly, despite histories of good mental health, the athletic group had a less favorable prognosis under treatment. Also, 73% of the patients in the athletic group experienced threats to their physical well-being in the form of illness or injury prior to their neurotic breakdowns, whereas the percentage was only 11 for the other group. The physical illness or injury seemed to represent a threat to the athlete's mortality, and this event presumably took the form of a "deprivation crisis."

IV. PHYSICAL FITNESS OF PSYCHIATRIC PATIENTS

It has been suggested by Layman (1955) that poor physical condition makes a person more susceptible to poor mental health. Findings of several investigators support this contention, and these studies will be reviewed.

A. Schizophrenia

Linton *et al.* (1934) reported that schizophrenic patients scored significantly lower than normals on a measure of cardiovascular fitness. This observation was corroborated by McFarland and Huddleson (1936) and Nadel and Horvath (1967).

Schizophrenics have also been reported to score significantly lower than normals on tests of muscular strength and endurance (Hodgdon and Reimer, 1960). Also, recently hospitalized schizophrenics do not differ from those hospitalized for prolonged periods (Rice *et al.* 1961), and, therefore, hospitalization per se does not seem to influence the physical fitness of such patients. Also, Rosenberg and Rice (1964) reported that schizophrenics score significantly lower on muscular strength and endurance than do normals or patients with diagnoses of psychoneurotic and personality disorder. However, the normals did not differ from the patients with either psychoneuroses or personality disorders.

B. Depression

More than half of all psychiatric patients have depressive disorders, and a large proportion of the adult patients seen by family physicians exhibit depressive symptoms (Morgan, 1970d). Furthermore, depression of clinical significance has been reported in approximately 10% of the nonhospitalized adult male population (Morgan *et al.*, 1970b). In short, depression represents one of twentieth century man's major health problems.

Physiological and psychomotor retardation are primary symptoms of the depressive illness, and depressed individuals often find it difficult to perform physical tasks that require minimal energy requirements. However, the role of physical fitness in the depressive illness is not entirely clear; that is, the question of whether or not the depressed patient lacks the physical working capacity to perform routine physical tasks has not been satisfactorily answered. The author and his associates have examined the interaction of physical competence and depression over the past five years, and these investigations will be summarized here.

In the first investigation, percent body fat, reaction time, strength of grip, finger ergometer endurance, hemoglobin, and hematocrit were evaluated in depressed and nondepressed psychiatric patients at the time of their admission to a state hospital. The only variable on which these groups were found to differ was finger ergometer endurance, which seemed to be more of a psychological than a physiological test (Morgan, 1968a). However, those patients who subsequently experienced long-term hospitalizations scored significantly lower on strength of grip, as well as finger ergometer endurance than short-term patients (Morgan, 1970b).

In a later study, depressed male patients were found to score significantly lower on the PWC_{150} than nondepressed patients, suggesting that physical working capacity is implicated in the pathogenesis of psychiatric depression (Morgan, 1969). However, this relationship was not observed in female patients; that is, depressed and nondepressed patients did not differ on strength of grip or physical working capacity tests (Morgan, 1970c).

The relationship of depression and variables such as age, height, weight, percent body fat, strength of grip and the PWC_{150} has been examined in normal adult males. Depression was not correlated significantly with any of these variables, and furthermore, the multiple correlation ($r = .28$) was quite low (Morgan et al., 1970b).

Morgan et al. (1970a) evaluated the relationship between depression and free fatty acid levels in 32 normal adult males. They observed a significant correlation ($r = .35$) between these variables. It may be that physical fitness tests simply are not sensitive enough to clearly delineate the physiological basis of depression.

The investigations reviewed in this section reveal that depression and physical working capacity interact in a very complex fashion. While these studies have demonstrated that psychiatric patients score significantly lower than normals on a wide variety of fitness measures, the relationship of *degree* of psychopathology and physical working capacity is not as clear. The physiological and psychomotor retardation that characterizes the depressed person may simply reflect his *affect* rather than actual physiological capacity. Our more recent work with hypnotic manipulation of perceived exertion in bicycle ergometry supports such a view (Morgan et al., 1973).

V. SUMMARY

In the present chapter, literature concerning the psychological effects of sport and physical activity, the athlete and mental health, and physical fitness correlates of the psychiatric patient has been reviewed. Aside from the subjective report of the "feeling better" sensation, there is very little objective evidence that supports the view that sport and physical activity improves psychic states in adult man. Furthermore, several recent reports suggest that physical activity may, in fact, evoke undesirable psychic states. Investigators have consistently reported that athletes are characterized by stability as opposed to neuroticism, and it is suggested that stability represents a prerequisite for high-level athletic performance. On the other hand, it should be emphasized that evidence exists that indicates that those athletes who develop psychological problems appear to be characterized by more severe disorders than are the nonathletes, and furthermore, prognosis for the athlete under treatment is generally less favorable. There is considerable evidence indicating that schizophrenia is associated with low levels of physical fitness. Also, a patient's muscular strength and endurance at the time of hospitalization have been demonstrated to influence length of hospital stay. There is some evidence suggesting that physical working capacity is implicated in the depression of psychiatric males, but this evidence is far from convincing. More recent research has revealed that acute physical activity designed to provoke anaerobic metabolism consistently reduces state anxiety in both normal adults and anxiety neurotics (Morgan, 1973).

REFERENCES

Beisser, A. R. (1967). 'The Madness In Sports." Appleton, New York.
Carmen, L. R., Zerman, J. L., and Blaine, G. B., Jr. (1968). Ment. Hyg. **52,** 134.
Hodgdon, R. E., and Reimer, D. (1960). J. Ass. Phys. Ment. Rehabil. **14,** 38.
Johnson, W. R., and Hutton, D. C. (1955). Res. Quart. **26,** 49.
Layman, E. M. (1955). "Mental Health Through Physical Education and Recreation." Burgess, Minneapolis, Minnesota.
Linton, J. M., Hamelink, M. H., and Hoskins, R. G. (1934). Arch. Neurol. Psychiat. **32,** 712.
Little, J. C. (1969). Acta Psychiat. Scand. **45,** 187.
Lukehardt, R., and Morgan, W. P. (1969). Abstr. Amer. Ass. Health, Phys. Educ. Recreation, 1969 Vol. 5, p. 122.
McFarland, R. A., and Huddelson, J. H. (1936). Amer. J. Psychiat. **93,** 956.

Morgan, W. P. (1968a). *Res. Quart.* 39, 1037.

Morgan, W. P. (1968b). *J. Sports Med.* 8, 212.

Morgan, W. P. (1969). *Res. Quart.* 40, 859.

Morgan, W. P. (1970a). *Int. J. Sport Psychol.* 1, 7.

Morgan, W. P. (1970b). *In* "Contemporary Psychology of Sport" (G. S. Kenyon, ed.), 1970. Athletic Institute, Chicago, Illinois.

Morgan, W. P. (1970c). *Amer. Corrective Ther. J.* 24, 14.

Morgan, W. P. (1970d). *In* "Integrated Development" (J. M. Cooper and A. H. Ismail, eds.), Indiana State Board of Health, Indianapolis.

Morgan, W. P. (1972). *In* "Psychomotor Domain: Movement Behaviors" (R. N. Singer, ed.), Lea & Febiger, Philadelphia, Pennsylvania.

Morgan, W. P. (1973). *Proc. Nat. Coll. Phys. Educ. Ass., Pittsburgh, Pennsylvania.*

Morgan, W. P., and Hammer, W. M. (1974). *Med. Sci. Sports* (in press).

Morgan, W. P., Horvath, S. M., and Batterton, D. L. (1970a). Institute of Environmental Stress, University of California, Santa Barbara. (unpublished research).

Morgan, W. P., Roberts, J. A., Brand, F. R., and Feinerman, A. D. (1970b). *Med. Sci. Sports* 2, 213.

Morgan, W. P., Roberts, J. A., and Feinerman, A. D. (1971). *Arch. Phys. Med. Rehabil.* 52, 422.

Morgan, W. P., Raven, P. B., Drinkwater, B. L., and Horvath, S. M. (1973). *Int. J. Clin. Exp. Hypnosis* 21, 86.

Nadel, E. R., and Horvath, S. M. (1967). *Int. J. Neuropsychiat.* 3, 191.

Naughton, J., Bruhn, J. G., and Lategola, M. T. (1968). *Arch. Phys. Med. Rehabil.* 49, 131.

Ogilvie, B. C., and Tutko, T. A. (1966). "Problem Athletes and How to Handle Them." Pelham, London.

Pierce, R. A. (1969). *J. Amer. Coll. Health Ass.* 17, 244.

Pitts, F. N., Jr., and McClure, J. N., Jr. (1967). *N. Engl. J. Med.* 277, 1329.

Rice, D. C., Rosenberg, D., and Radzyminski, S. F. (1961). *J. Ass. Phys. Ment. Rehabil.* 15, 143.

Rosenberg, D., and Rice, D. C. (1964). *J. Ass. Phys. Ment. Rehabil.* 18, 73.

Schendel, J. (1965). *Res. Quart.* 36, 52.

Werner, A. C., and Gottheil, E. (1966). *Res. Quart.* 37, 126.

Yanada, H., and Hirata, H. (1970). *Proc. Coll. Phys. Educ., Univ. Tokyo, 1970* Vol. 5, p. 1.

AUTHOR INDEX

Numbers in italics refer to the pages on which the complete references are listed.

SUBJECT INDEX

A

Abasement in baseball players versus norm values, 132

Abdominal cramps, avoidance, eating before contests, 158

Abdominal injury, 269–271

Abdominal muscle setting and rehabilitation of low back problems, 342

Ability
athletic, 133
level and personality, 132–134
psychological variables and, 132–134
sports success and, 237

Abortion, spontaneous, and activity level, 357–358

Abrasions
from artificial turf, 224
in wrestling, 191

Accidents
crowding and, 222
with physical activity and handicapped, 448
prevention by protective equipment, 161

Acclimatization, 34, see also Adaptation
altitude, 214, 228
effect on performance, 67, 214
heat, 212–213
with saunas, 227
sweat glands, number and, 224

Acetazolamide, 218

Acetylcholine, heart rate, effect on, 39

Achilles tendon
protection in ice hockey, 183
rupture, 240, 290, 292
strain, 294
tendonitis, retrocalcaneal bursitis, mistaken for, 295

Acid–base balance
at altitude, 216
buffers and, 150
minerals in diet and, 150–151

Acidosis, exercise in obese and, 576, 586

Acne, 377

Acromioclavicular joint
injury, 271–272
in ice hockey, 182
rehabilitation, 330–331
protection by shoulder pads, 177

Activity
physical
adaptive physical education and, 443–444
anxiety and, 673
catharsis theory of, 671
depression and, 674
evaluation, 5
handicapped
effect on, 467–468
reclassification for, 466–467
heat, metabolic, generated by, 206
human body, effect on, 37
mental health, maintaining, 671, 674
physical fitness, preservation of, 37
prescription, 5
psychological effects, 672–675
purposes, 39–40
supervised or unsupervised, 519–521
recreational
organization, 643
physical values, 642
psychosocial values, 641–642
tibia, for fractured, 668–669
sports and physical fitness, 48

Adaptation, 33–35
to air pollution, 3, 223
altitude, 214

693

G

Galvanometer, 22
Games
  lesson, 663–664
  rehabilitation
    selection, 663
    use of noncontact, 662
    use with musculoskeletal disorders,
      658–664
Ganglion, 295–296
Gangrene, leg contusions and, 287
Gastrointestinal distress, 217
  infection, 383–385
Genetics
  athlete's marriages, effect of, 70
  disorders, inclusion in adaptive physi-
    cal education, 422
  endowment, substrate oxidation and,
    156
  sexual abnormalities, 368
Genital injury, 270–271
Genitalia, examination of external, prior
  to competition, 26
Genitourinary infection, 385–386
Genotype
  adaptation and, 228
  mosaic, 26
Genu recurvatum, qualification for sports
  participation, 110
Genu valgum, qualification for sports participation, 110
Genu varum, qualification for sports participation, 110
Germicidal soaps, use with excessive
  perspiration, 397
Giantism, 60
Girth measurements, 459
Glands, secretion of nutrients, 143
Glenohumeral injury, 272–273
Gloves
  baseball, 199
  boxing, 193–194
  fencing, 194
  golf, 199
  ice hockey, 182–183
Glucose
  energy substrate, 574–575, 588
  muscle utilization, 156
Gluteal region, ischial avulsion, 279

Glycerin, prevention of swimmer's ear,
  380
Glycogen
  in anaerobic metabolism, 37
  carbohydrate intake and, 148
  muscle depletion and performance
    capacity, 156
  precontest meal, 158
  stores, 148
    increasing of, 156–158
Golf
  gloves, 199
  players' pain tolerance, 135
Goniometer, 319, 460
  in strength testing, 5
Grand mal seizure, 395
Gravity
  adaptation by muscle activity, 39–40
  performance, effect on, 67, 224
  stretch reflex and, 45
Greater multangular, fracture, 276
Greater trochanter, injury, 279–280
Grip strength
  in depressed individuals, 677
  index of physical maturity, 978
  of strength, 50
Griseofulvin, oral
  athlete's foot treatment, 379
  tinea curis treatment, 379
Groin pulls, 280
Groupement Latin de Médecine Physique
  et Sport, 9
Growth and development
  environmental impact, 33
  exercise, influence on young children,
    359
  genetic control, 33
  muscle activity, necessity of, 39
  nutrition status, effect of, 145
  protein, 147–148
  sexes, difference, 362–363
  vitamins and, 152
Growth hormone, difference in growth
  rate between sexes, 363
Growth spurt, cause in population, 39
Gymnastics, 19, 22
  height of participants, 59
Gynasium in rehabilitation, 554–555
Gymnastes, 14